Anesthesia and Critical Care Clinics–2

Declaration
The views and opinions expressed in this book are solely those of the original contributor(s)/author(s) and not that of Government, AIIMS.

Anesthesia and Critical Care Clinics–2

Editors

Puneet Khanna MD
Additional Professor
Department of Anesthesiology,
Pain Medicine and Critical Care
All India Institute of Medical Sciences
New Delhi, India

Abhishek Singh MD
Assistant Professor
Department of Anesthesiology,
Pain Medicine and Critical Care
All India Institute of Medical Sciences
New Delhi, India

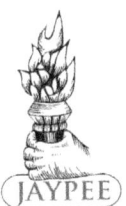

JAYPEE BROTHERS MEDICAL PUBLISHERS
The Health Sciences Publisher
New Delhi | London

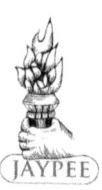 **Jaypee Brothers Medical Publishers (P) Ltd**

Headquarters

Jaypee Brothers Medical Publishers (P) Ltd
EMCA House, 23/23-B
Ansari Road, Daryaganj
New Delhi 110 002, India
Landline: +91-11-23272143, +91-11-23272703
+91-11-23282021, +91-11-23245672
Email: jaypee@jaypeebrothers.com

Corporate Office

Jaypee Brothers Medical Publishers (P) Ltd
4838/24, Ansari Road, Daryaganj
New Delhi 110 002, India
Phone: +91-11-43574357
Fax: +91-11-43574314
Email: jaypee@jaypeebrothers.com

Overseas Office

JP Medical Ltd
83 Victoria Street, London
SW1H 0HW (UK)
Phone: +44 20 3170 8910
Fax: +44 (0)20 3008 6180
Email: info@jpmedpub.com

Website: www.jaypeebrothers.com
Website: www.jaypeedigital.com

© 2023, Jaypee Brothers Medical Publishers

The views and opinions expressed in this book are solely those of the original contributor(s)/author(s) and do not necessarily represent those of editor(s) or publisher of the book.

All rights reserved. No part of this publication may be reproduced, stored or transmitted in any form or by any means, electronic, mechanical, photocopying, recording or otherwise, without the prior permission in writing of the publishers.

All brand names and product names used in this book are trade names, service marks, trademarks or registered trademarks of their respective owners. The publisher is not associated with any product or vendor mentioned in this book.

Medical knowledge and practice change constantly. This book is designed to provide accurate, authoritative information about the subject matter in question. However, readers are advised to check the most current information available on procedures included and check information from the manufacturer of each product to be administered, to verify the recommended dose, formula, method and duration of administration, adverse effects and contraindications. It is the responsibility of the practitioner to take all appropriate safety precautions. Neither the publisher nor the author(s)/editor(s) assume any liability for any injury and/or damage to persons or property arising from or related to use of material in this book.

This book is sold on the understanding that the publisher is not engaged in providing professional medical services. If such advice or services are required, the services of a competent medical professional should be sought.

Every effort has been made where necessary to contact holders of copyright to obtain permission to reproduce copyright material. If any have been inadvertently overlooked, the publisher will be pleased to make the necessary arrangements at the first opportunity.

Inquiries for bulk sales may be solicited at: jaypee@jaypeebrothers.com

Anesthesia and Critical Care Clinics–2

First Edition: **2023**

ISBN: 978-93-5465-691-0

Dedicated to
*The Teachers and Residents in Anesthesiology for their endeavor to
dissipate and acquire knowledge,
My parents for their blessings,
My daughter Ziva for her patience and tolerance
shown to loss of many precious moments and finally to
my wife Ishita for her understanding and encouragement*

–Puneet Khanna

My Parents, Wife, Teachers and Students

–Abhishek Singh

Contributors

Abhijit Kumar MBBS MD DESAIC
Senior Resident
Department of Anesthesiology
Vardhman Mahavir Medical College
and Safdarjung Hospital
New Delhi, India

Abhinav Prakash
Associate Consultant
Institute of Critical Care and Anesthesiology
Jai Prabha Medanta Super Specialty Hospital
Patna, Bihar, India

Abhishek Singh MD
Assistant Professor
Department of Anesthesiology,
Pain Medicine and Critical Care
All India Institute of Medical Sciences
New Delhi, India

Abhyuday Kumar
Assistant Professor
Department of Anesthesiology
All India Institute of Medical Sciences
Patna, Bihar, India

Ajay Singh
Assistant Professor
Department of Anesthesia
Postgraduate Institute of Medical Education
and Research
Chandigarh, India

Ajeet Kumar
Additional Professor
Department of Anesthesiology
All India Institute of Medical Sciences
Patna, Bihar, India

Ajit Kumar
Additional Professor
Department of Anesthesiology
All India Institute of Medical Sciences
Rishikesh, Uttarakhand, India

Akhilesh Gupta
Professor
Department of Anesthesia
Atal Bihari Vajpayee Institute of Medical Sciences
and Dr Ram Manohar Lohia Hospital
New Delhi, India

Amit Kohli
Professor
Department of Anesthesiology
Maulana Azad Medical College
New Delhi, India

Amit Kumar
Assistant Professor
Department of Anesthesiology,
Pain Medicine and Critical Care
All India Institute of Medical Sciences
New Delhi, India

Amitesh Chugh
Junior Resident
Department of Anesthesia and Intensive Care
Government Medical College and Hospital
Chandigarh, India

Anil Kumar
Senior Consultant and Head
Critical Care Medicine
Santosh Medical College Hospital
Ghaziabad, Uttar Pradesh, India

Anisha Singh MBBS MD (Anesthesiology)
Consultant
Santokba Durlabhji Memorial Hospital
Jaipur, Rajasthan, India

Anju Gupta
Assistant Professor
Department of Anesthesiology,
Pain Medicine and Critical Care
All India Institute of Medical Sciences
New Delhi, India

Contributors

Ankur Sharma
Associate Professor
Department of Trauma and Emergency
(Anesthesia and Critical Care)
All India Institute of Medical Sciences
Jodhpur, Rajasthan, India

Anshu Gupta
Associate Professor
Department of Anesthesia
Academic Block
Lady Hardinge Medical College
New Delhi, India

Arjun Balakrishnan
Senior Resident
Department of Neuroanesthesiology
and Critical Care
All India Institute of Medical Sciences
New Delhi, India

Arun A Bevoor
Senior Resident
Department of Anesthesia and Intensive Care
Government Medical College and Hospital
Chandigarh, India

Asim Ahmed
Senior Resident
Department of Anesthesiology,
Pain Medicine and Critical Care
All India Institute of Medical Sciences
New Delhi, India

Ayushi Mahajan MBBS MD (Anesthesiology)
Assistant Professor
Department of Anesthesiology
Maulana Azad Medical College
New Delhi, India

Baibhav Bhandari
Academic Senior Resident
Department of Anesthesiology
All India Institute of Medical Sciences
Rishikesh, Uttarakhand, India

Balaji Nagarajan
Senior Resident
Department of Anesthesiology,
Pain Medicine and Critical Care
All India Institute of Medical Sciences
New Delhi, India

Bhavna Kayarat
Senior Resident
Department of Critical Care Medicine
Sanjay Gandhi Postgraduate Institute
of Medical Sciences
Lucknow, Uttar Pradesh, India

Bhavya Krishna
Assistant Professor
Department of Anesthesia
Vardhman Mahavir Medical College
and Safdarjung Hospital
New Delhi, India

Chaitra TS
Junior Resident
Department of Anesthesia and Intensive Care
Government Medical College and Hospital
Chandigarh, India

Chandni Sinha
Additional Professor
Department of Anesthesiology
All India Institute of Medical Sciences
Patna, Bihar, India

Debyani Dey
Consultant Anesthesiologist
Department of Anesthesiology
Kailash Deepak Hospital
New Delhi, India

Deepak Kumar MBBS MD (Anesthesiology)
Senior Resident
Department of Anesthesia
Maulana Azad Medical College
New Delhi, India

Deepika Gupta
Assistant Professor
Department of Anesthesia and Intensive Care
Government Medical College and Hospital
Chandigarh, India

Devang Bharti
Assistant Professor
Department of Anesthesia
Atal Bihari Vajpayee Institute of Medical Sciences
and Dr Ram Manohar Lohia Hospital
New Delhi, India

Dhruv Jain
Assistant Professor
Department of Anesthesiology,
Pain Medicine and Critical Care
All India Institute of Medical Sciences
New Delhi, India

Gnanasekaran Srinivasan
Associate Professor
Department of Anesthesiology and Critical Care
Jawaharlal Institute of Postgraduate Medical
Education and Research
Puducherry, India

Gourav Mittal
Senior Resident
Department of Anesthesiology,
Pain Medicine and Critical Care
All India Institute of Medical Sciences
New Delhi, India

Himanshu Bhasin
Assistant Professor
Department of Anesthesia
Atal Bihari Vajpayee Institute of
Medical Sciences and
Dr Ram Manohar Lohia Hospital
New Delhi, India

Jyoti Singh
Associate Professor
Department of Anesthesia
Atal Bihari Vajpayee Institute of
Medical Sciences and
Dr Ram Manohar Lohia Hospital
New Delhi, India

Kiran Kumar Gudivada
Associate Professor
Department of Anesthesiology and Critical Care
All India Institute of Medical Sciences
Hyderabad, Telangana, India

Kirthiha Govindaraj
Assistant Professor
Department of Anesthesiology and
Critical Care
Jawaharlal Institute of Postgraduate
Medical Education and Research
Puducherry, India

Kunal Singh
Associate Professor
Department of Anesthesiology
All India Institute of Medical Sciences
Patna, Bihar, India

Magesh Parthiban
Senior Resident (Critical Care)
Department of Anesthesiology and Critical Care
Jawaharlal Institute of Postgraduate Medical
Education and Research
Puducherry, India

Manjula Sudhakar Rao
Assistant Professor
Department of Anesthesiology
Yenepoya Medical College
Yenepoya University
Mangaluru, Karnataka, India

Michelle Shirin Lazar
Senior Resident
Department of Anesthesia
Postgraduate Institute of Medical Education
and Research
Chandigarh, India

Mitchell Gullebani
Assistant Professor
Department of Anesthesia, Pain Medicine
and Critical Care
Guru Teg Bahadur Hospital
New Delhi, India

Nishant Sood MBBS MD (Anesthesiology)
Senior Consultant
Max Superspecialty Hospital
New Delhi, India

Nishkarsh Gupta
Professor
Department of Onco-Anesthesiology
and Palliative Medicine
All India Institute of Medical Sciences
New Delhi, India

Nitin
Assistant Professor
Department of Anesthesia
Atal Bihari Vajpayee Institute of Medical Sciences
and Dr Ram Manohar Lohia Hospital
New Delhi, India

Contributors

Parthodeep Jha
Junior Resident
Department of Anesthesiology,
Pain Medicine and Critical Care
All India Institute of Medical Sciences
New Delhi, India

Parul Sood
Junior Resident
Department of Anesthesia and Intensive Care
Government Medical College and Hospital
Chandigarh, India

Prachi Agrawal MBBS MD FIPM (Anesthesiology)
Senior Resident
Department of Anesthesiology
Maulana Azad Medical College
New Delhi, India

Pratik Singh
Junior Resident
Department of Anesthesiology
All India Institute of Medical Sciences
Patna, Bihar, India

Praveen Talawar
Additional Professor
Department of Anesthesiology
All India Institute of Medical Sciences
Rishikesh, Uttarakhand, India

Puja Saxena
Associate Professor
Department of Anesthesia and Intensive Care
Government Medical College and Hospital
Chandigarh, India

Puneet Khanna MD
Additional Professor
Department of Anesthesiology,
Pain Medicine and Critical Care
All India Institute of Medical Sciences
New Delhi, India

Rahil Singh MBBS DA DNB (Anesthesiology)
Associate Professor
Department of Anesthesiology
Maulana Azad Medical College
New Delhi, India

Revant Babu Chala
Academic Senior Resident
All India Institute of Medical Sciences
Rishikesh, Uttarakhand, India

Rajni Kalia
Senior Resident
Department of Anesthesia and Intensive Care
Government Medical College and Hospital
Chandigarh, India

Ranjitha N
Senior Resident
Department of Anesthesia
All India Institute of Medical Sciences
Mangaluru, Karnataka, India

Richa Saroa
Professor
Department of Anesthesia and Intensive Care
Government Medical College and Hospital
Chandigarh, India

Ridhima Bhatia MBBS DNB
Attending Consultant
Fortis Hospital
Faridabad, Haryana, India

Ridhima Sharma
Assistant Professor
Department of Anesthesiology
Superspecialty Pediatric Hospital and
Postgraduate Teaching Institute
Noida, Uttar Pradesh, India

Ripon Choudhary
Consultant
Department of Anesthesiology
ESI Hospital
Faridabad, Haryana, India

Samridhi Nanda
Associate Professor
Department of Anesthesia
Dhanwatri OT Complex
Sawai Man Singh Hospital
Jaipur, Rajasthan, India

Sangadala Priyanka
Junior Resident
Department of Anesthesiology
All India Institute of Medical Sciences
Rishikesh, Uttarakhand, India

Sangam Yadav MD
Senior Resident (Critical Care Medicine)
All India Institute of Medical Sciences
Jodhpur, Rajasthan, India

Sanjeev Palta
Professor
Department of Anesthesia and Intensive Care
Government Medical College and Hospital
Chandigarh, India

Saurabh Chandrakar
Academic Senior Resident
All India Institute of Medical Sciences
Rishikesh, Uttarakhand, India

Sayan Nath
Senior Resident (Critical Care Medicine)
All India Institute of Medical Sciences
New Delhi, India

Shivam Gupta
Additional Professor
Department of Anesthesiology
All India Institute of Medical Sciences
Rishikesh, Uttarakhand, India

Shubhi Singhal
Specialist
Department of Anesthesia
Cantonment General Hospital
New Delhi, India

Sudhansu Sekhar Nayak
Assistant Professor
Department of Anesthesiology
Atal Bihari Vajpayee Institute of Medical Sciences
and Dr Ram Manohar Lohia Hospital
New Delhi, India

Swati Jindal
Associate Professor
Department of Anesthesia and Intensive Care
Government Medical College and Hospital
Chandigarh, India

Swati Pandurangi
Senior Resident
Department of Anesthesia and Intensive Care
Vardhman Mahavir Medical College
and Safdarjung Hospital
New Delhi, India

T Nageswara Rao
Assistant Professor
Department of Anesthesiology,
Pain Medicine and Critical Care
All India Institute of Medical Sciences
New Delhi, India

Tanvi Meshram
Assistant Professor
Department of Anesthesia and Critical Care
All India Institute of Medical Sciences
Jodhpur, Rajasthan, India

Tazeen Khan
Senior Resident
Department of Anesthesiology,
Pain Medicine and Critical Care
All India Institute of Medical Sciences
New Delhi, India

Tenzin Nyima
Senior Resident
Department of Anesthesia and Intensive Care
Government Medical College and Hospital
Chandigarh, India

Umang Sharma
Junior Resident
Department of Anesthesia and Intensive Care
Government Medical College and Hospital
Chandigarh, India

Vadhan Prasanna S
Senior Resident (Critical Care Medicine)
Department of Anesthesiology
All India Institute of Medical Sciences
Rishikesh, Uttarakhand, India

Vrinda Chauhan
Senior Resident
Department of Anesthesiology,
Pain Medicine and Critical Care
All India Institute of Medical Sciences
New Delhi, India

Preface

Anesthesia and Critical Care Clinics-2 follows *Short and Long Cases in Anesthesiology* that was released in 2020. *Anesthesia and Critical Care Clinics-2* is a thoroughly updated and comprehensive textbook students in anesthesiology need in-depth knowledge of anesthesia workstation, monitoring, instruments and equipment as well as pharmacokinetics and pharmacodynamics of drugs in order to give safe anesthesia to the patient.

The art of giving safe anesthesia is so much dependent on technology of advanced monitoring gadgets as well as in-depth understanding of physics involved in it. Major part of the practical examination focuses on evaluating the examinee's knowledge of clinical case management but a substantial part also consists of testing the knowledge of the students in various aspect of instrument, understanding and interpreting chest X-ray, ECG, ventilator waveform and capnogram.

Very little books were available who can give students in-depth knowledge as well as being up-to-date covering complete Drugs, Instruments, Monitoring, CPR, ICU Equipment, PFT, ABG, ECG, X-ray, POCUS. In addition, judicious and liberal use of flowcharts, tables, boxes and figures make the content of book highly comprehensible.

The entire contributing faculties have paid special attention on gathering latest information about the subject and understanding the curriculum. All the faculties have utilized their clinical experience and academic knowledge for writing chapters in our book. I thank all our faculties for sparing their precious time as well as I thank our publisher for being patient, supporting and having complete faith on us.

We hope that the budding anesthetist will really benefit from this book and we are eagerly waiting for feedback, suggestion as well as criticism so that we can make next edition even better.

Puneet Khanna
Abhishek Singh

Acknowledgments

It was with great trepidation that we embarked upon our book, a hitherto uncharted territory in our academic career. Needless to say, that in an endeavor of this magnitude, we have piled up monumental debts. The least we can do to redeem ourself is to pay tributes to those whose efforts made it possible for our work to see the light of day.

We would like to thank Dr Gourav Mittal, Dr Vikas Saini and Dr Damarla Haritha who helped in proofreading the book.

We are extremely indebted to faculty, senior residents and junior residents for helping us to shape this book to its present form. Our special thanks to our friends for their support and faith. We would also like to thank our colleagues and juniors for their continuous support.

We are thankful to Shri Jitendar P Vij (Group Chairman), Mr Ankit Vij (Managing Director), Mr MS Mani (Group President), Ms Chetna Malhotra (Senior Director—Professional Publishing, Marketing and Business Development), Ms Pooja Bhandari (Production Head), and Ms Nikita Chauhan (Senior Development Editor) of M/s Jaypee Brothers Medical Publishers (P) Ltd., New Delhi, India, for giving the go-ahead at the very beginning and helping us in every way possible to bring out this book.

Nothing can be complete without extending our thanks and gratitude to the one who has powered us from within to complete this work—GOD ALMIGHTY.

Contents

SECTION 1: Anesthetic Pharmacology

1. Inhalational Agents 3
   Bhavya Krishna, Anju Gupta

2. Opioids 12
   Nishkarsh Gupta, Amit Kumar, Anju Gupta

3. Barbiturates 25
   Amit Kumar, Nishkarsh Gupta, Anju Gupta

4. Benzodiazepines 30
   Amit Kumar, Nishkarsh Gupta

5. Nonbarbiturate Intravenous Anesthetic Agents 38
   Anju Gupta, Asim Ahmed, Nishkarsh Gupta

6. Local Anesthetic 47
   Ridhima Sharma, Anju Gupta, Ripon Choudhary, Nishkarsh Gupta

7. Neuromuscular Blocking Agents 55
   Anju Gupta, Swati Pandurangi

8. Anticholinesterase Drugs and Cholinergic Agonists 60
   Dhruv Jain

9. Anticholinergic Medications 64
   Balaji Nagarajan, Puneet Khanna

10. Nonsteroidal Anti-inflammatory Drugs 69
    Balaji Nagarajan, Puneet Khanna

11. Sympathomimetics 74
    Magesh Parthiban, Puneet Khanna

12. Alpha and Beta Receptor Blockers 79
    Magesh Parthiban, Puneet Khanna

13. Antihypertensive Drugs 84
    Kiran Kumar Gudivada

14. Peripheral Vasodilators 86
    Kiran Kumar Gudivada

15. **Antiarrhythmic Drugs** 90
    Kiran Kumar Gudivada

16. **Calcium Channel Blockers** 94
    Debyani Dey, Anil Kumar, Vrinda Chauhan

17. **Histamine and Histamine Receptor Antagonist** 98
    Vrinda Chauhan, Puneet Khanna

18. **Insulin and Oral Hypoglycemic Drugs** 102
    Vrinda Chauhan, Puneet Khanna

19. **Diuretics** 106
    Vrinda Chauhan, Puneet Khanna

20. **Antacids and Prokinetics** 110
    Tanvi Meshram, Ankur Sharma

21. **Anticoagulants** 115
    Sangam Yadav, Ankur Sharma

22. **Chemotherapy** 125
    Tanvi Meshram, Ankur Sharma

23. **Enteral and Parenteral Nutrition** 130
    Vrinda Chauhan, Puneet Khanna

24. **Minerals and Electrolytes** 135
    Puneet Khanna, Vrinda Chauhan

25. **Intravenous Fluids** 147
    Anil Kumar, Debyani Dey, Vrinda Chauhan

26. **Anticonvulsants** 155
    Tanvi Meshram, Ankur Sharma

SECTION 2: Anesthesia Monitoring

27. **Arterial Blood Pressure Monitoring** 163
    Gnanasekaran Srinivasan, Kirthiha Govindaraj

28. **Central Venous Cannulation Technique and Central Venous Pressure Monitoring** 175
    Kirthiha Govindaraj, Gnanasekaran Srinivasan

29. **Pulmonary Artery Catheter Monitoring** 187
    Kirthiha Govindaraj, Gnanasekaran Srinivasan

30. **Perioperative Cardiac Output Monitoring** 198
    Sayan Nath, Abhishek Singh, Puneet Khanna

31. **Transcranial Doppler** 211
    Bhavana Kayarat, Arjun Balakrishnan, Puneet Khanna

32. **Cerebral Oximetry** 214
    Bhavana Kayarat, Puneet Khanna

33. **Electroencephalogram** 216
    Bhavana Kayarat, Puneet Khanna

34. **Somatosensory and Motor Evoked Potentials** 218
    Arjun Balakrishnan, Bhavana Kayarat, Puneet Khanna

35. **Bispectral Index** 222
    Bhavana Kayarat, Arjun Balakrishnan, Puneet Khanna

36. **Entropy** 224
    Sudhansu Sekhar Nayak, Arjun Balakrishnan

37. **Respiratory Monitoring** 227
    Vrinda Chauhan, Puneet Khanna, Abhishek Singh

38. **Pulse Oximetry** 234
    Abhishek Singh

39. **Capnometry and Capnography** 239
    Ajit Kumar, Baibhav Bhandari

40. **Patterns of Neuromuscular Stimulation** 245
    Anju Gupta, Mitchell Gullebani

41. **Nerve Stimulator** 253
    Anju Gupta, Manjula Sudhakar Rao

42. **Temperature Monitoring** 260
    Tazeen Khan, Parthodeep Jha, Puneet Khanna

43. **Acid–Base Status Evaluation** 266
    Ajit Kumar, Saurabh Chandrakar

44. **Pulmonary Function Test** 280
    Ajit Kumar, Shivam Gupta, Revant Babu Chala

SECTION 3: Anesthesia Instruments

45. **Medical Gas Cylinders** 289
    Ranjitha N, Puneet Khanna

46. **Gas Pipeline** 291
    Abhishek Singh

47. **Suction Apparatus** 293
    Ranjitha N, Puneet Khanna

48. **Anesthesia Machine** 295
    Richa Saroa, Sanjeev Palta, Swati Jindal, Rajni Kalia

49. **Vaporizers** 307
    Richa Saroa, Sanjeev Palta, Tenzin Nyima, Arun A Bevoor

50. **Breathing Circuits** 316
    Richa Saroa, Sanjeev Palta, Deepika Gupta, Chaitra TS

51. **Manual Resuscitators** 325
    Ajeet Kumar, Kunal Singh, Chandni Sinha

52. **Humidification Equipment** 328
    Chandni Sinha, Abhinav Prakash, Pratik Singh

53. **Circle System** 331
    Abhyuday Kumar, Chandni Sinha, Ajeet Kumar

54. **Face Masks and Airways** 335
    Prachi Agrawal, Amit Kohli

55. **Supraglottic Airway Devices** 342
    Deepak Kumar, Abhijit Kumar, Amit Kohli

56. **Laryngoscopes** 354
    Anisha Singh, Abhijit Kumar

57. **Endotracheal Tube** 362
    Rahil Singh, Nishant Sood

58. **Lung Isolation Devices** 371
    Ayushi Mahajan, Amit Kohli

59. **Devices for Difficult Airway Management** 377
    Ridhima Sharma, Ripon Choudhary

60. **Gas Monitoring Equipment** 386
    Abhishek Singh

61. **Spinal and Epidural Needles** 390
    Richa Saroa, Sanjeev Palta, Umang Sharma, Amitesh Chugh

62. **Patient-controlled Analgesia Pumps** 396
    Richa Saroa, Sanjeev Palta, Puja Saxena, Parul Sood

63. **Cleaning and Sterilization** 405
    Chandni Sinha, Abhinav Prakash, Ajeet Kumar

SECTION 4: ICU Instruments

64. **Percutaneous Tracheostomy** 413
    Akhilesh Gupta, Devang Bharti

65. **Oxygen Delivery Devices** 417
    Anshu Gupta, Akhilesh Gupta

66. **Ventilators, Modes of Ventilator, and Ventilator Graphics** 428
    Nitin, Akhilesh Gupta

67. **Deep Vein Thrombosis: Mechanical Pump** 432
    Devang Bharti, Akhilesh Gupta

68. **Jet Ventilation** 436
    Akhilesh Gupta, Shubhi Singhal

69. **Ultrasound Machine** 441
    Himanshu Bhasin, Akhilesh Gupta

70. **Rapid Infusion Pumps** 444
    Akhilesh Gupta, Jyoti Singh

71. **Automated Chest Compressor Machine** 447
    Jyoti Singh, Akhilesh Gupta

72. **Extracorporeal Membrane Oxygenation** 450
    Devang Bharti, Akhilesh Gupta

73. **Renal Replacement Therapy** 454
    Gourav Mittal

74. **Defibrillators** 465
    Shubhi Singhal, Akhilesh Gupta

75. **Intra-abdominal Pressure Monitoring** 469
    Anshu Gupta, Akhilesh Gupta

76. **Esophageal Pressure Manometry** 472
    Akhilesh Gupta, Himanshu Bhasin

SECTION 5: Resuscitation

77. **Cardiopulmonary Resuscitation** 479
    Ajay Singh, Michelle Shirin Lazar

SECTION 6: Miscellaneous

78. **Commonly Used Instruments in Chronic Pain** 503
    Samridhi Nanda

79. **Physics in Anesthesia** 510
    T Nageswara Rao

80. **Electrocardiogram and X-ray** 514
    Ridhima Bhatia, Puneet Khanna

81. **Point-of-care Ultrasonography for the Postgraduates** 528
    Praveen Talawar, Vadhan Prasanna S, Sangadala Priyanka

Index *541*

SECTION 1

Anesthetic Pharmacology

- **Inhalational Agents**
  Bhavya Krishna, Anju Gupta
- **Opioids**
  Nishkarsh Gupta, Amit Kumar, Anju Gupta
- **Barbiturates**
  Amit Kumar, Nishkarsh Gupta, Anju Gupta
- **Benzodiazepines**
  Amit Kumar, Nishkarsh Gupta
- **Nonbarbiturate Intravenous Anesthetic Agents**
  Anju Gupta, Asim Ahmed, Nishkarsh Gupta
- **Local Anesthetic**
  Ridhima Sharma, Anju Gupta, Ripon Choudhary, Nishkarsh Gupta
- **Neuromuscular Blocking Agents**
  Anju Gupta, Swati Pandurangi
- **Anticholinesterase Drugs and Cholinergic Agonists**
  Dhruv Jain
- **Anticholinergic Medications**
  Balaji Nagarajan, Puneet Khanna
- **Nonsteroidal Anti-inflammatory Drugs**
  Balaji Nagarajan, Puneet Khanna
- **Sympathomimetics**
  Magesh Parthiban, Puneet Khanna
- **Alpha and Beta Receptor Blockers**
  Magesh Parthiban, Puneet Khanna
- **Antihypertensive Drugs**
  Kiran Kumar Gudivada
- **Peripheral Vasodilator**
  Kiran Kumar Gudivada
- **Antiarrhythmic Drugs**
  Kiran Kumar Gudivada
- **Calcium Channel Blockers**
  Debyani Dey, Anil Kumar, Vrinda Chauhan
- **Histamine and Histamine Receptor Antagonist**
  Vrinda Chauhan, Puneet Khanna
- **Insulin and Oral Hypoglycemic Drugs**
  Vrinda Chauhan, Puneet Khanna
- **Diuretics**
  Vrinda Chauhan, Puneet Khanna
- **Antacids and Prokinetics**
  Tanvi Meshram, Ankur Sharma
- **Anticoagulants**
  Sangam Yadav, Ankur Sharma
- **Chemotherapy**
  Tanvi Meshram, Ankur Sharma
- **Enteral and Parenteral Nutrition**
  Vrinda Chauhan, Puneet Khanna
- **Minerals and Electrolytes**
  Puneet Khanna, Vrinda Chauhan
- **Intravenous Fluids**
  Anil Kumar, Debyani Dey, Vrinda Chauhan
- **Anticonvulsants**
  Tanvi Meshram, Ankur Sharma

Basic Questions

Q. 1. Define pharmacokinetics and pharmacodynamics?

Q. 2. Enumerate various routes of drug administration. Advantages of each and drawbacks?

Q. 3. What are phase I and phase II reactions? Describe pathways.

Q. 4. What is bioavailability and volume of distribution of drug?

Q. 5. Define redistribution, elimination and clearence. Significance?

Q. 6. What is plasma half life, context sensitive half time?

Q. 7. Enumerate and explain various pharmacokinetic modes?

Q. 8. With example explain (i) Partial agonist (ii) Agonist antagonist (iii) Inverse agonist.

Q. 9. Enumerate and describe various type of receptors.

Q. 10. Define potency and efficacy with examples (opioids).

Q. 11. How does genetic variation affect drugs i.e. (i) Opioids (ii) Succinylcholine?

CHAPTER 1

Inhalational Agents

Bhavya Krishna, Anju Gupta

Q. 1. What are inhalational agents? How are they classified? Describe an ideal anesthetic agent. Where can they be used?

Ans. Inhaled anesthetics are chemical compounds with general anesthetic properties that are delivered via inhalational route (e.g., via face mask, laryngeal mask airway, endotracheal tube).

They are primarily used for induction and maintenance of anesthesia, but can also be used for management of bronchospasm and status epilepticus, sedation in intensive care units (ICUs), and labor analgesia.

An ideal anesthetic agent will have: high potency, nonflammability, molecular stability, minimal systemic effects, low blood:gas solubility, good safety profile, inexpensive, and easy to store.

They can be classified as a volatile (sevoflurane, isoflurane, desflurane, methoxyflurane, enflurane, halothane, ether) or nonvolatile anesthetic agents (cyclopropane, nitrous oxide, xenon).

A few of the commonly used inhalational agents at present are shown in **Figure 1** (left to right) such as sevoflurane, desflurane, isoflurane.

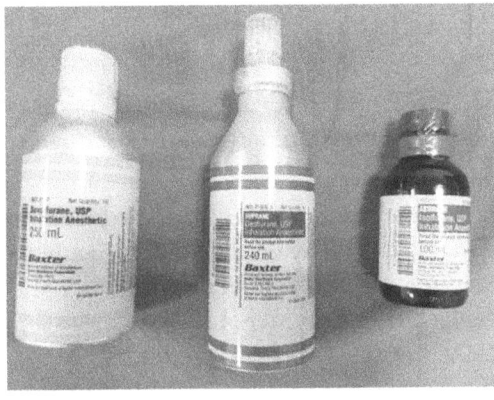

Fig. 1: Commonly used inhalational agents.

Q. 2. Explain their properties—chemical, physical, and biophysical.

Ans. *Vapor pressure:* When a liquid anesthetic agent (volatile) turns to gas, pressure is developed by the vaporization = vapor pressure (depends on temperature)

Solubility: Ratio of concentration in the blood to alveolar gas when partial pressures are the same.

The number of particles or volume of an individual gas in a mixture of gases $\propto$ partial pressure, and depend on solubility.

According to Henry's law: $V = S \times P$ (V = volume of gas, P = partial pressure of gas, S = solubility coefficient of gas in solvent)

For a poorly soluble agent in blood, equilibrium will be reached when relatively few molecules have dissolved and the partial pressure at which equilibrium occurs will be relatively high. When an agent is highly soluble in blood, there will be a large number of molecules in the liquid phase at an equilibrium and partial pressure will be relatively low.

Partition coefficient: A partition coefficient is the ratio of the concentration of the agent in one solvent to the concentration in another solvent at equilibrium. It is used to describe the solubility of inhalation anesthetics in a variety of different solvents like blood, oil, muscle, and gas.

Blood: Gas partition coefficient determines the speed of anesthetic induction and recovery.

Oil: Gas partition coefficient determines anesthetic potency, i.e., higher the coefficient, the more potent the agent.

High partition coefficient = high lipophilicity
= high potency = high solubility
High solubility = more anesthetic needs to be dissolved = slower onset

Physiochemical properties are described in **Table 1**.

Q. 3. What is minimum alveolar concentration (MAC)? What are the MAC derivatives? Mention the factors affecting MAC?

Ans. Minimum alveolar concentration (MAC) is defined as the minimum alveolar concentration of inhaled anesthetic at sea level required to prevent apparently purposeful movement in 50% of patients in response to surgical incision. (= ED50 for intravenous drugs). It is a measure of anesthetic potency. The values of MAC for specific anesthetic agents are mentioned in **Table 1**.

- *Minimum alveolar concentration derivatives:*
  MAC-awake: Anesthetic concentration required to suppress the voluntary response to verbal command in 50% of patients. Value = 0.15–0.5 MAC
  MAC-amnesia: Anesthetic concentration required to suppress explicit memory of noxious stimuli = 0.06–0.3 MAC.
  MAC-BAR: Anesthetic concentration that blocks autonomic changes to surgical incision = 1.5 MAC
  Other derivatives exist like MAC-EI (MAC-Endotracheal intubation), MAC-EX (MAC-extubation), and MAC-unawake.

- *Factors affecting minimum alveolar concentrations:*
  - *Physiological factors:*
    - Age. MAC peaks at 6 months of age then decreases every decade by 6%.
    - Pregnancy
    - Temperature
    - Sodium
    - Thyroid function
  - *Pharmacological factors:*
    - MAC additivity with other drugs
  - Pathological factors
  - Pharmacogenetic factors

Q. 4. Describe the mechanism of action of inhalational agents.

Ans. Inhaled anesthetics work on the central nervous system by enhancing postsynaptic inhibitory activity at gamma-aminobutyric acid (GABA-A) and glycine receptors and inhibiting presynaptic receptor activity at acetylcholine (muscarinic and nicotinic receptors), glutamate or N-methyl-D-aspartate (NMDA) receptors, and serotonin 5-hydroxytryptamine (5-HT) receptors. Various theories like Meyer-Overton hypothesis, lipid bilayer expansion theory, neuromodular theory, and Mullin's critical volume hypothesis explain the mechanism of action of inhaled anesthetics.

Q. 5. Explain pharmacokinetics of inhalational agents.

Ans. As shown in **Figure 2**, the pharmacokinetics of inhalational agents involves uptake, distribution, metabolism, and elimination.

Uptake and Distribution

Starts from the anesthesia machine vaporizer till the clinical effects of inhalational agents are visible once they reach therapeutic concentrations in the central nervous system (CNS). This occurs when there is equilibrium in Alveolar, blood, and brain partial pressures ($P_{CNS} = P_{blood} = P_{alveoli}$).

TABLE 1: Physicochemical properties of inhaled anesthetic agents.

Property	Sevoflurane	Desflurane	Isoflurane	Enflurane	Halothane	Nitrous oxide
Molecular structure	$C_4H_3F_7O$	$C_3H_2F_6O$	$C_3H_2ClF_5O$	$C_3H_2ClF_5O$	$C_2HBrClF_3$	N_2O
Odor	Nonirritant	Pungent	Irritant	Nonirritant	Nonirritant, sweet	Odorless
Boiling point (degree Celsius)	59	24	49	57	50	–88
Vapor pressure at 20°C (mm Hg)	157	669	238	172	243	38,770
Molecular weight (g)	200	168	184	184	197	44
Blood: Gas partition coefficient	0.65	0.42	1.46	1.9	2.5	0.46
Oil: Gas partition coefficient	47	19	91	97	224	1.4
Fat: Blood solubility	47.5	27.2	44.9	36	51.1	2.3
Muscle: Blood solubility	3.1	2.0	2.9	1.7	3.4	1.2
Brain: Blood solubility	1.7	1.3	1.6	1.4	1.9	1.1
Minimum alveolar concentration (MAC) in 100% Oxygen	1.8	6.6	1.17	1.63	0.75	104
MAC in 70% N_2O	0.66	2.38	0.56	0.57	0.29	
Preservative	Nil	Nil	Nil	Nil	Thymol	Nil
Stability in moist CO_2 absorber	No	Yes	Yes	Yes	No	Yes
% Biotransformation into metabolites	3.5	0.02	0.2	2	20, Hepatic cytochrome P450	<0.01
Metabolites	Inorganic and organic fluorides Compound A in the presence of soda lime and heat (Compounds B, C, D, and E)	Mainly excreted unchanged through exhaled air Trifluoroacetic acid	Trifluoroacetic acid and F	Inorganic and organic fluorides	Trifluoroacetic acid, Cl^-, Br^-	(N_2)

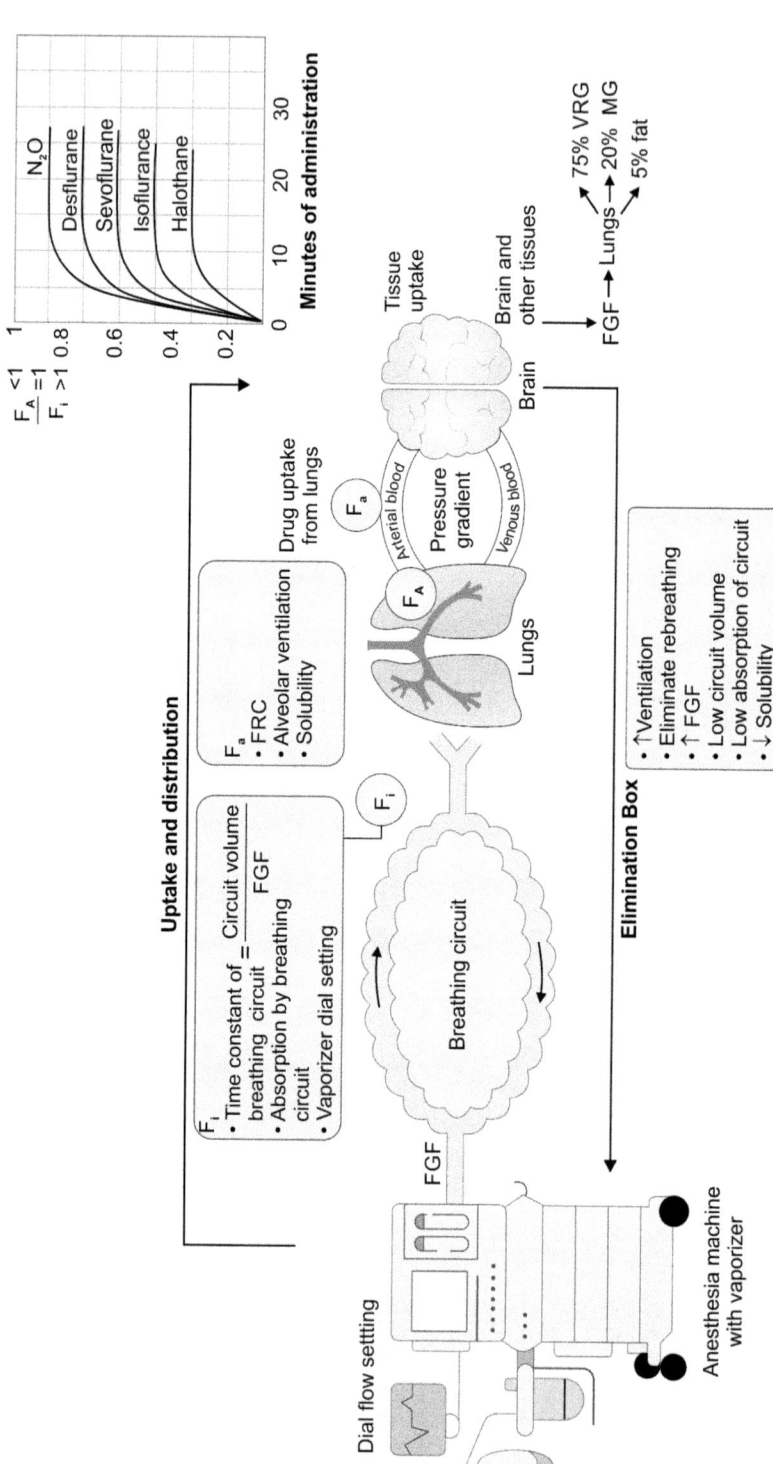

Fig. 2: Pharmacokinetics of inhalational anesthetics.
(F_a: arterial blood concentration; F_i: inspire concentration; F_A: alveolar concentration; FGF: fresh gas flow; FRC: functional residual capacity; MG: muscle group; VRG: vessel-rich group)

- *Alveolar concentration of inhalational agents depends on:*
  - The inspired concentration of agent: Concentration of inhaled anesthetic affects the rate of increase of the alveolar concentration (F_A) towards the inspired concentration (F_i). More the inspired concentration, the faster is the increase in the F_A/F_i ratio, hence the faster induction of anesthesia. Higher fresh gas flow, lower breathing system volume, higher vaporizer dial flow setting, and lower circuit absorption leads to higher inspired gas concentration and faster induction and emergence from anesthesia.
  - Alveolar ventilation: Increased alveolar ventilation leads to a faster increase in alveolar partial pressure by replacing the inhalation agent taken up by the pulmonary blood flow.
  - Functional residual capacity (FRC): Large FRC dilutes the inspired concentration of gas causing lower alveolar partial pressure and therefore slower onset of anesthesia.
- *Drug uptake from lungs:*

$$\text{Uptake} = \frac{\text{Blood gas partition coefficient} \times \text{Cardiac output} \times \text{Partial pressure (alveolar - mixed venous pressure)}}{\text{Barometric pressure}}$$

  - Solubility (blood gas solubility coefficient).
  - Pulmonary alveolar blood flow (cardiac output): Higher cardiac output leads to more uptake of anesthetic from the lungs hence more rapid delivery to the tissues. The equilibration of tissue anesthetic partial pressures and arterial blood is reached quicker. As the alveolar concentration is lowered by the high uptake of anesthetic, it doesn't lead to faster induction. In contrast, low cardiac output state results in the slow uptake of anesthetic agents and higher alveolar pressures (higher F_A/F_i ratio), and therefore faster induction of anesthesia.
  - Alveolar venous partial pressure gradient and tissue uptake as per the multicompartment kinetic model.
  - Effect of obesity and age, and second gas effect.
- *Elimination increased by:* Increasing ventilation, eliminating rebreathing, increasing FGF, low circuit volume, low absorption by circuit, decreased solubility.

Concentration Effect

Seen only with nitrous oxide, where increasing inspired concentration of the gas leads to its rise in alveolar concentration.

Second Gas Effect

Administrating anesthetic agent along with nitrous oxide increases the alveolar partial pressure of the agent, due to the rapid uptake of nitrous oxide by lungs owing to its increased solubility and hence faster induction time. The loss of volume associated with the uptake of nitrous oxide, concentrates the inhaled anesthetic. It is due to the concentration effect.

Diffusion hypoxia: Due to the reverse of concentration effect, when nitrous oxide delivery is stopped, it displaces oxygen from the alveoli and leads to diffusion hypoxia.

Tissue uptake depends upon the tissue/blood partition coefficient (tissue solubility), the tissue blood flow, and the tissue anesthetic concentration. Brain, liver, kidneys, heart, endocrines, splanchnic beds are a vessel-rich group and will be saturated first by the inhalational agents followed by vessel poor regions such as skin, fat, etc.

Metabolism, breakdown, and toxicity are mentioned in **Table 1**.

Q. 6. Explain pharmacodynamics of inhalational agents.

Ans. **Table 2** explains the pharmacodynamics of inhalational anesthetic agents and the system-wise effects.

TABLE 2: System wise effects of anesthetic agents.

	Sevoflurane	Desflurane	Isoflurane	Enflurane	Halothane	Nitrous oxide
Suitability for induction	Suitable	Potent odor, not suitable	Not recommended	–	Can be used	–
Cardiac output	↔	↔	↓↓	↓↓	↓	↓
Systemic vascular resistance	↓	↓↓	↓↓	↓	↓	↑, also increases Pulmonary vascular resistance
Mean arterial pressure	↓	↓↓	↓↓	↓↓	↓↓	↔
Heart rate	↔, can prolong QT interval	↑↑	↑↑↑	↑	↓↓	↑
Contractility	↓	Minimal	↓	↓↓	↑↑↑, Has high arrhythmogenic potential with even 1.1–1.3 mcg/kg/min at 0.7–1.3 MAC	
Coronary steal	Nil	Nil	Possibly	Nil	Nil	
Splanchnic blood flow	Unchanged	Unchanged	Unchanged	↓	↓	
Sensitization to catecholamines	Nil	Nil	↑	↑	Arrhythmogenic potential: Halothane > Isoflurane > Desflurane > Sevoflurane	
Respiratory rate	↑↑	↑↑	↑↑	↑↑	↑↑	
Tidal volume	↓	↓↓	↓↓	↓↓↓	↓	
Airway resistance	↓	↔	↓		↓	
Respiratory center	The threshold of the respiratory center for hypercarbia and hypoxia is decreased					
Hypoxic pulmonary vasoconstriction (HPV) response	↓↓	↓↓	↓↓	↓↓	↓↓	↓↓
$PaCO_2$	↑	↑↑	↑↑	↑↑↑	Unchanged	

Contd...

Chapter 1: Inhalational Agents

Contd...

	Sevoflurane	Desflurane	Isoflurane	Enflurane	Halothane	Nitrous oxide
Cerebral blood flow	↑↑↑	↑, increases cerebrospinal fluid (CSF) production without decreasing reabsorption	↑, least cerebral vasodilation, maintains cerebral autoregulation better than others	↑	↑	
CMRO₂	↓	↓	↓	↓	↓	
Increased intracranial pressure (ICP)	↓	↓	↓	↑, increases CSF production and reduces the reabsorption	↓	↑
Motor-evoked potentials (MEPs) Sensory evoked potentials (SSEPs)	↓	All are cerebral vasodilators and may potentially increase ICP	↓	↓	↓	
Electroencephalogram (EEG)	Burst suppression	Burst suppression	Burst suppression	Epileptiform activity	Burst suppression	Burst suppression
Glomerular filtration rate (GFR)	↓	↓	↕			
Hepatic blood flow	↓	↓	↓, Causes hepatic arterial vasodilatation. Oxygen delivery preserved.	↓	↓	→
Effect on uterus	Some relaxation	Some relaxation	Some relaxation	Some relaxation	Some relaxation	Some relaxation
Analgesia	Some	Some	Some	Some	Some	Some
Potentiation of muscle relaxation	Significant	Significant	Significant	Significant	Some	Significant

Works by postsynaptic effect at the nicotinic acetylcholine receptor located at the neuromuscular junction

Contd...

Contd...

	Sevoflurane	Desflurane	Isoflurane	Enflurane	Halothane	Nitrous oxide
Specific mention	Higher incidence of postoperative agitation in children	Due to the low boiling point (23°C), needs Tec 6 vaporizer, has a fast onset and offset of action, therefore suitable in long procedures where rapid wake up is required	Coronary steal phenomenon—normally responsive coronary arterioles are dilated and divert blood away from areas supplied by diseased and unresponsive vessels, resulting in ischemia		Maximum bronchodilatory effect	"Laughing gas"
Contraindications	Genetic disorders like *malignant hyperthermia*. To be used with caution in severe *hypovolemia*.				Heart failure with reduced EF, pheochromocytoma, avoid repeat exposure within 3 months	Venous/arterial air embolism, Pneumothorax, intestinal obstruction, intraocular and middle ear surgeries
Adverse effects	Metabolism produces increased levels of inorganic fluoride—causes renal impairment in rats, not reported in humans yet, but recommended to avoid in preexisting renal dysfunction undergoing extensive procedures, compound A formation	Carbon monoxide (CO) toxicity seen with desflurane > enflurane > isoflurane, occurs when the volatile agent comes in contact with anhydrous soda-lime or baralyme "Monday morning phenomenon"			Halothane hepatitis—fulminant hepatic necrosis—caused by its metabolite trifluoroacetyl chloride	Exposure of few hours may cause megaloblastic changes in bone marrow; prolonged exposure may result in agranulocytosis and neurological syndromes due to chronic vitamin B_{12} inactivation. Teratogenicity has been seen in rats, may be avoided in the first trimester in humans. *Diffusion hypoxia*

Overdose of any inhalational agent can lead to cardiovascular depression. Postoperative nausea and vomiting.

Q. 7. Mention the adverse effects and other nonanesthetic effects of inhalational agents, contraindications.

Ans. It is described in **Table 2**.

Q. 8. Explain about pharmacoeconomics and environment.

Ans.
- Formula for consumption of inhalational agent:

$$\text{Fluid volatile agent (in mL)} = \left(\text{FGF}\left(\frac{mL}{min}\right) \times \text{VA conc. (vol\%)} \times \text{duration}\right) \div \left(\text{Saturated gas vol}\left(in\,\frac{mL}{mL}\right) \times 100\right)$$

Where FGF = Fresh gas flow, VA conc. is a dial flow percentage, saturated gas volume is a constant for the various volatile anesthetics = Sevoflurane (184), isoflurane (195), desflurane (210), halothane (229). Useful for calculating costing as well as conservation of gases.

- Greenhouse effect: WAG (Waste anesthetic gases) accounts for 6% of total greenhouse gases and is comprised mostly of nitrous oxide and halogenated anesthetics (isoflurane, sevoflurane, desflurane), can cause ozone depletion.

Q. 9. Describe individual agents which are summarized in Table 1.

Ans. Isoflurane, desflurane, sevoflurane, enflurane, halothane, and nitrous oxide.

Q. 10. What are recent advances?

Ans. The recent advances are as follows:
- *Xenon:* Closest to an ideal anesthetic agent. The blood gas coefficient is 0.12—rapid onset and rapid recovery. Not metabolized in liver or kidney—does not trigger malignant hyperthermia. Potent intraoperative analgesic. Nonflammable. Does not deplete ozone or cause environmental pollution. MAC 71%
- *Anesthetic conserving device (AnaConDa):* It is an anesthetic delivery system developed for the administration of volatile anesthetics to invasively ventilated patients especially in ICU with ventilators.
- *Cognitive dysfunction* and *neurotoxicity* with the use of inhalational agents are being evaluated in preclinical data, more studies are required.
- *Enhanced recovery after anesthesia (ERAS)* protocols suggest avoiding inhalational agents and nitrous oxide.
- The *ENIGMA-II* trial showed that nitrous oxide does not increase the risk of death or cardiovascular complications.

QUESTIONS

Q. 1. Historical milestones of inhalation anesthesia.

Q. 2. Enumerate arrhythmogenic doses of epinephrine with inhalation anesthetic activities at various MACs.

Q. 3. Enumerate and explain MOA by (i) Lipid based theories (ii) Protein based theories.

Q. 4. Scavenging, advantages. Difference between active and passive scavenging.

Q. 5. What is MIRUS?

Q. 6. Inference of GAS and PANDA studies.

FURTHER READING

1. Barash PG, Cullen BF, Cahalan MK, Stock MC, Ortega R, Sarhar SR, et al. Clinical Anesthesia Fundamentals: Print + Ebook with Multimedia, 7th edition. Philadelphia: Lippincott Williams and Wilkins; 2015.
2. Gropper MA, Eriksson LI, Fleisher LA, Wiener-Kronish JP, Cohen NH, Leslie K. Miller's Anesthesia, 9th edition. Philadelphia: Elsevier-Health Sciences Division; 2019. pp. 3112.

CHAPTER 2: Opioids

Nishkarsh Gupta, Amit Kumar, Anju Gupta

INTRODUCTION

- Opioids are naturally occurring or synthetic drugs which have stereospecific action on opioid receptors and their actions can be reversed by antagonist naloxone **(Table 1)**.
- Opium is obtained from the capsule of unripe *Oriental Poppy (Papaver somniferum)*.
- Initially used for antidiarrheal properties later analgesic, sedative, and antitussive properties were recognized.
- *Diamorphine* or *diacetylmorphine (heroin)* was produced to cure morphine dependence but itself became the powerful drug of addiction.
- *Pethidine* was used for antispasmodic properties but later found to have analgesic properties.
- *Phenylpropylamine* or *methadone* was developed and used as a morphine alternative during the Second World War.
- All of the effective opioids have a tendency of drug dependence.
- These drugs are more effective for reactive pain components (e.g., anxiety, fear, suffering, etc.) and the pain threshold is minimally affected.

MECHANISM OF ACTION

- There exist three major classes of opioid receptors (μ, κ, δ) and one orphan receptor (ORL_1).
- The opioid drugs act on these receptors.
- Receptor downregulation may be the reason for opioid tolerance with prolonged use. Receptor up-regulation may also be seen.

The mechanism of action of opioids is shown in **Flowchart 1**.

ENDOGENOUS OPIOID PEPTIDES (BOX 1)

- Enkephalins
- Endorphins
- Dynorphins
- Nociceptin/Orphanin-FQ
- Endomorphins
- Other peptides—β-casomorphins, hemorphins, cytochrophins, dermorphins, and deltorphins
  - *Enkephalins*
    - Selective affinity for δ receptors.
    - Two similar pentapeptides, methionine (Met)-enkephalin and leucine (Leu)-enkephalin, have been isolated from brain extracts.
    - Wide distribution in the central nervous system (CNS)—spinal cord, hypothalamus, posterior pituitary, the globus pallidus, the limbic system, and cerebrospinal fluid (CSF). Also found in sympathetic ganglia, adrenal medulla, and gastrointestinal tract.

TABLE 1: Opioid drugs and their common receptors.

Receptors	Other names	Effects	Agonist	Partial agonist	Antagonist
μ-receptor ($μ_1, μ_2$)	OP_3/MOR/ MOP	Supraspinal analgesia ($μ_1$), Spinal analgesia ($μ_2$), euphoria, nausea, and vomiting, bradycardia, respiratory depression ($μ_2$), miosis, inhibition of gut motility, pruritus	• β-Endorphin • Endomorphins • Morphine • Pethidine • Methadone • Fentanyl Prototypical agonist- morphine	• Buprenorphine	• Naloxone • Naltrexone • Pentazocine • Nalorphine
κ-receptor ($κ_1, κ_2, κ_3$)	OP_2/KOR/ KOP	• Analgesia • Sedation • Dysphoria • Diuresis	• Dynorphin • Morphine • Pentazocine • Nalorphine Prototypical agonist- ketocyclazocine		• Naloxone • Naltrexone
δ-receptor ($δ_1, δ_2$)	OP_1 DOR/ DOP	Spinal analgesia	• (Met)-enkephalin • (Leu)-enkephalin • Deltorphin-II Prototypical agonist-N-allyl- normetazocine		• Naloxone
N/OFQ receptor	ORL_1/OP_4/ NOR/NOP	• Structurally similar to classical opioid receptors. • Does not specifically bind endogenous opioid peptides and opioid analgesics			
σ-receptor		• No longer classified as opioid receptors (as they lack stereoselectivity or antagonism of classical receptors) • Receptor site for phencyclidine and ketamine			

- Seen in CSF after placebo analgesia, acupuncture, and electrical stimulation of periaqueductal gray.
- Rapid hydrolysis by specific peptidases (e.g., enkephalinase), action may be prolonged by enzyme inhibitors (D-phenylalanine).
- Synthetic analogs are produced but have issues of tolerance and dependence.

- *Endorphins:*
  - Act primarily on μ and δ receptors.
  - Distributed mainly in the hypothalamus and pituitary gland.
  - More potent than enkephalins and produce long-lasting analgesia.
- *Dynorphins:*
  - Primarily bound on κ-receptors.
  - Distributed in posterior pituitary and hypothalamus.

Section 1: Anesthetic Pharmacology

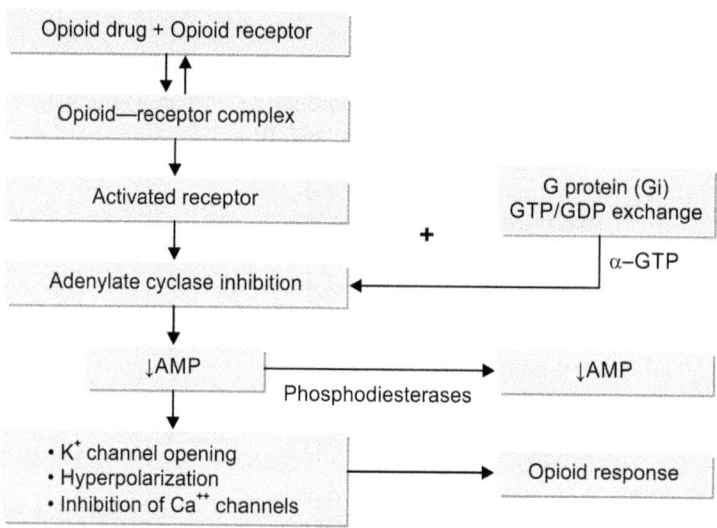

Flowchart 1: Mechanism of action of opioids.

(GTP: guanosine triphosphate; GDP: gastroduodenal perforation; AMP: adenosine monophosphate)

BOX 1: Clinical significance of endogenous opioids.

- Body temperature regulation
- Immune function
- Gastrointestinal mobility
- Renal and hepatic physiology
- Cardiac and respiratory physiology
- Extrapyramidal activity
- Stress response
- Appetite and thirst regulation
- Behavioral role
- Hypothalamus and pituitary function
- Autonomic function

- Modulate the effect of other opioids, have no analgesic effect on the brain or spinal cord.
- They have a role in the pathophysiology of spinal cord injuries; their administration may improve neurological outcomes and prolong survival in cerebrovascular events.
• *Nociceptin/Orphanin FQ:*
  - This peptide is bound to an opioid-like orphan receptor (ORL$_1$).
  - It has no significant activity on μ-, κ- or δ- receptors.
  - Distributed in the dorsal horn, sensory pathways of the trigeminal nerve, periaqueductal gray, dorsal raphe, hippocampus, and amygdaloid nuclei.
  - It is involved in analgesic, hyperalgesic, and biphasic response.
• *Endomorphins:*
  - Primarily bound to μ receptors to produce spinal and supraspinal analgesia.
  - Two isolated forms—(1) *endomorphin-I* and (2) *endomorphin-II*

OPIOID ANALGESIC DRUGS

Opioid analgesic drugs are described in **Table 2**.

PURE OPIOID AGONIST

Morphine (Tables 3 and 4)

- Its name is derived from the name of the Greek God of dreams—"Morpheus."
- It is the standard opioid analgesic agent. All opioid agents are compared against morphine.

TABLE 2: Opioid analgesic drugs.

Agonists	Mixed agonist-antagonist	Antagonist
Phenanthrene alkaloids of opium		
• Codeine		Methylnaltrexone
• Morphine		
• Papaveretum		
• Thebaine	Buprenorphine	
Semisynthetic alkaloids		
• Diamorphine		
• Dihydrocodeine		
• Dihydromorphinone		
• Oxycodone		
• Oxymorphone	Nalbuphine	Naloxone
Synthetic agents		
• Morphinans		
• Levorphanol	• Butorphanol	
• Benzomorphinans	• Dezocine	
	• Meptazinol	
	• Pentazocine	
Phenylpiperidine derivative		
• Alfentanil		
• Fentanyl		
• Pethidine		
• Phenoperidine		
• Remifentanil		
• Sufentanil		
• Tramadol		
Diphenylheptane derivative		
• Dipipanone		
• Dextromoramide		
• Methadone		
• Piritramide		
• Propoxyphene		

- Its actions are mostly mediated by μ receptors in CNS.

Pharmacokinetics

The pharmacokinetics of different opioid analgesic drugs are given in **Table 5**.
- It has hydrophilic opioid to avoid confusion and remembering easily and slow permeability to the blood-brain barrier causing latency in the action of the drug after administration.
- It undergoes extensive first-pass metabolism, only 10–30% of the orally administered dose reaches systemic circulation. Also available as extended-release and suppository form.
- On intramuscular injection peak effect comes around 30–60 minutes, duration of action is approximately 15–30 minutes.
- The subcutaneous route of administration gives blood concentrations comparable to intravenous dose but is susceptible to aberrant and slow absorption in cases with hypovolemia, hypotension, hypothermia, or severe pain.
- After intravenous administration, plasma level decay occurs in a triexponential manner. Initial rapid decrease in plasma concentration due to distribution, followed by a slower decrease due to gradual penetration into the central nervous system and lastly exponential decrease reflecting terminal half-life.
- Morphine has a terminal half-life of around 3 hours but the duration of action is longer explained by lower lipid solubility causing a slow decline of CNS concentration and active metabolite (morphine-6-glucuronide).
- Morphine metabolism is reduced by half in severe liver disease and its terminal half-life is doubled **(Flowchart 2)**. With liver cirrhosis, glucuronidation is largely unaffected and may not affect morphine clearance.

Papaveretum

- A semisynthetic mixture of morphine (65%), codeine, and papaverine.
- It is rarely used clinically, can be used in premedication and postoperative pain.

TABLE 3: Pharmacological effects of morphine.

Pharmacological effects	Remarks
Analgesia	• Most effective in continuous, dull aching, poorly localized pain arising from visceral and deeper organs • Effective when fear and anxiety are dominant features • Pain threshold is not decreased in many patients but patients are more comfortable
Sedation	• Sleep is not commonly induced • The shift of EEG more toward increased voltage and lower frequencies and suppression of REM sleep • *Euphoria* and *dysphoria* may be seen if given to patients without symptoms of pain
Respiratory depression	• Rate and depth of respiration are decreased by a direct effect on centers in the brainstem • Decreased CO_2 responsiveness as evident by flattening of curve and shift of PCO_2—ventilation curve to the right • Fetal respiratory centers are highly sensitive to morphine
Nausea and vomiting	• Caused primarily due to dopamine and $5-HT_3$ receptors stimulation in chemoreceptor trigger zone (CTZ) in area postrema of the medulla • Other mechanisms may be action on the vestibular apparatus and gastrointestinal smooth muscle cells
Cardiovascular effects	• It decreases the sympathetic drive. It also has a direct vagal stimulatory effect by acting on vagal nuclei • Hypotension may occur due to decreased sympathetic tone and histamine release from mast cells • Its sedation properties help in paroxysmal nocturnal dyspnea
Histamine release	• Histamine release from mast cells may result in bronchospasm, hypotension, generalized pruritus, and nasal itching
Gastrointestinal effects	• Sphincter tone is increased with morphine, resulting in increased gastric emptying time, constipation • Sphincter of *Oddi spasm* may be seen • The tone and amplitude of uterine contractions are also increased • Lower esophageal sphincter tone is decreased in patients with gastroesophageal reflux disease
Ocular effects	• Miosis is characteristic of morphine overdose • It results from Edinger-Westphal nucleus stimulation, supranuclear pathway suppression, or decreased central sympathetic activity
Hormonal effects	• The dopamine receptors stimulation in the hypothalamus may cause decreased ACTH, prolactin, and gonadotrophic hormonal release • ADH secretion is increased
Muscle rigidity	• It can produce rigidity due to the effects of dopaminergic and GABA pathways on receptors in substantia nigra and corpus striatum (more common with fentanyl)
Tolerance	• May be due to a negative feedback system causing decreased production of endogenous opioids along with downregulation of opioid receptors • Also increased glutamate pathway transmission via NMDA receptors is attributed to tolerance

Contd...

Contd...

Pharmacological effects	Remarks
Dependence	• Physical and psychological dependence is known • Withdrawal symptoms constitute restlessness, irritability, excessive sweating, lacrimation, yawning, painful abdominal cramps, severe vomiting, diarrhea, and urination

(ACTH: adrenocorticotropic hormone; ADH: antidiuretic hormone; CTZ: chemoreceptor trigger zone; EEG: electroencephalogram; GABA: gamma-aminobutyric acid; NMDA: N-methyl-D-aspartate; REM: rapid eye movement)

TABLE 4: Morphine milligram equivalents.

Opioid	Conversion factor
Codeine	0.15
Fentanyl transdermal (in µg/hour)	2.4
Hydrocodone	1
Hydromorphone	4
Methadone	
1–20 mg/day	4
21–40 mg/day	8
41–60 mg/day	10
≥61–80 mg/day	12
Morphine	1
Oxycodone	1.5
Oxymorphone	3
Tapentadol	0.4

Diamorphine (Heroin)

- It is a morphine analog formed with diacetylation.
- It does not have an affinity for opioid receptors.
- It has a rapid onset of action, 1.5–2 times more potent, and has a slightly shorter duration of action compared to morphine.
- Diamorphine is metabolized by red cells and tissue esterases into monoacetylmorphine. Monoacetylmorphine and diamorphine both readily cross the blood-brain barrier to get converted to morphine in CNS.
- Equivalent larger doses of diamorphine can be administered in smaller volumes compared to morphine.

TABLE 5: Pharmacokinetics of opioids.

	Relative lipid solubility	Terminal half-life	Context-sensitive half-life (4 hour infusion) min	Clearance (mL/min/kg)	Volume of distribution	pK_a	% non-ionized
Morphine	1	3		15	3.5	7.9	24
Pethidine	28	4		12	4.0	8.7	5
Fentanyl	580	3.5	260	13	4.0	8.4	9
Alfentanil	90	1.6	60	6	0.8	6.5	89
Remifentanil	50	0.06	4	50	0.4	7.1	65
Tramadol	1	5		6	3.1	4.5	99

Flowchart 2: Morphine metabolism.

```
Codeine ← Morphine —Demethylated→ Normorphine (5%)
         (Liver, Kidneys) │                        │ Glucuronyl transferase
                          ↓                        ↓
          Morphine-3-glucuronide        Morphine-6-glucuronide
                (75–85%)                       (5–10%)
                   ↓                              ↓
        • Physiologically inactive     • Physiologically active
        • Partly excreted in bile      • Analgesia and respiratory depression
                                       • Analgesic potency 650 folds of morphine
                                       • Accumulates in renal failure
```

Codeine

- It is formed by the methylation of morphine.
- It has analgesic and antitussive properties. Its large doses are excitatory and have low abuse potential.
- 3-methyl group renders it less susceptible to conjugation in the liver.
- The action of CYP2D6 metabolizes codeine by O-demethylation to form morphine. This enzyme exhibits genetic polymorphism. More important are the rapid metabolizers who are more susceptible to overdose leading to black box warning regarding usage of codeine in cough syrups.
- Dihydroxycodeine and oxycodone are related compounds. They are useful in chronic pain and analgesia management in terminal patients. Oxycodone has higher abuse potential.

Pethidine

- Also called as Meperidine. Chemically it is an antimuscarinic drug with dissimilarities to morphine. Due to structural relationship with atropine, it is a phenylpiperidine derivative and agonist at mu and kappa receptors.
- Have similar analgesia, tolerance, and dependence profile as of morphine and is one tenth as potent as morphine. Side effects of respiratory depression, nausea, and vomiting profile are also similar.
- It has a rapid onset and shorter duration of action as it is more lipid-soluble.
- Contraindicated in patients on monoamine oxidase (MAO) inhibitors, it can cause serotonin toxicity.
- Metabolized to norpethidine, pethidinic acid, and pethidine-N-oxide in the liver. 5–10% of pethidine and norpethidine excreted in the urine. In renal failure, pethidine and norpethidine accumulates to cause neurological toxicity.
- It is used for labor analgesia though pethidine crosses the placenta readily. Pethidine is the only opioid which can produce surgical anesthesia when given in intrathecal route.
- Elimination of pethidine and norpethidine is significantly prolonged in neonates due to reduced clearance.
- It was the drug of choice in treatment of postoperative shivering due to its agonism at kappa and alpha 2 receptors before tramadol.

Fentanyl (Table 6)

- It is a phenylpiperidine derivative and highly potent opioid analgesic (100 times of morphine) due to high lipid-solubility.

TABLE 6: Equianalgesic dose (in mg).

Drug	Parenteral	Oral
Morphine	10	25
Fentanyl	0.15	N/A
Hydrocodone	N/A	25
Hydromorphone	2	5
Oxycodone	10	20

- Rapid onset, short duration of action (20–30 min), and mild sedation at low dose.
- At a higher dose, it decreases stress response and causes sedation and unconsciousness. Slower recovery after higher doses is dependent on the elimination rate.
- Muscular rigidity can be caused at higher doses; rapid bolus can result in cough reflex.
- It causes dose-dependent cardiorespiratory depression.
- After the bolus dose, its plasma concentration decreases rapidly due to redistribution (distribution half-life is around 13 min) and has a terminal half-life of 3–4 hours.
- It is metabolized in the liver by N-dealkylation and hydroxylation. Inactive metabolites are excreted in urine over several days.
- Available as injectable, lozenges, transdermal patches. It is one of the most frequent perioperative opioids used in India.

Alfentanil (Table 7)

- It is a synthetic opioid related to fentanyl having 10–20% potency and is given for similar indications.
- More rapid onset with a shorter duration of action though has less lipid solubility compared to fentanyl.
- It is used as a continuous infusion (0.2–2.0 μ/kg/min) following a loading dose (35–70 μ/kg).

TABLE 7: Alfentanil pharmacokinetics.

Distribution half-life	10–12 min
Terminal half-life	90–120 min
Context-sensitive half-life	30–60 min

- Similar cardiorespiratory effects may cause unpredictable apnea.
- Extensive hepatic metabolism by CYP3A4 and have a hepatic extraction ratio of 0.3–0.5.
- It has a smaller volume of distribution and clearance of approximately half of fentanyl.
- Its clearance is prolonged in hepatic cirrhosis and the presence of CYP3A4 inhibitors.

Remifentanil

- It is piperidine ester which is susceptible to red cell and tissue esterase and metabolized into remifentanilic acid which is inactive.
- Its metabolism is not affected by plasma cholinesterases (butyrylcholinesterase).
- It has a rapid onset of action as it equilibrates rapidly with CNS (half time = 1.3 min)
- Remifentanil has a low volume of distribution (400 mL/kg) while clearance is high (4–45 mL/kg/min). So, the elimination half-life of remifentanil is short (8–10 min).
- It has a context-sensitive half-life of 3–5 min. Due to this rapid offset of action; it is always used as a continuous intravenous infusion. Loading dose of 50–100 μ over 10 min followed by infusion of 0.5–1 μ/kg/min.
- Severe muscle rigidity requiring muscle relaxant has been seen with remifentanil, fentanyl, and alfentanil.
- Due to its organ-independent metabolism, it is well suited to be given in patients with hepatic and renal failure.

Methadone

- It has high oral bioavailability due to insignificant first-pass metabolism.

- Its onset of action is slower but the duration of action is long with a terminal half-life of 15–20 hours.
- Methadone is extensively plasma protein bound (90%). It may have a cumulative effect on repeated dosage due to avid tissue protein binding.
- It has been used in the treatment of morphine dependence as it does not precipitate withdrawal symptoms. But it also has comparable abuse potential to morphine.

Dipipanone

- It is a methadone-related piperidine derivative. It has high oral bioavailability.
- It has been used in the management of malignancy-related chronic pain treatment.

Tramadol

- It is a cyclohexanol-derived racemic mixture of centrally acting opioid with two enantiomers.
- It has significant agonistic activity on μ-receptors while it also weakly binds with κ- and δ-receptors.
- Tramadol indirectly activates central descending monoaminergic pathways by inhibiting nor-adrenaline and 5-HT neuronal reuptake.
- It has high oral bioavailability (70–80%) with an oral dose approximately similar to intravenous dosages.
- It has hepatic metabolism by CYP2D6 to N- and O-demethylated metabolites, its O-desmethyltramadol has more affinity for μ receptors.
- Its dosage must be reduced in chronic liver and renal diseases by 50%. Enzyme inducer drugs may decrease the plasma concentration and analgesic efficacy.
- It has similar efficacy and potency as pethidine. But it is less effective in severe postoperative pain and neuropathic pain.
- Tramadol is contraindicated in patients with MAO inhibitors.
- Its metabolite laudanosine may get accumulated in renal failure and result in a decreased seizure threshold.

Agonist-Antagonists

- These drugs exhibit full agonism on all opioid receptors. Two distinct types are:
    1. *Mixed agonist-antagonist*: They produce analgesia by their agonist effect at κ-receptors whereas antagonist at μ receptors.
        a. K-agonist or partial agonist activity predominates—pentazocine, meptazinol
        b. μ-antagonist activity predominates-Nalorphine.
    2. *Essentially partial agonist*: Their low intrinsic activity may result to produce agonist or antagonist effects at μ receptors—Buprenorphine.

Pentazocine

- It is a mixed agonist-antagonist, has an agonistic action on κ- and δ-receptors while weak antagonist action on μ receptor. It has one-fourth analgesic potency of morphine.
- It is a derivative of piperidine, is classified as benzomorphan.
- There is a hypertensive and tachycardiac response with pentazocine due to an increase in serum catecholamine levels. Pulmonary vascular resistance is also increased with pentazocine.
- Due to the above reasons, this drug should not be used in the patients who are susceptible to major adverse cardiac events (e.g., myocardial infarction, systemic or pulmonary hypertension, heart failure, etc.).

- May cause acute withdrawal in patients with other opioid drug dependence. This drug itself has low abuse potential.
- It may also precipitate acute porphyria in susceptible patients.

Meptazinol

- It has a high μ receptor affinity and is an antagonist at the receptor. So, it may precipitate acute withdrawal symptoms in morphine-addicted patients.
- It also exhibits central cholinergic action which may contribute to its analgesic effects, lesser respiratory depression.
- It has side effects of nausea and vomiting which may be reduced by antimuscarinic drugs.

Buprenorphine (Table 8)

- It is a partial agonist at μ-receptors and has lesser effects on κ- and δ- receptors.
- Its analgesic effects are predominantly due to partial agonistic action on the μ-receptor and partly due to κ-receptor agonistic activity.
- Buprenorphine has very low oral bioavailability due to extensive first-pass metabolism in the liver.
- Sublingual route has radial absorption of the preferred route of administration due to high lipid solubility through intravenous and intramuscular routes can also be used.
- It has a long duration of action as buprenorphine has strong avidity for μ- receptors and it dissociates slowly.
- Interactions with other opioid analgesics depend upon the relative doses involved of both drugs. Buprenorphine along with naloxone is used in de-addiction drug regimens for opioid dependence.
- Buprenorphine is 30 times more potent than morphine and has a duration of action of approximately 6–8 hours.
- It is less susceptible to naloxone or naltrexone for reversal of effects due to high affinity to μ-receptors. Its dependence is known but it has low potency for abuse and it is classified as a controlled drug.

TABLE 8: Transdermal opioids.

Fentanyl patch (μg/hour)	Buprenorphine patch (μg/hour)	24 hour oral morphine dose (mg)	Breakthrough oral morphine (mg)
12		<60	5–10
25	35	61–90	10–15
37	52.5	91–134	15–20
50	70	135–224	30
75	105	225–314	40
100	140	315–404	60
125	This is debated	405–494	80
150		495–584	90
175		585–674	100
200		675–764	120
225		765–854	130
250		855–944	150

SPINAL OPIOID ANALGESIA

- Opioid receptors in the spinal cord are located in the dorsal horn in lamina I and substantia gelatinosa.
- Opioid analgesia is mediated via pre-and post-synaptic receptors of interneurons and C-fibers in the dorsal horn.
- Spinal administration of opioid drugs have predominantly two advantages, they are:
  1. Relatively low doses are needed for the analgesic effects and have prolonged analgesia due to the absence of metabolizing enzymes in the site of neuraxial opioid deposition.
  2. The supraspinal activity is minimal, so are the common adverse effects.
- Intrathecal administration of morphine results in rapid attachment of morphine in the lamina of the dorsal horn.
- A small dose of intrathecal opioid (10% of systemic parental dose) produces effective analgesia for a prolonged period.
- Fentanyl (5–25 µg), morphine (100–300 µg), or diamorphine (100–250 µg) are used intrathecally along with local anesthetic to increase the intensity and prolong analgesic effects.
- The high lipophilicity of fentanyl results in a decreased duration of action of fentanyl (1-6 hours) whereas morphine and diamorphine have a longer duration of action.
- Morphine use increases the incidence of delayed respiratory depression, pruritus, and urinary retention. These are attributed to decreased lipophilicity of morphine and delayed respiratory depression is due to convection of morphine upwards in the intrathecal space.
- Preservative-free opioid drugs must be given in the intrathecal space to avoid neurological sequelae.

EPIDURAL OPIOIDS

- The dosage of opioids in the epidural route is significantly increased compared to the intrathecal route, especially in drugs with low lipid solubility (e.g., morphine).
- The mechanism of action predominantly is the uptake of drugs from extradural to intrathecal space.
- There are additive effects of opioids with local anesthetic drugs which are frequently given together, this result in a decrease in dose requirement for both the drugs and diminution of adverse effects of individual drugs.
- The absorption of opioids in the systemic circulation through epidural veins, peridural fat and CSF is dependent on the lipophilicity of the drug and is minimally affected by molecular weight as molecular.
- The hydrophilic nature of morphine results in less systemic absorption post epidural administration and delayed onset of action, CSF levels peak after 1-2 hours.
- Due to its hydrophilic nature, morphine stays in CSF for a prolonged period and this results in the rostral spread of morphine via convection. This phenomenon might explain the thoracic analgesia after lumbar extradural injection and also the late-onset respiratory depression, urinary retention, and pruritus.
- As fentanyl is highly lipophilic, there is rapid absorption across the dura mater with fast spinal analgesic action. Simultaneously high absorption of fentanyl through epidural veins results in early increased plasma levels. So, there is early onset of respiratory depression, urinary retention, or pruritus.
- Diamorphine, when administered via epidural route has a rapid onset of action but a longer duration of action. This is

caused due to high lipid solubility of diamorphine compared to morphine whereas it is hydrolyzed rapidly to monoacetylmorphine and morphine has low lipophilicity and is spread by convection method. These metabolites result in prolonged action.

OPIOID ANTAGONISTS

Nalorphine (N-allyl-normorphine)

- This is the first opioid antagonist recognized (μ-receptor antagonist). This drug shows antagonistic action for analgesic as well as respiratory effects.
- It also has intrinsic analgesic properties but is not clinically used for these properties due to psychotomimetic side effects. These effects are κ-receptors mediated.

Naloxone (N-allyl-oxymorphone)

- It is a pure opioid antagonist and has no agonistic activity. It has the highest affinity for μ-receptors among opioid receptors.
- Long-acting opioids such as buprenorphine are only partially reversed by naloxone.
- It has intrinsic antanalgesic effects in susceptible opioid-naive patients and can also cause hypo- or hypertensive response, pulmonary edema, and ventricular arrhythmias.
- Naloxone is readily absorbed in oral administration; it is extensively metabolized in the liver by glucuronide conjugation. It is excreted in bile. Due to high

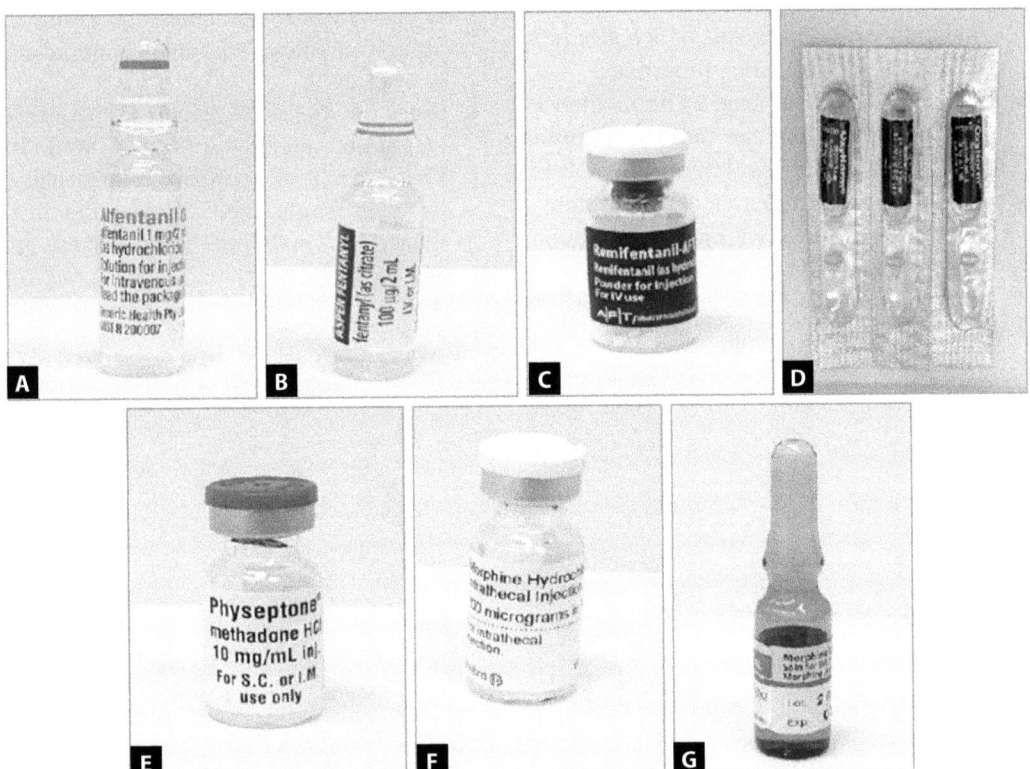

Figs. 1A to G: (A) Alfentanil ampoule; (B) Fentanyl ampoule; (C) Remifentanil vial; (D) Oxycodone ampoule; (E) Methadone vial; (F) Morphine vial; (G) Morphine ampoule.

metabolism on oral administration, it has to be given parentally, and also it has a short terminal half-life (0.5–2 hours).
- Naloxone is the drug of choice for opioid overdose. A dose of 0.5–1 µ/kg may be sufficient for reversing respiratory depression without reversal of analgesic effects.
- Severe opioid overdose may need a higher dose (1–2 mg) to antagonize adverse effects.
- Mild to moderate opioid overdose may be treated with 100–400 µg naloxone but the dose needs to be repeated or an infusion has to be started as µ-agonistic effects last longer than naloxone duration of action.

Naltrexone

- Naltrexone is longer acting and has low first-pass metabolism on oral administration.
- It has a terminal half-life of 7–9 hours. Its metabolite is 6β-naltrexol, which also has some (5%) antagonistic properties.
- It is sufficient for at least 24 hours after a single oral dose and can cause severe and prolonged withdrawal symptoms. It is used in the maintenance of opioid detoxified patients. Also, it will block the euphoric effects of opioids in relapsing cases.

QUESTION

Q. 1. Opioid-free anesthesia, advantages and disadvantages.

FURTHER READING

1. Azzam AAH, McDonald J, Lambert DG. Hot topics in opioid pharmacology: mixed and biased opioids. Br J Anaesth. 2019;122(6): e136-45.
2. Calvey N, Williams N. Principles and Practices of Pharmacology for Anaesthetists, 5th edition. New Jersey: Wiley-Blackwell; 2008.
3. Chong WS, Johnson DS. Update on opioid pharmacology. ATOTW. 2012:1-7.
4. Flood P, Rathmell JP, Shafer MD. Stoelting's Pharmacology and Physiology in Anesthetic Practice, 5th edition. Philadelphia: Lippincott Williams and Wilkins; 2014. pp. 960.
5. Grooper MA, Eriksson LI, Fleisher LA, Wiener-Kronish JP, Cohen NH, Leslie K. Miller's Anesthesia, 9th edition. Amsterdam: Elsevier; 2019.
6. Gupta DK, Krejcie TC, Avram MJ. Pharmacokinetics of opioids. In: Evers A, Maze M, Kharasch E (Eds). Anesthetic Pharmacology: Basic Principles and Clinical Practice. Cambridge: Cambridge University Press. pp. 509-30.

CHAPTER 3

Barbiturates

Amit Kumar, Nishkarsh Gupta, Anju Gupta

INTRODUCTION

- This class of drugs was one of the earliest anesthetic drugs which revolutionized the practice of general anesthesia. Thiopentone was introduced in 1934.
- Before the use of barbiturates, induction of anesthesia was slow, frequently unpleasant, and more hazardous with diethyl ether.
- It has been used as a constituent of "lethal injection" or "Cocktail" for capital punishment which includes an anesthetic agent, muscle relaxant, and potassium chloride as the sole agent or in combination.
- This group of agents has prototype pharmacokinetics and pharmacodynamics and all newer anesthetic drugs at some point have been compared against the barbiturate group **(Tables 1, 2 and Figs. 1A to C)**. Barbiturates have bacteriostatic property and also most of are incompatible with other solution because of alkalinity. All the commercial preparations of barbiturates contain six parts of sodium carbonate to prevent precipitation from atmospheric carbon dioxide.

MECHANISM OF ACTION

- These act by partially potentiating the $GABA_A$ channel activity and partially

TABLE 1: Classification of barbiturates.

Long-acting (≥8 hours)	• Phenobarbitone • Mephobarbital
Intermediate-acting (4–8 hours)	• Amobarbital • Aprobarbital • Butabarbital sodium
Short-acting (<4 hours)	• Pentobarbitone • Secobarbitone
Ultra-short-acting (minutes)	• Thiopentone • Methohexital

TABLE 2: Barbiturates drugs (are derived from barbituric acid).

Substitution	Drugs		Remarks
Oxygen at second position	Oxybarbiturate	• Pentobarbital • Secobarbital	Enzyme induction
Replacement of oxygen with sulfur	Thiobarbiturate	Thiopental, thiamylal	Lipid soluble, greater hypnotic potency
Phenyl group at fifth position	Phenobarbital		Increases the anticonvulsant potency
Methyl group on the nitrogen	Methohexital		• Increases the hypnotic potency but lowers the seizure threshold • Myoclonus during induction

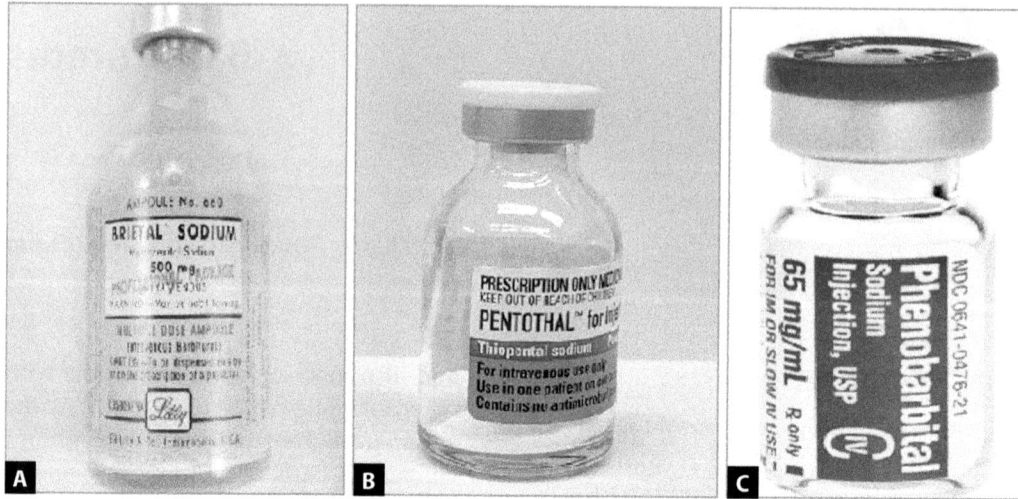

Figs. 1A to C: (A) Methohexital vial; (B) Thiopental sodium vial; (C) Phenobarbital vial.

acting on glutamate, adenosine, and neuronal nicotinic acetylcholine receptors. Barbiturates also act by mimicking gamma-aminobutyric acid (GABA) at higher doses to directly activate $GABA_A$ receptors.
- $GABA_A$ has specific binding sites for benzodiazepine, barbiturates, and steroids.
- Barbiturates increase the affinity of GABA for its receptors by allosteric interaction to increase the time duration of $GABA_A$ activated opening of chloride channels. This results in hyperpolarization, reduced neuronal excitability, and postsynaptic inhibition.

PHARMACOLOGY

- Thiopental is 5-ethyl-5-(1-methyl butyl)-2-thiobarbituric acid. It is the sulfur analog of phenobarbital. The clinically used drug is a racemic mixture of two stereoisomers.
- It has a garlic-like odor and bitter taste. Thiopental is available as pale yellow-white powder kept under nitrogen-filled vials.
- Thiopental solution is diluted to 2.5%, w/v (pH—10.5) for intravenous injection.

TABLE 3: Pharmacokinetic properties of thiopental.

Terminal half-life (min)	Clearance (mL/min/kg)	The volume of distribution (L/kg)
300–600	1.4–5.7	1.0–4.0

It remains stable for 2 weeks after the constitution but is usually used up to 48 hours after preparation. The solution should be discarded if it becomes cloudy.
- Thiopental is bacteriostatic due to its alkaline pH. It must not be mixed with other drugs.

PHARMACOKINETICS

- Thiopental has a rapid onset and rapid awakening after a single intravenous dose and reaches the maximum brain uptake within 30 seconds but it decreases rapidly over next 5 minutes due to rapid redistribution **(Table 3)**.
- It is a highly lipophilic drug. Elimination of thiopental depends exclusively on metabolism as only <1% is excreted unchanged in the urine.

- Due to high lipophilicity, this drug is sequestrated in the fat and skeletal muscles and has a long context-sensitive half-life after prolonged infusion.
- Metabolism of thiobarbiturates occurs in hepatocytes, also minimally in kidneys and CNS **(Flowchart 1)**.
- Thiopental has a low hepatic extraction ratio and capacity-dependent elimination. But severe hepatic dysfunction is needed before the prolonged duration of action of thiopental is evident as the liver has a huge reserve capacity to oxidize barbiturates.
- Pediatric patients have rapid clearance of thiopental. Whereas pregnant patients have increased elimination half-time because of elevated protein binding of thiopental.

PHARMACODYNAMICS AND CLINICAL USE (TABLE 4)

- Thiopental has rapid induction after a normal induction dose of 3–5 mg/kg, it is partly due to the high vascularity of brain tissue and partly due to high lipid solubility at pH—7.4 (due to its tautomerism with oil-water solubility coefficient = 500–700).
- Their use for premedication has been replaced by benzodiazepines. These drugs have a short period of drowsiness but a longer residual hangover effect.
- These drugs are useful in grand mal seizures, but benzodiazepines have a specific site of action in the CNS and are preferred.
- Barbiturates are also used in the treatment of raised ICP but can cause hypotension leading to compromised perfusion. They were popularly used for cerebral protection after cardiac arrest because they can produce an isoelectric EEG.
- Minimal effect on cardiac, skeletal, and smooth muscles. The cardiac effects may be more pronounced in hypovolemic

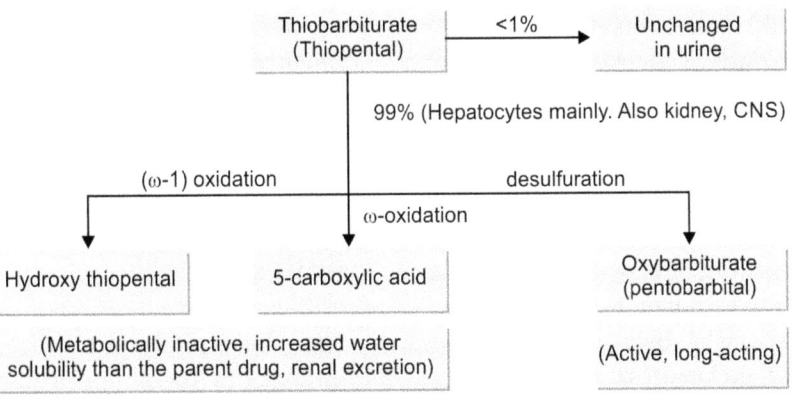

Flowchart 1: Metabolism of thiobarbiturates.

(CNS: central nervous system)

TABLE 4: Pharmacodynamics of different barbiturates.		
Drugs	**Relative potency of the drug**	**% Nonionized at 7.4 pH**
Thiopental	1	61%
Thiamylal	1.1	
Methohexital	2.5	76%

- patients and patients with significant cardiovascular disease.
- Thiopental may cause a decrease in stroke volume and cardiac output with compensatory increased systemic vascular resistance. High doses may cause direct cardiac depression due to membrane stabilizing effects and may be problematic in patients with fixed cardiac output states.
- Thiopental causes decreased renal blood flow resulting in decreased glomerular filtration rate, renal plasma flow, and excretion of electrolytes and water.
- Anesthesia induction dose for thiopental is decreased with age. Also, pregnancy causes a decrease in thiopental induction dose by 18%.
- Thiopental has long context-sensitive half-time and prolonged recovery time and so is not an agent of choice for daycare procedures.
- Methohexital has different pharmacodynamic effects compared to thiopental. Methohexital decreases the seizure threshold and is useful in inducing seizures during epilepsy surgery.
- Methohexital is also useful in electroconvulsive therapy and cardioversion.
- Methohexital has an excitatory phenomenon (e.g., involuntary skeletal muscle contraction- myoclonus or hiccough). These are seen on a higher dose and can be decreased with opioid pretreatment.
- Methohexital has been used in anesthesia for dental procedures.
- Barbiturates can be used to decrease intracranial pressure in refractory patients. It decreases cerebral blood flow mostly due to systemic hypotension.
- Thiopental decreases the cerebral blood flow as well as cerebral metabolism but there is an increase in the cerebral perfusion to metabolism ratio. This helps in protecting poorly perfused areas of the brain.
- It is seen that patients given barbiturates during cardiopulmonary bypass recover rapidly from neuropsychiatric complications.
- The efficacy of barbiturate in cerebral ischemia and elevated increased intracranial pressure (ICP) remains unproven.
- Therapeutic hypothermia (33–34°C) appears to be more effective compared to barbiturates during cardiac surgery or after stroke. So, routine administration of these agents is not recommended.
- Thiopental can be used when somatosensory evoked potential monitoring is planned.
- Thiopental is the drug of choice in refractory status epilepticus not responding to conventional treatment (Airway management plan has to be kept in mind).
- Among barbiturates, phenobarbital has liver enzyme induction properties after 2–7 days of use. This results in increased metabolism of tricyclic antidepressants, phenytoin, and anticoagulants. Also, the metabolism of endogenous substances such as corticosteroids, bile salts, and vitamin K is increased.

ADVERSE EFFECTS OF BARBITURATES

- Thiopental is a relatively cardiostable drug, but it produces a decrease in blood pressure by 10–20 mm Hg and increased heart rate by 15–20 beats/min after an intravenous dose of 5 mg/kg. This effect is due to peripheral vasodilation which is a result of decreased sympathetic outflow from CNS and depression of the medullary vasomotor center. Also, a mild direct myocardial depressant effect may contribute to the above effects.

- There is decreased sensitivity of respiratory centers in pons and medulla to carbon dioxide in presence of barbiturates due to direct action on these centers. This may result in an increase in $PaCO_2$, acidosis, and apnea.
- On recovery from barbiturates, there is slow and shallow breathing.
- Large doses of barbiturates are required to depress laryngeal and cough reflexes. May result in laryngospasm and bronchospasm during reversal of anesthesia or airway stimulation at lower doses.
- Allergic reactions such as anaphylaxis may be associated with IV administration of thiopental. It can also cause signs of allergic reaction without prior exposure; few of them can be classified as anaphylactoid reactions.
- Methohexital causes localized pain on injection, excitatory adverse effects, and a tendency to cause tachycardia.
- Extravasation of the thiopental causes extensive tissue necrosis due to insoluble thiopental precipitation at 7.4 pH. It may be treated with local hyaluronidase injection and topical application of demulcents.
- The enzyme induction results in increased heme production, which in susceptible individuals may precipitate an acute attack of porphyria. All forms of porphyria should contraindicate the use of barbiturates.
- *Accidental intra-arterial injection of thiopental:*
  - This results in severe vasoconstriction with excruciating pain. The pain radiates along the path of the artery.
  - These are produced due to the crystallization of thiopental at 7.4 pH. These crystals block the progressive narrowed vascular bed.
  - The severe vasoconstriction results in blanching of limbs distal to injection, absent distal pulse. This is followed by cyanosis, arterial thrombosis, permanent nerve damage, and gangrene.
- Its treatment includes:
  - The needle/cannula is left in situ
  - Attempt for immediate dilution of the drug should be done
  - Injection of arterial dilator such as lidocaine or papaverine to prevent vasoconstriction should be done
  - Continuous axillary block or repeated stellate ganglion block causes sympathetic blockade to increase collateral circulation. Also, heparin may be useful
  - General measures to maintain adequate limb blood flow should be taken

QUESTIONS

Q. 1. Current status of thiopentone in anesthesia.
Q. 2. Thiofol, Thiodex and Thioketal uses, advantages and disadvantages of combinations.
Q. 3. Explain ceiling effect with respect to barbiturates.

FURTHER READING

1. Calvey TN, Williams NE. Principles and Practices of Pharmacology for Anaesthetists, 5th edition. England: Blackwell Science Ltd; 2009. pp. 376.
2. Dowd FJ, Johnson B, Mariotti A. Pharmacology and Therapeutics for Dentistry 7th edition. St Louis: Mosby; 2017. pp. 864.
3. Dumps C, Halbeck E, Bolkenius D. Drugs for intravenous induction of anesthesia: barbiturates. Anaesthesist. 2018;67(7): 535-52.
4. Dundee JW, McIlroy PD. The history of barbiturates. Anaesthesia. 1982;37(7):726-34.
5. Flood P, Rathmell JP, Shafer SL. Stoelting's Pharmacology and Physiology in Anesthetic Practice, 5th edition. Philadelphia: Lippincott Williams and Wilkins; 2014. pp. 960.
6. Grooper MA, Eriksson LI, Fleisher LA, Wiener-Kronish JP, Cohen NH. Miller's Anesthesia, 9th edition. Philadelphia: Elsevier; 2019. pp. 3122.

CHAPTER 4

Benzodiazepines

Amit Kumar, Nishkarsh Gupta

INTRODUCTION

- This class of drugs produces sedation, anxiolysis, hypnosis, anterograde amnesia, anticonvulsion, and centrally produced muscle relaxation. They do not have any analgesic properties.
- The most common intravenous benzodiazepines administered in the perioperative setting are midazolam, diazepam, and lorazepam **(Figs. 1A to D)**.
- These groups of drugs are frequently used for premedication, conscious sedation, and also for induction of general anesthesia in high doses.
- These drugs cause drowsiness, disorientation, unsteadiness, and acute confusional states. Also, postoperative cognitive dysfunction is seen especially in elderly patients.
- Side effects are rare (except for drowsiness and central depression), and may cause nightmares, nausea, skin rashes, and an increase in body weight when used for a prolonged duration. All of these drugs impair judgment, affect psychomotor behavior, increase reaction time, and may cause hangover effect on the day after their administration.
- These drugs alter the pattern of physiological sleep to increase stage 2 while decreasing stage 3, 4, and rapid eye movement REM sleep. There is a rebound phenomenon on stopping these drugs to compensate for earlier loss of REM sleep and associated with unpleasant dreams and nightmares.
- They do not induce hepatic microsomal enzymes and do not usually interact with

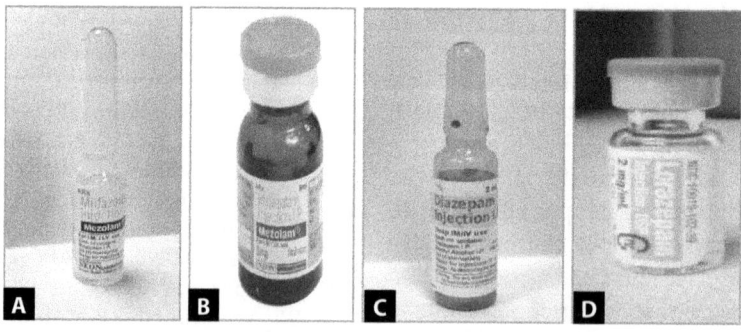

Figs. 1 to D: (A) Midazolam ampoule; (B) Midazolam vial; (C) Diazepam ampoule; and (D) Lorazepam ampoule.

other drugs other than sedatives and hypnotics including alcohol use.
- Greater than 2–3 weeks of use may be associated with a significant risk of tolerance and drug dependence. Hypnotic effects get tolerance after 3–14 days of continual use. Physical dependence can be seen in up to 15% of patients on chronic use. In recent years, there is an increasing incidence of drug abuse for this group of drugs.
- There is a *benzene ring* in the chemical structure with a seven-member *diazepine ring*. Various substitutions on the rings distinguish individual drugs.
- Midazolam is water-soluble at low pH (3.5) and has aqueous preparations due to the imidazole ring; it increases lipid solubility at physiological pH by intramolecular rearrangement. The preserving agent, propylene glycol can cause venoirritation sometimes and can explain the pain on injection with midazolam. While intravenous diazepam and lorazepam contain propylene glycol which is water-insoluble and is associated with venous irritation.
- In supraclinical dosage, midazolam has antitumorigenic properties in certain types of cancers.
- Remimazolam an ultra-short acting $GABA_A$ agonist may be useful in future anesthesia practice.

MECHANISM OF ACTION

- Benzodiazepines act by enhancing γ-aminobutyric acid type A ($GABA_A$) receptors mediated inhibitory neurotransmission. These receptors are most numerous in the cerebral cortex, the cerebellar cortex, corpus striatum, and limbic system. Also, these receptors are present in the brainstem and spinal cord.
- $GABA_A$ receptors are transmembrane proteins with five subunits surrounding the intrinsic ion pore which is selective chloride ion permeable. These five subunits are derived from seven families and constitute 18 different types (α_{1-6}, β_{1-3}, γ_{1-3}, δ, ε, θ, and ρ_{1-3}).
- In the human brain >60% of GABA receptors contain three subunits in combination α_1, α_2, β_2, β_2, and γ_2. The receptors also contain barbiturates, steroids, and proconvulsive drug binding sites.
- Sedation, anterograde amnesia, and anticonvulsant effects are mediated via α_1 subunits of $GABA_A$ receptors. Anxiolysis and muscle relaxation are mediated via the α_2 subunits.
- Benzodiazepine binding site is at the interface between α and γ subunit close to histidine residue. Replacing histidine with arginine results in 1,000-folds decreased benzodiazepine affinity for the $GABA_A$ receptor.
- Benzodiazepines enhance and facilitate the effect of GABA by increasing affinity of GABA for the receptors. This increases the frequency of opening of a chloride channel in response to a given stimulus without increasing (or slight increase) the duration of channel opening resulting in neuronal hyperpolarization and inhibition.
- Depression of activity between the limbic system and reticular system causes decreased alertness and arousal reactions. Anticonvulsant effects occur due to inhibition of amygdaloid nuclei. Midazolam, diazepam, and lorazepam increase the seizure initiation threshold.
- Indirectly benzodiazepines may affect other neurotransmitters in central nervous system (CNS). They decrease 5-hydroxytryptamine (5-HT) and dopamine in specific regions of brain and prevent increase of stress-induced noradrenaline turnover.
- Intrathecal midazolam decreases the excitatory GABA mediated neurotransmission

- leading to a decrease in spinal dorsal horn neuron's excitability.
- The order for receptor affinity is lorazepam > midazolam > diazepam. Effects are dose-dependent. Receptor saturation can produce a ceiling effect.
- Flumazenil reverses the effects of benzodiazepines by acting as an antagonist on these same receptors.
- $GABA_B$ receptors which are mainly located in presynaptic sites in CNS and peripheral autonomic nerve terminals do not have high-affinity binding sites for benzodiazepines.
- The benzodiazepines preserve cerebral blood flow (CBF) to cerebral oxygen consumption ($CMRO_2$) ratio while decreasing the $CMRO_2$.
- Inverse agonist—some drugs when bind to benzodiazepine receptors may have proconvulsant effects (e.g., β-carboline esters) due to antagonism of spontaneous activity of benzodiazepine receptors. Benzodiazepine antagonist flumazenil may occasionally produce similar effects.

PHARMACOKINETICS

- These drugs are nonpolar and highly lipid-soluble. So, these are well-absorbed after oral administration, and have a large volume of distribution with high bioavailability.
- These are extensively bound to plasma proteins, but only an unbound fraction can cross the blood-brain barrier to have CNS effects.
- These drugs may be divided into hypnotics and sedatives/tranquilizers according to duration of action due to variation of half-lives. Hypnotics are with relatively short terminal half-life and sedatives/tranquilizers with relatively long half-lives.
- Diazepam and midazolam readily cross blood-brain barrier due to high lipid solubility and have onset of CNS effects within 2–3 minutes. Lorazepam has a slightly longer onset of action as it is moderately lipid-soluble. The effects of single dose are terminated within 3–10 minutes by redistribution **(Table 1)**.
- Metabolism of benzodiazepines via oxidation and glucuronide conjugation takes place in liver to transform these into water-soluble end products and minimal amounts are excreted unchanged. All benzodiazepines (except midazolam) have low intrinsic hepatic clearance which is not affected by liver blood flow.

TABLE 1: Physiochemical properties.

	Molecular weight (Da)	pKa	Water solubility (g/L)	Lipid solubility (logP)
Diazepam	284.7	3.4	0.051	2.801
Lorazepam	321.2	1.3	0.12	2.382
Temazepam	300.7	1.6, 11.7	0.28	2.188
Midazolam	325.8 (hydrochloride 362.2)	6.0	0.004 (7.5, pH-1)	3.798
Remimazolam	439.3 (besylate 597.5)	5.3	0.008 (7.5, pH-1)	3.724
Flumazenil	303.3	0.86	0.042	2.15

Lipid solubility: Midaz > Remimazolam > diazepam > lorazepam > temazepam

Water solubility: Midazolam = Remimazolam (at pH-1) > temazepam > lorazepam > diazepam > remimazolam > midazolam

- Midazolam has perfusion limited clearance due to a higher liver extraction ratio, whereas lorazepam and diazepam are cleared with dependence on enzymatic activity (capacity limited clearance).
- The metabolism of benzodiazepines may be impaired in liver function impairment and in presence of hepatic enzyme inhibitors. Cimetidine reduces metabolism of diazepam by binding to cytochrome P450. Erythromycin decreases the metabolism of midazolam. Heparin increases the unbound diazepam by displacing diazepam from protein binding sites.
- *Midazolam*:
  - Postoral ingestion, complete absorption. Peak plasma concentration achieved in 30–80 minutes.
  - Significant first-pass metabolism—> bioavailability <50%. Hepatic extraction ratio—0.30–0.40, metabolic clearance may be susceptible to hepatic blood flow.
  - Distribution half-life 6–15 minutes after intravenous administration.
  - 94–98% plasma protein binding.
  - Elimination half-life 1.7–3.5 hours.
  - Plasma clearance is 5.8–9.0 mL/kg/min— > higher compared to other benzodiazepines due to rapid oxidization of the fused imidazole ring.
  - It has pH dependent ring opening phenomenon. The commercial preparation has a pH of 3.5 in which the imidazole ring is closed making it water soluble but at pH of the blood which is more than 4, its ring opens and makes it highly lipophilic.
  - Factors affecting pharmacokinetics of midazolam include obesity, age, and hepatic cirrhosis.
  - It is metabolized by CYP3A4 and CYP3A5 to 1-hydroxymethylmidazolam and 4-hydroxymidazolam. 1-hydroxymidazolam has 60% less affinity to receptors than the parent compound.
  - These metabolites are rapidly conjugated and renally excreted. Profound sedation may be seen in patients with renal impairment.
- *Diazepam*:
  - Postoral ingestion has around 94% bioavailability. Peak concentration after around 60 minutes.
  - It is extensively protein bound and has a volume of distribution of 0.7–4.7 L/kg.
  - Plasma clearance ranges between 0.2 and 0.5 mL/kg/min.
  - Obesity, liver dysfunction, and age affect pharmacokinetics.
  - It is metabolized by CYP2C19 and CYP3A4 producing metabolite N-desmethyldiazepam which is further metabolized to oxazepam. Also, diazepam is metabolized to temazepam which is conjugated to temazepam glucuronide. A smaller part of temazepam is demethylated to oxazepam which gets conjugated to oxazepam glucuronide. N-desmethyldiazepam has similar characteristics to diazepam but has a prolonged elimination half-life of 200 hours.
  - It is not eliminated with hemodialysis making its overdose very toxic.
  - It shows a secondary peak in plasma concentration at 6–12 hours with possible resedation due to enterohepatic circulation.
- *Temazepam*:
  - Orally active BZD used for insomnia owing to its less tolerance potential and almost complete absorption after oral administration.
  - Major part (90%) is conjugated by the liver to 3-oxy glucuronide which is inactive and excreted in the urine.

- Minor amounts demethylated to oxazepam. It is eliminated as a glucuronide conjugate.
- *Lorazepam*:
  - High oral bioavailability of around 90%. Peak plasma concentration around 120 minutes after oral ingestion.
  - Elimination half-life ranges from 8 to 25 hours with a mean of 15 hours.
  - It is >90% plasma protein bound with a higher volume of distribution from 0.8 to 1.3 L/kg.
  - Its clearance is 0.8-1.8 mL/kg/min, clearance decreases with liver dysfunction.
  - Conjugated in liver to inactive conjugate and is excreted in urine.
- *Remimazolam*:
  - New short-acting $GABA_A$ agonist which degrades by nonspecific esterases to its carboxylic acid metabolite. It has first-order pharmacokinetic elimination.
  - It has a more rapid onset of action, greater depth of sedation, and more rapid recovery than midazolam with no accumulation after prolonged infusion.
  - It has a large volume of distribution of 34.8 ± 9.4 L and has a rapid clearance of 70.3 ± 13.9 L/hour.
  - Possible benefit of safe administration by endoscopists compared with propofol.

PHARMACODYNAMICS
Cardiovascular System
- Under normal circumstances, sympathetic nervous system is tonically inhibited dependent on GABAergic signaling.
- Slight reduction in arterial blood pressure resulting from a decrease in systemic vascular resistance.
- Induction of anesthesia with benzodiazepine preserves the heart rate, ventricular filling pressure and cardiac output. Heart rate may rise due to preservation of homeostatic reflex mechanism or vagolysis.
- Combination with an opioid will produce a greater decrease in systemic blood pressure and reduce sympathetic tone.
- There is a plateau plasma drug effect above, which there is little change in arterial blood pressure.

Respiratory System
- These drugs affect muscular tone resulting in upper airway obstruction.
- Depresses ventilatory response to carbon dioxide.
- Depress the hypoxic ventilatory response.
- Dose-related central respiratory depression [more pronounced in patients with chronic obstructive pulmonary disease (COPD), old age, debilitating diseases] and additive synergistic effect in combination with opioids.
- Depresses swallowing reflex and upper airway reflex activity.

Cerebral
- Moderate reduction of CBF which parallel reductions CMR. (Narcotics< benzodiazepines < barbiturates).
- With 15 mg diazepam, a 25% reduction in CBF and $CMRO_2$ was seen in head injury patients.
- Midazolam 0.15 mg/kg to healthy volunteers decreased CBF by 30-34%.
- Dose-related reduction in $CMRO_2$ and cerebral blood flow CBF.
- Normal ratio of $CMRO_2$ to CBF.
- Preserves cerebral vasomotor responsiveness to carbon dioxide (CO_2).
- Potent anticonvulsant but not neuroprotective.
- Safe to administer in intracranial hypertension provided that respiratory

depression [associated increase in partial pressure of carbon dioxide ($PaCO_2$)] or hypotension do not occur.
- Increases the seizure threshold to local anesthetic.
- Does not produce a burst suppression isoelectric pattern on electroencephalography (EEG).
- At lower doses, these behave like propofol causing consolidation failure while leaving encoding intact, whereas at higher doses significant encoding impairment emerges. These may reduce REM sleep when used as sedation in intensive care unit (ICU).

USES

Premedication

- Midazolam, diazepam, and lorazepam are frequently used drugs for premedication **(Table 2)**. Given for anxiolysis, sedation, amnesia, sympathicolysis, and reduction of postoperative nausea and vomiting (PONV). Amnesia caused is anterograde and no retrograde memory is affected.
- Midazolam is commonly used short-acting sedative anxiolytic, whereas lorazepam is used when prolonged and intense anxiolysis is pursued.
- Respiration and oxygen saturation are affected minimally with midazolam even with doses up to 1.0 mg/kg with a maximum of 20 mg.

Sedation

- It causes anxiety relief and possibility of recall of unpleasant event during diagnostic which actually accounts for prerequisite for sedation.
- Midazolam has a peak effect at around 2–3 minutes, whereas diazepam takes slightly longer and lorazepam even longer for peak effect. Recovery is similar with midazolam and diazepam due to similar early plasma redistribution patterns while lorazepam has longer-lasting effects.
- Compared to propofol for sedation, midazolam has a similar profile except that propofol has a rapid recovery.
- Remimazolam is a newer agent useful for procedural sedation especially upper gastrointestinal endoscopy.
- Studies found single dose midazolam may be safe for cesarean section as minimal fraction is transferred to 24 hours breast milk.
- It has been used for ICU sedation due to its suitable profile of hemodynamic stability and amnesia but is not without disadvantages of potential lingering sedative effect and high prevalence of delirium.

TABLE 2: Frequently used drugs for premedication.

		Midazolam	Diazepam	Lorazepam
Oral premedication (usual adult dose)		7.5–15 mg	5–10 mg	2–4 mg
Intravenous	Sedation*	0.5–1 mg repeated dose	2 mg repeated dose	0.25 mg repeated dose
	Induction	0.05–0.15 mg/kg	0.3–0.5 mg/kg	0.1 mg/kg
	Maintenance	0.05 mg/kg PRN 1 µg/kg/min	0.1 mg/kg PRN	0.02 mg/kg PRN

*Sedation is given for anxiety relief and for lack of recall of unpleasant events during a diagnostic procedure or minor surgical procedure

Induction and Maintenance of Anesthesia

- Among benzodiazepines, midazolam is induction agent of choice with a dose of 0.1–0.2 mg/kg in premedicated patients and up to 0.3 mg/kg in unpremedicated patients. This single anesthetic dose gives amnesia for a period of around 1–2 hours.
- It has onset of anesthesia within 30–60 seconds.
- It has synergistic effects with other anesthetic agents and opioids. Emergence time depends on the dose of midazolam and adjuvant anesthetic agents.
- Benzodiazepines do not possess analgesic properties so must be combined with analgesic agents.
- After continuous infusions, the recovery time is prolonged with benzodiazepines due to accumulation especially diazepam and lorazepam compared to midazolam (as midazolam has a shorter context-sensitive half-life).

Nausea and Vomiting Prophylaxis

- Intravenous midazolam 2 mg, 30 minutes before end of surgery has been shown to reduce the incidence of PONV comparable to ondansetron 4 mg.
- Children (4–12 years) posted for strabismus surgeries when given intravenous midazolam 0.05 mg/kg reduced PONV compared to placebo or intravenous dexamethasone.
- However, midazolam is not recommended due to sedation-related adverse effects.

Side Effects and Toxicity

- Respiratory depression is the major side effect. Diazepam and lorazepam also have venous irritation and thrombophlebitis related to poor aqueous solubility and propylene glycol vehicles for dissolution.
- Benzodiazepines have limited allergenic effects and do not suppress adrenal gland.
- It can cross placenta to cause neonatal depression.
- The incidence of cleft palate may be increased with administration during first trimester of pregnancy.
- When used for sedation or for induction and maintenance of anesthesia, benzodiazepines may cause undesirable postoperative sedation, amnesia, and less frequent respiratory depression. Flumazenil may be used to reverse the residual effects.

Flumazenil

- It is a competitive antagonist for benzodiazepines at GABA receptors and is highly specific.
- Reversal occurs in 2 minutes and it has a peak effect at 10 minutes and duration of action of 30 minutes.
- It is short-acting with a half-life of 1 hour and is rapidly metabolized in liver. Rebound sedation can be seen with respiratory suppression, but is less likely when it is used to reverse midazolam which has more rapid clearance compared to other benzodiazepines.
- When flumazenil is used in small dosage in presence of large dose of agonist, it attenuates deep CNS depression (loss of consciousness and respiratory depression) without reducing the agonist effect that occurs at low fractional occupancy of receptors (drowsiness, amnesia).

Dose: 0.2 mg/kg IV bolus followed by 0.1 mg/kg subsequently at an interval of 60 seconds.

- The CBF, cerebral metabolic rates (CMR), and intracranial pressure (ICP) lowering actions of midazolam are reversed with this agent.

- It should not be given to reverse benzodiazepine when benzodiazepines are used to treat convulsions. Also, in head injury patients with poor ICP control can get severe increase in ICP with flumazenil and so it should be used with caution in patients with impaired intracranial compliance.

QUESTION

Q. 1. Various routes of administration of benzodaizepines.

FURTHER READING

1. Calvey TN, Williams N. Principles and Practice of Pharmacology for Anaesthetists, 5th edition. United States: Wiley-Blackwell; 2008.
2. Flood P. Stoelting's Pharmacology and Physiology in Anesthetic Practice, 5th edition. Haryana: Wolters Kluwer India Pvt. Ltd; 2015.
3. Griffin CE, Kaye AM, Bueno FR, Kaye AD. Benzodiazepine pharmacology and central nervous system–mediated effects. Ochsner J. 2013;13(2):214-23.
4. Gropper MA, Eriksson LI, Fleisher LA, Wiener-Kronish JP, Cohen NH, Leslie K. Miller's Anesthesia, 2-Volume Set, 9th edition. Amsterdam: Elsevier; 2019.
5. Kilpatrick G. J. Remimazolam: Non-clinical and clinical profile of a new sedative/anesthetic agent. Front Pharmacol. 2021;12: 690875.
6. Olkkola KT, Ahonen J. Midazolam and other benzodiazepines. Handb Exp Pharmacol. 2008;(182), 335-60.
7. Rudolph U, Davies FM, Barr J. Benzodiazepines. In Evers A, Maze M, Kharasch ED (Eds). Anesthetic Pharmacology: Basic Principles and Clinical Practice. United Kingdom: Cambridge University Press; 2011. pp. 466-77.

CHAPTER 5

Nonbarbiturate Intravenous Anesthetic Agents

Anju Gupta, Asim Ahmed, Nishkarsh Gupta

INTRODUCTION

Intravenous induction of anesthesia has been widely accepted and practiced since the introduction of thiopentone in 1934. Since then the number of nonbarbiturate drugs have been introduced thereafter in an attempt to overcome the undesirable properties of barbiturates. Most commonly used nonbarbiturate intravenous induction agents are propofol, etomidate, ketamine, dexmedetomidine, and benzodiazepines (BZDs). In this chapter, we summarize the properties of nonbarbiturate intravenous anesthetic agents and their clinical uses.

PROPOFOL

- First introduced in 1977 but was initially retracted owing to anaphylactic reactions.
- It was reformulated and launched in 1986.

Physical Properties

Structure

It is lipid-soluble drug and belongs to the alkylphenol group. It is chemically described as 2, 6-diisopropylphenol.

Composition

It is a milky white viscous solution. It contains propofol (1% or 2%), soybean oil (10%), purified egg lecithin as emulsifier (1.2%), glycerol for tonicity (2.25%), and sodium hydroxide for pH.

- For bacteriostatic action, ethylenediaminetetraacetic acid (EDTA) or disodium editate, or sodium metabisulfite is added.
- Fospropofol is a water-soluble prodrug, painless at the injection site and metabolized by alkaline phosphatase in liver, which releases propofol, formaldehyde, and phosphate.

Pharmacokinetics (Flowchart 1)

- Mainly metabolized in liver.
- Extrahepatic site of metabolism—kidneys (30%) and lungs.
- Propofol is a cytochrome 3A4 inhibitor, thereby decreasing hepatic blood flow and drug metabolism.
- *Elimination half-life:* 4–7 hours
- *Distribution half-life:* 2–8 minutes
- Context-sensitive half-life after 8 hours of infusion is 40 minutes and 10 minutes for <3 hours infusion.

Flowchart 1: Pharmacokinetics of propofol.

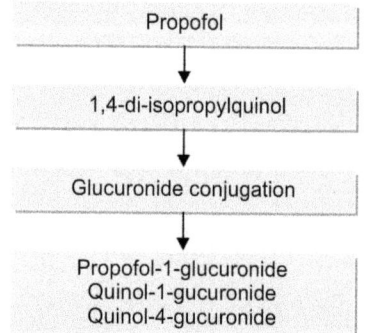

- Pharmacokinetics is affected by age, gender, weight, comorbidities, and drug interactions

Pharmacodynamics

Central Nervous System

- Propofol has a central nervous system (CNS) depressant and hypnotic action.
- *Indirect action:* Acts on γ-aminobutyric acid type A (GABA$_A$) receptors and increases chloride channel current.
- Inhibits acetylcholine release in the hippocampus.
- *Direct action:* Depressant action on neurons of the spinal cord.
- Increases dopamine concentration in nucleus accumbens—sense of well-being and abuse tendency.
- Decreases serotonin in area postrema, providing antiemetic action.
- Onset of hypnosis—11 seconds (one arm brain circulation).
- *Peak effect:* 90-100 seconds.
- Propofol has a tendency to develop tolerance so dosage needs to be adjusted upwards to maintain the same effect in intensive care unit (ICU).
- Propofol decreases intracranial pressure and cerebral perfusion pressure (CPP).

Respiratory System

- Propofol decreases tidal volume and rate frequency. It blunts airway reflexes and helps prevent intubation response.
- Apnea after injection depends on dose, speed of injection, and concomitant premedication.
- Decreases ventilatory drive to hypoxia and hypercarbia.
- Chronic obstructive pulmonary disease (COPD)—it has a bronchodilatory effect.
- But causes vagal and methacholine-mediated bronchoconstriction in low doses.
- Propofol preserves hypoxic pulmonary vasoconstriction.

Cardiovascular System

- Propofol causes peripheral vasodilation, hence decreasing systemic vascular resistance (SVR) and systolic blood pressure (SBP). These effects are more pronounced in patients with hypovolemia, compromised LV function and elderly population.
- Propofol decreases cardiac output and stroke volume.
- Also inhibits baroreceptor reflex hence tachycardic response to hypotension is abolished.

Other Actions

- *Antiemetic effect:* 10-20 mg, can repeat every 5-10 minutes
- *Antipruritic (for cholestatic jaundice):* 10 mg
- Decreases polymorphonuclear leukocyte chemotaxis
- Inhibits phagocytosis and killing of *Staphylococcus aureus*.

Uses

- *Induction and maintenance of anesthesia:*
  - Propofol has a rapid onset of action and quicker recovery. The dose needs to be titrated according to age, lean body mass, and central blood volume.
  - Hypotension after induction can be treated with IV fluids; therefore, careful titration is required in induction of shock patients.
    - *Dosing:*
      - *Induction of anesthesia:* 1-2.5 mg/kg (dose reduction with increasing age is advised)
      - *Maintenance of anesthesia:* 50-150 µg/kg/min

- *Sedation*:
  - *Sedation dose with regional anesthesia:* 25–75 µg/kg/min
  - Early recovery of psychomotor function, hence drug of choice for daycare anesthesia

Side Effects

- Pain on injection site which can be offset with premixing with lignocaine, injection in a larger vein, or premedication with opioids
- Myoclonus
- Hypotension and apnea
- Allergic reactions
- Bronchoconstriction in low dosing and inadequate plane of anesthesia
- Hypertriglyceridemia
- Infections with the use of prolonged open vials
- Pancreatitis
- *Propofol infusion syndrome:* It is a rare but lethal complication. Prolonged infusions of propofol >4 mg/kg/hour for >48 hours in susceptible individuals
  - *Risk factors:* Pediatric age group, sepsis, poor oxygen delivery, low glucose stores in liver, high dosage for a prolonged duration, and genetic predisposition which impairs fatty acid metabolism.
  - *Signs and symptoms:*
    - Cardiac arrhythmias, cardiomyopathy
    - Rhabdomyolysis
    - Acute kidney injury
    - Hypertriglyceridemia
    - Hepatomegaly
    - Skeletal myopathy.
  - Specific lab findings—metabolic acidosis, hyperkalemia, raised lactates, high urea, creatinine and creatine kinase (CK), hyperlipidemia.
  - Prevention—carefully titrated dosing of infusions, use of alternative drugs for sedation, ensuring adequate carbohydrate nutrition, and monitoring regular investigations.
  - Treatment—stop propofol, use of alternative drugs, supportive measures such as inotropes, pacing, extracorporeal membrane oxygenation (ECMO), and renal replacement therapy.

ETOMIDATE

- Introduced into clinical practice in 1972.
- Better clinical profile in terms of hemodynamic stability, minimal respiratory depression, cerebral protection, and rapid recovery.

Chemical Structure

- Imidazole derivative
- R – (+) – pentylethyl – 1H – imidazole – 5 carboxylate sulfate
- At physiological pH, it is hydrophobic, therefore formulated either in 35% propylene glycol or in lipid emulsion.

Pharmacokinetics

- Distribution half-life—2.7 minutes
- Redistribution half-life—29 minutes
- Elimination half-life—2.9–5.3 hours
- In plasma, it is 75% protein-bound
- Metabolism—in liver by ester hydrolysis
  - Metabolites are excreted mainly by kidneys and less fraction via bile.
  - 2% excreted in unchanged form.
- Diseases that alter serum protein (hepatic and renal diseases) affect the free unbound fraction and may exaggerate the pharmacodynamic effects on patients.

Pharmacodynamics

- CNS
- Produces hypnosis through GABA-A receptor via direct (in high dose) and indirect action (low dose)

- Decreases cerebral blood flow and cerebral metabolic rate of oxygen ($CMRO_2$) through vasoconstriction
- Transient decrease in intracranial pressure (ICP) postinduction
- Increases cerebral oxygen supply-demand ratio
- No alterations in mean arterial pressure (MAP), therefore CPP is maintained or increased
- In epileptogenic areas, increases electroencephalogram (EEG) activity.

Respiratory System
- Has minimal respiratory depressant action
- Induction follows transient hyperventilation may or may not be accompanied by apnea.
- It is a nonhistamine-releasing drug both in COPD and normal individuals.
- Dampens the ventilatory drive to blood CO_2 levels.

Cardiovascular System
- Because it has no effect on the sympathetic nervous system and on baroreceptor functioning therefore it is a hemodynamically stable drug. It has minimal change in heart rate but can cause decrease in MAP by 15% due to reduction of systemic vascular resistance.
- The preferred drug in cases of valvular heart disease, ischemic heart disease, patients with active heart failure, patients with hemorrhagic shock, and in patients with inflammatory sepsis.
- Nonanalgesic properties may precipitate tachycardia and high blood pressure (BP) during induction which can be managed with prior administration of opioids.

Endocrine System
- *Dose-dependent reversible inhibition of enzyme:* 11-beta-hydroxylase, leading to decreased cortisol, and mineralocorticoids.
- As per studies, the dose needed for adrenal suppression (10 ng/mL) is far less than that needed for hypnosis (200 ng/mL).
- However, inhibition of steroidogenesis is reversible and lasts for 72 hours.

Uses
- *Induction of anesthesia:*
  - *Dose:* 0.2–0.6 mg/kg IV (mostly administered 0.3 mg/kg).
  - Takes one arm brain circulation time.
  - Obliterated for maintenance of anesthesia as infusions.
  - Advantageous in the induction of patients with cardiovascular diseases, heart failure, reactive airway disease, trauma patients, critically septic patients, and patients with raised ICP.
  - Maintains MAP.
  - In electroconvulsive therapy (ECT), prolongs seizure duration.
- It can be a pharmacological treatment adjuvant in patients with endogenous hypercortisolemia.

Side Effects
- Postoperative nausea and vomiting
- Pain on injection site—lesser with lipid formulation, alleviates on a prior administration of lidocaine 20–40 mg
- Myoclonic movements—less with premedication with midazolam or magnesium.
- Hiccups
- Emergence delirium
- Adrenal suppression
- Allergic reactions.

Derivative
- Methoxycarbonyl-etomidate (MOC)—showed no suppression of steroid synthesis in preclinical studies.
- Carboetomidate—showed decreased emetogenic potential and less adrenal suppression in rat models.

- Newest—may prove useful in infusions up to 2 hours
  - Cyclopropyl-methoxycarbonyl metomidate (CPMM)
  - Dimethyl-methoxycarbonyl metomidate (DMMM).

KETAMINE

- First used by Corssen and Domino in 1965
- First released for clinical use in 1970
- Structurally, it is a phencyclidine derivative and is a racemic mixture of R and S isomers. Out of which, S isomer is a more potent analgesic, and has faster clearance and recovery with few psychomimetic side effects, whereas R isomer has psychotropic effects and cognitive impairment.
- It produces dissociative anesthesia—cataleptic state where eyes remain open with slow nystagmus but the person is unaware of the surroundings and non-communicative.
- It also produces analgesia at subclinical doses.

Mode of Action

Antagonizes the phencyclidine site on N-methyl-D-aspartate receptors (NMDAR). Also inhibits reuptake of catecholamines at the postganglionic sympathetic nerve endings. Other effects on sigma opioid receptors, muscuranic receptors producing anticholinergic symptoms such as bronchodilation, sympathpomimmetic action and voltage sensitive sodium and L-type calcium receptors exhibiting mild local anesthetic properties is also seen.

Chemical Characteristics

- Lipid-soluble phencyclidine derivative
- High first-pass metabolism—oral bioavailability is 20% only and intranasally 40%
- 12% protein-bound
- *Molecular weight:* 238kDa—hence can cross blood-brain barrier.

Pharmacokinetics

- Metabolized in liver by hepatic microsomal enzymes into norketamine which is one fifth to one-third potent as ketamine
- *Distribution half-life:* 11–16 minutes
- *Elimination half-life:* 2–3 hours.

Pharmacodynamics

Central Nervous System

- Produces dose-dependent unconsciousness and analgesia.
- Raises ICP, cerebral blood flow (CBF), $CMRO_2$.
- Acts on various receptors namely, NMDR receptors, opioid receptors, and monoaminergic receptors.
- Dissociative anesthesia—a cataleptic state with open eyes, profound analgesia, and maintained airway reflexes.
- Onset of action in 30–60 seconds.
- Effects—pupillary dilatation, lacrimation, salivation, nystagmus, and purposeless movements of arms, legs, and trunk.
- Duration of anesthesia after a dose of 2 mg/kg is 10–15 minutes.
- *Full recovery:* 15–30 minutes.
- Prevents opioid-induced hyperalgesia by antagonizing NMDAR actions. It inhibits nociceptive central hypersensitization, provides postoperative analgesia, and prevents long-lasting enhancement in pain sensitivity as induced by opioids.
- Neuroprotection by its antiapoptotic mechanism.

Respiratory System

- Bronchial smooth muscle relaxant
- Transient decreases in minute ventilation but airway reflexes are preserved
- Minimal alteration in CNS respiratory drive
- It leads to excessive salivation, therefore co administrated with anticholinergics.

Cardiovascular System

- Increases heart rate, cardiac output, blood pressure, and myocardial oxygen consumption.
- Directly has of cardiodepressant action which is prominent when there is depletion of all presynaptic catecholamine stores.
- Indirectly has a stimulatory action on sympathetic nervous system which increases catecholamine release. In general, this action overrides its direct cardiodepressant effects.
- It enhances the arrhythmogenic effects of adrenaline.

Uses

- *Induction and maintenance of anesthesia*:
  - Favored for its sympathomimetic and bronchodilator action.
  - Preferred drug for induction in patients with hypovolemic shock, cardiovascular instable patients with sepsis, trauma patients with blood loss, cardiac tamponade, restrictive pericarditis, and congenital heart disease (prevents right to left shunt)
  - In patients with depleted catecholamine stores such as in sepsis or trauma, the cardio-depressant action of ketamine may manifest. Therefore, preoperative intravascular volume resuscitation is must.
  - Total intravenous anesthesia (TIVA)—propofol along with small doses of ketamine provides minimal respiratory depression and stable hemodynamics.
- *Pain management*:
  - Low-dose ketamine 0.2 to 0.5 mg/kg perioperatively decreases the postoperative analgesic consumption
  - Part of multimodal analgesia regimen
  - Effective in chronic pain states, phantom limb, fibromyalgia, cancer pain, complex regional pain syndrome
- *Sedation*:
  - As an adjunct to regional anesthesia with dose of 0.2–8 mg/kg
  - Preferred for pediatric patients undergoing short procedures
- Antidepressant effects
- Also used for reversal of opioid tolerance, restless leg syndrome.

Doses and Routes of Administration

Ketamine can be administered orally, nasally, intramuscular, and as intravenous (IV) bolus or infusion, for premedication, induction or maintenance of anesthesia, multimodal pain management, and in chronic pain. The various indications of ketamine and its routes and doses are mentioned in **Table 1**.

Side Effects

- Increases ICP, more in spontaneously breathing head injury patients.
- Contraindicated in open eye injury, as it raises intraocular pressure (IOP).
- Tachycardia and hypertension, careful, and titrated dosing in ischemic heart disease patients. Avoid using as sole anesthetic agent in these patients.
- High BP during induction unfavorable in vascular aneurysms.

TABLE 1: Uses and doses of ketamine.

Premedication	*Oral:* 4–8 mg/kg IM: 2–4 mg/kg
Induction of general anesthesia	0.5–2 mg/kg IV 4–6 mg/kg IM
Maintenance of anesthesia	30–90 µg/kg/min
Sedation and analgesia	0.2–0.8 mg/kg IV (over 2–3 minutes) 2–4 mg/kg IM
Component of multimodal analgesia	0.15–0.25 mg/kg IV

(IV: intravenous; IM: intramuscular)

- Lacrimation, salivation, nystagmus, purposeless movements.
- Emergence delirium—can be attenuated with concomitant use of BZDs.
- Preservative in ketamine—chlorobutanol, is neurotoxic, this formulation contraindicated in epidural and subarachnoid blocks.
- Inhibits platelet aggregation through suppressed formation of inositol 1,4,5 - triphosphate and cytosolic free calcium concentrations.

DEXMEDETOMIDINE

- Selective α-2 agonist, having sedative, analgesic, hypnotic, anxiolytic, sympatholytic effects
- Introduced in clinical practice in 1999 in USA
- Receptor affinity ratio for α-2 receptor versus α-1 receptor is 1600:1, compared to clonidine which has a lesser selectivity, i.e., 220:1
- Atipamazole—specific and selective alpha 2 receptor antagonist which causes rapid reversal of hemodynamic effects of dexmedetomidine.

Chemical Properties

- S-enantiomer of medetomidine, isotonic solution.
- Water-soluble, pKa 7.1.

Pharmacokinetics

- Metabolized by glucuronidation mainly, and also mediated via cytochrome (CYP450).
- 94% protein-bound.
- Clearance decreases as hepatic impairment worsen, not influenced by renal diseases.
- Elimination half-life 2–3 hours.
- Context-sensitive half-life after 10 minutes of infusion is 4 minutes, and 250 minutes after 8 hours of infusion.

Mode of Action

- Nonselective α-2 adrenoceptor agonist.
- Location—α2B and α2C in brain and spinal cord, α2A in the periphery.
- It causes sympatholysis, antinociception, and sedation.
- Action reversed with alpha-antagonist—atipamezole, not yet approved for human use.

Dose

- *Intravenous*:
  - Loading dose: 0.5–1 µg/kg
  - Maintenance: 0.2–0.7 µg /kg/h
- *Intranasal or buccal route*: Dose 3–4 µg/kg, 1 hour prior to induction.

Pharmacodynamics

Central Nervous System

- Acts on locus coeruleus produce hypnosis and sedation.
- Does not act on GABA system unlike propofol and other induction agents.
- Acts on endogenous sleep-promoting pathways and hence produces conscious sedation.
- Lessens occurrence of delirium in ICU patients.
- Provides analgesia by inhibiting pain transmission along spinal cord by inhibiting release of substance P and glutamate.
- Neuroprotection is attributed by reduction of glutamate and modulation of anti-apoptotic proteins.

Respiratory System

- Mild decrease in minute ventilation, but preserves hypercapnic ventilatory response.
- Minimal respiratory depression.
- Maintains airway reflexes and other respiratory parameters.

Cardiovascular System

- Produces bradycardia, initial transient hypertension followed by hypotension.
- Initially increasing arterial BP can be attributed to α2-mediated vasoconstriction.
- Administration of large intravenous loading dose should be avoided to prevent bradycardia and hypotension or slowly administer loading dose over 20 minutes.

Uses

- Sedation and premedication especially in the pediatric group, as it has high bioavailability through nasal and buccal routes.
- Adjuvant in regional blocks.
- Hypnotic agents in neurosurgical procedures, such as awake craniotomy, deep brain stimulation.
- Opioid sparing effects in bariatric surgery or patients with risk of postoperative respiratory compromise.
- Facilitates awake-fiberoptic intubation as it decreases salivation in addition to sedation and anxiolysis.
- Decreases shivering episodes.
- Helpful in ICU sedation as well as during graded weaning.
- This is the only FDA approved use for dexmedetomidine that too only for <24 hours duration.

QUESTIONS

Q. 1. What is egg less any advantages?

Q. 2. (i) Ketofol (ii) Ketodex (iii) Thiofol (iv) Thiodex.

Q. 3. TIVA with propofol.

FURTHER READING

1. American Academy of Emergency Medicine. (2008). Procedural Sedation Consensus Statement. [online] Available from: https://www.aaem.org/resources/statements/position/procedural-sedation-consensus-statement [Last accessed May, 2022].
2. American Dental Association. (2007). Guidelines for the Use of Sedation and General Anesthesia by Dentists. [online] Available from: https://www.ada.org/-/media/project/ada-organization/ada/ada-org/files/publications/cdt/anesthesia_guidelines.pdf [Last accessed May, 2022].
3. American Society of Anesthesiologists. (1999). Continuum of Depth of Sedation: Definition of General Anesthesia and Levels of Sedation/Analgesia. [online]. Available from: https://www.asahq.org/standards-and-guidelines/continuum-of-depth-of-sedation-definition-of-general-anesthesia-and-levels-of-sedationanalgesia [Last accessed May, 2022].
4. Andolfatto G, Willman E. A prospective case series of single-syringe ketamine-propofol (ketofol) for emergency department procedural sedation and analgesia in adults. Acad Emerg Med. 2011;18(3):237-45.
5. Bhatt-Mehta V, Rosen DA. Sedation in children: current concepts. Pharmacotherapy. 1998;18(4):790-807.
6. Black E, Campbell SG, Magee K, Zed PJ. Propofol for procedural sedation in the emergency department: a qualitative systematic review. Ann Pharmacother. 2013; 47(6):856-68.
7. Coté CJ, Wilson S, American Academy of Pediatrics, American Academy of Pediatric Dentistry. Guidelines for Monitoring and Management of Pediatric Patients before, during, and after Sedation for Diagnostic and Therapeutic Procedures: Update 2016. Pediatrics. 2016;138 (1):e20161212.
8. David H, Shipp J. A Randomized controlled trial of ketamine/propofol versus propofol alone for emergency department procedural sedation. Ann Emerg Med. 2011; 57(5):435-41.
9. Devlin JW, Skrobik Y, Gélinas C, Needham DM, Slooter AJC, Pandharipande PP, et al. Clinical Practice Guidelines for the Prevention and Management of Pain, Agitation/Sedation, Delirium, Immobility, and Sleep Disruption in Adult Patients in the ICU. Crit Care Med. 2018;46(9):e825-73.

10. Doyle L, Colletti JE. Pediatric procedural sedation and analgesia. Pediatr Clin North Am. 2006;53(2):279-92.
11. Drown MB. Integrative review utilizing dexmedetomidine as an anesthetic for monitored anesthesia care and regional anesthesia. Nurs Forum. 2011;46(3):186-94.
12. Dumps C, Bolkenius D, Halbeck E. [Etomidate for intravenous induction of anaesthesia]. Anaesthesist. 2017;66(12):969-80.
13. Dyck JB, Maze M, Haack C, Azarnoff DL, Vuorilehto L, Shafer SL. Computer-controlled infusion of intravenous dexmedetomidine hydrochloride in adult human volunteers. Anesthesiology. 1993;78(5):821-8.
14. Ebert TJ, Hall JE, Barney JA, Uhrich TD, Colinco MD. The effects of increasing plasma concentrations of dexmedetomidine in humans. Anesthesiology. 2000;93(2):382-94.
15. Godwin SA, Caro DA, Wolf SJ, Jagoda AS, Charles R, Marett BE, et al. Clinical policy: procedural sedation and analgesia in the emergency department. Ann Emerg Med. 2005;45(2):177-96.
16. Jewett J, Phillips WJ. Dexmedetomidine for procedural sedation in the emergency department. Eur J Emerg Med. 2010;17(1):60.
17. Krauss B, Green SM. Procedural sedation and analgesia in children. Lancet. 2006; 367(9512):766-80.
18. Lemoel F, Contenti J, Giolito D, Boiffier M, Rapp J, Istria J, et al. Adverse events with ketamine versus ketofol for procedural sedation on adults: a double-blind, randomized controlled trial. Acad Emerg Med. 2017;24(12):1441-9.
19. Maze M, Tranquilli W. Alpha-2 adrenoceptor agonists: defining the role in clinical anesthesia. Anesthesiology. 1991;74(3): 581-605.
20. Miller RD, Eriksson LL, Fleisher LA, Wiener-Kronish JP, Young WL. Miller's Anesthesia 2 volume set, 7th edition. London: Churchill Livingstone Elsevier; 2009.
21. Mistry RB, Nahata MC. Ketamine for conscious sedation in pediatric emergency care. Pharmacotherapy. 2005;25(8):1104-11.
22. Nejati A, Moharari RS, Ashraf H, Labaf A, Golshani K. Ketamine/Propofol versus midazolam/fentanyl for procedural sedation and analgesia in the emergency department: a randomized, prospective, double-blind trial. Acad Emerg Med. 2011;18(8):800-6.
23. Practice Guidelines for Moderate Procedural Sedation and Analgesia 2018: A Report by the American Society of Anesthesiologists Task Force on Moderate Procedural Sedation and Analgesia, the American Association of Oral and Maxillofacial Surgeons, American College of Radiology, American Dental Association, American Society of Dentist Anesthesiologists, and Society of Interventional Radiology. Anesthesiology. 2018;128(3):437-79.
24. Sener S, Eken C, Schultz CH, Serinken M, Ozsarac M. Ketamine with and without midazolam for emergency department sedation in adults: a randomized controlled trial. Ann Emerg Med. 2011;57(2):109-114.e2.
25. Shankar V, Deshpande JK. Procedural sedation in the pediatric patient. Anesthesiology Clin North Am. 2005;23:635-54.
26. Stark RD, Binks SM, Dutka VN, O'Connor KM, Arnstein MJ, Glen JB. A review of the safety and tolerance of propofol ('Diprivan'). Postgrad Med J. 1985;61(Suppl 3):152-6.
27. Strayer RJ, Nelson LS. Adverse events associated with ketamine for procedural sedation in adults. Am J Emerg Med. 2008; 26(9):985-1028.
28. Valtonen M, Iisalo E, Kanto J, Rosenberg P. Propofol as an induction agent in children: pain on injection and pharmacokinetics. Acta Anaesthesiol Scand. 1989;33(2):152-5.
29. Valtonen M, Iisalo E, Kanto J, Tikkanen J. Comparison between propofol and thiopentone for induction of anaesthesia in children. Anaesthesia. 1988;43(8):696-9.
30. Venn RM, Karol MD, Grounds RM. Pharmacokinetics of dexmedetomidine infusions for sedation of postoperative patients requiring intensive caret. Br J Anaesth. 2002;88(5): 669-75.
31. Virtanen R, Savola JM, Saano V, Nyman L. Characterization of the selectivity, specificity and potency of medetomidine as an alpha 2-adrenoceptor agonist. Eur J Pharmacol. 1988;150(1-2):9-14.
32. Wakai A, Blackburn C, McCabe A, Reece E, O'Connor G, Glasheen J, et al. The use of propofol for procedural sedation in emergency departments. Cochrane Database Syst Rev. 2015;2015(7):CD007399.

6

Local Anesthetic

Ridhima Sharma, Anju Gupta, Ripon Choudhary, Nishkarsh Gupta

INTRODUCTION

Local anesthetics (LA) agents are comprised of drugs that can produce localized anesthesia, along with reversible loss of sensation in the body. It can be used as a sole anesthetic agent or in amalgam with general anesthesia, and/or, to bestow postoperative analgesia. In the regional anesthesia technique, local anesthetics are applied or injected very near to their required site of action; therefore, their pharmacokinetic profiles are additionally more important determinants of toxicity and elimination, than their desired clinical action.

Local anesthetics agents impede the nerve impulse conduction in the central and peripheral nervous system without central nervous system depression and alteration in the mental state. Furthermore, there occurs sequential blockade, depending upon the volume and concentration of the local anesthetic used, i.e., autonomic block followed by sensory block and finally motor blockade.

DEFINITION

Local anesthesia is defined as the loss of sensation in a circumscribed/localized part of the body due to depression of nerve endings excitation or inhibition of nerve conduction in the peripheral nerves (Stanley F Malames; 1980).

HISTORICAL PERSPECTIVE

In 1532, Europeans found the anesthetic properties of coca leaves from the natives of Peru (who considered coca leaves as a *stimulant* when chewed). The saliva after chewing the leaves of coca was frequently used by the natives for the alleviation of pain in the wounds. In 1860, Niemann discovered the active principle of the leaf (coca) and coined the term cocaine, and recorded its anesthetic properties on the tongue. In 1884, Koller (an Austrian ophthalmologist) reported the first successful use of cocaine surgically. Furthermore, leading to the rapid evolution of neo-local anesthetic agents and anesthesia techniques.

Q. 1. Describe the chemical structure of local anesthetic.

Ans. Local anesthetic is comprised of three vital structures namely: (1) An aromatic ring; (2) An alkyl chain (intermediate); and (3) A tertiary amine **(Fig. 1)**. The aromatic ring (lipophilic component) of the drug helps to determine the potency of the drug. Noteworthy LA with high potency may contribute to enhance toxicity. The aromatic ring and tertiary amine are linked together by the intermediate alkyl chain.

Q. 2. What is the classification of local anesthetics and how they are differentiated?

Ans. The LAs are broadly classified as follows:
- *Based on mode of application:* They are divided as topical and injectable. The topical LAs are further classified as soluble—cocaine, lidocaine, tetracaine,

Section 1: Anesthetic Pharmacology

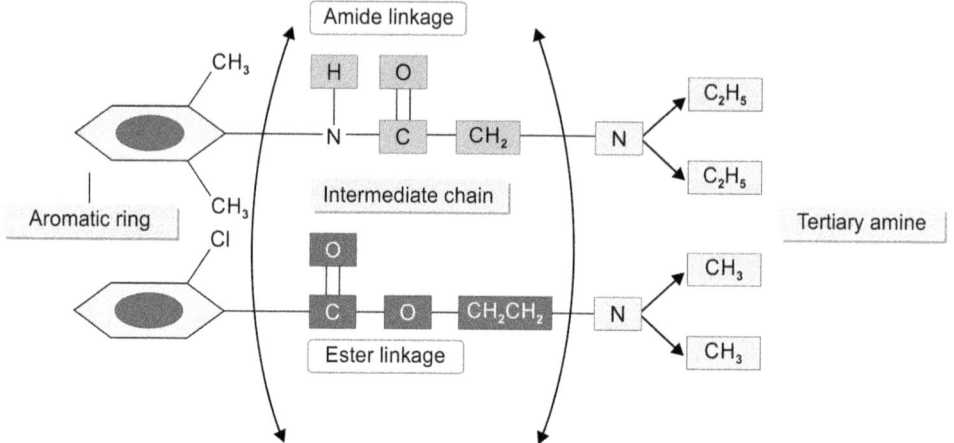

Fig. 1: Chemical structure of local anesthetic.

benoxinate, and insoluble—benzocaine, butylamino-benzoate. Injectable are classified as lidocaine, mepivacaine, bupivacaine, and dibucaine.

- *Based on the duration of action:* They are classified as ultra-short acting (chloroprocaine, procaine), short-acting (lidocaine, prilocaine), and medium-acting (mepivacaine, articaine), and long-acting (bupivacaine, etidocaine).
- *Based on potency:* They are classified as low potent—procaine and chloroprocaine, intermediate potent—lidocaine, mepivacaine, and high potent—tetracaine, bupivacaine, and dibucaine.
- *Based on chemical structure attachment:* The intermediate chain linkage as an ester or amide, binding the aromatic ring to the rest of the molecule allows the classification of local anesthetics as either amino-esters or amino-amides **(Table 1)**.

Q. 3. What is the mechanism of local anesthetic action?

Ans. Local anesthetics block voltage-gated sodium channels, preventing sodium influx intracellularly, and thereby blocking the nerve impulse transmission.

TABLE 1: Esters and amides local anesthetics.

Esters	Amides
Benzocaine	Bupivacaine
Chloroprocaine	Etidocaine
Cocaine	Levobupivacaine
Procaine	Lidocaine
Tetracaine	Mepivacaine
	Prilocaine
	Ropivacaine

The voltage-gated sodium channel is a membrane-bound protein, composed of one large α-subunit (through which Na passes) and one or two small β-subunits. Neurons have a resting membrane potential of -60 to -70 mV across the cell membrane. The electrogenic Na^+-K^+-ATPase pump couples the transfer of Na ions outside the cell, in exchange for K ions movement inside the cell (3Na ions in exchange for 2K ions). This causes an ionic disequilibrium and thus favoring the movement of intracellular K ions to extracellular sites. The cell membrane compared to Na^+-ions is more freely permeable to K ions (leaky), causing accumulation of relatively excess of negatively charged ions (anions) intracellularly. This accounts for the negative resting membrane potential (−70 mV). Impulse generation leads to the rapid influx of Na ions inwards and K ions outwards through the ion channels. An increase in the membrane potential to a threshold of −50 mV causes the generation of an action potential by the rapid influx of Na^+ ions through voltage-gated Na channel, peaking at +40 mV. Repolarization of the nerve impulse again to its resting state is achieved via the Na^+ channel inactivation and efflux of K^+ ions. Therefore, the electrochemical gradient of the resting membrane potential is restored through the Na^+/K^+ pump.

Local anesthetics bind α-subunit (specific site) and inhibit voltage-gated Na-channel. Thereby, preventing the channel activation and influx of Na associated with the membrane depolarization. There exist three conformational forms of Na^+ channel: (1) Resting; (2) Open; and (3) inactivated. Local anesthetics do not alter the resting membrane potential and have a great affinity for the open or inactivated state of channels than in the resting state.

Q. 4. Explain the use-dependent block phenomenon.

Ans. The fraction of Na channels bound to LAs increases during trains of impulses (with frequent depolarization); this is termed as a use-dependent block. In another way, LAs inhibition is voltage and frequency-dependant and is more in rapidly firing nerve fibers than with infrequent depolarization.

Q. 5. Explain the clinical implication of ionized and nonionized forms of local anesthetics.

Ans. Local anesthetics are commercially prepared as water-soluble hydrochloride salts (pH 6–7). In commercially prepared solutions containing epinephrine, the local anesthetic solutions are made more acidic (pH 4–5) compared with solutions lacking epinephrine, due to instability of the epinephrine in the alkaline environment. Due to this, these epinephrine-containing commercial preparations have decreased concentration of free base and consequently, are slow-onset than the epinephrine added at the time of use. To hasten the clinical onset, a carbonated solution of epinephrine containing the LAs is used instead of hydrochloric acid (HCl) solutions. Alternatively, sodium bicarbonate 1 mL (8.4% sodium bicarbonate) per 10 mL of local anesthetic can hasten/speed the onset and increase the amount of free base and thereby improving the quality of the block. Also, it has been found that alkalinization decreases pain with subcutaneous infiltration. Similarly, the extracellular base-to-cation ratio is decreased and onset is delayed when LA's are used in infected tissues (acidic).

Q. 6. What are the factors determining the physiological activities of the local anesthetics?

Ans.
- *pH:* In an acidic milieu (low pH), the potency is less because of the predomination of the ionized fraction in the acidic conditions. Because of less availability of the unionized form, less of the LA available can cross the lipid bilayer and thereby, block the voltage-gated sodium channels. This background can be used to understand the decreased efficacy of the LAs in infected tissues (abscess) in reducing pain, as the pH of these tissues is much lower than the physiological pH of the body.
- *pKa:* The pKa is the pH at which the fraction of ionized and unionized drugs are in equilibrium. The LAs with pKa closer to the physiological pH will have a more

unionized fraction and hence the faster onset of action. In other words, the lower the pKa, the more the unionized drug fraction is present for any given pH and faster the onset of action.

- *Potency:* The longer the intermediate chain, the more potent the LA drug. Bupivacaine is 3–4 times more potent than lignocaine because of the longer intermediate chain.
- *Lipid-solubility:* The more lipids-soluble the local anesthetic is, the faster the onset of action, the higher the potency, and the longer the duration of action. This can be explained by the presence of more drugs able to cross the neuronal membrane lipid bilayer and thus creating a depot of the drug within the axoplasm.
- *Protein-binding:* Local anesthetics with high-protein binding to α-1 glycoprotein exhibit a longer duration of action. Hypoxia, hypercarbia, and acidemia increase the risk of toxicity, due to decreased protein binding. Pediatric age groups younger than 6 months have less protein-binding capacity.

Q. 7. Explain differential blockade.
Ans. The nerve fibers with different functions have different sensitivities to blockade due to local anesthetics; this clinical phenomenon is known as "differential block." The sensitivity of nerve fibers to local anesthetics depends on two major factors including (1) nerve fiber diameter and (2) myelination. Thinner nerve fibers are most sensitive than thick fibers and myelination fibers are more sensitive than nonmyelinated ones. Thus, Aα (larger, faster) fibers are less susceptible to local anesthetics than Aδ (small, slow conducting). On the contrary C fibers (small, unmyelinated) are relatively resistant to inhibition by local anesthetics compared with large unmyelinated fibers. The sequence of the blockade is autonomically followed by sensory and motor in spinal nerve local anesthetic inhibition **(Table 2)**.

Q. 8. Describe the pharmacokinetics of local anesthetics?
Ans.
- *Absorption:* Intact skin needs a high concentration of local anesthetic base (lipid-soluble) to ensure better permeation and analgesia. The mucous membrane provides a minimum barrier to local anesthetic, causing rapid onset of action. Eutectic mixture of local anesthetics (EMLA) cream consists of—5% of

TABLE 2: Local anesthetic sensitivity depending upon nerve fiber diameter, presence of myelination, a phenomenon known as a differential blockade.

Fiber type	Function	Diameter (mm)	Conduction velocity (m/s)	Myelination	LA sensitivity
Aα	Motor proprioception	Largest 12–20	70–120	Yes	+
Aβ	Touch pressure	5–15	30–70	Yes	++
Aγ	Motor	3–6	15–30	Yes	++
Aδ	Pain, temperature, touch	2–5	12–30	Yes	+++
B	Preganglionic autonomic fibers	<3	3–4	Yes	++++
C	Pain, temperature, postganglionic sympathetic fibers	0.4–1.2	0.5–2.3	Yes	+++

lignocaine and 5 % of prilocaine (1:1) base in an oil-in-water emulsion and requires a contact period of at least 1 hour under occlusive dressing. (1–2 g/10 cm² area of skin), the maximum area of 2,000 cm² in an adult (In children <10 kg, 100 cm² maximum application area).

- *Factors affecting systemic absorption:* It depends upon the blood flow, which is further determined by the following factors:
  - *Site of injection:* The rate of systemic absorption is intravenous > tracheal > intercostal > paracervical > epidural > brachial plexus > sciatic > subcutaneous (related to the vascularity of the site of the drug).
  - *Presence of vasoconstrictors:* The addition of vasoconstrictors (epinephrine) causes vasoconstriction at the site of administration, decreases absorption, and prolongs the duration of action.
  - *Local anesthetic agent:* More lipid-soluble local anesthetics are slowly absorbed (highly tissue bound).
- *Distribution:* The LAs uptake depends on organ uptake and is determined by the following factors:
  - The highly perfused organs (brain, lung, liver, kidney, heart) have the initial high uptake (phase-α) followed by a redistribution (slow, β-phase) to moderately perfused organs (muscle, gut).
  - Blood/tissue partition coefficient—increased lipid solubility (tissue) is associated with increased protein binding and increased tissue uptake.
  - Tissue mass—increased muscle mass provides a great reservoir for the distribution of LAs in the bloodstream.
- *Biotransformation/excretion:* The biotransformation depends upon the chemical linkage of the LAs.
  - *Esters:* The LAs with ester linkages are predominately metabolized by pseudocholinesterase (butyrylcholinesterase or plasma cholinesterase). Ester hydrolysis is fast, and the water-soluble metabolite is excreted in the urine. Benzocaine and procaine are metabolized by p-aminobenzoic acid (PABA) and have been associated with anaphylactic reactions (rare).
  - *Amides:* They are metabolized by the P-450 microsomal enzyme in the liver. The rate of metabolism is agent-specific (prilocaine > lidocaine > mepivacaine > ropivacaine > bupivacaine. Impairment in the liver function or blood flow (cirrhosis, congestive heart failure, β-blockers, H_2-receptor blocker) will reduce the metabolic rate and potentially predisposes the patient to increased risk of systemic toxicity. Prilocaine is the only anesthetic metabolized to ortho-toluidine (o-toluidine), producing methemoglobinemia in a dose-dependent manner. Benzocaine (common in topical LAs spray), may also cause toxic levels of methemoglobinemia. Treatment of methemoglobinemia is methylene blue (1–2 mg/kg of 1% solution over 5 minutes). It reduces methemoglobin (Fe^{3+}) to hemoglobin (Fe^{2+}).

Q. 9. Enumerate indications and contraindications of local anesthetics.

Ans. Indications and contraindications of local anesthetics are listed in **Table 3**.

TABLE 3: Indications and contraindications of LAs.

Indications	Contraindications
• Nerve block • Cavity preparation especially in deep painful cavities • Dental procedures • Periodontal surgery and gingival surgery • Cyst marsupialization or enucleation • Removal of residual infection, small neoplastic • Growths and salivary stones, etc. • Treatment of trismus and trigeminal neuralgia	• Patient refusal • Acute infection • Allergy to the local anesthetic solution • Mentally retarded and uncooperative children • Anatomic anomalies, preventing sodium influx into the cell and blocking impulse transmission

Q. 10. Describe the clinical use of local anesthetics and their maximum recommended dose.

Ans. The clinical use of a local anesthetic is recommended in **Table 4**.

Effect of Local Anesthetics on Different Organs

Neurological

The CNS is vulnerable to local anesthetic toxicity. Early symptoms include circumoral numbness, tongue paresthesia, dizziness, tinnitus, and blurred vision. Excitatory signs encompass—restlessness, agitation, nervousness, feeling of impending doom, and garrulousness. Higher doses may cause central nervous system depression. Treatment includes benzodiazepines, barbiturates, and supportive oxygen. In the previous era, unintentional injection of chloroprocaine (large volume) into the subarachnoid space produced total spinal anesthesia and prolonged neurological deficits. The presence of preservative sodium bisulfite and the low pH of chloroprocaine were considered responsible for this neurotoxicity. Later, this formulation has been replaced by ethylenediaminetetraacetic acid (EDTA). Also, 5% lidocaine has been associated with cauda equina syndrome. Transient neurological symptoms dysesthesia, burning pain, and aching in the lower extremities and buttocks, have also been reported with many local anesthetics, especially lidocaine.

Cardiovascular

Decreased myocardial automaticity decreased refractory period, decreased contractility, and decreased conduction velocity, arrhythmias, or circulatory collapse. Inadvertently intravascular injection of bupivacaine can lead to severe cardiac toxicity; atrioventricular heart block left ventricular depression and life-threatening arrhythmias. Resuscitation from bupivacaine-induced cardiotoxicity is often difficult. Intralipid 20% injection (1.5 mL/kg over 1 minute, may repeat bolus in 5 minutes (maximum dose of 10 mL/kg in 30 minutes).

Immunological

- Esters are more likely to induce allergic reactions (IgG/IgE antibodies).
- p-aminobenzoic acid derivatives (procaine, benzocaine) are especially known as allergen.

Musculoskeletal

Direct injection of local anesthetics in Skelton's muscle is mildly myotoxic. It takes 3–4 weeks to regenerate after direct injection into the muscle.

Hematological

Lidocaine may reduce thrombosis and decrease platelet aggregation.

Drug Interactions

Local anesthetics may potentiate nondepolarizing muscle relaxant. Histamine

TABLE 4: Clinical use of local anesthetic is recommended.

Agent	Clinical use	Concentration	Maximum dose (mg/kg)
Esters			
Benzocaine	Topical	20%	NA
Chloroprocaine	Epidural, spinal, peripheral nerve block	1%, 2%, 3%	12
Cocaine	Topical	4%, 10%	3
Procaine	Local infiltration, spinal	1%, 2%, 10%	12
Tetracaine	Spinal, topical (eye)	0.25%, 0.3%, 0.5%, 1%, 2%	3
Amides			
Bupivacaine	Epidural, spinal, peripheral nerve block, infiltration	0.25%, 0.5%, 0.75%	3
Lidocaine	Topical, epidural, spinal, peripheral nerve block, intravenous regional	0.5%, 1%, 1.5%, 2%, 4%, 5%	4.5 / 7 (with epinephrine)
Mepivacaine	Epidural, spinal, peripheral nerve block, infiltration	1%, 1.5%, 2%, 3%	4.5 / 7 (with epinephrine)
Prilocaine	Topical eutectic mixture of local anesthetics (EMLA), epidural, intravenous regional	0.5%, 2%, 3%, 4%	8
Ropivacaine	Epidural, spinal, peripheral nerve block, infiltration	0.2%, 0.5%, 0.75%, 1%	3

receptor and β-blockers decreased hepatic blood flow and lidocaine clearance.

KEY POINTS

- Local anesthetic block Na^+ channel from inside of the cell membrane and raises the threshold of channel opening.
- The minimum concentration of LA needed to block a nerve fiber is Cm (thick, myelinated fiber has greater cm).
- Esters local anesthetics are predominantly metabolized by pseudocholinesterase.
- Amide LAs are metabolized by microsomal enzyme P-450 enzyme in the liver.
- Duration of action correlates with potency and lipid-solubility.
- Highly lipid soluble local anesthetics have a longer duration of action.
- Speed of onset, potency, and duration depends on the pKa, lipid solubility, and protein-binding, respectively.
- The rate of systemic absorption is related to the vascularity of site of injection; intra-arterial > tracheal > intercostal > paracervical > epidural > brachial plexus > sciatic > subcutaneous.
- Local anesthesia systemic toxicity (LAST) is increased by hypoxia, hypercapnia, and acidosis.

QUESTIONS

Q. 1. What is eutectic mixture of local anesthetics?

Q. 2. Management of local anesthetic systemic toxicity (LAST).

Q. 3. Adjuvants to local anesthetics in peripheral nerve blocks.

Q. 4. Mechanism of action by which local anesthetic reduce cancer recurrence?

Q. 5. Advantages of liposomal bupivacaine over traditional local anesthetic?

Q. 6. What are (a) Buffered local anesthetics, (b) Extended release local anesthetics?

Q. 7. Effect of local anesthetics and wound healing.

Q. 8. Local anesthetic allergy.

Q. 9. Anti-inflammatory and antimicrobial properties of anesthetics.

Q. 10. Local anesthetic patches for pain releaf.

FURTHER READING

1. Becker DE, Reed KL. Local anesthetics: review of pharmacological considerations. Anesth Prog. 2012;59(2):90-103.
2. Calatayud J, Gonzalez A. History of the development and evolution of local anesthesia since the coca leaf. Anesthesiology. 2003;98(6):1503-8.
3. Catterall WA, Swanson TM. Structural basis for pharmacology of voltage-gated sodium and calcium channels. Mol Pharmacol. 2015;88:141-50.
4. Colvin LA. Physiology and pharmacology of pain. In: Thompson JP, Wiles MD, Moppett IG (Eds). Smith and Aitkenhead's Textbook of Anaesthesia, 7th edition. St Louis: Elsevier; 2019. pp. 100-21.
5. de Lera Ruiz M, Kraus RL. Voltage-gated sodium channels: structure, function, pharmacology, and clinical indications. J Med Chem. 2015;58(18):7093-118.
6. Ehrenström Reiz GM, Reiz SL. EMLA—a eutectic mixture of local anaesthetics for topical anaesthesia. Acta Anaesthesiol Scand. 1982;26(6):596-8.
7. Fozzard HA, Lee PJ, Lipkind GM. Mechanism of local anesthetic drug action on voltage-gated sodium channels. Curr Pharm Des. 2005;11(21):2671-86.
8. Gitman M, Marina MD, Weinberg GL, Neal JM, Barrington MJ. Local anesthetic systemic toxicity: a narrative literature review and clinical update on prevention, diagnosis, and management. Plast Reconst Surg. 2019;144:783-95.
9. Guay J. Methemoglobinemia related to local anesthetics: a summary of 242 episodes. Anesth Analg. 2009;108(3):837-45.
10. Liljestrand G. The historical development of local anesthesia in local anesthetics. In: Lechat P (Ed). International Encyclopedia of Pharmacology and Therapeutics. Oxford: Pergamon Press; 1971. pp. 1-38.
11. Miller RD, Eriksson LI, Fleisher LA, Wiener-Kronish JP, Young WL. Miller's Anesthesia, 7th edition. Philadelphia: PA: Churchill Livingstone/Elsevier; 2010. pp. 263-5.
12. Morgan GE, Mikhail MS, Murray MJ. Clinical Anesthesiology. New York: Lange Medical Books/McGraw Hill; 2006.
13. Ruetsch YA, Böni T, Borgeat A. From cocaine to ropivacaine: the history of local anesthetic drugs. Curr Top Med Chem. 2001;1(3):175-82.
14. Swain A, Nag DS, Sahu S, Samaddar DP. Adjuvants to local anesthetics: current understanding and future trends. World J Clin Cases. 2017;5(8):307-23.
15. Vandam LD: Some aspects of the history of local anesthesia. In: Strichartz GR (Ed). Local Anesthetics: Handbook of Experimental Pharmacology. Germany: Springer-Verlag; 1987. pp. 1-19.

CHAPTER 7

Neuromuscular Blocking Agents

Anju Gupta, Swati Pandurangi

Q. 1. Describe the adult mammalian neuromuscular junction in brief.

Ans.
- The mammalian neuromuscular junction consists of pre- and postjunctional nicotinic ACh receptors (NAChR).
- Prejunctional receptors are alpha 3 beta-2 complexes. They are responsible for the modulation of Ach release in the neuromuscular junction.
- Postjunctional receptors have alpha-2 beta delta epsilon complexes. The subunits are arranged in such a way to form a transmembranous pore and have binding sites for *acetylcholine* and its agonists **(Fig. 1)**. Alpha subunit has four domains, i.e., M1–M4.

Q. 2. What are neuromuscular blocking agents and how are they classified?

Ans.
- Neuromuscular blocking agents (NMBAs) are drugs that act at the peripheral neuromuscular junction to reduce muscle tone and cause muscle paralysis.
- They can be broadly classified into nondepolarizing muscle relaxants, and depolarizing muscle relaxants.

Q. 3. Outline the mechanism of action of nondepolarizing muscle relaxants and depolarizing muscle relaxants.

Ans.
- Nondepolarizing muscle relaxants compete with acetylcholine at the postjunctional alpha subunits.

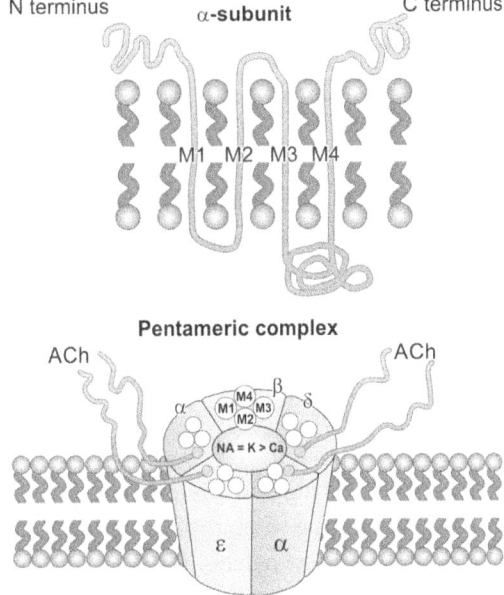

Fig. 1: Nicotinic acetylcholine receptor.

- Succinylcholine is the only depolarizing muscle relaxant currently being used in clinical practice. It produces muscle paralysis by causing prolonged depolarization of the postsynaptic NACh receptors, leading to inhibition of propagation of action potential across the membrane.

Q. 4. Explain structure, pharmacodynamics and pharmacokinetics succinylcholine.

Ans.
- Succinylcholine is composed of two molecules of acetylcholine linked through the acetate methyl group.

- Succinylcholine is rapidly acted upon by the enzyme pseudocholinesterase present in the plasma.
- Only around 10% of the administered drug reaches the neuromuscular junction.
- Succinylcholine is hydrolyzed into succinic acid and choline.
- Little or nil pseudocholinesterase is there at the junction, so entry into recirculation terminates action of scoline.
- The dose of succinylcholine is given in **Table 1**.

Q. 5. What is dibucaine number?
Ans.
- Dibucaine is an ester local anesthetic agent that inhibits pseudocholinesterase.
- When a standard dose of dibucaine is given, the unchanged percentage of pseudocholinesterase is determined, which gives the dibucaine number.
- Atypical pseudocholinesterase is dibucaine resistant and is not inhibited by dibucaine.
- *Normal dibucaine number:* 70–80.

The relation between dibucaine number and duration of succinylcholine block is given in **Table 2**.

Q. 6. What are the other factors that decrease pseudocholinesterase activity?
Ans.
- Advanced liver disease
- Malnutrition
- Pregnancy
- Burns
- Oral contraceptives
- Drugs—monoamine oxidase (MAO) inhibitors, cytotoxic drugs, anticholinesterase drugs, metoclopramide.

Q. 7. What are the side effects of succinylcholine?
Ans.
- *Cardiovascular effects:*
  - Sinus bradycardia, junctional rhythm (due to action on M2 receptors)
  - Tachycardia, increase BP (autonomic ganglion stimulation)
- *Hyperkalemia:*
  - Increase in K^+ by 0.5 mEq/dL
  - Severe hyperkalemia is associated with burns, closed head injury, metabolic acidosis.
- *Myoglobinuria:* Pediatric patients are more susceptible.
- Increased intraocular, intragastric, and intracranial pressures.

TABLE 1: Dose of succinylcholine.

Dose	Effect	Onset of action	Duration of action	Remarks
1.0 mg/kg	Tracheal intubation	60 seconds	9–13 minutes	Dose of 1.5 mg/kg has no advantage over 1 mg/kg in RSI

(RSI: rapid sequence intubation)

TABLE 2: Relation between dibucaine number and duration of succinylcholine block.

Type	Genotype	Incidence	Dibucaine number	Duration of such action
Homozygous typical	$E_1^u E_1^u$	Normal	70–80	Normal
Heterozygous atypical	$E_1^u E_1^a$	1/480	50–60	↑ by 50–60%
Homozygous atypical	$E_1^a E_1^a$	1/3200	20–30	↑ to 4–8 hours

- *Myalgias:*
  - Mechanism of postoperative myalgia is not fully understood
  - Two factors are postulated—fasciculations or the possible role of prostaglandin and cyclo-oxygenase release.
- *Masseter spasm:*
  - Triggers malignant hyperthermia
  - Inadequate dosage in children.

Q. 8. Classify nondepolarizing muscle relaxants.
Ans. The classification of nondepolarizing muscle relaxants is given in **Table 3**.

The metabolism and elimination of commonly used nondepolarizing neuromuscular blocking drugs are described in **Table 4**.

Q. 9. What is the relation between the potency of nondepolarizing muscle agents and speed of onset?
Ans.
- Potency can be described as the dose required to produce an effect. ED 95 is the dose of the drug which produces 95% reduction in the force of contraction or amplitude of the EMG at adductor pollicis following ulnar nerve stimulation.

TABLE 3: Nondepolarizing muscle relaxants.

Class of blocker	Long acting (>50 minutes)	Intermediate acting (20–50 minutes)	Short acting (10–20 minutes)
Steroidal compounds	Pancuronium	• Vecuronium • Rocuronium	
Benzylisoquinolinium compounds	Tubocurarine	• Atracurium • Cisatracurium	Mivacurium

TABLE 4: Metabolism and elimination of commonly used nondepolarizing neuromuscular blocking drugs.

Drug	Metabolism	Elimination	Remarks
Pancuronium	Liver (10–20%)	• Renal (85%) • Liver (15%)	• Vagolytic action. Blocks norepinephrine reuptake • –OH metabolite is responsible for long duration of action
Vecuronium	Liver (30–40%)	• Renal (40–50%) • Liver (50–60%) • Metabolites eliminated in urine and bile	Similar structure to pancuronium but lacks N-methyl group making it less potent, reduction in vagolytic properties, and molecular instability
Rocuronium		• Renal (10–25%) • Liver (>70%)	Faster onset of action makes it a good choice for RSI
Atracurium	Hofmann elimination	• Renal (10–40%) • Metabolites eliminated in urine and bile	Laudanosine is the metabolite that has CNS stimulating properties
Cisatracurium	Hofmann elimination	Renal (77%)	Less laudanosine
Mivacurium	Psuedocholinesterase	Renal (<5%)	Inactive metabolites

(RSI: rapid sequence intubation)

- Usually, onset of action is inversely proportional to potency of nondepolarizing NMBA.
- This explains faster onset of action of rocuronium (13% of potency of vecuronium)
- The exception is atracurium.

Q. 10. What is buffered diffusion?
Ans. It is seen with high potency NMBAs. There is repetitive binding and unbinding from the receptors, increasing the concentration of the drug in the area of effector sites and increasing the duration of action.

Q. 11. Describe the factors that affect increase potency of nondepolarizing neuromuscular blocking agents.
Ans. Factors that affect increase potency of NMBAs are given in **Table 5**.

Q. 12. Mention the factors that reduce potency of nondepolarizing neuromuscular blocking agents.
Ans. The factors that reduce potency of nondepolarizing neuromuscular blocking agents are given in **Table 6**.

Q. 13. What are the adverse effects of nondepolarizing muscle relaxants?
Ans.
- Autonomic effects due to interaction with N and M receptors can be seen. Pancuronium has vagolytic properties.
- Histamine release is associated with benzylquinolium compounds except for cisatracurium.
- Allergic reactions including anaphylactic and anaphylactoid reactions are a rare occurrence associated with these drugs.

Q. 14. What is Hofmann elimination?
Ans.
- Spontaneous degradation in the body at physiological pH and temperature that is organ-independent is known as *Hofmann elimination*.
- Cisatracurium and atracurium undergo Hofmann elimination to form laudanosine and a monoquaternary acrylate metabolite. The monoquaternary acrylate metabolite undergoes hydrolysis by nonspecific plasma esterases to form a monoquaternary alcohol.
- Hydrolysis of cisatracurium by plasma esterases is not an important pathway for its elimination; in contrast, atracurium is eliminated by Hofmann degradation and hydrolysis by nonspecific esterases.

Q. 15. Describe the doses of some commonly used neuromuscular blocking agents.
Ans. Doses of some commonly used neuromuscular blocking agents are described in **Table 7**.

TABLE 5: Factors that affect increase potency of NMBAs.

Agent	Mechanism that causes potentiation
Inhalational agents Desflurane > sevoflurane > isoflurane > halothane > nitrous oxide	• Central effect on alpha motor neurons • Increases affinity at a receptor site • Inhibit postsynaptic NACh receptors
Antibiotics Aminoglycosides, polymyxins, clindamycin, lincomycin	• Inhibit prejunctional release of ACh • Reduce postjunctional receptor sensitivity to ACh
Hypothermia	
Magnesium sulfate	Inhibits calcium channels at presynaptic junction, so prevents release of ACh

TABLE 6: Factors that reduce potency of nondepolarizing neuromuscular blocking agents.

Agent	Mechanism that reduces potency
Antiepileptic drugs	• Increased clearance of drug • Increased binding of drug to alpha 1 acid glycoproteins • Upregulation of ACh receptors
Hypercalcemia	• Decreased sensitivity to atracurium, pancuronium

TABLE 7: Doses of some commonly used neuromuscular blocking agents.

Drug	ED 95	Intubating dose (mg/kg)	Onset of action (min)	Duration (min)	Maintenance dose bolus (mg/kg)	Maintenance dose (infusion (µg/kg/min)
Succinylcholine	0.5	1.0	0.5	5–10	0.15	2–15 mg/kg/min
Rocuronium	0.3	0.8	1.5	35–75	0.15	9–12
Atracurium	0.2	0.5	2.5–3.0	15–20	0.05	4–15
Cisatracurium	0.05	0.2	2.0–3.0	40–75	0.02	1–2
Vecuronium	0.05	0.12	2.0–3.0	45–90	0.01	1–2
Pancuronium	0.07	0.12	2.0–3.0	60–120	0.01	–

QUESTIONS

Q. 1. What will be the effect if succinylcholine is given after nondepolarizing muscle relaxant?

Q. 2. What will be effect if nondepolarizing muscle relaxant is given after succinylcholine?

Q. 3. What will be the effect if reversal agent is given after succinylcholine?

Q. 4. Total intravenous anesthesia (TIVA) and muscle relaxants used and concerns with them.

Q. 5. Advantage of cisatracurium over atracurium and sugammadex over neostigmine/glycopyrrolate?

Q. 6. Baricity? Advantages of isobaric bupivacaine.

FURTHER READING

1. De Wolf AM, Freeman JA, Scott VL, Tullock W, Smith DA, Kisor DF, et al. Pharmacokinetics and pharmacodynamics of cisatracurium in patients with end-stage liver disease undergoing liver transplantation. Br J Anaesth. 1996;76(5):624-8.
2. Larijani GE, Gratz I, Silverberg M, Jacobi AG. Clinical pharmacology of the neuromuscular blocking agents. DICP. 1991;25(1):54-64.
3. Naguib M, Lien CA, Meistelman C. Pharmacology of Neuromuscular Blocking Drugs. Miller's Anesthesia, 9th edition. Gurugram, India: Elsevier; 2019.
4. Naguib MA. Neuromuscular-Blocking drugs and Reversal Agents. Stoelting's Pharmacology and Physiology in Anesthetic Practice, 6th edition. Philadelphia; Wolters Kluwer Health; 2021.

Anticholinesterase Drugs and Cholinergic Agonists

Dhruv Jain

INTRODUCTION

Acetylcholine is an important neurotransmitter of the body and nervous system. It is an ester of acetic acid and choline. It is the primary neurotransmitter of the parasympathetic system, the preganglionic sympathetic nervous system, and sweat glands. In addition to the autonomic nervous system, it is the chief chemical released at the motor end-plates of the neuromuscular junction resulting in the activation of skeletal muscles. The action of acetylcholine is mediated by two kinds of receptors—(1) muscarinic and (2) nicotinic. Muscarinic receptors are present on various parasympathetic innervated tissues and mediate the action of acetylcholine.

- *Heart:* Bradycardia, reduced contraction, decreased atrioventricular (AV) conduction
- Smooth muscle contraction, increased secretions, and bronchoconstriction
- Vasodilatation
- *Central nervous system (CNS):* Learning, memory, and attention.

NICOTINIC RECEPTORS

Nicotinic receptors are the predominant receptors found at the neuromuscular junction. On the generation of action potential in motor nerve, acetylcholine is released from presynaptic terminals which bind to nicotinic receptors leading to muscle contraction. These receptors are also present in autonomic ganglia and the central nervous system.

The drugs which mimic the action of acetylcholine are called *cholinergic drugs*. The drugs may act directly on the acetylcholine receptors and are termed as *cholinergic agonist*. They may act indirectly by inhibiting the enzyme known as acetylcholinesterase involved in the breakdown of acetylcholine at the terminals and are called *anticholinesterases*. The classification of cholinergic drugs is summarized in **Flowchart 1**.

ANTICHOLINESTERASES

These are indirectly acting parasympathomimetic drugs which inhibit enzyme acetylcholinesterase resulting in increased accumulation of acetylcholine at synaptic cleft with increased activity on nicotinic and muscarinic receptors. There are three classes of drugs in this group, they are as follows:

1. *Quaternary ammonium alcohol—edrophonium:* It binds electrostatically to the anionic site of enzyme and is strengthened by hydrogen bonds at the esteratic site. This bond is weak and therefore, the inhibition is reversible with a short duration of action.
2. *Carbamates—neostigmine, physostigmine, and pyridostigmine:* These drugs bind to esteratic site of an enzyme by forming a stronger carbamyl ester complex. This results in the inactivation of an enzyme with longer duration of action. Neostigmine and pyridostigmine have

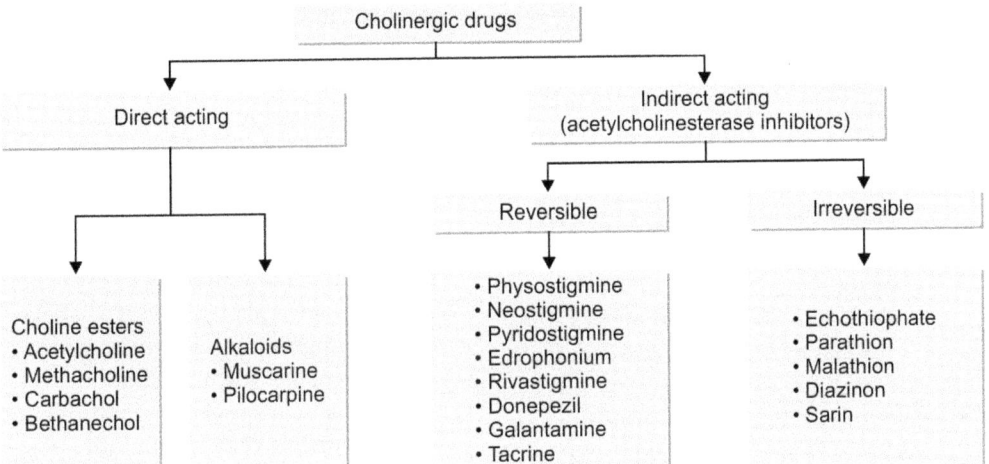

Flowchart 1: Classification of cholinergic drugs.

quaternary structures and are unable to penetrate lipid-rich layers like the blood-brain barrier. On the other hand, physostigmine is a tertiary amine that can penetrate blood-brain barrier producing various CNS effects.

3. *Organophosphates:* They bind to the esteratic site to form a stable complex that produces irreversible inhibition of the enzyme. This causes overstimulation of muscarinic and nicotinic receptors, producing toxic and CNS effects.

Clinical Uses

- *Reversal of neuromuscular blockade:*
  - This is the most common use of anticholinesterases in anesthesia practice. During neuromuscular blockade by nondepolarizing neuromuscular blockers, nicotinic receptors are occupied by the drug. Anticholinesterases such as edrophonium, neostigmine, and pyridostigmine increase the concentration of acetylcholine at the junction which competes with neuromuscular blocking drugs to bind with a nicotinic receptor, thereby causing muscle contraction and reversal of blockade. However, there is a "ceiling effect" of these drugs and excessive dosage of drugs does not lead to faster reversal of neuromuscular blockade.
  - *Edrophonium* (0.5–1 mg/kg) is a rapid and short-acting agent with an effect lasting for 10 minutes. This can lead to recurarization if spontaneous recovery was not present. *Neostigmine* (50–70 µg/kg) has an intermediate duration of action lasting for 20–30 minutes and therefore is the most commonly used reversal agent. The duration of action of pyridostigmine is 6 hours and is not used for reversal of neuromuscular blockade.
  - The *dose* and *timing* of reversal of neuromuscular blockade should be appropriate to reduce the chances of residual blockade. With the deep blockade, administration of reversal should be avoided, as there is a ceiling effect to anticholinesterases and acetylcholine would not be able to displace the muscle relaxant. The use of

neuromuscular monitoring can guide to the dosage of anticholinesterases.
- Train-of-four (TOF) count 2 or 3—administer neostigmine at a dose of 70 µg/kg
- TOF ratio >0.4—administer neostigmine at a dose of 50 µg/kg
- TOF ratio between 0.4 and 0.7—administer neostigmine at a dose of 20 µg/kg
- TOF ratio >0.7—avoid anticholinesterase as it may lead to muscle weakness.

• All the cholinesterase inhibitors in addition to increasing concentration of acetylcholine at nicotinic receptors increase the concentration at muscarinic receptors which can produce various adverse effects such as bradycardia, hypotension, bronchospasm, and increased secretions. To counter these effects, the administration of anticholinesterases is always accompanied by an anticholinergic drug like atropine or glycopyrrolate (10 µg/kg). The choice of an anticholinergic is based upon the pharmacologic profile of anticholinesterase used **(Table 1)**. As the onset and duration of action of glycopyrrolate closely match with neostigmine, both of these drugs are frequently combined.

- *Myasthenia gravis:* Neostigmine and pyridostigmine are used in the symptomatic management of this autoimmune neuromuscular disease. By increasing the concentration of acetylcholine, they increase the response of skeletal muscles. *Oral pyridostigmine* is most commonly used due to its long half-life. Edrophonium is used to diagnose and assess the anticholinesterase therapy in myasthenia gravis. Improvement in muscular weakness after edrophonium injection suggests the diagnosis of myasthenia gravis.
- *Alzheimer's disease:* The pathogenesis of Alzheimer's disease includes loss of cholinergic neurons. Centrally acting cholinesterase inhibitors (tacrine, rivastigmine, donepezil) are used for this condition.
- *Central anticholinergic syndrome:* Physostigmine is used to antagonize CNS effects of anticholinergic drugs (atropine and hyoscine) such as hallucinations, thought impairment, ataxia, and delirium.
- *Glaucoma:* Echothiophate and physostigmine are used for both narrow and wide-angle glaucoma by increasing the drainage of aqueous humor causing a decrease in intraocular pressure.
- *Postoperative analgesia:* Neostigmine has been used intrathecally (50–100 µg) or epidurally (1–4 µg/kg) to produce analgesia for postoperative period. It is used as an adjuvant to local anesthetics and opioids. It acts by increasing the

TABLE 1: Pharmacological properties of anticholinesterases.

Drug	Edrophonium	Neostigmine	Pyridostigmine
Dose	0.5–1 mg/kg	50–70 µg/kg	0.1 mg/kg (myasthenia gravis)
Onset (minutes)	1	1–2	>15
Duration of action (minutes)	10	20–30	360
Elimination half-life (minutes)	110	77	112
Renal contribution to clearance (%)	66	54	76
Recommended anticholinergic dose	Atropine (7 µg/kg)	Glycopyrrolate (10 µg/kg)	Glycopyrrolate (10 µg/kg)

concentration of acetylcholine in dorsal horn of spinal cord which mediates analgesia. It may produce adverse effects such as nausea, vomiting, pruritus, and prolonged motor blockade.

Adverse Effects

- *Muscle weakness:* Though anticholinesterases antagonize the neuromuscular blockade, they can also cause muscle weakness when given in large doses or if the neuromuscular blockade has completely recovered
- Nausea and vomiting
- Bronchoconstriction
- Bradycardia, increased salivation, complete heart block, and hypotension
- CNS side effects of centrally acting anticholinesterases—confusion, ataxia, seizures, depression of ventilation
- *Organophosphorus poisoning:* Due to irreversible inhibition, these agents are highly toxic and can cause death from bradycardia, bronchoconstriction, and convulsions. Atropine is used to antagonize the muscarinic effects, while oximes are used to reactivate the acetylcholinesterase enzyme.

CHOLINERGIC AGONISTS

- These synthetic analogs of acetylcholine have their primary site of action on muscarinic receptors. They have more selective effects and a longer duration of action than acetylcholine.
- Methacholine, carbachol, and bethanechol have some clinical utility; however, they are not commonly used because of other systemic side effects.
- Carbachol and bethanechol are used as stimulants for the gastrointestinal and urinary tract. Stimulation of peristalsis helps in gastric atony and ileus. Contraction of detrusor muscle and urethral peristalsis helps in the condition of neurogenic bladder.
- Pilocarpine is an alkaloid with strong muscarinic action. It is used topically as eye drops and causes miosis, cycloplegia and a decrease in intraocular pressure. It is also used to treat dry mouth in Sjogren's syndrome by stimulating the secretion of saliva.

POINTS TO REMEMBER

- Anticholinesterases are indirect-acting cholinergic drugs that inhibit the breakdown of acetylcholine and increase its concentration to stimulate the nicotinic and muscarinic receptors.
- Most common use of anticholinesterases in anesthesia practice is reversal of neuromuscular blockade.
- Neostigmine (50-70 µg/kg) is most commonly used because of its intermediate duration of action and devoid of central effects (does not cross blood-brain barrier because of quaternary structure). Its administration is accompanied by anticholinergic (glycopyrrolate) to counter muscarinic side effects.
- Cholinergic agonists are seldomly used because of widespread muscarinic actions. Pilocarpine is used topically as eye drops for miosis and reducing intraocular pressure.

FURTHER READING

1. Flood P, Rathmell JP, Shafer SL. Stoelting's Pharmacology & Physiology in Anesthetic Practice, 5th edition. Philadelphia: Lippincott Williams and Wilkins; 2014.
2. Miller RD. Miller's Anesthesia, 8th edition. San Diego: Churchill Livingstone; 2015.
3. Nair VP, Hunter JM. Anticholinesterases and anticholinergic drugs. Cont Edu Anaesth Crit Care Pain. 2004;4(5):164-8.

CHAPTER 9

Anticholinergic Medications

Balaji Nagarajan, Puneet Khanna

Q. 1. What are anticholinergic drugs and their classification?

Ans. Anticholinergic drugs are those drugs that block the actions of acetylcholine exerted through the muscarinic receptors on the autonomic and central nervous system. Acetylcholine is the principal neurotransmitter secreted at:

- Neuromuscular junctions (acting at nicotinic receptors).
- Preganglionic nerve fibers of the autonomic nervous system (acting at muscarinic receptors).
- Postganglionic nerve fibers of all parasympathetic and few sympathetic fibers (acting at muscarinic receptors).

Classification of antimuscarinic agents is shown in **Flowchart 1**.

Q. 2. Explain the pharmacokinetics of commonly used anticholinergics.

Ans. Pharmacokinetics of commonly used anticholinergics is tabulated in **Table 1**.

Q. 3. Explain the pharmacodynamics of anticholinergic drugs.

Ans. Anticholinergic drugs work by competitively antagonizing the effects of the

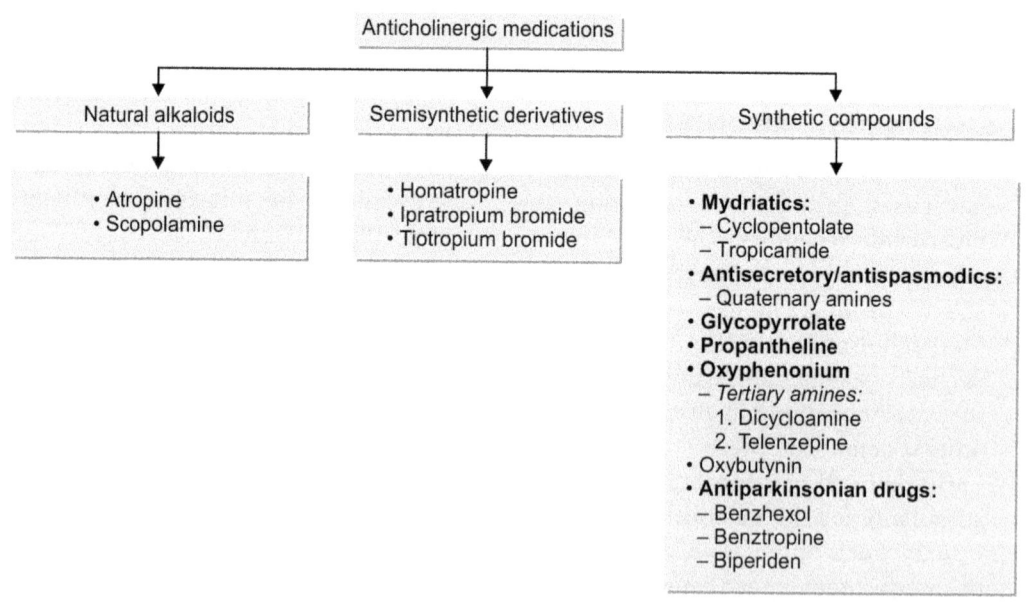

Flowchart 1: Classification of antimuscarinic agents.

TABLE 1: Pharmacokinetics of commonly used anticholinergics.

	Atropine	*Glycopyrrolate*	*Scopolamine*
Chemical	Tertiary amine; ester of tropic acid and tropine	Quaternary ammonium compound	Ester of tropic acid and scopine
Absorption	Rapid and well absorbed from all dosage forms (oral bioavailability: 10–25%)	Oral bioavailability: 5%; absorbed in comparable amounts when administered by either IM or IV route	Poor oral absorption (oral bioavailability: 10%); well absorbed following SC or IM administration
Distribution	14–44% protein-bound	4% protein-binding property; rapidly disappears from plasma	Only 4–11% protein bounds
Metabolism	Enzymatic hydrolysis particularly in the liver (major) and tissues to tropine and tropic acid	Only negligible biotransformation occurs	Metabolized in liver and tissues to scopine and scopic acid
Excretion	94% of the drug is excreted in urine (13–50% as unchanged drug); elimination half-life is 2.5 hours	More than 85% of the drug is excreted in urine; remaining in bile; elimination half-life is 0.5–1 hours	40–60% of drug is excreted in urine and the remaining is excreted in feces; elimination half-life is 4.5 hours

neurotransmitter acetylcholine at receptor sites within the cholinergic system. The cholinergic system involves two types of receptors:
1. *Muscarinic receptor*—present on target organs of the parasympathetic nervous system and sweat glands.
2. *Nicotinic receptor*—present in postganglionic dendrites, motor endplates.

Anticholinergic drugs are those that predominantly affect the muscarinic receptors, e.g., atropine and glycopyrrolate. Drugs that affect preferentially the nicotinic receptors are called *ganglion blockers* or *neuromuscular blockers*.

Q. 4. What are the adverse effects of commonly used anticholinergic drugs?
Ans. Effects of anticholinergic drugs on various systems are given in **Table 2**.

Comparison between anticholinergic drugs is given in **Table 3**.

Q. 5. What are the doses of commonly used anticholinergic drugs?
Ans. The doses of commonly used anticholinergic drugs are described in **Table 4**.

TABLE 2: Effects of anticholinergic drugs on various systems.

Central nervous system	Impairs memory; causes agitation, delirium, hallucinations; fever
Peripheral vasculature	Vasoconstriction
Cardiovascular system	Tachycardia; increased AV conduction
Gastrointestinal system	Decreases motility and decreases the gastric acid secretion
Respiratory system	Bronchodilation
Eye	Dilates pupil, increases intraocular pressure, and causes loss of accommodation
Skin	Decreases sweat production, causes vasodilation
Others	Decreases saliva production, causes dryness of mucous membranes, decreases bladder activity, and promotes urine retention

TABLE 3: Comparison between anticholinergic drugs.

	Atropine	Glycopyrrolate	Scopolamine
Antisialagogue	+	++	+++
Heart rate	+++	++	+
Sedation	+	0	+++
Mydriasis/cycloplegia	+	0	+++
Prevention of motion sickness	+	0	+++

TABLE 4: Doses of commonly used anticholinergic drugs.

	Atropine	Glycopyrrolate	Scopolamine
Dose	IM/IV For adults: 0.5–1 mg For children <12 years: 20 µg/kg repeated every 4–6 hours; maximum total dose is 1 mg >2 years: 20 µg/kg repeated every 4–6 hours; maximum total dose is 2 mg	IM: 4–9 µg/kg IV: 3–10 µg/kg (Maximum dose 100 µg/dose for Pediatrics)	IM or IV: 0.3–0.5 mg (8–15 µg/kg) Oral: 20 mg
Onset	IM: Within 30 min Maximum effect: 30–60 min IV: Immediately	IM: 15–30 min IV: Within 1 minute; peak effect within 3 min	IM: 20 min approximately IV: 15 min Oral: 2 hours Transdermal: 6–8 hours
Duration	Antisialagogue action: <4 hours Antivagal effect: Up to 1–2 hours	Antisialagogue action: Up to 7 hours Antivagal effect: Up to 2–3 hours	IV or IM: 4 hours Transdermal: 72 hours

Peripheral muscarinic effects of anticholinesterase agents are given in **Table 5**.

To counter bradycardia due to increased vagal tone, effects of drugs are given in **Table 6**.

Q. 6. What are the special considerations in the perioperative usage of anticholinergic medications?

Ans. *Glaucoma patients:* Anticholinergic drugs when administered systemically usually have little effect on intraocular pressure except in patients with narrow-angle glaucoma [where it causes an acute rise in intraocular pressure (IOP)]. Anticholinergic drugs can be used safely in open-angle

TABLE 5: Peripheral muscarinic effects of anticholinesterase agents.

Atropine	Glycopyrrolate
Used with edrophonium since both of them have similar onset and peak	Used along with neostigmine since both of them have similar pharmacokinetics
Dose: 5–7 µg/kg	Dose: 10 µg/kg. In general, a dose equivalent to one-fourth the dose of neostigmine can be used to have minimal effects on the cardiovascular system

TABLE 6: Effects of drugs.

Atropine	Glycopyrrolate
• More preferred agent • *Dose:* 0.5–1 mg every 3–5 min; maximum total dose—3 mg • *For pediatric:* 20 µg/kg; maximum dose—0.5 mg/dose	• Less preferred • *Dose:* 0.1 mg as a single dose; can be repeated at 2–3 min intervals • *For pediatrics:* 4 µg/kg; maximum dose—100 µg/dose

glaucoma, particularly if the patient's IOP is adequately controlled with appropriate miotic agents.

Heart transplant recipients: Anticholinergic drugs are ineffective in the treatment of bradycardia due to the lack of parasympathetic innervation by vagal fibers. Cholinergic innervation of the transplanted heart may occur over time. Hence, the management should be by direct-acting sympathomimetic agents.

Cardiovascular-diseased patients: Anticholinergic drugs particularly atropine and glycopyrrolate should be used with caution in patients with coronary artery disease, arrhythmias, heart failure, uncontrolled hypertension, or in patients with tachycardia. Scopolamine can be considered as a premedicant for its antisialagogue and sedative as it has a very minimal effect on the cardiovascular system than other anticholinergic drugs. Restrict total dose to 0.03–0.04 mg/kg in patients with ischemic heart disease.

Elderly patients: These drugs should be used with caution with elderly patients as they are associated with increased risk for anticholinergic effects, confusion, and hallucinations.

Prostatic hyperplasia: Since these drugs reduce bladder activity and promote urine retention, they should be used with caution in patients with prostatic hyperplasia or bladder neck obstruction. Dosage reduction should be considered.

Q. 7. What are the concerns of anticholinergic drug usage in pregnancy?

Ans. Atropine crosses the placenta and is present in breast milk, while glycopyrrolate being a quaternary ammonium compound is found in negligible amounts in breast milk and umbilical vein. Anticholinergic drugs are used with anticholinesterase agents to reverse the neuromuscular blockade; most commonly neostigmine is used in combination with glycopyrrolate since the onset and peak effect of these drugs are relatively the same. But in those, who are undergoing surgery during their pregnancy, it is recommended to use anticholinesterase agents along with atropine to reverse the neuromuscular blockade since neostigmine crosses the placenta and glycopyrrolate does not lead to fetal bradycardia.

Q. 8. What is an anticholinergic syndrome?

Ans.

Anticholinergic syndrome: Anticholinergic syndrome is due to the competitive antagonism of acetylcholine at central and peripheral muscarinic receptors. Inhibition of central muscarinic receptors leads to—delirium, hallucinations, agitation, confusion, disorientation, seizures, and coma, while the peripheral muscarinic receptor antagonism leads to hot, dry skin, tachycardia, mydriasis, urinary retention and decreased or absent bowel sounds. Perioperative incidence is more common in patients who are on psychotropic agents or other classes of medications with anticholinergic properties such as antihistamines, antiparkinson agents, spasmolytics, and inhaled bronchodilators).

Diagnosis is mainly based on the clinical signs and symptoms of antimuscarinic toxicity. Presence of only peripheral symptoms is less concerning, while the presence of central symptoms and signs are consistent with more severe toxicity.

Initial management includes securing the airway, breathing, and circulation. Definite therapy in the management of patients with central anticholinergic toxicity includes treatment with physostigmine (adult dose— 0.5-2 mg; pediatrics—0.02 mg/kg, up to a maximum dose of 0.5 mg per dose), given by slow IV push. Benzodiazepines can be used to treat seizures.

Q. 9. Explain the use of anticholinergic medications in organophosphorus poisoning.

Ans. Organophosphates, which have been used as insecticides, are potent cholinesterase inhibitors. On exposure to these agents, it causes a syndrome of cholinergic excess. The clinical features include muscarinic signs which can be remembered by mnemonics— Salivation, Lacrimation, Urination, Defecation, Gastric Emesis (SLUDGE) and Bronchorrhea, Bronchospasm, Bradycardia (BBB). Diagnosis of organophosphate poisoning is generally based on clinical grounds, however, if doubt exists, then the trial dose of atropine 1 mg for adults (10-20 µg/kg for pediatrics) is administered; absence of anticholinergic signs strongly suggests poisoning with organophosphates.

Once the diagnosis is confirmed, then further atropine doses of 2-5 mg IV bolus for adults (50 µg/kg for pediatrics) is given and double the dose every 3-5 minutes if bronchial secretions and wheezing persist. Inhaled ipratropium bromide along with parenteral atropine can also be used for relieving bronchospasm.

Since atropine is ineffective in treating neuromuscular dysfunction (as it does not antagonize the effect of increased acetylcholine on nicotinic receptors), cholinesterase reactivating agents such as pralidoxime at the dose of 30 mg/kg in adults and 25-50 mg/kg for children are used as bolus injections over 30 minutes. If severe, continuous infusions of 8 mg/kg/hour in adults and 10 mg/kg/hour in children are used.

Q. 10. Clinical uses of anticholinergic drugs.

Ans.
1. Premedication—to prevent bradycardia and reduce secretions
2. Mild sedation—scopolamine
3. Antisialogogue effects—visibility in fibreoptic examination
4. Treatment of bradycardia—atropine in ACLS algorithm
5. Combination with cholinesterase inhibitors during reversal of neuromuscular blockade
6. Bronchodilation—ipatropium and tiotropium
7. Release of sphincter spasm
8. Prevention of motion sickness
9. Treatment of Parkinson's disease— benzotropine and trihexyphenydyl
10. Treatment of hiccups.

FURTHER READING

1. Calvey N, Williams N. Principles and Practice of Pharmacology for Anaesthetists, 5th edition.
2. Miller RD. Miller's Anesthesia, 5th edition.

CHAPTER 10

Nonsteroidal Anti-inflammatory Drugs

Balaji Nagarajan, Puneet Khanna

Q. 1. What are nonsteroidal anti-inflammatory drugs?

Ans. NSAIDs are nonsteroidal anti-inflammatory drugs. NSAIDs refer to a group of drugs possessing anti inflammatory, antipyretic and analgesic properties. These are simple, over-the-counter analgesic compounds with a wide variety of clinical applications. They are used increasingly in the perioperative period for treating mild-to-moderate pain and for reducing opioid consumption. Unlike opioids, NSAIDs exhibit a "ceiling effect" with respect to maximum analgesic effects.

Q. 2. What are the different classes of drugs among NSAIDs?

Ans. Nonsteroidal anti-inflammatory drugs (NSAIDs) are broadly classified into two groups—(1) selective and (2) nonselective NSAIDs. These nonselective NSAIDs are further classified based on the chemical structure into five types **(Flowchart 1)**.

Q. 3. What is the mechanism of action?

Ans. Nonsteroidal anti-inflammatory drugs (NSAIDs) act by inhibiting the cyclooxygenase (COX) enzyme, leading to

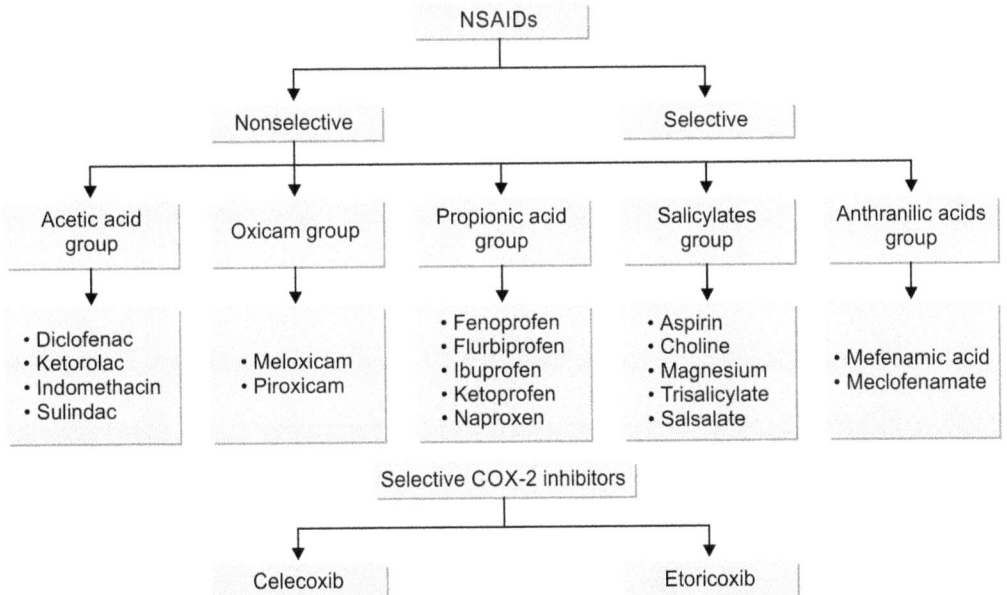

Flowchart 1: Classification of nonsteroidal anti-inflammatory drugs (NSAIDs).

the decreased production of various types of prostaglandins. There are three isoforms of COX enzymes, which are as follows:
1. *COX-1:* Constitutively present in many tissues; helps in maintaining gastric mucosal protection, platelet aggregation, vascular homeostasis, and renal blood flow.
2. *COX-2:* Inducible enzyme, its function is increased during states of inflammation and tissue injury. Prostaglandin E2 and Prostaglandin F2a result in sensitization of peripheral nociceptive nerve fibers to painful stimuli following tissue injury **(Flowchart 2 and Table 1)**.
3. *COX-3:* Recently discovered; believed to be the site of action of paracetamol.

Many of the NSAIDs act by reversibly inhibiting the COX enzyme except aspirin which inhibits the enzyme irreversibly.

Q. 4. Explain the pharmacokinetics of NSAIDs?
Ans. NSAIDs are weak organic acids and are absorbed rapidly in the stomach and small intestine, because the stomach has a lower pH and a more unionized form of the drug, is available for absorption and the small intestine has a larger surface area.

They have a high bioavailability due to their negligible first-pass hepatic metabolism. They are highly protein-bound (more than 90%). Most of the drugs undergo hepatic metabolism either by oxidation or by glucuronidation and the metabolites are excreted in the urine (majority) and bile.

Q. 5. What are the doses of commonly administered NSAIDs?
Ans. Some commonly administered NSAIDs doses are enlisted in **Table 2**.

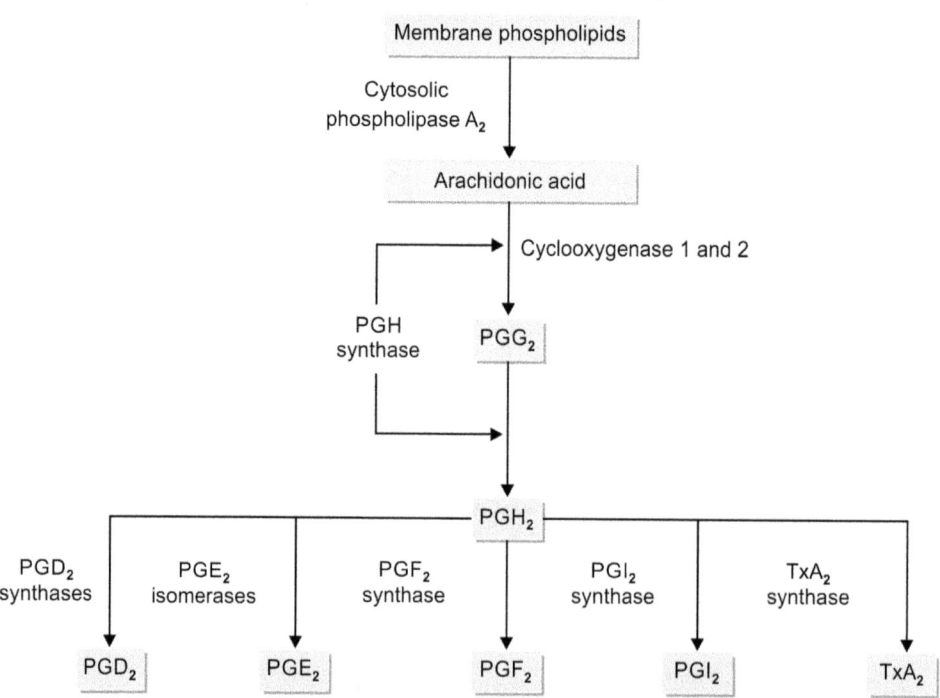

Flowchart 2: Prostaglandin and thromboxane synthesis.

Chapter 10: Nonsteroidal Anti-inflammatory Drugs

TABLE 1: Effects of various prostaglandin subtypes.

PGE_2	Sensitize nerve endings to bradykinin, increase body temperature, vasodilation, gastroprotection
$PGF2_\alpha$	Bronchoconstriction, uterine contractions
PGD_2	Bronchoconstriction
PGI_2 (prostacyclin)	Vasodilatation (vasoconstriction in pulmonary epithelium), decreased platelet aggregation, gastroprotection
TXA_2	Platelet aggregation, vasoconstriction

Q. 6. What are the significant drug interactions in the perioperative period?

Ans. NSAIDs are highly protein-bound substances that can result in the displacement of other protein-bound medications such as warfarin, anticonvulsants such as phenytoin/valproic acid—leading to the increased free drug concentration and increased risk of adverse events.

Concurrent administration of NSAIDs and drugs such as lithium/digoxin—results in the decreased clearance of these drugs resulting in accumulation and potential digoxin and lithium toxicities.

TABLE 2: Commonly administered NSAIDs doses.

Aspirin	PO: 325–650 mg q4–6 hours For pediatrics: 10–15 mg/kg MDD: 4 g	Avoid use in children <12 years due to the risk of Reye's syndrome
Diclofenac	PO: 50 mg every 8 hours For pediatrics: 0.5–1 mg/kg MDD: 150 mg	Also available in topical patch, solution, IV, gel formulations
Ketorolac	IV: 30 mg initially f/b 15–30 mg q6–8 hours not to exceed 5 days For pediatrics: 0.5 mg/kg Loading dose f/b 0.2–0.5 mg/kg MDD: 120 mg	Decrease the dose in renal failure and in elderly (>65 years)
Ibuprofen	PO: 400 mg q4–6 hours For pediatrics: 5–10 mg/kg MDD: 3,200 mg	10 mg/kg dose is used in newborns to close —PDA
Meloxicam	PO: 7.5–15mg q24 hours MDD: 15 mg	Slow onset; long duration (other NSAIDs are preferred for treating acute pain) Relatively COX-2 selective
Naproxen	PO: Loading dose—500 mg f/b 250–500 mg every 12 hours For pediatrics: 5–10 mg/kg MDD: 1500 mg	
Indomethacin	PO: 25–50 mg q8–12 hours MDD: 200 mg	Potent inhibitory effects on renal prostaglandin synthesis; associated with CNS side effects compared with other NSAIDs
Celecoxib	PO: Loading dose—400 mg f/b 100–200 mg every 12 hours For pediatrics: 10–25 kg—50 mg BD >25 kg—100–200 mg BDMDD—400 mg	Avoid this drug in patients with coronary heart disease, cerebrovascular disease, or in patients allergic to sulfonamides

(CNS: central nervous system; f/b: followed by; MDD: maximum daily dose; PDA: patent ductus arteriosus)

For patients who are on antithrombotic medications, concurrent use of nonselective NSAIDs will result in additive inhibition of platelet aggregation and an increased risk of bleeding.

Patients who are on angiotensin-converting enzyme (ACE) inhibitors or angiotensin receptor blockers (ARBs) are at increased risk of developing hyperkalemia with the concurrent NSAID use, however, the data are conflicting.

Q. 7. What are the special considerations in the use of nonsteroidal anti-inflammatory drugs?

Ans.

Gastrointestinal system: Patients with a history of peptic ulcer, *Helicobacter pylori* infection, or those with concurrent use of low dose aspirin, anticoagulants are at high risk of developing NSAIDs induced gastroduodenal toxicity. Therefore, it is recommended to use selective COX-2 inhibitors or to use a combination of nonselective NSAIDs and some gastroprotective agents such as proton pump inhibitors.

Hepatic system: Since NSAIDs are highly protein-bound, conditions such as hypoalbuminemia due to liver failure/nephrotic syndrome/active rheumatoid arthritis may have a higher free serum concentration of the drug. Moderate to severe liver disease affects the NSAIDs metabolism thereby increasing the potential for toxicity.

Cardiovascular system: Irrespective of the cardiovascular status of the patient, the use of NSAIDs (both selective and nonselective) are found to be associated with increased risk of adverse events such as MI, heart failure, stroke, and death. The risk increases several folds when patients already have cardiovascular comorbidities. For patients without any cardiovascular diseases, it is reasonable to use any of the NSAIDs available whereas, in patients who are at risk of cardiovascular diseases or a known cardiovascular disease patient, it is advisable to use naproxen (NSAID of choice) as it does not affect the vascular homeostasis.

Renal system: Synthesis of prostaglandins in the renal afferent and efferent arterioles helps in maintaining the renal perfusion, interfering with this protective response, NSAIDs can cause renal ischemia and decreased GFR. This risk is further increased in patients who are on ACE inhibitors, diuretics, or a known *renal disease patient*. NSAIDs should be avoided in patients with an estimated GFR < 30 mL/min/1.73 m^2 or in stage 4 or 5 chronic kidney disease (CKD) or patients with hypovolemia.

Q. 8. What are the various adverse effects of nonsteroidal anti-inflammatory drugs?

Ans. The various adverse effects of NSAIDs are given in **Table 3**.

TABLE 3: Various adverse effects of nonsteroidal anti-inflammatory drugs.

Cardiovascular	Hypertension, increased risk of thrombotic events leading to MI, stroke; can exacerbate or induce heart failure
Respiratory	Bronchospasm, angioedema, pulmonary infiltrates with eosinophilia
Gastrointestinal	Dyspepsia, peptic ulcer disease, gastric bleeding
Central nervous system	Aseptic meningitis, psychosis, tinnitus, hearing loss
Hematologic	Neutropenia, antiplatelet effects
Dermatology	Urticaria, rash, Stevens-Johnson syndrome rarely
Hepatic	Hepatitis
Renal	Interstitial nephritis, renal insufficiency

Q. 9. What are the concerns of NSAID use in pregnant patients?

Ans. The use of NSAIDs and moderate to high dose aspirin during the first trimester is associated with an increased rate of spontaneous abortions due to impaired implantation resulting from inhibition of prostaglandin production, hence should be avoided. However, in 2020, the US Food and Drug Administration (FDA) suggested that if NSAID treatment is necessary for some medical reasons, it can be used between 20 and 30 weeks of pregnancy at the lowest effective dose and for the shortest duration and monitoring by ultrasound be considered for those treated for more than 48 hours and should be discontinued if oligohydramnios occurs.

Use of these agents in the third trimester carries a greater risk of premature closure of ductus arteriosus and should be avoided. Among NSAIDs, indomethacin and ibuprofen have greater ductal effects.

Regarding aspirin, use of low dose (e.g., aspirin 75 mg for obstetrical indications such as preeclampsia, antiphospholipid syndrome, etc.), is compatible with pregnancy and lactation, while the use of moderate to high doses should be avoided in pregnant women and during lactation, as it is associated with intrauterine growth retardation, abnormal bleeding, neonatal metabolic acidosis, and fetal mortality.

Transfer of NSAIDs to breast milk is very low and can be safely administered in the first 24–72 hours postpartum when low volumes of breast milk are produced. Among NSAIDs, ibuprofen is the NSAID of choice since a very small amount of the drug is secreted in breast milk. However, it should be cautiously used in breastfeeding mothers of infants with duct-dependent cardiac lesions.

Q. 10. What are the concerns of NSAID use and regional anesthesia?

Ans. In patients not taking any antithrombotic medications, the use of NSAIDs and aspirin is not associated with an increased risk of spinal epidural hematoma.

While in patients who are on other antithrombotic medications, aspirin should be stopped 7–10 days before neuraxial anesthesia if clinically appropriate, since aspirin irreversibly inhibits COX enzyme causing dysfunction for the life of platelets. Other NSAIDs which reversibly inhibit the enzyme should be stopped 3 days before the procedure. The use of selective COX-2 inhibitors has minimal effects on platelet function and may be used together with other antithrombotic medications, except for warfarin.

The use of neuraxial techniques in patients on aspirin and other NSAIDs should be better avoided if early postoperative use of other antihemostatic drugs is anticipated.

Q. 11. What are the concerns of NSAID use in orthopedic surgeries?

Ans. The use of both selective and nonselective NSAIDs has shown a theoretical risk of reducing bone healing rates leading to increased rates of nonunion. However, recent evidence showed that is no increased risk of nonunion with NSAIDs exposure. Thus, a short-term NSAID regimen can be used for treating fracture pain and in perioperative settings.

FURTHER READING

1. Flood P, Rathmell JP, Shafer S. Stoelting's Pharmacology and Physiology in Anesthetic Practice, 6th edition.
2. Katzung BG. Basic and Clinical Pharmacology, 14th edition.

CHAPTER 11

Sympathomimetics

Magesh Parthiban, Puneet Khanna

Q. 1. How do you classify sympathomimetics?
Ans.
They can be classified based on their mechanism of action into the following:
- *Directly-acting:*
  - Catecholamines:
    - Endogenous—adrenaline, noradrenaline, and dopamine
    - Synthetic—dobutamine, dopexamine, fenoldopam, Isoprenaline
  - Noncatecholamines:
    - α-1 agonist: nasal decongestants → xylometazoline, oxymetazoline
    - α-2 agonist: Clonidine and dexmedetomidine
    - β-2 agonist: bronchodilators → salbutamol, salmeterol; tocolytics → isoxsuprine
- *Indirectly-acting:* By Inhibiting reuptake or metabolism → tricyclic antidepressants
- *Mixed action:* Ephedrine and mephentermine.

Q. 2. What are the various effects of sympathomimetics in the body?
Ans.
- *Cardiovascular effects:*
  - *Heart rate*—drugs with β-agonist action increase the heart rate while noradrenaline which has more alpha selectivity will cause reflex bradycardia. However, in critically ill patients who require noradrenaline, there are many other factors that alter the heart rate and thus this effect may not be seen.
  - *Blood pressure*—Alpha-1 receptors are stimulated by neuronally released catecholamines which result in vasoconstriction. Alpha-2 receptors present in blood vessels are extrajunctional and are stimulated only by circulating catecholamines. Their stimulation also causes vasoconstriction. While β-2 receptors present in the blood vessels cause vasodilation. Drugs with predominantly β action like isoprenaline can decrease the diastolic blood pressure (DBP) by decreasing systemic vascular resistance (SVR) while increasing the mean arterial pressure (MAP) and systolic blood pressure (SBP) because of direct cardiac stimulation. While drugs that have minimal β action such as phenylephrine and noradrenaline increase SBP, MAP, and DBP.
  - *Cardiac output*—all drugs except pure alpha agonists like phenylephrine increase cardiac output.
  - *Pulmonary artery pressure*—all sympathomimetics increase pulmonary artery pressure and are to be used with caution in right heart failure.

- Central venous pressure—although there is an increase in venomotor tone in the central venous circulation, there is no change in CVP.

- Blood flow:

	Phenylephrine	Adrenaline	Isoprenaline
Skin and mucous membrane	↓	↓	Nil
Renal	↓	↓	↑
Splanchnic	↓	Variable	↑
Cerebral	↓	↓	↑
Venous tone	↑	↓	↑
Skeletal muscle	↓	Variable	↑

- **Respiratory:** β-2 agonists such as isoprenaline, adrenaline, and other inhaled agents like salbutamol cause bronchodilation.
- **Ocular:** Mydriasis due to contraction of pupillary dilator muscle (α-1) and reduces aqueous humor formation.
- **Gastrointestinal tract:** It decreases peristalsis and increases sphincter tone. Although it does not have much of a clinical significance.
- **Bladder:** It relaxes detrusor muscle (β-3 receptor)
- **Metabolic:** The stimulation of α-1 and β-3 receptors results in glycogenolysis and lipolysis. While α-2 receptor stimulation reduces insulin release and β-2 receptor stimulation results in release of glucagon.
- **Uterus:** Beta receptor stimulation results in uterine relaxation. Beta-agonists like isoxsuprine are used as tocolytics for this reason.

Q. 3. Why are noradrenaline and adrenaline preserved in an acidic solution?

Ans. Noradrenaline and adrenaline if stored an alkaline solution get oxidized and become inactive, especially at room temperatures. Similarly, it was previously thought that diluting them in saline would result in oxidative degradation. However, there seems to be no difference when diluted with either dextrose or saline.

Q. 4. Can we administer vasopressors through peripheral access?

Ans. Central venous administration for potent vasopressors such as adrenaline and noradrenaline is safer because they can cause blanching and ischemic damage to the vein by causing constriction of vasa vasorum. This then results in extravasation and ultimately necrosis. However, in resource-poor settings peripheral administration can be justified for a short period of time owing to the rare occurrence of such side effects. Other less potent agents such as ephedrine and phenylephrine can be given safely through a peripheral access.

Q. 5. What is the effect of acidosis on the adrenoreceptor sensitivity of catecholamines?

Ans. Acidosis can decrease the sensitivity of adrenoreceptors to catecholamines. This is more for α-2 receptors than α-1 receptors. Alpha-2 receptors are present in the precapillary arterioles. Acidosis also decouples vasomotor tone from catecholamines, thereby resulting in increasing noradrenaline requirement during moderate to severe acidosis.

Q. 6. What are the various indications of sympathomimetics and which is the preferred agent for each scenario?

Ans.
- *Undifferentiated shock:* Noradrenaline is the preferred agent in situations when the cause of shock is still unknown because of fewer adverse events.
- *Septic shock:* Previously dopamine was the choice owing to the deleterious effects suspected of noradrenaline because of its vasoconstrictor properties. However, all recent evidence suggests that noradrenaline is the vasopressor of choice in septic shock.
- *Cardiogenic shock:* Again noradrenaline is the preferred agent due to reduced mortality and fewer adverse events as compared to other agents.
- *Hypotension following subarachnoid block or drug-induced:* Ephedrine, mephentermine phenylephrine, metaraminol, and noradrenaline have all been used to treat hypotension following subarachnoid block with similar clinical efficacy and similar adverse outcomes. Phenylephrine is the agent of choice to treat hypotension where an increase in heart rate is to be avoided like in patients with coronary artery disease. In obstetric settings, ephedrine is the agent which appears to cause worse maternal and fetal outcomes, and phenylephrine can cause bradycardia, however, with very minimal fetal complications. Hence, the preferred agent is still debatable until more RCTs especially multidrug trials are conducted.
- *Cardiac arrest:* Adrenaline is the preferred agent; however, the agent of choice after the return of spontaneous circulation is still not conclusive.
- *Anaphylaxis:* 0.5 mg adrenaline (1:1,000) intramuscular injection should be administered in anaphylaxis.
- *Adjuvant with local anesthetic:*
  - Adrenaline—it reduces the diffusion of local anesthetics from the site and also reduces the blood flow. Therefore, it prolongs the duration of action and a lower dose of local anesthetic can be used.
  - Clonidine and Dexmedetomidine—both α-2 agonists have been used as adjuvants to local anesthetics in peripheral nerve blocks and subarachnoid blocks to prolong their duration of action.
- *Bronchodilator:* Inhaled β-2 agonists such as salbutamol and salmeterol are used for acute treatment of bronchospasm, bronchial asthma, and chronic obstructive pulmonary disease.
- *Hyperkalemia:* Inhaled salbutamol is also used for the treatment of hyperkalemia. A higher dose of 10–20 mg is used for hyperkalemia management.
- *Ophthalmic:* The topical phenylephrine is used as a mydriatic and α-2 agonist such as apraclonidine and brimonidine are used for the treatment of glaucoma.
- *Nasal decongestants:* Xylometazoline and oxymetazoline are used as nasal decongestants.
- *Tocolytics:* Beta-2 agonists such as isoxsuprine and terbutaline are used as tocolytics.
- *Sedation:* Dexmedetomidine an α-2 agonist is one of the agents for sedation in intensive care.
- *Antihypertensive:* clonidine, an α-2 agonist decreases sympathetic outflow and is a potent antihypertensive.

- *Central muscle relaxant:* Tizanidine again an α-2 agonist is a useful central muscle relaxant for treating muscle spasms.

Q. 7. What are the contraindications?
Ans. There are very few relative contraindications:
- Takotsubo cardiomyopathy
- Hypertrophic obstructive cardiomyopathy
- Catecholaminergic polymorphic ventricular tachycardia.

Q. 8. How does adrenaline cause hyperlactatemia?
Ans. Stimulation of β-2 receptor results in increased activity of Na-K ATPase which results in increased lactate production in skeletal muscles despite the presence of adequate oxygen as an alternative source of fuel during times of stress. Salbutamol administration can also cause hyperlactatemia.

Q. 9. What are the various routes adrenaline can be administered?
Ans.
- Intravenously
- Intramuscular (anaphylaxis)
- Subcutaneous (with a local anesthetic)
- As an inhaled agent (postextubation stridor)
- Topically, as a spray vasoconstrictor for bronchoscopy
- As eye drops, (glaucoma)
- Endotracheal tubes (ETT), in a cardiac arrest (when no other route is available).

Q. 10. How are catecholamines synthesized and metabolized?
Ans.
- *Synthesis:* All catecholamines are synthesized from phenylalanine and tyrosine hydroxylase is the rate-limiting enzyme. All adrenergic neurons produce dopamine and noradrenaline. While adrenaline is only produced in the adrenal medulla by methylation of noradrenaline.
- *Metabolism:* About 75–90% of noradrenaline released is taken up by axonal and vesicular reuptake for termination of the action. While the remaining are metabolized by monoamine oxidase (MAO) and catechol-o-methyl transferase (COMT). The major metabolites excreted after conjugation with glucuronic acid or sulfate are vanillylmandelic acid (VMA), metanephrines, and normetanephrines. Exogenous catecholamines are metabolized by COMT.

Q. 11. What is racemic epinephrine? Where can it be used?
Ans. Adrenaline which is commonly available has 99% levo-isomer of adrenaline with 1% dextro-isomer. The L-isomer is 15 times more potent, hence more prone to adverse events. A racemic mixture is one that has equal proportions of both levo and dextro-isomers. It is available as 2.25% racemic solution (1.125% levo-isomer and 1.125% dextro-isomer) for nebulization. It can be used for acute treatment of asthma, postextubation stridor, and croup in children.

Q. 12. What is renal dose dopamine?
Ans. It refers to the administration of dopamine as a continuous infusion at low doses of 1–3 µg/kg/min for its presumed renal protective effects. It was postulated that at low doses, stimulation of D1 and D2 receptors in the proximal tubule, ascending loop of Henle, and cortical collecting tubule leads to inhibition of Na-K ATPase and stimulation of prostaglandin E2 resulting in natriuresis and diuresis. However, all evidence so far has shown no beneficial effect of dopamine at such doses in preventing renal failure. Moreover, it has been shown to cause far more deleterious consequences than anticipated. Hence, until further evidence to prove otherwise, the use of renal dose dopamine is not recommended **(Table 1).**

TABLE 1: Summary of selected sympathomimetics.

	Receptors stimulated and their order of affinity	Mechanism of action	Half-life (hours)	Metabolism
Natural catecholamines				
Adrenaline	$\alpha_1 = \alpha_2; \beta_1 = \beta_2$	Activation of adenylyl cyclase	2–3 minutes	COMT and MAO
Noradrenaline	$\alpha_1 = \alpha_2; \beta_1 >>> \beta_2$	Activation of adenylyl cyclase	2–3 minutes	COMT and MAO
Dopamine	$D_1 = D_2 >>> \beta >> \alpha$	Activation of adenylyl cyclase	2–3 minutes	COMT and MAO
Synthetic catecholamines				
Isoprenaline	$\beta_1 = \beta_2 >>>>>>> \alpha$	Activation of adenylyl cyclase	2–3 minutes	Largely unchanged in urine and COMT
Dobutamine	$\beta_1 > \beta_2 >>>>>>> \alpha$	Activation of adenylyl cyclase	2 minutes	COMT
Synthetic noncatecholamines				
Ephedrine	$\alpha > \beta_1 = \beta_2$	Release of NA and direct activation of adenylyl cyclase	3–6 hours	Excreted unchanged in urine
Mephentermine	$\alpha > \beta_1 = \beta_2$	Release of NA and direct activation of adenylyl cyclase	Onset is 5–10 minutes, $T_{1/2}$: 10–12 hours	Excreted unchanged in urine
Phenylephrine	$\alpha_1 > \alpha_2 >>>>> \beta k$	Activation of adenylyl cyclase	2.5 hours	MAO

(COMT: catechol-O-methyltransferase; MAO: monoamine oxidase A)

FURTHER READING

1. Brunton L, Parker K, Lazo J, Buxton I, Blumenthal D. Goodman and Gilman's Pharmacological Basis of Therapeutics, 11th edition. New York: McGraw-Hill; 2005.
2. Fagerholm V, Haaparanta M, Scheinin M. α2-adrenoceptor regulation of blood glucose homeostasis. Basic Clin Pharmacol Toxicol. 2011;108(6):365-70.
3. Hoellein L, Holzgrabe U. Ficts and facts of epinephrine and norepinephrine stability in injectable solutions. Int J Pharm. 2012;434(1-2): 468-80.
4. Katzung B. Basic & Clinical Pharmacology, 14th edition. New York: McGraw-Hill; 2018.
5. Singh PM, Singh NP, Reschke M, Ngan Kee WD, Palanisamy A, Monks DT. Vasopressor drugs for the prevention and treatment of hypotension during neuraxial anaesthesia for Caesarean delivery: a Bayesian network meta-analysis of fetal and maternal outcomes. Br J Anaesth. 2020;124(3):e95-e107.
6. Tian DH, Smyth C, Keijzers G, Macdonald SPJ, Peake S, Udy A, et al. Safety of peripheral administration of vasopressor medications: a systematic review. Emerg Med Australas. 2020;32(2):220-7.

CHAPTER 12

Alpha and Beta Receptor Blockers

Magesh Parthiban, Puneet Khanna

ALPHA RECEPTOR BLOCKERS

Q. 1. How do you classify α-receptor blockers?
Ans. They can be classified based on their selectivity for receptors into:
- α-1 blockers—prazosin, indoramin, urapidil
  - α-1A subtype—terazosin, doxazosin, and alfuzosin
- α-2 blockers—Yohimbine and idazoxam
- Nonselective blockers—phenoxybenzamine, phentolamine, and tolazoline

Q. 2. What are the indications for the use of α-blockers?
Ans. Alpha-1 blockers and nonselective blockers have been used to treat hypertensive crisis and pheochromocytoma. Prazosin is used in the treatment of hypertension and scorpion stings. Selective α-1A blockers like tamsulosin are used in the management of benign prostatic hypertrophy (BPH) because of the absence of their effect on blood pressure. Yohimbine has been used to treat male sexual dysfunction; however, its efficacy is not established.

Q. 3. What are the various routes of administration for α-receptor blockers?
Ans. *Oral:* All selective α-1 blockers and phenoxybenzamine.

IV: Phentolamine.

Q. 4. Why phentolamine cannot be given orally?
Ans. Phentolamine has a very good oral bioavailability and initial trials involved oral administration for its evaluation and the result showed it has an oral antihypertensive. However, it had to be stopped prematurely because of severe diarrhea associated with its use.

Q. 5. Why is the duration of action prolonged with phenoxybenzamine?
Ans. Phenoxybenzamine binds covalently to α-1 receptors rendering it an irreversible antagonist. Therefore, the duration of action is prolonged to 3–4 days until new α-receptors are synthesized.

Q. 6. Why is there no reflex tachycardia with the use of prazosin?
Ans.
Prazosin is a selective α-1 receptor blocker with no to minimal effect on α-2 receptors. However, other nonselective blockers block the α-2 receptors in addition to α-1 receptors, thereby increasing the central sympathetic outflow. This increased central sympathetic outflow will cause reflex tachycardia and increased cardiac output.

Q. 7. What are the adverse effects of α-blockers?
Ans. Adverse effects seen with nonselective α-blockers include hypotension, weakness,

tachycardia, and tremulousness. Hypotension is seen due to direct blockade of α-1 receptor whereas the other side effects are due to increased noradrenaline release following blockade of α-2 receptors. Selective α-1 blockers are associated with orthostatic hypotension, light-headedness, syncope, and first dose effect. All these unwanted effects are more pronounced in the elderly.

Q. 8. What are the contraindications of α-blockers?

Ans. Any previous hypersensitivity reaction to any of the α-blockers makes it a contraindication. In addition, the use of α-1-blockers must be used with caution in patients who need to undergo cataract surgery, where the iris may prolapse due to relaxation of iris dilator muscle, a condition known as "intraoperative floppy iris syndrome (IFIS)". Nonselective α-blockers need to be used with caution in patients with renal dysfunction, cerebrovascular accidents, coronary artery disease, and active pulmonary infections.

Q. 9. How are α-blockers metabolized?

Ans. All α-blockers are primarily metabolized by hepatic conjugation or demethylation. Phentolamine is excreted 80% by the kidney

TABLE 1: Summary of α-blockers.

	Prazosin	Phenoxybenzamine	Phentolamine
Chemical structure	Quinazoline derivative	Haloalkylamine	Imidazoline
Route of administration	Oral only	Oral only	IV only
Solubility and protein binding	Moderate lipid solubility to allow BBB penetration; V_d 42 L/kg and highly protein-bound 92%	Highly lipid-soluble, V_d—large	Highly lipid-soluble, V_d—large and 50% protein-bound
Half-life	2–3 hours	24 hours	20 minutes
Metabolism	Primarily metabolized in the liver and excreted in the bile	Mostly metabolized in the liver	After hepatic metabolism, 80% is excreted by kidneys and 20% in stools. 13% in excreted unchanged in the urine
Duration of action	6–8 hours, onset after 1–3 hours	Duration is prolonged because of irreversible binding for 3–4 days. Onset after 1 hour	Onset and offset are within minutes
Side effects	Postural hypotension (first dose effect) can be seen	Tachycardia, drowsiness, fatigue, nasal congestion, dry mouth, miosis, nausea, vomiting, and rarely seizures are the possible side effects	Reflex tachycardia and increased cardiac output due to α-2 blockade
Clinical use	Refractory hypertension, hypertensive crisis, scorpion sting, Raynauld's phenomenon, PTSD	Pheochromocytoma	Pheochromocytoma

(BBB: blood-brain barrier; PTSD: posttraumatic stress disorder; V_d: volume of distribution)

(13% in unchanged form) and 20% by the fecal route **(Table 1)**.

BETA RECEPTOR BLOCKERS

Q. 1. How do you classify β-blockers?
Ans. Beta-blockers can be classified based on different properties:
- *Selectivity of receptors:*
  - Nonselective β-blockers (first generation)—***propranolol***, timolol, nadolol, pindolol
  - β-1 blockers/cardioselective (second generation)—atenolol, metoprolol, bisoprolol, nebivolol, esmolol, and sotalol
  - α and β-blockers/vasodilator property (third generation): labetalol and carvedilol
- Presence of membrane-stabilizing effect—propranolol, metoprolol, and sotalol
- Presence of intrinsic sympathomimetic activity—labetalol, acebutolol, and pindolol

Q. 2. What makes some β-blockers selective for β-1-receptor?
Ans. All β-blockers are made from the parent molecule aryloxypropanolamine to which are added various side chains and aromatic rings. The presence of the side chain aryl ring in the "p" para position makes the β-blockers cardio-selective. If they are present at meta or ortho position it renders them less selective for β-1 receptor.

Q. 3. What are the clinical uses of β-blockers?
Ans.
- *Cardiac uses:*
  - Hypertension
  - Coronary artery disease
  - Chronic congestive cardiac failure
  - Supraventricular arrhythmias
  - Mitral valve prolapse
  - Hypertrophic obstructive cardiomyopathy
  - Tetralogy of Fallot

- *Noncardiac uses:*
  - Pheochromocytoma
  - Thyroid storm
  - Migraine
  - Prophylaxis for variceal bleed (portal hypertension)
  - Tremors
  - Performance anxiety
  - Glaucoma
  - Alcohol and opioid withdrawal.

Q. 4. What is the mechanism of action?
Ans. All β-blockers bind to β-receptors which are G_s protein-coupled receptors and act by decreasing cyclic adenosine monophosphate (cAMP).

Q. 5. What are the various clinical effects?
Ans.
- *Cardiovascular system:*
  - Heart rate—it inhibits the IF (funny current) channels by decreasing the levels of cAMP, thereby slowing the rate of pacemaker activity. (negative chronotropy)
  - Contractility—by convention decrease in cAMP should decrease the contractility but by decreasing the heart rate, end-diastolic volume is higher due to increased filling time. Hence, contractility is only slightly decreased.
  - Myocardial oxygen demand—as heart rate and afterload to a lesser extent are reduced with β-blockade, myocardial oxygen demand is decreased.
  - Blood pressure—there is a decrease in blood pressure, although not significant. More so with combined α and β-blockers.
  - Myocardial relaxation—there is a increase in the rate of myocardial relaxation (lusitropy). However, the total diastolic phase is increased because of a decrease in heart rate.

- Arrhythmogenicity—the ectopic pacemakers are decelerated and there is an increase in the refractory period.
- Other systemic effects:
  - Decreased production of aqueous humor through β-2 action.
  - Inhibits release of renin from kidneys.
  - Dyslipidemia due to β-3 blockade will cause a decrease in high-density lipoprotein (HDL) and an increase in low-density lipoprotein (LDL).
  - Bronchoconstriction through the β-2 blockade (nonselective blockers).
  - Inhibits tremors through the β-2 blockade.
  - Increases contraction of gastrointestinal (GIT), bladder, and pregnant uterus.
  - Inhibits gluconeogenesis, glycogenolysis, and insulin release.

Q. 6. What are the adverse effects of β-blockers?
Ans. Hypotension and bradycardia are the most common side effects. Fatigue, nausea, constipation, erectile dysfunction, and dizziness are other adverse effects that can be observed. Bronchospasm especially in patients with bronchial asthma and exacerbation of Raynaud phenomenon can be seen with nonselective blockers. Some adverse effects like QT prolongation and edema can occur with the use of sotalol and carvedilol, respectively. The lipophilic β-blockers which can cross over to the central nervous system (CNS) can cause less common adverse effects such as insomnia and nightmares. All β-blockers carry the inherent risk of precipitating a heart block.

Q. 7. What are the contraindications?
Ans. Nonselective β-blockers are contraindicated in asthmatics (reactive airway disease) and patients with the Raynaud phenomenon. Patients with QT prolongation or torsades de pointes should avoid sotalol. Acute or chronic bradycardia and hypotension are relative contraindications.

Q. 8. Which drugs require precaution in renal failure?
Ans. Atenolol and sotalol are the only two β-blockers that are excreted through the kidneys. Hence their dose has to be modified as per the renal clearance.

Q. 9. Which drugs require precaution in hepatic failure?
Ans. Excluding atenolol, esmolol, and sotalol all other β-blockers are metabolized extensively by the liver. Hence, should be used with caution in liver failure.

Q. 10. What is the membrane-stabilizing effect and what is its clinical relevance?
Ans. Propranolol, carvedilol, labetalol, metoprolol, and sotalol have Na channel blocking activity which contributes to the membrane-stabilizing effect (class I antiarrhythmics). However, none of these drugs have a clinically significant effect on Na channels at their usual dose. Sotalol also blocks K channels, therefore used as class III antiarrhythmic.

Q. 11. Which drugs are dialyzable and what is the clinical significance?
Ans. Atenolol, metoprolol, and acebutolol are highly dialyzable, whereas carvedilol, propranolol, and labetalol have low dialyzability. Hence, in patients on maintenance hemodialysis, carvedilol or labetalol are preferred over the dialyzable ones.

Q. 12. What are the clinical manifestations of β-blocker toxicity?
They usually present with the triad of hypotension, altered mental status, and bradycardia. At levels causing toxicity, even the β-1 selective blockers will cause pulmonary manifestations such as bronchospasm. Hypoglycemia and hyperkalemia are also seen with BB overdose.

TABLE 2: Characteristics of selected β-blockers.

	Selectivity	Lipid-solubility	Protein-binding	Half-life (hours)	Metabolism
Propranolol	0.52	Highest lipid-solubility	93%	2–6	Mainly hepatic
Labetalol	0.4	Lipid-soluble	50%	3–4	Hepatic
Atenolol	20.89	Poor solubility	3%	6–9	Renal excretion
Bisoprolol	102.33	Limited	30%	9–12	Both renal and hepatic
Metoprolol	58.88	Poor	12%	3–4	Hepatic
Carvedilol	0.62	Highly lipid-soluble	95%	7–10	Hepatic
Nebivolol	138.04	Highly lipid-soluble	98%	10–30	Hepatic
Esmolol	52.48	Very poor	60%	9 minutes	Hepatic

Although calcium channel blocker toxicity can mimic beta-blocker (BB) overdose, the presence of hypoglycemia and altered mental status can help us in identifying the drug.

Q. 13. How do you treat β-blocker toxicity?
Ans. Beta-blocker toxicity can cause CNS depression; hence, the airway may need to be secured in patients with poor sensorium. Patients who present early can be given gastric lavage, activated charcoal, and bowel irrigation with polyethylene glycol. Careful monitoring is required for at least 6 hours in BB overdose and in the case of propranolol and sotalol 12 hours and 24 hours, respectively.

If there is QRS widening it can be treated with sodium bicarbonate and magnesium sulfate for QT prolongation. Beta-blocker toxicity causing seizures responds well to benzodiazepines, hence are the first line. Glucagon acts through G protein-coupled receptors and increases cAMP levels to counteract the effects of BB. In refractory cases, high dose insulin euglycemia has been tried to augment cardiac contractility **(Table 2)**.

FURTHER READING

1. Brunton L, Parker K, Lazo J, Buxton I, Blumenthal D. Goodman and Gilman's Pharmacological Basis of Therapeutics, 11th edition. New York: McGraw-Hill; 2005.
2. Cruickshank JM. The clinical importance of cardioselectivity and lipophilicity in beta-blockers. Am H J. 1980;100(2):160-78.
3. Gould L, Reddy CV. Phentolamine. Am Heart J. 1976;2(3):397-402.
4. Graham RM. Selective alpha 1-adrenergic antagonists: therapeutically relevant antihypertensive agents. Am J Cardiol. 1984;53(3):16A-20A.
5. Jaillon P. Clinical pharmacokinetics of prazosin. Clin Pharmacokinet. 1980;5(4):365-76.
6. K atzung B. Basic & Clinical Pharmacology, 14th edition. New York: McGraw-Hill; 2018.
7. López-Sendón J, Swedberg K, McMurray J, Tamargo J, Maggioni AP, Dargie H, et al. Expert consensus document on beta-adrenergic receptor blockers. Eur Heart J. 2004;25(15):1341-62.
8. McDevitt DG. Comparison of pharmacokinetic properties of beta-adrenoceptor blocking drugs. Eur Heart J. 1987;8 Suppl M:9-14.
9. Oliver E, Mayor F Jr, D'Ocon P. Beta-blockers: Historical perspective and mechanisms of action. Rev Esp Cardiol (Engl Ed). 2019;72(10):853-62.
10. Tsuchihashi H, Nagatomo T. Alpha-blocking potencies of antihypertensive agents (prazosin, terazosin, bunazosin, SGB-1534 and ketanserin) having with quinazoline or quinazolinedione as assessed by radioligand binding assay methods in rat brain. J Pharmacobiodyn. 1989;12(3):170-4.

CHAPTER 13: Antihypertensive Drugs

Kiran Kumar Gudivada

Q. 1. How do you classify antihypertensive drugs?

Ans. Antihypertensive drugs are broadly classified as follows **(Table 1)**.

Q. 2. What are the causes of hypertension?

Ans.
- Essential (primary)
- Secondary
  - Obstructive sleep apnea
  - Renal disease
    - Renal parenchymal disease
    - Renal artery stenosis
  - Endocrine disease
    - Pheochromocytoma
    - Primary aldosteronism
    - Cushing disease
    - Hyperparathyroidism
    - Hyper- and hypothyroidism
  - Medications
    - Oral contraceptives
    - Chronic NSAID use
    - Antidepressants
    - Alcohol
  - Aortic coarctation.

TABLE 1: Antihypertensive drugs.

S. No.	Antihypertensive category
1.	Sympathetic system blockers • Alpha-blockers • Beta-blockers • Alpha + beta-blockers • Central sympatholytic
2.	Calcium channel blockers • Phenyl alkylamine • Benzothiazepine • Dihydropyridine
3.	RAAS inhibitors • ACE inhibitors • Angiotensin receptor blockers • Direct renin inhibitors
4.	Vasodilators • Pure arteriolar dilators • Arteriolar + venodilators
5.	Diuretics • Thiazide • Loop diuretics • Potassium-sparing

(ACE: angiotensin-converting enzymes; RAAS: renin-angiotensin-aldosterone system)

Q. 3. What are renin-angiotensin-aldosterone system (RAAS) inhibitors? Describe their mechanism of action.

Ans. Angiotensin-converting enzymes inhibitor (ACEI) and angiotensin II receptor blocker (ARB) are two major RAAS inhibitors commonly used in clinical practice.

Mechanism of action:
- Angiotensin-converting enzymes then convert angiotensin I to its physiologically active form, angiotensin II. The ACE inhibitor blocks the conversion of angiotensin I to angiotensin II. ACE inhibitors block the vasoconstrictive actions of angiotensin II.
- Angiotensin II receptor blockers block the effects of angiotensin II thereby promoting vasodilatation.

Q. 4. How do angiotensin-converting enzyme (ACE) inhibitors/angiotensin receptor blockers (ARBs) are different from other antihypertensive drugs?

Ans.

- These drugs are free from central nervous system side effects associated with other antihypertensive drugs such as depression, insomnia, and sexual dysfunction.
- Cardiovascular system (CVS) adverse effects, such as congestive heart failure, bronchospasm, bradycardia, and exacerbation of the peripheral vascular disease, are not seen with ACE inhibitors/ARBs either. Rebound hypertension is also not with ACE inhibitors/ARBs.

Q. 5. What is the side effect profile of these drugs?

Ans.

- Cough, upper respiratory congestion, rhinorrhea, allergic-like symptoms and angioedema are the side effects of ACE inhibitors, while ARBs are devoid of these side effects.
- Decreases in glomerular filtration rate, Hyperkalemia is possible due to decreased production of aldosterone.
- The risk of hyperkalemia is greatest in patients with recognized risk factors (congestive heart failure with renal insufficiency)
- Hypotension following induction of anesthesia has been observed in patients being treated with ACE inhibitors and angiotensin II receptor blockers.
- However, the 2014 American College of Cardiology/American Heart Association (AHA) guidelines for perioperative management suggest it is "reasonable" to continue these drugs until the time of surgery.
- Treatment for exaggerated hypotension attributed to ACE inhibitor therapy is a crystalloid fluid infusion and/or administration of a catecholamine.

Q. 6. Discuss the mechanism of action and side effects of hydralazine?

Ans.

- Hydralazine is a direct systemic arterial vasodilator.
- Hydralazine hyperpolarizes smooth muscle cells and activates guanylate cyclase to produce vasorelaxation.
- This drug produces reflex sympathetic nervous system stimulation, increasing heart rate and myocardial contractility. Hence, Hydralazine is not recommended for patients with myocardial ischemia or coronary disease.
- A combination of hydralazine and nitrates is commonly used for outpatient treatment of congestive heart failure.
- *Side effects:* Long-term hydralazine use is associated with drug-induced lupus and antineutrophil cytoplasmic antibody-associated vasculitis.

■ QUESTION

Q. 1. ACE/ARB to be continued or stopped on day of surgery. Guidelines and consensus?

■ FURTHER READING

1. Flood P, Rathmell JP, Shafer S. Stoelting's Pharmacology and Physiology in Anesthetic Practice, 6th edition.
2. Katzung BG. Basic and Clinical Pharmacology, 14th edition.

14

Peripheral Vasodilators

Kiran Kumar Gudivada

Q. 1. What are nitrodilators?
Ans.
- *Sodium nitroprusside (SNP), nitroglycerin compounds*, and *isosorbide dinitrate* are the commonly used nitrodilators.
- These agents work through the generation of nitric oxide (NO), which then augments cyclic guanosine monophosphate (cGMP) in vascular smooth muscle, leading to vasodilation of both arteries and veins.

Q. 2. What is sodium nitroprusside (SNP) and how does it works?
Ans.
- The SNP is a direct-acting, nonselective peripheral vasodilator that causes the relaxation of both arterial and venous vasculature.
- SNP contains 44% cyanide by weight. Its onset of action is immediate, transient, and equipotent on both arteries and veins. It requires continuous infusion and close monitoring of blood pressure.

  Mechanism of action: When given IV, SNP interacts with oxyhemoglobin, and immediately dissociates and forms methemoglobin while releasing cyanide and NO. NO activates *guanylate cyclase* and increases intracellular cGMP. cGMP inhibits calcium uptake by vascular smooth muscles and produces vasodilatation. Additionally, NO can directly mediate vasodilatation. SNP can spontaneously generate NO, this is in contrast with *nitroglycerin* which requires thio-containing compounds to generate NO.

Q. 3. How is SNP metabolized?
Ans.
- Metabolism of SNP involves the transfer of electrons from oxyhemoglobin to SNP, thereby producing methemoglobin and unstable SNP radicle.
- Unstable SNP radicle breaks down into cyanide ions which in turn react with methemoglobin to form *cyanmethemoglobin*.
- The remaining cyanide ions are metabolized by the liver and kidney into less toxic thiocyanate. *Rhodanese* is an enzyme that uses thiosulfate ions as *sulfur donors*. Most adults can detoxify approximately 50 mg of SNP using existing sulfur stores **(Flowchart 1)**.

Q. 4. Why is SNP always covered with aluminum foil?
Ans.
Sodium nitroprusside, upon exposure to light can rapidly get converted to aquapentacynoferrate and release hydrogen cyanide. Hence, it is recommended to dilute it only 5% dextrose and prevent exposure to sunlight.

Flowchart 1: Sodium nitroprusside metabolism.

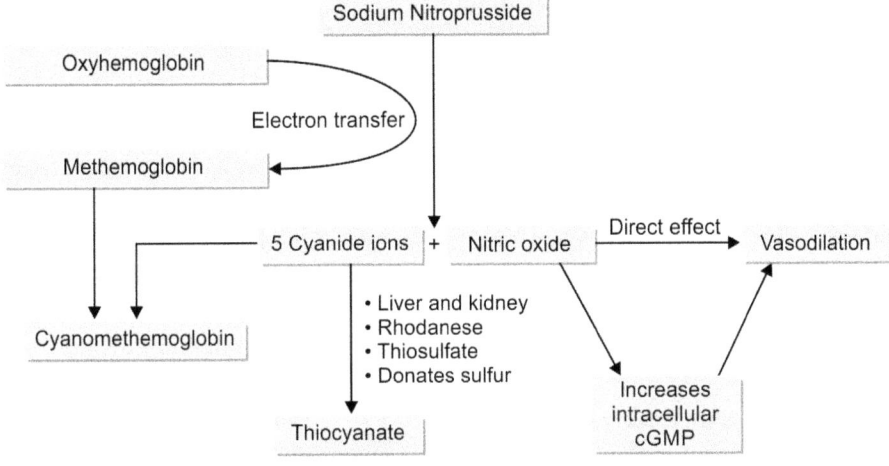

(cGMP: cyclic guanosine monophosphate)

Q. 5. Describe the dosage and administration of SNP.

Ans.

- Recommended initial dose of SNP is 0.3 µg/kg/minute IV titrated to a maximum rate of 10 µg/kg/minute IV, with the maximum rate not to be infused longer than 10 minutes.
- The SNP infusion rates of greater than 2 µg/kg/minute IV result in dose-dependent accumulation of cyanide, and the risk of cyanide toxicity must be considered.

Q. 6. What are the organ-specific effects of SNP?

Ans. *Cardiovascular:*

- Baroreceptor-mediated reflex responses—tachycardia and increased myocardial contractility.
- The net effect is an increase in cardiac output due to reflex-mediated increases in peripheral sympathetic nervous system activity and decreased impedance to the left ventricular ejection.

- *Coronary blood flow:* In myocardial infarction (MI), SNP may increase the area of damaged myocardium through a phenomenon called "coronary steal." A decrease in diastolic BP produced by SNP also contributes to the decrease in coronary perfusion.

Renal:

- Decreases in systemic blood pressure induced by SNP may result in decreases in renal function and release of renin. This release of renin may contribute to rebound Hypertension (HTN) observed while discontinuation of SNP.

Hepatic:

- Despite 20–60% decreases in systemic blood pressure produced by SNP, hepatic blood flow will not change when cardiac output is maintained in anesthetized patients.

Cerebral:

- The SNP increases cerebral blood flow and cerebral blood volume thereby increasing intracranial pressure.

- However, when SNP induced mean arterial pressure decreases greater than 30%, then intracranial pressure (ICP) may tend to decrease.

Pulmonary:
- Attenuation of hypoxic pulmonary vasoconstriction by peripheral vasodilators may lead to decreased PaO_2.

Hematologic:
- Increased intracellular concentrations of cGMP are shown to inhibit platelet aggregation. Vasodilatation can also prolong bleeding time.

Q. 7. What are the toxic effects of SNP and describe their management?

Ans. Toxicity of SNP may manifest as follows:
- Cyanide toxicity
- Thiocyanate toxicity
- Methemoglobinemia
- *Cyanide toxicity:*
  - Cyanide toxicity may become evident when SNP infusion is greater than 2 µg/kg/minute or when sulfur donors and methemoglobin are exhausted.
  - Free cyanide radical may bind to cytochrome oxidase and prevent oxidative phosphorylation. This precipitates tissue hypoxia, lactic acidosis and cell death.
  - *Signs and symptoms:* Lactic acidosis, increased cerebral venous oxygen content, increased mixed venous partial pressure of oxygen (PvO_2). The patient may have mental status changes, seizures, and coma.
  - *Treatment:* Immediate discontinuation of SNP and administration of 100% oxygen despite the normal oxygen saturation.
    - *Sodium thiosulfate,* 150 mg/kg IV administered over 15 minutes: Thiosulfate acts as a sulfur donor to convert cyanide to thiocyanate a less toxic compound.
    - *Hydroxocobalamin* (vitamin B12a), a 5-g initial dose, binds cyanide to form cyanocobalamin (vitamin B12).
    - *Note:* Hydroxocobalamin may produce a reddish discoloration of the skin and mucous membranes and interfere with co-oximetry blood gas analysis.
    - In severe cases: Sodium nitrate, a 5 mg/kg, converts hemoglobin to methemoglobin, which acts as an antidote by converting cyanide to cyanmethemoglobin.
- *Thiocyanate toxicity:*
  - Thiocyanate is 100-fold less toxic compound than cyanide. It is eliminated by kidneys, with an elimination half-time of 3–7 days. However, a prolonged infusion of 7–14 days at 2–5 µg/kg/minute range may be required to produce toxicity.
  - Toxicity may occur early in presence of renal failure that is not on renal replacement therapy.
  - *Signs and symptoms:* Fatigue, tinnitus, nausea, and vomiting. Hyperreflexia, confusion, psychosis, and miosis. Hypothyroidism due to inhibition of uptake of iodine by thyroid gland by thiocyanate.
  - Dialysis can effectively eliminate thiocyanate.
- *Methemoglobinemia:*
  - It is very rare since the dose required to produce 10% methemoglobinemia exceeds 10 mg/kg of SNP. Methemoglobin can be measured via co-oximetry.

Q. 8. What are the clinical uses of SNP?

Ans.
- Controlled hypotension for hypotensive anesthesia
- Hypertensive emergencies

- Reducing left ventricular afterload in left ventricular failure, MR, and AR
- To reduce hypertension caused to crossclamping of aorta in aortic surgeries
- During rewarming phase of cardiopulmonary bypass to permit high flow rates and increased delivery of heat to peripheries.

Q. 9. What is nitroglycerin (NTG), describe the mechanism of action and clinical use of NTG.

Ans.
- Nitroglycerin (NTG) is an organic nitrate that acts principally on venous capacitance vessels and large coronary arteries. NTG decreased cardiac ventricular wall tension.
- As the dose increases, it will produce arterial and pulmonary vasodilation.
- *Mechanism of action:* NTG generates NO, which stimulates the production of cGMP to cause peripheral vasodilation.
- In contrast to SNP, which spontaneously produces NO, NTG requires the presence of thio-containing compounds.
- The nitrate group of NTG is biotransformed to NO through a glutathione-dependent pathway by glutathione and glutathione S-transferase.
- *Route of administration:* Sublingual, oral tablet, buccal or transmucosal tablet, sublingual spray, transdermal ointment, or a continuous IV infusion.
- Only about 15% of the blood flow from the sublingual area passes through the liver.
- *Side effects:* NTG is capable of oxidizing the ferrous ion in hemoglobin to the ferric state with the production of methemoglobin.
- A limitation to the use of all nitrates is the development of tolerance to their vasodilating effects. Tolerance is dose-dependent and duration-dependent, usually manifesting within 24 hours of sustained treatment.
- A drug-free interval of 12–14 hours is recommended to reverse tolerance.
- *Clinical use:* Perioperatively, NTG is used to treat suspected myocardial ischemia.
- Preload reduction in setting of heart failure. Systemic antihypertensive.

Q. 10. What is isosorbide dinitrate? Describe its uses and side effects.

Ans.
- Isosorbide dinitrate is an oral nitrate, used for the prophylaxis of angina pectoris and preload reduction in patients with heart failure.
- Isosorbide dinitrate is well-absorbed from the gastrointestinal tract, has minimal first-pass metabolism.
- Metabolite of isosorbide dinitrate, isosorbide-5-mononitrate, is more active than the parent compound. At a usual dose of 60–120 mg effect may last for 6 hours.
- *Side effects:* Orthostatic hypotension, however, tolerance develops over time.

FURTHER READING

1. Flood P, Rathmell JP, Shafer S. Stoelting's Pharmacology and Physiology in Anesthetic Practice, 6th edition.

CHAPTER 15

Antiarrhythmic Drugs

Kiran Kumar Gudivada

Q. 1. What is arrhythmia?
Ans.
- Arrhythmia is a condition where the heartbeat is either irregular or heartbeats at an abnormal rate. This may be due to abnormality in conduction or origin of the site of impulse.
- If the origin of arrhythmia is from the sinoatrial (SA) node, atrioventricular (AV) node, or atria, then it is called *supraventricular arrhythmia* and if it arises from ventricles, then it is called *ventricular arrhythmia*.

Q. 2. What are the most common causes of arrhythmia?
Ans.
- In general arteriosclerosis, coronary artery spasms, myocardial infarction, and heart block are common causes of arrhythmias.
- In the perioperative period, acid-base disturbances, electrolyte abnormalities, hypoxia, myocardial ischemia, and abnormal sympathetic nervous system activity are the important causes of arrhythmias. Additionally, hypokalemia and hypomagnesemia may predispose to ventricular arrhythmias.

Q. 3. What are the common types of arrhythmias?
Ans.

Supraventricular	Ventricular
Sinus tachycardia	Ventricular premature beats

Contd...

Contd...

Supraventricular	Ventricular
Atrial tachycardia	Ventricular tachycardia
Paroxysmal atrial tachycardia	Ventricular fibrillation
Atrial flutter	Ventricular flutter
Atrial fibrillation	

Q. 4. What are the goals of antiarrhythmic drug therapy?
Ans.
- Revert back to normal sinus rhythm.
- Avoid lethal arrhythmias from occurring.
- Rate control.

Q. 5. How do you classify antiarrhythmic drugs?
Ans. Vaughan–Williams classification is the most commonly used classification system to categorize drugs. This classification is based primarily on the ability of the drug to control arrhythmias by blocking specific ion channels and currents during the cardiac action potential.

Class of action	Drugs
Class I (inhibit fast sodium ion channels)	
Class IA	Quinidine, procainamide disopyramide, moricizine
Class IB	Lidocaine, tocainide, mexiletine
Class IC	Flecainide, propafenone
Class II (decrease rate of depolarization)	Esmolol, propranolol, acebutolol
Class III (inhibit potassium ion channels)	Amiodarone, sotalol, ibutilide, dofetilide, bretylium

Contd...

Chapter 15: Antiarrhythmic Drugs

Contd...

Class of action	Drugs
Class IV (inhibit slow calcium channels)	Verapamil, diltiazem
Class V	Others

Q. 6. What is the mechanism of action of various antiarrhythmics drugs?
Ans.

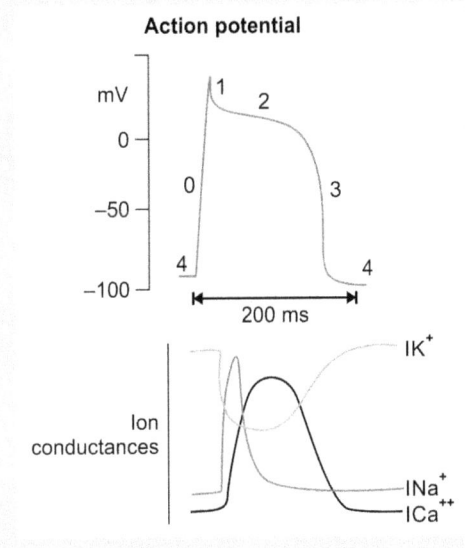

Antiarrhythmic drugs work by blocking the passage of ions across the following channels—sodium, potassium, and calcium ion channels which are present in the cell membrane of the heart.

Phase 0: Rapid depolarization resulting from the opening of Na^+ channels and closing of K^+ channels.

Phase 1: Initial repolarization resulting from the closure of Na^+ and opening of K^+ channels.

Phase 2: Plateau phase that results from the sustained Ca^{++} current.

Phase 3: Repolarization due to opening of K^+ and closure of Ca^{++} channels.

Phase 4: Resting potential during which time K^+ channels are open and Na^+ and Ca^{++} channels are closed.

Q. 7. What are the electrophysiologic and electrocardiographic effects of various antiarrhythmic drugs?
Ans.

	Class IA	Class IB	Class IC	Class II	Class III	Class IV
Depolarization rate (Phase 0)	↓	0	↓↓	0	0	0
Conduction velocity	↓	0	↓↓	↓	↓	0
Effective refractory period	↑↑	↓	↑	↓	↑↑	0
Action potential duration	↑	↓	↑	↑	↑↑	↓
Automaticity	↓	↓	↓	↓	↓	0
P-R duration	0	0	↑	0/↑	↑	0/↑
QRS duration	↑	0	↑↑	0	↑	0
QTc duration	↑↑	0/↓	↑	↓	↑↑	0

Q. 8. Which group of antiarrhythmic drugs predisposes to further arrhythmias?
Ans.
- Class IA drugs (quinidine and disopyramide) and class III drugs (amiodarone) block potassium channels and increase QTc interval which predisposes the patient to the torsades de pointes.
- Class IA and class IC drugs may precipitate ventricular tachycardia by slowing the conduction of cardiac impulses, especially in patients with a previous history of

sustained ventricular tachycardia or poor left ventricular function.
- Class IC drugs in the background of structural heart disease may predispose to wide complex ventricular arrhythmias
- Class IA and class IC drugs are better avoided in patients with congestive heart failure.

Q. 9. What is the role of prophylactic use of antiarrhythmic drugs?
Ans.
- Amiodarone is known to reduce the risk of sudden cardiac death in patients with heart failure.
- It is a reasonable alternative for patients who don't have access to or are not eligible for an implanted cardiac defibrillator.
- Prophylactic therapy with β-blockers, magnesium, amiodarone, and sotalol has a role in decreasing episodes of atrial fibrillation after heart surgery

Q. 10. Highlight a few important points about each antiarrhythmic drug.
Ans.
- *Quinidine:* Class IA drug, used for the treatment of acute and chronic supraventricular arrhythmia. Also, for tachyarrhythmias associated with Wolff-Parkinson-White syndrome.
  - *Side effects:* Hypotension, heart block, and proarrhythmic potential along with a low therapeutic ratio are some of the side effects.
- *Lidocaine:* Class IB drug, used for suppression of ventricular arrhythmias. Lidocaine for IV administration should not contain a preservative.
  - At a plasma concentration of <5 μg/mL lidocaine is devoid of effects on the cardiovascular system.
  - At levels >5–10 μg/mL results in myocardial depression and peripheral vasodilation leading to hypotension and seizures.
  - At levels >10 μg/mL, producing central nervous system (CNS) depression, apnea, and cardiac arrest.
- *Phenytoin:* Class IB drug is effective in the treatment of ventricular arrhythmias associated with digitalis toxicity.
  - The usual intravenous dose is 1.5 mg/kg every 5 minutes till cardiac arrhythmia is controlled up to the maximum of 1,000 mg.
  - Phenytoin can precipitate in 5% dextrose in water, hence to be diluted in normal saline.
  - *Side effects:* Cerebellar disturbances, hyperglycemia, leukopenia, granulocytopenia, and thrombocytopenia.
- *Beta-adrenergic antagonist:* This class of drug is effective in treating arrhythmias arising due to increased activity of the sympathetic nervous system.
  - In patients with prolonged QTc intervals, propranolol is very effective in controlling torsades de pointes.
  - *Side effects:* Bradycardia, hypotension, myocardial depression, and bronchospasm
- *Amiodarone:* It is a wide spectrum antiarrhythmic drug with good activity against refractory ventricular and supraventricular tachyarrhythmias.
  - Amiodarone 300 mg IV is recommended for ventricular tachycardia or fibrillation which is resistant to electrical defibrillation.
  - After starting therapy with amiodarone, a reduction in ventricular tachyarrhythmias is noted to occur within 72 hours.
  - *Mechanism of action:*
    - Prolongs the effective refractory period in all cardiac tissues
    - Noncompetitive blockade of α and β-receptors
    - Antianginal activity by dilating coronary arteries and increasing coronary blood flow.

- Side effects:
  - *Pulmonary alveolitis:* Approximately 5–15% of chronically treated patients have pulmonary toxicity. The proposed mechanism is the enhanced production of free oxygen radicals in the lungs.
  - *Cardiovascular:* Prolongation of the QTc interval, increased incidence of ventricular tachyarrhythmias. Bradycardia is often resistant to treatment with atropine.
  - Other uncommon side effects are corneal microdeposits, optic neuropathy, mild increases in plasma transaminase, and fatty liver infiltration.
  - Amiodarone contains iodine; therefore, it can result in either hyperthyroidism or hypothyroidism in 2–4% of the patients.
- *Verapamil:* Class IV drug, effective in terminating paroxysmal supraventricular tachycardia, controls reentrant tachycardia, and helps in controlling ventricular rate in patients with atrial fibrillation and flutter.
  - *Side effects:* Atrioventricular heart block, direct myocardial depression, peripheral vasodilation.

Q. 11. Explain the uses and side effects of digoxin.
Ans.
- Digoxin is a digitalis preparation that is effective in preventing as well as treating atrial tachyarrhythmias.
- Digoxin has a vagomimetic effect which results in slowing of cardiac impulse through the AV node and subsequently helps in slowing the ventricular rate.
- *Dose:* 0.5–1 mg in divided doses over 12–24 hours.
- *Side effects:* Toxicity may lead to any cardiac arrhythmia (most commonly atrial tachycardia with block). Digoxin can enhance the conduction of cardiac impulses through the accessory tracts and can dangerously increase the ventricular response rate in patients with Wolff-Parkinson-White syndrome (WPW syndrome).

Q. 12. Describe the uses and side effects of adenosine.
Ans.
- Adenosine works by decreasing the conduction of cardiac impulses through the AV node.
- *MOA:* Electrophysiologic effects of adenosine are similar to those of diltiazem and verapamil. It activates myocardial adenosine receptors to increase potassium ion currents, reduces the action potential duration, and hyperpolarizes the cardiac cell membranes.
- Effective in the acute treatment of paroxysmal supraventricular tachycardia, including tachycardias of accessory pathways (WPW syndrome).
- It is not effective in treating atrial fibrillation, flutter or ventricular tachycardia.
- *Dose:* 6 mg IV followed by a push of 6–12 mg IV about 3 minutes later, if needed.
- *Side effects:* Headache, chest discomfort, flushing, bronchospasm, transient atrioventricular block, etc.

Q. 13. What is Class 0 drug?
Ans. Ivabradine a "Class 0" drug was approved by Food and Drug Administration (FDA) in 2015.
- Ivabradine selectively inhibits the current in the sinoatrial node and slows the heart rate. It does not have other hemodynamic effects other than reducing heart rate.
- Ivabradine reduces heart rate and this property is used in patients with heart failure who have decreased ejection fraction and are on maximal doses of β-blockers.
- It has also been used as an isolated bradycardia agent in patients with sepsis with tachycardia.

FURTHER READING
1. Flood P, Rathmell JP, Urman RD. Stoelting's Pharmacology & Physiology in Anesthetic Practice, 6th edition. Philadelphia: Wolters Kluwer Health; 2021.

CHAPTER 16

Calcium Channel Blockers

Debyani Dey, Anil Kumar, Vrinda Chauhan

INTRODUCTION

Calcium ions have an important role in the electrical excitation of cardiac cells and vascular smooth muscle cells. Calcium channel blockers (CCBs) interfere with the inward movement of calcium ions across the myocardial and vascular smooth muscle cells. They are classified on the basis of chemical structure as phenylalkylamines, dihydropyridines, and benzothiazepines.

CLASSIFICATION OF CALCIUM CHANNEL BLOCKERS

Phenylalkylamine
Verapamil.

Dihydropyridines
- Nifedipine
- Nicardipine
- Nimodipine
- Isradipine
- Felodipine
- Amlodipine.

Benzothiazepine
Diltiazem.

MECHANISM OF ACTION

Phenylalkylamines and benzothiazepines act on AV node whereas dihydropyridines act on arteriolar beds. Calcium channel blockers (CCBs) act on voltage-gated calcium channels (L type-long lasting, N-neural type, T-transient type) and maintain these channels in an inactive/closed state **(Tables 1 to 3)**.

L type channel has five subunits—α_1, α_2, β, γ, δ out of which α_1 forms the core of the channel. Calcium channel blockers (CCBs) bind at unique sites on the $\alpha 1$ subunit of the channel, which forms the main entry pathway for calcium entry.

Voltage-gated calcium ion channels are present in the cell membranes of skeletal muscle, vascular smooth muscle, cardiac muscle, mesenteric muscle, glandular cells, and neurons.

Calcium ion influx through L-type calcium channels is responsible for phase 2 of the cardiac action potential, which is important in excitation-contraction coupling, so the blockade of these channels causes—slowing of the heart rate, reduction in myocardial contractility, decreased speed of conduction of cardiac impulses through the atrioventricular node, and vascular smooth muscle relaxation.

INTERACTION WITH VARIOUS DRUGS

Neuromuscular Blocking Agents

They potentiate the effect of nondepolarizing muscle relaxants. Verapamil and diltiazem due to their local anesthetic properties,

TABLE 1: Pharmacokinetics of calcium channel blockers.

	Verapamil	Nifedipine	Nicardipine	Nimodipine	Diltiazem
Dosage					
– Oral	80–160 mg every 8 h	10–30 mg every 8 h	20 mg every 8 h	30–60 mg every 4–6 h	60–90 mg every 8 h
– Intravenous	75–150 µg/kg	5–15 µg/kg		10 µg/kg	75–150 µg/kg
Absorption (%)					
– Oral	>90	>90		>90	
– Bioavailability (%)	10–20	65–70	30	5–10	40
Onset of effect (min)					
– Oral	<30	<20	20–60	30–90	30
– Sublingual		3			
– Intravenous	1–3	1–3	1–3	1–3	
First-pass hepatic extraction after oral administration (%)	75–90	40–60	20–40	90	70–80
Protein binding (%)	83–93	92–98	95	99	98
Clearance					
– Renal (%)	70	80	55	20	35
– Hepatic (%)	15	<15	45	80	60
Active metabolites	Yes	No		Yes	
Therapeutic plasma concentration (ng/mL)	50–250	10–100	5–100	10–30	100–250
Elimination half time (h)	3–7	3–7	3–5	2	4–6

Source: Reves JG, Kissin I, Lell WA, Tosone S. Calcium entry blockers: uses and implications for anesthesiologists. Anesthesiology. 1982;57(6):504-18.
Durand PG, Lehot JJ, Foex P. Calcium-channel blockers and anaesthesia. Can J Anaesth. 1991;38(1):75-89.

TABLE 2: Calcium channel blocker, their uses, and side effects.

Calcium channel blocker	Uses	Side effects

• **Verapamil**
  – Binds to the intracellular portion of the L-type channel a1 subunit when the channel is in an open state and occludes the channel
  – Dextroisomer—devoid of calcium channel blocking property/acts on fast sodium channels
  – Levoisomer—acts on slow calcium channels
	• Treatment of supraventricular tachydysrhythmias
	• Used for treating vasospastic angina, essential hypertension (mild vasodilating action)
	• Treatment of symptomatic HOCM with/without LV outflow obstruction
	• Treatment of maternal and fetal tachydysrhythmias as well as premature labor
		• Caution in view of negative chronotropic effects, not to be used in patients with heart failure, or patients with severe bradycardia, or SA or AV node dysfunction
		• To be avoided with concomitant beta-blockade
		• Can cause ventricular dysrhythmias in WPW syndrome

Contd...

Contd...

Calcium channel blocker	Uses	Side effects
• Nifedipine – Produces greater coronary and peripheral arterial vasodilator properties – It has little/no depressant properties on SA or AV node	Treatment of angina pectoris due to coronary artery vasospasm	• Flushing, vertigo, and headache • Less common side effects include peripheral edema (venodilation), hypotension, paresthesias, and skeletal muscle weakness • May induce renal dysfunction • Abrupt discontinuation is associated with coronary artery vasospasm
• Nicardipine – Greatest vasodilating properties especially that of coronary arteries and peripheral arterioles – Minimal myocardial depression	• Treatment of patients with residual hypertension, despite beta-blockade • As a tocolytic • Immediately before electroconvulsive therapy to blunt the hemodynamic response to treatment	
• Nimodipine – Highly lipid-soluble analog of nifedipine facilitates entry into CNS, blocks the contraction of cerebral arteries by blocking the calcium influx	• Preventing and treating cerebral vasospasm in subarachnoid hemorrhage • Cerebral protection after global ischemia associated with cardiac arrest	
• Amlodipine – Minimal myocardial depressant effects – Provides anti-ischemic effects comparable to beta-blockers	• Treatment of hypertension • Is more effective when used in combination with beta-blockers in the treatment of myocardial ischemia	
• Diltiazem – Blocks the calcium channels of predominantly AV node	• Chronic control of essential hypertension • Treatment of angina pectoris • Diltiazem is also used for rate control in atrial fibrillation and flutter	

(AV: atrioventricular; CNS: central nervous system)

by sodium channel blockade, contribute to potentiation of the neuromuscular blockade.

Local Anesthetics

Increased chances of local anesthetic toxicity, due to the local anesthetic properties of verapamil and diltiazem.

Potassium-containing Solutions

Increased chances of hyperkalemia, due to slowing of inward movement of potassium ions by CCBs.

Dantrolene

Increased chances of hyperkalemia due to slow inward movement of potassium ions by

TABLE 3: Comparative pharmacologic effects of calcium channel blockers.

	Verapamil	Nifedipine	Nicardipine	Diltiazem
Systemic blood pressure	Decrease	Decrease	Decrease	Decrease
Heart rates	Decrease	Increase to no change	Increase to no change	Decrease
Myocardial depression	Moderate	Moderate	Slight	Moderate
Sinoatrial node depression	Moderate	None	None	Slight
Atrioventricular node conduction	Marked	None	None	Moderate depression
Coronary artery dilation	Moderate	Marked	Greatest	Moderate
Peripheral artery dilation	Moderate	Marked	Marked	Moderate

CCBs along with dantrolene-induced trigger of potassium release from cells.

Platelet Function

Calcium channel blockers interfere with platelet function.

Digoxin

Increases the concentration of digoxin, by reducing its plasma clearance.

Antagonists

By altering the enzyme activity or hepatic blood flow, they increase the plasma concentrations of CCBs.

QUESTIONS

Q. 1. What are the contraindications for use of CCB?

Q. 2. Compare amlodipine with clinidipine.

Q. 3. Clinical features and treatment in CCB.

Q. 4. What are the advantages with clinidipine?

FURTHER READING

1. Flood P, Rathmell JP, Shafer S. Stoelting's Pharmacology and Physiology in Anesthetic Practice, 6th edition.

CHAPTER 17

Histamine and Histamine Receptor Antagonist

Vrinda Chauhan, Puneet Khanna

INTRODUCTION

- Histamine was first prepared synthetically from ergot extract and was later on it was found as a natural constituent of mammalian tissues.
- It consists of an imidazole ring and an amino acid group connected by an ethylene group, decarboxylation of histidine leads to the formation of histamine.
- Histamine receptors belong to the G protein-coupled receptor (GPCR) group which are activated by different analogs of histamine and inhibited by specific antagonists. They are mainly four types of histamine receptors.
- It is formed by the decarboxylation of histidine by the enzyme L-histidine decarboxylase. Histamine is synthesized by *mast cells* and *basophilic granules*, stored in secretory granules, and is released as a result of the interaction of antigen with immunoglobulin E (IgE) antibodies on the mast cell surface **(Tables 1 to 4)**.

TRIPLE RESPONSE OF LEWIS

- A localized "reddening" around the injection site, appears within a few seconds, and a maximal at about one minute.
- A "flare" or red flush extends about 1 cm beyond the original red spot and develops more slowly.
- A "wheal" or swelling that is discernible in 1–2 minutes at the injection site.

TABLE 1: Major physiologic actions of histamine.

Tissue	Effect of histamine	Clinical manifestations	Receptor subtype
Lungs	Bronchoconstriction	Asthma-like symptoms	H_1
Vascular smooth muscle	• Postcapillary venule dilation • Terminal arteriole dilation • Vasoconstriction	Erythema	H_1
Vascular endothelium	Contraction and separation of endothelial cells	Edema, wheal response	H_1
Peripheral nerves	Sensitization of afferent nerve terminals	Itch, pain	H_1
Heart	Minor increase in contractility and heart rate	Minor	H_2
Stomach	Increased gastric acid secretion	Peptic ulcer disease, heartburn	H_2
CNS	Neurotransmitter	Circadian rhythms, wakefulness	H_3

(CNS: central nervous system)

TABLE 2: Characteristics of histamine receptors.

	H_1	H_2	H_3^a	H_4
Size (amino acids)	487	359	329–445	390
G protein coupling (second messengers)	$G_{q/11}$ ($\uparrow Ca^{+2}$; $\uparrow$ NO and $\uparrow$ cGMP)	G_s ($\uparrow$ cAMP)	$G_{i/o}$ ($\downarrow$ cAMP; $\uparrow$ MAP kinase)	$G_{i/o}$ ($\downarrow$ cAMP; $\uparrow Ca^{2+}$)
Distribution	Smooth muscle, endothelial cells, CNS	Gastric parietal cells, cardiac muscle, mast cells, CNS	CNS: pre- and post-synaptic	Cells of hematopoietic origin
Representative agonist	2-CH_3-histamine	Amthamine	(R)-α-CH_3-histamine	4-CH_3-histamine
Representative antagonist	Chlorpheniramine	Ranitidine	Tiprolisant	JNJ7777120

[a]At least 20 alternately spliced H_3 isoforms have been detected at the mRNA level. Eight of these isoforms, ranging in size from 329 to 445 residues, were found to be functionally competent by binding or signaling assays (see Esbenshade et al., 2008).

(cAMP: cyclic adenosine monophosphate; cGMP: cyclic guanosine monophosphate)

TABLE 3: Classification of H1-blockers.

First-generation agents	Second-generation agents
• Diphenhydramine	• Cetirizine
• Dimenhydrinate	• Levocetirizine
• Promethazine	• Azelastine
• Cinnarizine	• Mizolastine
• Cyclizine	• Loratadine
• Meclizine	• Desloratadine
• Hydroxyzine	• Fexofenadine
• Pheniramine	• Ebastine
• Chlorpheniramine maleate	• Rupatadine
• Cyproheptadine	
• Clemastine	
• Triprolidine	

Clinical Uses

- Treatment of allergic rhinoconjunctivitis, urticarial lesions.
- As adjunctive treatment in anaphylaxis.
- Preanesthetic medication-promethazine.
- Prophylaxis of motion sickness-Promethazine, diphenhydramine, dimenhydrinate.
- To control tremor, rigidity (central action), and sialorrhea of parkinsonism due to their anticholinergic and sedative properties.
- *Vertigo in Meniere's disease:* Cinnarizine, dimenhydrinate, and meclizine.

Adverse Effects

- Common adverse effects are sedation, drowsiness, lack of concentration, headache, fatigue, weakness, lassitude, and psychomotor incoordination.
- Gastrointestinal side effects include nausea, vomiting, loss of appetite, and epigastric discomfort.
- Anticholinergic side effects such as dryness of mouth, blurring of vision, constipation, and urinary retention.

H_2-RECEPTOR ANTAGONISTS (TABLE 5)

They produce selective and reversible inhibition of H_2 receptor-mediated secretion of hydrogen ions by parietal cells in the stomach, e.g., cimetidine, ranitidine, famotidine, and nizatidine.

TABLE 4: Pharmacokinetics.

	Time to peak plasma level (h)	Elimination half-time (h)	Clearance rate (mL/kg/min)
First-generation receptor antagonists			
Chlorpheniramine	2.8	27.9	1.8
Diphenhydramine	1.7	9.2	23.3
Hydroxyzine	2.1	20	98
Second-generation receptor antagonists			
Loratadine	1.0	11	202
Acrivastine	0.85–1.4	1.4–2.1	4.56
Azelastine	5.3	22	8.5

TABLE 5: Pharmacokinetics of H_2-receptor antagonists.

	Cimetidine	Ranitidine	Famotidine	Nizatidine
Potency	1	4–10	20–50	4–10
EC_{50} (µg/mL)[a]	250–500	60–165	10–13	154–180
Bioavailability (%)	60	50	43	98
Time to peak plasma concentration (hours)	1–2	1–3	1.0–3.5	1–3
Volume of distribution (L/kg)	0.8–1.2	1.2–1.9	1.1–1.4	1.2–1.6
Plasma protein binding (%)	13–26	15	16	26–35
Cerebrospinal fluid: plasma	0.18	0.06–0.17	0.05–0.09	Unknown
Clearance (mL/min)	450–650	568–709	417–483	667–850
• Hepatic clearance (%)				
– Oral	60	73	50–80	22
– Intravenous	25–40	30	25–30	25
• Renal clearance (%)				
– Oral	40	27	25–30	57–65
– Intravenous	50–80	50	65–80	75
Elimination half-life (hours)	1.5–2.3	1.6–2.4	2.5–4	1.1–1.6
Decrease dose in presence of renal dysfunction	Yes	Yes	Yes	Yes
Hepatic dysfunction	No	No	No	No
Interfere with drug metabolism by cytochrome P450 enzymes	Yes	Minimal	No	No

[a]EC_{50} denotes the plasma concentration of the drug necessary to inhibit the pentagastrin-stimulated secretion of hydrogen ions by 50%.

Source: Feldman M, Burton ME. Histamine-2-receptor antagonists. N Engl J Med. 1990;323:1672-80.

Mechanism of Action

The presence of histamine on H_2-receptors activates adenylate cyclase which increases concentrations of cyclic adenosine monophosphate (cAMP) which further activates the proton pump of gastric parietal cells (an enzyme designated as hydrogen-potassium-ATPase) to secrete hydrogen ions against a large concentration gradient in exchange for potassium ion.

H_2-receptor antagonists competitively and selectively inhibit the binding of histamine to H_2-receptors, thereby decreasing the intracellular concentrations of cAMP and the subsequent secretion of hydrogen ions by the parietal cells.

Clinical Uses

Most commonly used for the treatment of duodenal ulcer disease.

Side Effects of H_2-Receptor Antagonists

- Cerebral symptoms—headache, somnolence, confusion
- Cardiac symptoms—bradycardia, hypotension, heart block
- Hyperprolactinemia
- Acute pancreatitis
- Increased hepatic transaminase levels
- Alcohol dehydrogenase dehydration
- Thrombocytopenia
- Agranulocytosis
- Interstitial nephritis
- Interference with drug metabolism by cytochrome P450.

H_3-RECEPTOR ANTAGONISTS

They are presynaptic autoreceptors on histaminergic neurons that originate in the tuberomammillary nucleus in the hypothalamus and project throughout the central nervous system (CNS), mostly to the hippocampus, and amygdala, nucleus accumbens, globus pallidus, striatum, hypothalamus, and cortex.

The H_3 antagonists/inverse agonists have a wide range of central effects, they promote wakefulness, improve cognitive function and reduce food intake.

Nonimidazole H_3 antagonists/inverse agonists like tiprolisant have been developed and some are in phase 2 and 3 clinical trials.

H_4-RECEPTOR ANTAGONISTS

H_4-receptors are expressed on cells with inflammatory or immune functions. They mediate histamine-induced chemotaxis, secretion of cytokines, and upregulation of adhesion molecules. They also have a role in pruritus and neuropathic pain.

The H_4-specific antagonist JNJ-39758979 has been tested in phase 1 and 2 clinical trials for the treatment of persistent asthma, pruritus, dermatitis, and rheumatoid arthritis.

FURTHER READING

1. Flood P, Rathmell JP, Shafer S. Stoelting's Pharmacology and Physiology in Anesthetic Practice, 6th edition.

CHAPTER 18

Insulin and Oral Hypoglycemic Drugs

Vrinda Chauhan, Puneet Khanna

INTRODUCTION

Insulin is naturally secreted from pancreatic β-cells as a single polypeptide chain, preproinsulin which is further converted to proinsulin and then to insulin and C peptide.

The basal rate of insulin secretion is 1 U/hours which becomes 5–10 folds after food intake, with total daily secretion of approximately 40 units. It has a t½ of 5–6 minutes due to extensive hepatic clearance.

Insulin secretion is under the control of various pancreatic hormones, gastrointestinal (GI) hormones, and autonomic neurotransmitters. Glucose being the primary insulin secretagogue, insulin secretion is tightly regulated by extracellular glucose concentration.

Stimulation of the α_2-adrenergic receptors in the islets or activation of sympathetic nervous system inhibits insulin secretion whereas β_2-adrenergic receptor agonists and vagal nerve stimulation increases insulin release.

The insulin response to glucose is greater after oral ingestion because of glucose dependent insulinotropic polypeptide release and augmentation of β-cell response (Flowchart 1).

INSULIN PREPARATIONS (TABLE 1)

Nowadays human insulin is mostly manufactured using recombinant deoxyribonucleic acid (DNA) technology replacing the previous use of extracts from beef and pork pancreas, thus decreasing the associated allergic reactions.

Insulin Lispro

It parallels physiological insulin secretion and needs. It decreases postprandial hyperglycemia and less risk of hypoglycemia.

Insulin Aspart and Glulisine

They are synthetic rapid acting analogs with profile of action similar to lispro.

Regular Insulin

Fast acting, only form that can be given IV as well as subcutaneously. It is preferred for the abrupt onset hyperglycemia or the appearance of ketoacidosis.

Neutral Protamine Hagedorn

This insulin is conjugated with protamine due to which absorption from the subcutaneous site is delayed.

Glargine, Detemir, and Degludec

Long-acting preparations used for basal insulin requirements, they have late onset and less pronounced peak. They can be administered at bedtime as a single injection to provide basal insulin for 24 hours.

Chapter 18: Insulin and Oral Hypoglycemic Drugs

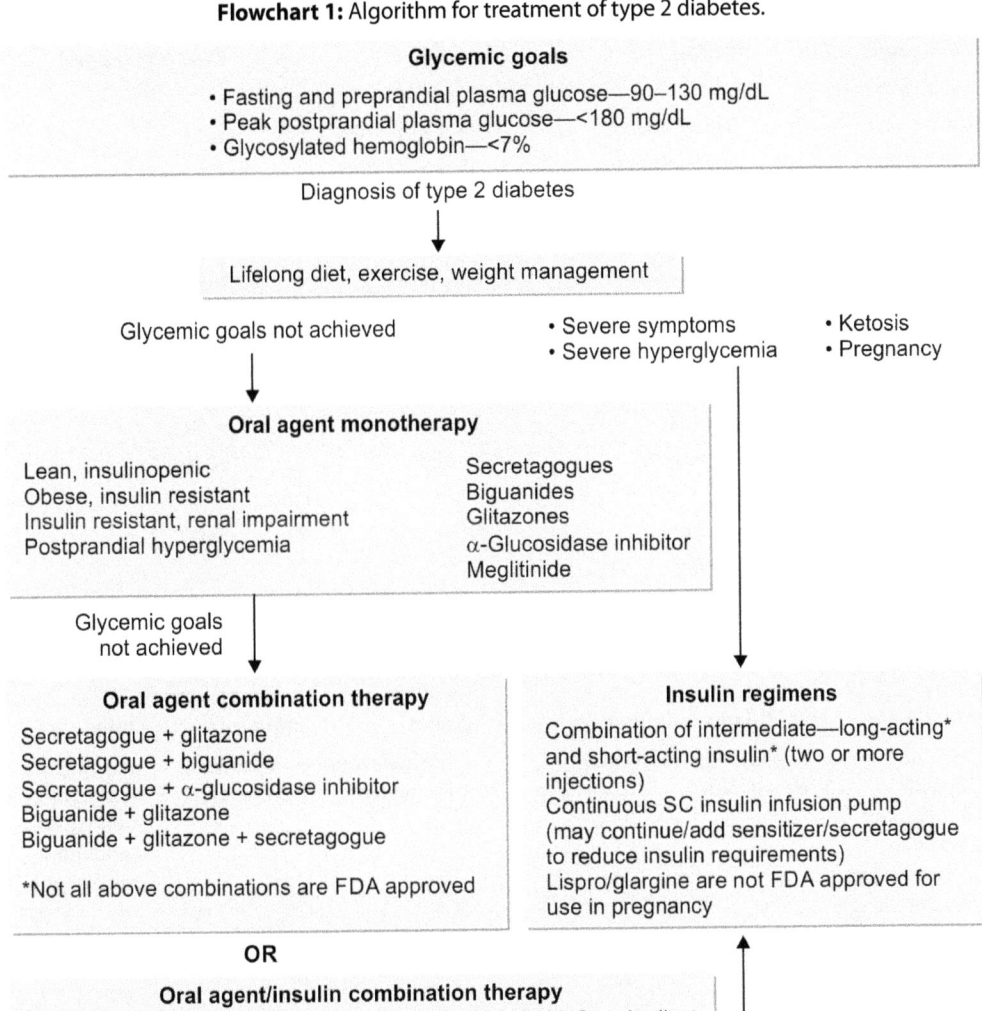

Flowchart 1: Algorithm for treatment of type 2 diabetes.

(FDA: Food and Drug Administration; FPG: fasting plasma glucose level; SC: subcutaneous)

Side Effects

The side effects are as follows:
- Hypoglycemia
- Allergic reactions—to animal preparations or protamine.
- Lipodystrophy
- Insulin resistance.

ORAL HYPOGLYCEMIC DRUGS (TABLES 2 AND 3)

Oral hypoglycemic drugs are of various type used mainly in patients with type 2 diabetes mellitus. Often one single drug is not able to control hyperglycemia, so a combination of

TABLE 1: Insulin preparations.

Insulin preparation	Onset	Peak	Duration (hours)
Very rapid acting			
Lispro	5–15 minutes	45–75 minutes	2–4
Insulin aspart	5–15 minutes	45–75 minutes	2–4
Glulisine	5–15 minutes	45–75 minutes	2–4
Rapid acting			
Regular	30 minutes	2–4 hours	6–8
Intermediate acting			
NPH or Lente	2 hours	4–12 hours	18–28
Long acting			
Detemir	2 hours	3–9 hours	6–24
Glargine	1.5 hours	None	20 to >24
Ultralong acting			
Degludec	2 hours	None	>40

(NPH: neutral protamine hagedorn)

TABLE 2: Oral hypoglycemic drugs.

Sulfonylureas	Meglitinides	Biguanides	Thiazolidine-diones	α-glucosidase inhibitors	DPP-4 inhibitors
• Glyburide • Glipizide • Glimepiride • Gliclazide • Tolbutamide • Tolazamide • Chlorpropamide • Acetohexamide	• Repaglinide • Nateglinide	Metformin	• Rosiglitazone • Pioglitazone	• Acarbose • Miglitol	Saxagliptin, sitagliptin, linagliptin, alogliptin, vildagliptin
Mechanism of action					
• β-cell function is required for its action • Inhibition of ATP sensitive K ion channels on pancreatic β-cells leads to calcium ion influx and release of insulin	Action similar to sulfonylureas act on pancreatic β-cells to stimulate insulin release	• Suppress glucose production hepatic by decreasing gluconeogenesis and glycogenolysis • Decreasing gastrointestinal glucose absorption, increasing	• Act on skeletal muscle, liver, and adipose tissue via peroxisome proliferator activator receptor-γ (PPAR-γ) to decrease insulin	• Decrease carbohydrate digestion and absorption of disaccharides by interfering with intestinal glucosidase activity	• Enhance the incretin effect via inhibition of native GLP-1 degradation increase insulin secretion from α cells (glucose

Contd...

Contd...

Sulfonylureas	Meglitinides	Biguanides	Thiazolidine-diones	α-glucosidase inhibitors	DPP-4 inhibitors
		insulin sensitivity in peripheral tissues, and enhancing synthesis of glucagon-like peptide-1 (GLP-1) in the ileum	resistance and hepatic glucose production and to increase use of glucose by the liver • Act in the presence of insulin • Useful in obese patients • Clinical effect takes 4–12 weeks	• Slow release and absorption of glucose from GIT	dependent) and reduce pancreatic a cell secretion of glucagon • Duration of action 12–24 hours
Highest risk of hypoglycemia, not recommended for patients with liver dysfunction Close K_{ATP} channels and Inhibit ischemic preconditioning		• Causes anorexia, nausea, diarrhea • Associated with lactic acidosis, vitamin B_{12} deficiency	Contraindicated in liver failure and congestive heart failure		

TABLE 3: Classification and pharmacokinetics of sulfonylurea oral hypoglycemics.

	Equivalent daily dose (mg)	Daily dose range (mg)	Doses/day	Duration of action (hours)	Elimination half-time (hours)[a]
Glyburide	2.5–5	2.5–20	1–2	18–24	4.6–12
Glipizide	5–10	5–40	1–2	12–24	4–7
Glimepiride	2	2–4	1	24+	5–8
Tolbutamide	1,000	500–1,000	2–3	6–12	4–8
Tolazamide	250	200–1,000	1–2	16–24	7
Acetohexamide	500	250–1,500	2	12–18	1.3–6
Chlorpropamide	100–250	100–750	1	36	30–36

[a]Approximate.

one or more drugs is required to adequately control the blood sugar. Insulin is also combined with oral hypoglycemic agents to control the blood sugar.

FURTHER READING

1. Flood P, Rathmell JP, Shafer S. Stoelting's Pharmacology and Physiology in Anesthetic Practice, 6th edition.

Diuretics

Vrinda Chauhan, Puneet Khanna

INTRODUCTION

Diuretics are the group of drugs used mainly for the treatment of hypertension or heart failure that cause decrease in the intravascular fluid volume in such patients and promote renal excretion of excess salt and water or diuresis. These drugs promote delivery of sodium to the distal parts of the nephron by blocking the sodium reabsorption proximally at various parts of nephron. This results in secretion of potassium in exchange for sodium reabsorption in the distal parts of renal tubules and thus causing hypokalemia.

CLASSIFICATION (TABLES 1 AND 2; FLOWCHART 1)

Carbonic Anhydrase Inhibitors

Hypoxia at high altitudes is normally counteracted by hyperventilation, which leads to respiratory alkalosis which depresses ventilation. Acetazolamide induced metabolic acidosis reverses this hypoventilation, so is used for the treatment of high altitude sickness. It can also cause fatigue, decreased appetite, paresthesias, and depression.

Furosemide

It is the first line diuretics in patients with renal insufficiency. Dose may vary from 0.5 to 1 mg/kg. It produces rapid onset diuresis within 5-10 minutes and peak effect at 30 minutes and duration of action 2-6 hours. Dosing should be increased in patients with chronic renal insufficiency; bolus doses up to 200 mg may be required. It should be only administered in the presence of normal or raised intravascular volume. Tolerance may develop with chronic use due to compensatory hypertrophy of tubular area involved in sodium reabsorption thiazide diuretic can be added in such situation. Acute tolerance can also develop due to activation of renin-angiotensin-aldosterone system (RAAS) in the presence of volume contracted state. It also potentiates the nondepolarizing neuromuscular blockade.

Thiazide Diuretics

They cause diuresis, natriuresis and vasodilation often used for long term treatment of essential treatment. They have long half-life 8-12 hours. They are also used to mobilize edema fluid in renal, hepatic, cardiac dysfunction. They are also used for the treating diabetes insipidus and hypercalcemia. Thiazide induced peripheral vasodilation is responsible for sustained effects in hypertension which often takes several weeks to establish. These are not effective in renal insufficiency. They can cause glucose intolerance when used in combination with beta blockers.

TABLE 1: Major uses of various diuretics.

	Receptors	Site of action	Uses	Side effects
Carbonic anhydrase inhibitors	Carbonic anhydrase	Proximal convoluted tubules	Glaucoma	Metabolic acidosis
Loop diuretics	Na-K-2Cl cotransport	Medullary thick ascending loop of Henle	Treatment of raised ICP	• Ototoxicity • Alkalosis • Hypokalemia
Thiazides	Na-Cl cotransport	Cortical ascending loop of Henle	Therapy for hypertension	• Alkalosis • Hypokalemia • Diabetes and dyslipidemia • Hyperuricemia • Hyponatremia
Osmotic diuretics		Proximal convoluted tubule and loop of Henle	Raised ICP Oxygen free radical scavenging	Volume overload in congestive heart failure, hypokalemia, hyponatremia, hypomagnesemia
Potassium sparing diuretics	Epithelia Na channel	Collecting duct	Adjuncts to loop or thiazide diuretics	Hyperkalemia
Aldosterone blockers	Na-K-ATPase	Collecting duct	Heart failure with low ejection fraction	Hyperkalemia
Dopamine and fenoldopam	D1	Proximal tubule and loop of Henle	Renal protection and treatment of hypertension in critically ill patients	Effectiveness not substantiated
Brain natriuretic peptide	Na-K-ATPase	Collecting duct	Management of decompensated heart failure	
Vasopressin	V2	Collecting duct	SIADH, Cirrhosis	
Aquaporins	AQP	Collecting duct	CHF	

(AQP: aquaporin; CHF: congestive heart failure; ICP: increased intracranial pressure; SIADH: syndrome of inappropriate antidiuretic hormone secretion)

Osmotic Diuretics

Triphasic response to mannitol—initial hypertension due to mobilization of the extracellular fluid into intravascular compartment, the second phase—hypotension due to the diuretic effect and the final phase—return of hemodynamic parameters to baseline. Mannitol begins to exert its effect within 10-15 minutes, with a peak effect at 30-45 minutes and duration of action of 6 hours. Effect on ICP is dose dependent with larger dose producing longer effect. It requires an intact blood brain barrier for its action. It causes vasodilation of the renal vessels mediated by prostaglandins, which increases renal blood flow and thus has renoprotective effect.

Section 1: Anesthetic Pharmacology

TABLE 2: Pharmacokinetics and pharmacodynamics of diuretics.

Drug	Relative potency	Oral bioavailability	T½ (hours)	Route of elimination
Acetazolamide	1	100%	6–9	Renal
Furosemide	1	60%	1.5	65% renal excretion, 35% metabolism
Bumetanide	40	80%	0.8	62% renal excretion, 38% metabolism
Ethacrynic acid	0.7	100%	1	67% renal excretion, 33% metabolism
Thiazide diuretic				
Chlorothiazide	0.1	9–56%	1.5	Renal excretion
Hydrochlorothiazide	1	70%	2.5	Renal excretion
Thiazide-like diuretic				
Chlorthalidone	1	65%	47	65%—renal, 10%—bile, 20% unknown pathway
Indapamide	20	93%	14	Metabolized
Spironolactone		65%	1.6	Metabolized

Flowchart 1: "Brater's algorithm" for diuretic therapy of chronic renal failure, nephrotic syndrome, CHF and cirrhosis. Follow algorithm until adequate response is achieved. If adequate response is not obtained, advance to the next step. For illustrative purposes, the thiazide diuretic used is HCTZ. An alternative thiazide-type diuretic may be substituted with dosage adjusted lo be pharmacologically equivalent to the recommended dose of HCTZ. *Do not combine, two K$^+$ sparing diuretics due to the risk of hyperkalemia.* CrCl indicates creatinine clearance in milliliters per minute, and ceiling dose refers to the smallest dose of diuretic that produces a near-maximal effect.

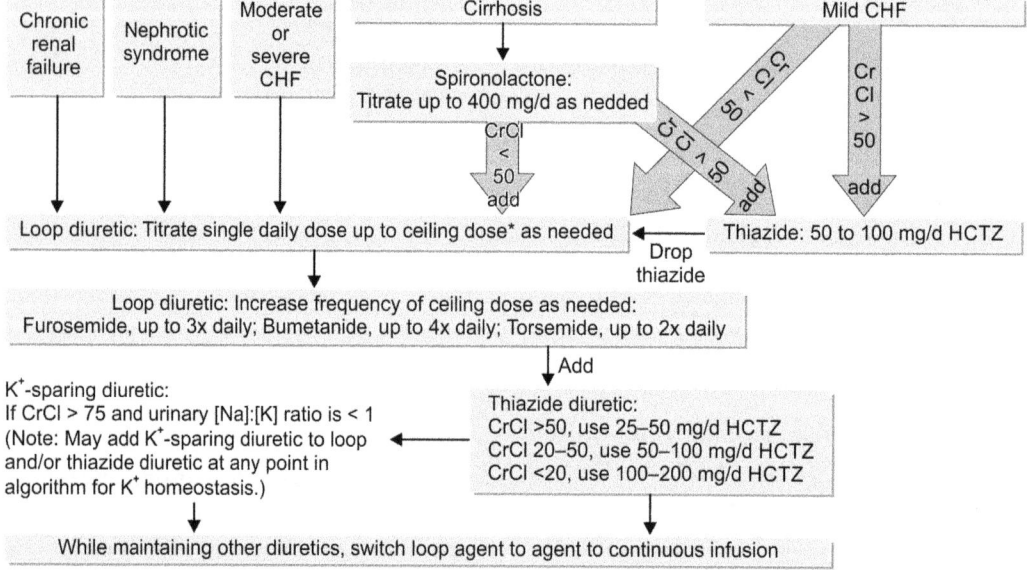

*Ceiling doses of loop diuretics and dosing regimens for continuous intravenous infusions of loop diuretics are disease-state specific. Doses are for adults only.
(CHF: congestive heart failure; HCTZ: hydrochlorothiazide)

Potassium Sparing Diuretics

Used in combination with loop or thiazide diuretics to avoid their side effects such as hypokalemia and augment diuresis.

Natriuretic Peptides

Currently only nesiritide, a recombinant brain natriuretic peptide is available for IV use, used as a continuous infusion with a half-life of about 18 minutes.

Vasopressin Receptor Antagonist

They inhibit V2 receptors in the collecting duct thereby decreasing the water reabsorption. Currently only tolvaptan is the US Food and Drug Administration (USFDA) approved drug for the treatment of euvolemic and hypervolemic hypernatremia associated with syndrome of inappropriate antidiuretic hormone secretion (SIADH), congestive heart failure (CHF), and, cirrhosis.

Neprilysin Antagonists

It is a membrane bound metalloproteinase found mainly in cardiovascular and renal tissue. Natriuretic peptides increase renal water secretion and are broken down by neprilysin (NEP). In conditions such as heart failure, increased release of natriuretic peptides occurs and use of NEP antagonists in such situation can prevent their breakdown, thus promoting natriuresis. They also reduce CVS remodeling that occurs with end stage heart failure.

FURTHER READING

1. Flood P, Rathmell JP, Shafer S. Stoelting's Pharmacology and Physiology in Anesthetic Practice, 6th edition.

20

Antacids and Prokinetics

Tanvi Meshram, Ankur Sharma

Q. 1. Describe the physiology of gastric acid secretion.

Ans. The stomach is a digestive organ involved in handling and preparing food for absorption. Gastric function is defined by the propensity to secrete hydrogen ions in the form of hydrochloric acid. The total daily stomach output is around 2 L with a pH ranging from 1.0 to 3.5. Hydrochloric acid, pepsinogen, intrinsic factor, and mucus are the most important secretions. Mucus secretion protects the stomach mucosa from mechanical and chemical damage. Alcohol and medicines that limit prostaglandin formation are examples of substances that disturb the mucosal barrier and produce stomach discomfort (aspirin, nonsteroidal anti-inflammatory drugs). About 1 billion parietal cells are located in the walls of oxyntic glands, the major secretory unit of the gastric mucosa. The glands may be found throughout the majority of the stomach's fundus and corpus. Histamine, acetylcholine (vagal stimulation), and gastrin all stimulate receptors in the membrane of parietal cells, resulting in hydrochloric acid secretion. These receptors enhance the hydrogen-potassium adenosine triphosphatase (ATPase) enzyme system's transport of hydrogen ions into the stomach lumen **(Fig. 1)**.

Prostaglandins (PGE2) engage receptors to activate stimulatory guanine proteins (Gs), which enhance adenylate cyclase (AC)

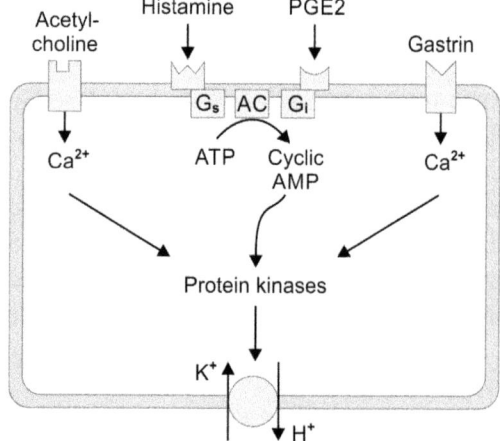

Fig. 1: Hydrochloric acid secretion in the gastric lumen after stimulation of parietal cells.
(AMP: adenosine monophosphate; ATP: adenosine triphosphate; PGE2: prostaglandin E2)

activity, while histamine activates inhibitory guanine proteins (Gi), which reduce AC activity. Cyclic adenosine monophosphate (cyclic AMP) and calcium promote hydrogen ion transport into the stomach lumen through protein kinases.

Parietal cells generate intrinsic factor, which is essential for ileum vitamin B_{12} absorption. Pepsinogen, proteolytic enzymes required for protein breakdown, is secreted by the chief cells. In the presence of hydrochloric acid, it cleaves to pepsin. Gastrin is produced into the blood by gastric antral cells (G cells), which transport it to receptive receptors in parietal cells to increase gastric hydrogen ion production.

Gastric fluid volume and gastric-emptying time are substantially influenced by neural and humoral systems. Gastric fluid production and motility are increased when the parasympathetic neural system is stimulated, while sympathetic nervous system activation has the opposite effect.

Aspiration occurs when the contents of the stomach or oropharynx are inhaled into the lungs. As a result, medications that increase the pH of gastric contents (antacids) and decrease the volume of gastric contents (prokinetic drugs) help to lower the severity of aspirating stomach contents sequelae.

Q. 2. What are antacids and describe them?
Ans. Antacids are weak bases that react with the hydrochloric acid in the stomach to produce salt and water. Their primary mode of action is to reduce intragastric acidity. Around 45 mEq/hour of hydrochloric acid is released after a meal. A single dosage of 156 mEq of antacid given 1 hour after a meal successfully neutralizes gastric acid for up to 2 hours.

Sodium bicarbonate: The most quickly acting antacid is sodium bicarbonate. It forms sodium chloride, carbon dioxide, and water when combined with hydrochloric acid. Excess bicarbonate is absorbed rapidly in the small intestine. Due to the absence of endogenous bicarbonate in the small intestine, dosages of sodium bicarbonate may cause a mild metabolic alkalosis with urine alkalinization. Due to the rapid formation of carbon dioxide, sodium bicarbonate may cause stomach distension, belching, and flatulence. It results in a prompt and quick antacid action causing a raised pH leading to acid rebound. Because of the high sodium load and the mentioned side effects, it is not recommended for use.

Magnesium hydroxide: It is distinguished by a strong laxative effect. It causes immediate neutralization of stomach acid but does not cause acid rebound. In individuals with renal disease, systemic magnesium absorption may result in neurologic, neuromuscular, and cardiovascular damage. Some people may develop metabolic alkalosis as a result of renal impairment.

Calcium carbonate: It reacts with hydrochloric acid in the stomach to generate calcium chloride, carbon dioxide, and water. In the small intestine, over 90% of the calcium chloride produced is converted into insoluble calcium salts, mostly calcium soaps, and is not absorbed. Constipation may be caused by calcium salts. The use of calcium carbonate-containing antacids may cause hypophosphatemia. Another downside is the gritty taste of calcium carbonate. Eructation and flatulence may result from CO_2 emission in the stomach.

Aluminum hydroxide: Aluminum hydroxide and aluminum oxide dissolve slowly in the stomach. They react with gastric acid to form aluminum chloride and water. Aluminum chloride is 17–30% bioavailable in the small intestine and is eliminated by the kidneys. Aluminum is retained when renal function is compromised. Aluminum excess in the urine has been linked to dementia. Aluminum compounds induce constipation and delay stomach emptying.

Sodium citrate: In the stomach, aluminum hydroxide and aluminum oxide dissolve slowly. Aluminum chloride and water are formed when they combine with stomach acid. Aluminum chloride is 17–30% accessible in the small intestine and is excreted through the kidneys. When renal function is impaired, aluminum is retained. Excess aluminum in the blood has been related to dementia. Aluminum compounds cause constipation and cause stomach emptying to be delayed.

Q. 3. Describe different histamine receptor antagonist.

Ans. Drugs are categorized as H1, H2, H3, or H4 receptor antagonists depending on the histamine responses they decrease. The central nervous system (CNS), mast cells, and T lymphocytes all have H3 and H4 receptors.

H1-receptor antagonist: There are two types of receptor antagonists: (1) first-generation and (2) second-generation antagonists. Antagonist to H1 receptor is highly selective, having minimal effect on H2, H3, or H4 receptors. Compared to second-generation antagonists, first-generation H1-receptor antagonists may activate muscarinic, cholinergic, and 5-hydroxytryptamine receptors, producing more significant sedation.

- *First-generation:*
  - Chlorpheniramine
  - Diphenhydramine
  - Hydroxyzine
- *Second-generation:*
  - Loratadine
  - Acrivastine
  - Azelastine.

H1 antagonists of the first-generation often have adverse effects on the CNS, such as somnolence, reduced alertness, delayed reaction time, and cognitive function impairment. Anticholinergic symptoms such as dry mouth, decreased eyesight, urine retention, and impotence may occur due to cross-reactivity with muscarinic receptors. Tachycardia is common, and it has been linked to QTc interval prolongation, heart block, and cardiac arrhythmias.

H2-receptor antagonist (Table 1): Cimetidine, ranitidine, famotidine, and nizatidine are H2-receptor antagonists that selectively and reversibly inhibit the H2-mediated release of hydrogen ions by stomach parietal cells. In response to baseline and meal-stimulated acid secretion, H2 antagonists competitively block the parietal cell H2-receptor and diminish acid production in a linear, dose-dependent manner. They are very selective and have no effect on H1 or H3 receptors. Acid production caused by histamine, gastrin, and cholinomimetic drugs is inhibited by H2 antagonists. Despite the fact that H2-receptors are found all throughout the body, the principal impact of H2-receptor antagonists is to inhibit histamine binding to the receptors on stomach parietal cells.

Adverse reactions

Central nervous system: Headache, somnolence, confusion, and hallucination.

Cardiovascular system (CVS): Bradycardia, hypotension, and heart block.

Cimetidine inhibits dihydrotestosterone binding to androgen receptors, slows estradiol

TABLE 1: Pharmacokinetics of H2-receptor antagonist.

	Cimetidine	Ranitidine	Famotidine	Nizatidine
Potency	1	4–10	20–50	4–10
Bioavailability (%)	60	50	43	98
Time to peak plasma concentration (hours)	1–2	1–3	1–3.5	1–3
Elimination half-life (hours)	1.5–2.3	1.6–2.4	2.5–4	1.1–1.6
Dose to achieve >50% acid Inhibition for 10 hours	400–800 mg	150 mg	20 mg	150 mg
• Interfere with drug metabolism by cytochrome P450 enzymes	Yes	Minimal	No	No

metabolism, and causes hyperprolactinemia. When used in excess or over an extended period, it may induce gynecomastia or impotence in males and galactorrhea in women.
- Acute pancreatitis
- Increased hepatic transaminase levels
- Alcohol dehydrogenase dehydration
- Thrombocytopenia
- Agranulocytosis
- Interstitial nephritis.

Q. 4. Elaborate different proton pump inhibitors (PPIs) and describe them.
Ans. Six PPIs are available for clinical use: omeprazole, esomeprazole, lansoprazole, dexlansoprazole, rabeprazole, and pantoprazole. They block the membrane enzyme proton pump (hydrogen potassium-ATPase), which moves hydrogen ions across the stomach parietal cell membranes for exchange of potassium ions **(Table 2)**.

Proton pump inhibitors, unlike H2 antagonists, diminish both fasting and meal-stimulated secretion. Proton pump inhibitors inhibit 90-98% of 24-hour acid secretion by inhibiting the common route of acid secretion.

Adverse effects:
- In general, diarrhea, headache, and stomach pain are reported in 1-5% of people. Proton pump inhibitor usage has been associated to acute interstitial nephritis and long-term renal impairment.
- *Nutrition*: Acid is required for vitamin B_{12} absorption from food. When the proton pump is turned off, cyanocobalamin absorption may decrease somewhat. PPIs have the potential to impair osteoclast function and reduce calcium absorption.
- *Respiratory and enteric infections*: Gastrointestinal acid is essential in preventing germs from invading and infecting the stomach and intestine. Individuals on PPIs had higher bacterial concentrations in their stomach.
- *Potential side effects of high serum gastrin levels*: Acid suppression alters normal feedback inhibition, causing serum gastrin levels to rise. Serum gastrin levels over a certain threshold might cause parietal cell hyperplasia, resulting in brief rebound acid hypersecretion with exacerbated dyspepsia or heartburn following drug discontinuation.

Q. 5. Describe various gastrointestinal prokinetic agent.
Ans. Motility-modulating medications work by raising the tone of the lower esophageal

TABLE 2: Pharmacokinetics of proton pump inhibitors.

Drugs	Bioavailability	T1/2 (hours)	Protein binding	Hepatic metabolism	Interference with cytochrome P450	The usual dosage for peptic ulcer or GERD
Omeprazole	60%	0.5-1	>90%	Yes	Minimal	20-40 qd
Esomeprazole	60%	1.5	>90%	Yes	Minimal	20-40 mg qd
Lansoprazole	85%	1.0-2.0	97%	Yes	Minimal	30 mg qd
Dexlansoprazole	NA	1.0-2.0	97%	Yes	Minimal	30-60 mg qd
Pantoprazole	77%	1.0-1.9	98%	Yes	No	40 mg qd
Rabeprazole	85%	1.0-2.0	96%	Yes	No	20 mg qd

(GERD: gastroesophageal reflux disease)

TABLE 3: Pharmacokinetics of dopamine blockers.

	Bioavailability	T1/2	Protein binding	Dose
Metoclopramide	75%	2–4 hours	30%	10 mg
Domperidone	17%	7.5 hours	92%	40–120 mg

sphincter, boosting peristaltic contractions, and increasing the pace of gastric emptying.

Dopamine blockers (Table 3): Dopamine D2 receptor antagonists include metoclopramide and domperidone. They inhibit cholinergic smooth muscle stimulation, resulting in increasing lower esophageal sphincter pressure and greater gastric emptying but no effect on small intestine or colonic motility. They also inhibit D2 receptors in the medulla's chemoreceptor trigger zone (area postrema), resulting in a strong antiemetic effect. Domperidone, unlike metoclopramide, does not readily pass the blood–brain barrier and has no anticholinergic effect.

Adverse effects: In 10–20% of patients, CNS symptoms such as restlessness, sleepiness, insomnia, anxiety, and agitation occur. Due to central dopamine receptor blockade, extrapyramidal symptoms occur in 5% of patients undergoing long-term treatment and in patients receiving higher dosages. Tardive dyskinesia has been reported in individuals receiving extended metoclopramide therapy.

Prolactin elevations may result in galactorrhea, gynecomastia, impotence, and menstrual irregularities.

With domperidone, neuropsychiatric and extrapyramidal symptoms are rare.

Macrolide antibiotics: The prokinetic characteristics of macrolides are linked to their binding to motilin receptors, as well as secondary cholinergic stimulatory activities. In patients with diabetic gastroparesis, patients awaiting emergent surgery, and ICU patients with food intolerance, erythromycin and other macrolide antibiotics raise lower esophageal sphincter tone, and facilitate gastric emptying.

5-HT4-receptor agonists: Cisapride, mosapride, tegaserod, and prucalopride.

5-HT4 receptor activation promotes proximal bowel contraction and distal bowel relaxation. Cisapride reverses opioid-induced gastric stasis. Tegaserod increases small and large intestine transit and alleviates constipation. Cisapride and mosapride are related with QT prolongation due to their relative nonselectivity.

FURTHER READING

1. Katzung B. Basic and Clinical Pharmacology, 14 edition. New York: Lange Medical Books/McGraw-Hill; 2018.
2. Maton PN, Burton ME. Antacids revisited: a review of their clinical pharmacology and recommended therapeutic use. Drugs. 1999;57(6):855-70.
3. Reddymasu SC, Soykan I, McCallum RW. Domperidone: review of pharmacology and clinical applications in gastroenterology. Am J Gastroenterol. 2007;102(9):2036-45.
4. Shafer SL, Rathmell JP, Flood P. Stoelting's Pharmacology and Physiology in Anesthetic Practice, 5th edition. Philadelphia: Wolters Kluwer Health; 2015.

CHAPTER 21

Anticoagulants

Sangam Yadav, Ankur Sharma

INTRODUCTION

Hemostasis is a physiological response to any insult on the blood vessels to prevent excessive blood loss. There are two phases of hemostasis:
1. *Primary:* It involves constriction of the blood vessel and formation of a platelet plug.
2. *Secondary:* It involves the activation of the extrinsic, intrinsic, and common pathway of coagulation.

MECHANISM (FIGS. 1 TO 3)

Whenever there is a vessel wall injury, the following sequence of events is set into motion:
- Vasoconstriction
- Platelet aggregation—primary hemostasis—weak plug
- Coagulation and fibrin formation—secondary hemostasis
- Fibrin clot
- Clot retraction
- Invasion by fibroblasts leads to scar formation

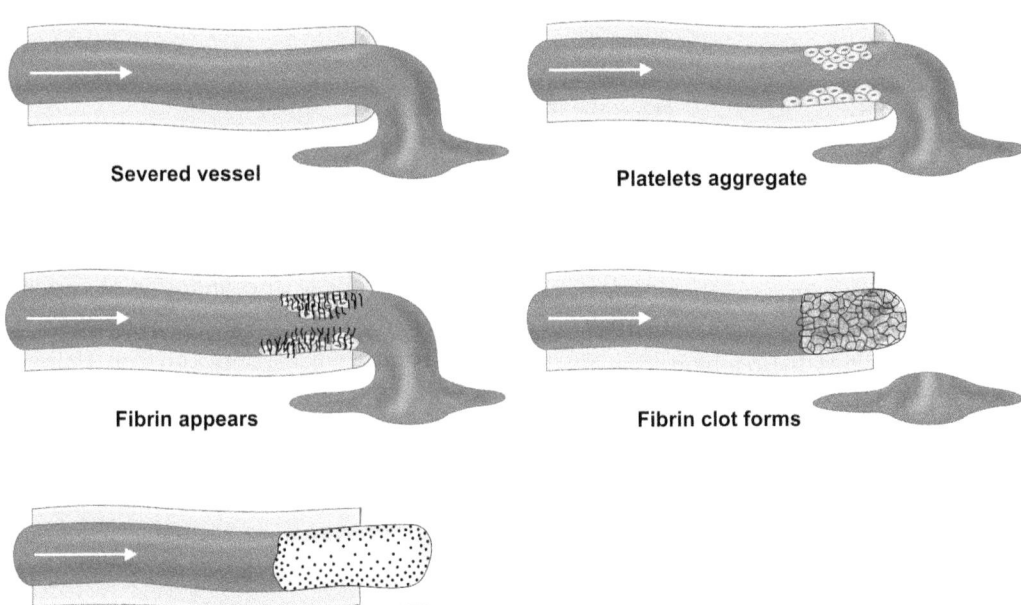

Fig. 1: Mechanism of coagulation.

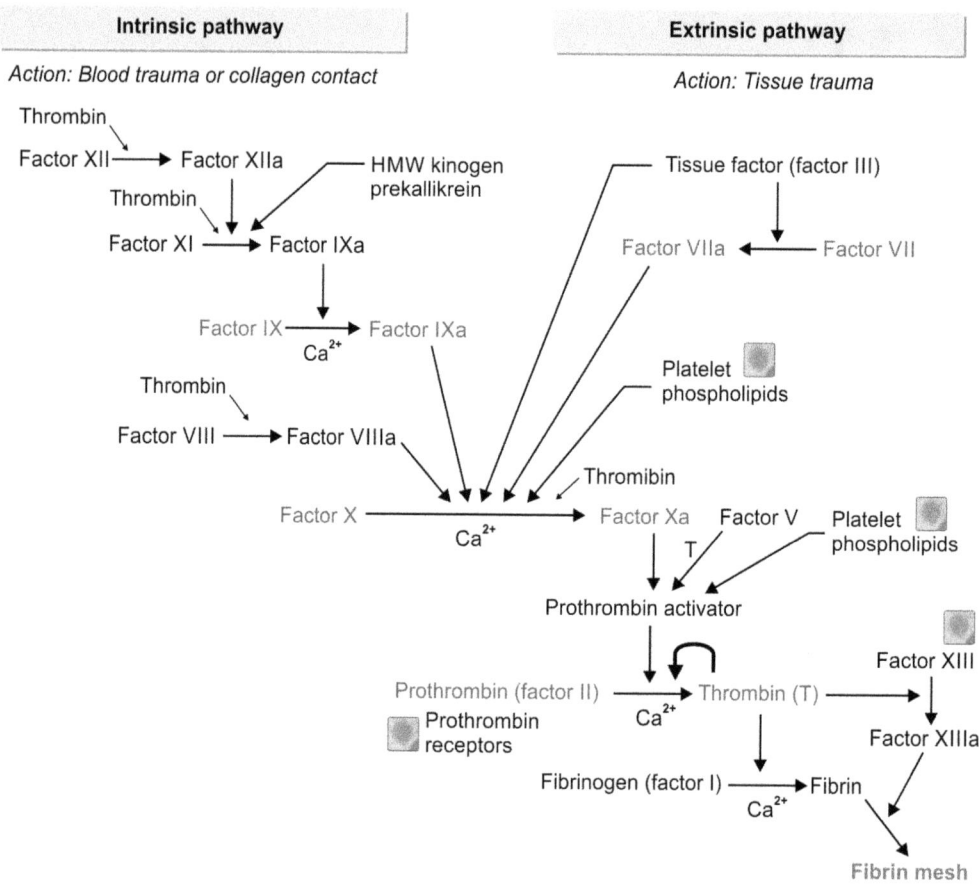

Fig. 2: The coagulation pathway.

DRUGS

Heparin

Heparin was the first anticoagulant to be discovered in 1922. Heparin requires a cofactor, antithrombin III (ATIII), to inhibit coagulation. Heparin and ATIII directly inhibits coagulation factors IX, X, XIa, XIIa, and indirectly suppresses thrombin-induced activation of factors V and VIII by binding to thrombin. It is present intrinsically in basophils, mast cells, and liver. One unit is defined as volume of heparin solution that can prevent 1 mL of citrated sheep blood from clotting for 1 hour after adding 0.2 mL of $CaCl_2$.

Pharmacokinetics

Distribution is limited by large molecular size to vascular space and endothelial system. Eliminated by kidneys or by metabolism in reticuloendothelial system and liver. Half-life ($t\frac{1}{2}$) dose-dependent:

- Low doses, 100–150 U/kg, 1 hour
- Cardiopulmonary bypass (CPB) dose 350–400 U/kg 2 hours; may persist 4–6 hours without neutralization
- Average time 1–2 hours but increased with liver/renal disease or dose >100 U/kg
- Activated clotting time (ACT) is used to monitor effect and reversal during CPB.

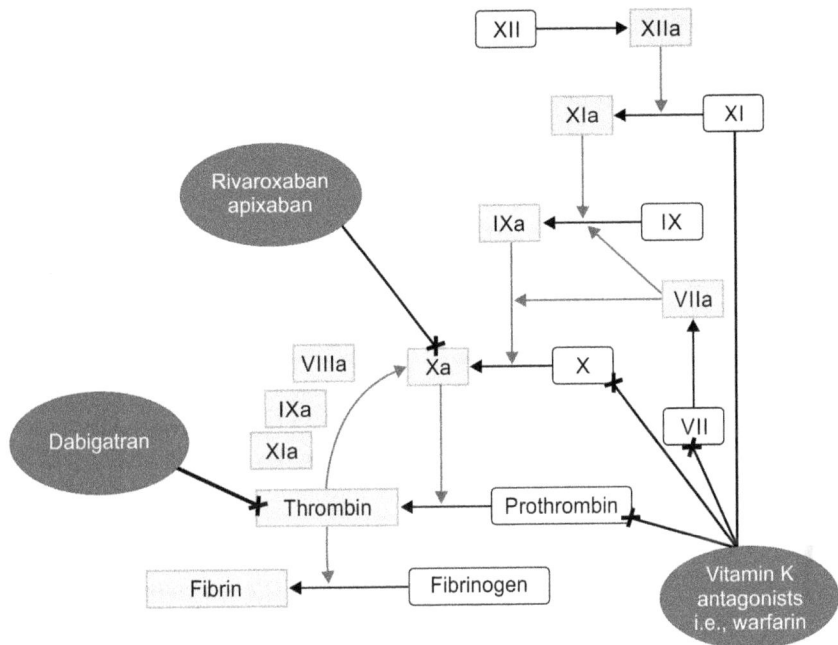

Fig 3: A brief overview of the action site of different anticoagulants.

The onset of action is 1 minute with the intravenous route, while it is 20–60 minutes in the subcutaneous route. It is not absorbed through the gastrointestinal tract (GI) tract.

Uses
- Treatment/prevention of deep vein thrombosis (DVT)
- Unstable angina—aPTT 1.5–2.5 × control
- Angioplasty, stenting—ACT 350 s
- CPB (cardiac surgery)—ACT 480 s.

Substantial Variability in Patient Response
- Heparin resistance due to ATIII deficiency.
- Population at risk—cardiac surgery, nitroglycerin infusion, nephrotic syndrome, cirrhosis, prolonged heparin infusion, disseminated intravascular coagulation (DIC).
- Four-fold variation in heparin sensitivity; three fold variation in rate in which it is metabolized.

Monitoring
Test of intrinsic pathway: aPPT; aPTT 1.5–2.5 control correlated with heparin levels of 0.2–0.7 U/mL.

Side Effects
- Main and most frequent complication is bleeding due to improper titration and over dose.
- Boluses decrease systemic vascular resistance, usually small (10–20%).
- Rarely anaphylaxis.
- During CPB, ACT values for heparin anticoagulation can be misleading due to hypothermia, hemodilution.

Heparin-induced Thrombocytopenia
It is seen in 0.1–5% of patients and denoted by a marked fall in platelet count after exposure to heparin. It has two subtypes, namely Type1 and Type II **(Table 1)**.

TABLE 1: Comparison between heparin-induced thrombocytopenia (HIT) type I and type II.

HIT Type I	HIT Type II
Rapid onset: 2–4 days	Occurs after more than 5 days of administration (average 9 days)

Characterized by a mild decrease in platelet count without thrombosis or immune response	Considerably more severe
	• High morbidity:
	  – Incidence of thrombosis: 20–50%
	  – Mortality after thrombosis: 20–30%

Results from heparin's proaggregatory effect on platelets	• Antibody binding between heparin-platelet complex • Causes platelet activation, complement activation, white clot

Investigation for Heparin-induced Thrombocytopenia

Complete blood count (CBC) to assess platelet count, ELISA for anti-IgG antibody, serotonin release assay.

Management

Immediate discontinuation of heparin, use of alternative agents such as bivalirudin, argatroban, lepirudin, desirudin, dabigatran (oral direct thrombin inhibitor).

Reversal of Heparin: Protamine

It was commercially prepared from fish sperm.

Mechanism:
- Produces strong ionic bond with heparin devoid of anticoagulant effects
- 1 mg protamine neutralizes 100 U of heparin
- Neutralization of heparin occurs in 5 minutes

Heparin rebound: Protamine is cleared by the reticuloendothelial system in 10–20 minutes which is quicker than heparin clearance.

Heparin rebound is bleeding 30 min to 9 hours after protamine administration related to the extravascular release of heparin from protein binding sites. Management is by clinical monitoring and small doses of protamine as indicated.

Adverse effects of protamine:
- Hypotension with rapid administration—due to pulmonary vasoconstriction and decreased cardiac output.
- Noncardiogenic pulmonary edema.
- Anaphylactoid reaction.
- Excessive dose (600–800) is associated with antiplatelet activity and has a risk of increased bleeding.

Warfarin (Coumarin)

It interferes with the production of vitamin K-dependent factors: II, VII, IX, X. Among the factors—II and X, are most important for antithrombotic activity. The onset of action is 8–12 hours, whereas the peak effect occurs in 36–72 hours. Normal hemostasis is achieved within 1–3 days after stopping the drug.

Laboratory tests done to assess the response include:
- Prothrombin time (PT) and international normalized ratio (INR) most sensitive.
- PT + INR—reflect primarily factor VII and X activity.
- INR >1.2—factor VII less 55%.

A factor activity level of 40% is needed for normal hemostasis. Recovery factor VII rapid; II, X slower.

Emergent situations require reversal: Vitamin K, fresh frozen plasma (FFP), four factor prothrombin complex concentrate (PCC).

Prothrombin Complex Concentrate

It contains factors II, VII, IX, X plus protein C and S. It was Food and Drug Administration (FDA) approved on April 30, 2013.

It is indicated to reverse coumarin in patients with the following:
- INR >8
- Prolonged PT
- Raised D-dimer
- Emergency operation in a patient on coumarin
- Deficiency of one of II, VII, IX, X factors.

Prothrombin complex concentrate is made of pooled plasma and requires a lower volume than FFP to reverse *coumarin*. Also, the rate of complication is lower than FFP owing to lesser volume. However, PCC may be associated with thromboembolic events. Earlier, it was believed that it is contraindicated in DIC, but PCC may restore the deficient factors if coagulation factors are low.

LOW MOLECULAR WEIGHT HEPARINS

It is a fraction of heparin with a molecular weight of 2000–6000 Daltons. It has better bioavailability and a longer duration. Dosing is once or twice daily. For example, enoxaparin, dalteparin.

Mechanism

Binds to ATIII to inhibit factor X while having a minor effect on thrombin.

Pharmacokinetics

Effect prolonged in patients with renal failure. Half-life (t½) is approximately 3–6 hours; however, the activity may persist for 24 hours.

Monitoring

It requires measurement of anti-Xa activity. Anti-Xa levels peak at 3–5 hours, but significant anti-Xa activity remains 12 hours after injection.

Antagonist

Only partially antagonized by *protamine*, which reverses only IIa activity.

Pharmacological Properties

Pharmacological properties differ from unfractionated heparin (UFH):
- Lack of monitoring of anticoagulant effect.
- Prolonged half-life
- Irreversibility with protamine
- Less risk of heparin-induced thrombocytopenia.

NEWER FACTOR X INHIBITORS

Rivaroxaban

It has been approved for use in the US, Canada, and Europe. It is the first available oral direct factor Xa inhibitor. The onset of action is within 30 minutes, and maximum inhibition occurs 4 hours after administration. The effect lasts 8–12 hours post-administration though the factor Xa activity does not return to normal till 24 hours.

Pharmacokinetics

It undergoes hepatic metabolism and renal excretion. So should be avoided when CrCl <30 mL/min or severe liver disease is present.

Advantages

- Predictable pharmacokinetics.
- Low potential for interaction with diet or alcohol.
- No routine monitoring is required.

Antidote

Reversibility occurs after cessation for 24 hours, depending on plasma concentration and elimination half-life. No antidote is available.

Apixaban

It is a direct factor Xa inhibitor which was FDA approved in December 2012. It is used for the prevention of thromboembolism. It is highly protein-bound, reaches peak plasma concentration 2–3 hours after administration. Like rivaroxaban, it also has limited drug interactions. Half-life in healthy subjects is 8–15 hours.

Dosage

2.5 mg BID orally.

Note: Andexanet—this drug reversed anticoagulant activity of apixaban and rivaroxaban in healthy older patients within minutes of bolus and infusion.
- *Apixaban:* 400 mg bolus; infusion 4 mg/min 2 hours
- *Rivaroxaban:* 800 mg bolus; 8 mg/min for 2 hours.

Andexanet is a specific, rapidly acting antidote being developed for urgent reversal factor Xa inhibitors.

Fondaparinux

It acts by antithrombin III inhibition of factor Xa. It is administered subcutaneously or intravenously once a day. It is rapidly and completely absorbed with a peak steady-state reaching within 3 hours. It is 94% bound to ATIII, eliminated unchanged in the urine in 72 hours with normal renal function.

It should be discontinued two days before surgery; a more extended period may be required with a renal disease.

Direct Thrombin Inhibitors (Tables 2 to 4)

Argatroban

This is a synthetic direct thrombin inhibitor, indicated for prophylaxis or Rx thrombus in patients at risk for HIT undergoing PCI. It is available for intravenous use only.

TABLE 2: Warfarin versus dabigatran.

	Coumadin	Pradaxa
Dosage	Varies with INR	150 mg BID CrCl >30; 75 mg BID CrCl 15–30
Administration	Tablet	Capsule
Onset	12–24 hours	Within few hours
Half-life	36 hours	12–17 hours
Excretion	Hepatic	Renal
Monitoring	Yes; INR	No
Dietary considerations	No leafy green vegetables or food high in vitamin K	No
Antidote	Vitamin K	Paxabind
Drug interactions	Several	• Avoid St John's wart, quinidine, rifampicin • Verapamil, amiodarone, • Clarithromycin
Side effects	Bleeding, SOB, edema, allergic reactions	Bleeding, GI disturbances, >risk MI, <risk intracranial bleed
Cost	50 cents day, $15 month + INR cost	$7 day, $210 month
Procedural points	DC 5–6 days before	Skip 2–8 doses depending on renal function
Age considerations	>75 increased risk cerebral bleed	Caution in those <age 15 or over 75

(INR: international normalized ratio; MI: myocardial infarction)

TABLE 3: Summary of new oral anticoagulants.

	Dabigatran	Rivaroxaban	Apixaban
Mechanism	Direct thrombin inhibitor	Factor Xa inhibitor	Factor Xa inhibitor
Time to peak effect (h)	1–3	2–4	1–3
Half-like (h)	14–17	5–9	8–15
Dialyzable	Yes	No	No
Metabolism/excretion	80% renal excreted	30% hepatic; 35% renal excretion	15% hepatic; 25% renal excretion
Coagulation tests affected	• aPTT • Ecarin clotting time • Thrombin time	• PT • Antifactor X levels	• PT • Antifactor X levels
Oral activated charcoal	Yes	Likely	Likely
Dialysis	Yes	No	No
Vitamin K	No	No	No
Fresh frozen plasma	Minimal	Minimal	Minimal
Recombinant FVII	Possible	Possible	Possible
3-Factor PCC	Possible	Possible	Possible
4-Factor PCC	Possible	Possible	Possible

TABLE 4: Summary of direct thrombin inhibitors.

Drug	Dose	Clinical status	Indication	Monitoring
Bivalirudin	IV	Available in the US	HIT; PTCA	ACT
Argatroban	IV	Available US and Europe	HITPCT in HIT patients	aPTT or ACT
Lepirurdin	IV	Available in the US and Europe	HIT, prevention VTE	aPTT
Desurdin	SQ	US and Europe	Hip surgery	aPTT
Dabigatran	Oral	US and Europe	Hip knee surgery; VTE, A-fib	Thrombin times, aPTT

(ACT: activated clotting time; A-fib: atrial fibrillation; HIT: heparin-induced thrombocytopenia; PTCA: percutaneous transluminal coronary angioplasty; PTT: partial thromboplastin time; SQ: subcutaneous; VTE: venous thromboembolism)

Half-life is 40–50 minutes and duration of 4 hours. Argatroban is eliminated via the liver compared to other replacements for heparin in patients at risk for HIT, which are eliminated by the kidney. Monitoring is done by aPTT or ACT. It should be stopped 4–6 hours before surgery.

Lepirudin
This is an analog of hirudin approved for use in patients with HIT which irreversibly inhibits thrombin. Heparin-induced thrombocytopenia (HIT) patients receiving this drug develop antibodies requiring close monitoring of a PTT to avoid bleeding complications. Drug action is prolonged in patients with renal dysfunction and stopped 24 hours before surgery.

Desirudin
It is also an analog of hirudin which is administered subcutaneously. It has been

approved to prevent DVT after total hip or knee replacement surgery and is being studied in patients with acute coronary syndrome or percutaneous coronary angioplasty.

Anaphylaxis has been reported though the risk is low. Primarily eliminated by kidney and monitoring is done by aPTT. It needs to be stopped 24 hours before surgery.

Dabigatran (Pradaxa)

It is a direct oral competitive, reversible thrombin inhibitor. It has a low potential for interaction with diet or alcohol. Proton pump inhibitors inhibit its absorption.

The onset of anticoagulation—30 minutes, duration: 24-36 hours, reversibility after cessation—24-36 hours depending on the plasma concentration. It has predictable pharmacokinetics and no hepatic metabolism, so safe in patients with liver disease. It is metabolized by esterase-catalyzed hydrolysis and has renal and GI clearance.

There is no routine monitoring required, but aPTT and thrombin time can be used **(Table 2)**.

It should be stopped 48 hours before surgery in patients with normal renal function; 72-96 hours in patients with abnormal renal function.

Dose
If: CrCl. ≥30 mL/min 150 mg PO BID
CrCl <15 mL/min 75 mg PO BID

Antidote: Idarucizumab (Praxbind) is a humanized antibody fragment that binds to the pradaxa molecule, reversing the effect without interfering with the coagulation cascade.

It has been approved for:
- Emergency surgery/urgent procedures
- Life-threatening or uncontrolled bleeding.

Following administration of 5 g, a complete reversal occurs within minutes.

ANTIPLATELET DRUGS (TABLE 5)

Flowchart 1 describes the different antiplatelet drugs.

Mechanism of Action

- Inhibit thromboxane by blocking cyclooxygenase
- Thromboxane A_2 stimulator of platelet aggregation
- Aspirin irreversibly inhibits the enzyme.

Toxicity

- GI bleeding
- CNS effect
- Enhance effects other anticoagulants.

Types of Antiplatelet Agents

- Glycoprotein IIB/IIIA receptor inhibitor agents
- Aspirin preparations
- Platelet-ADP-receptor antagonist agents
- Platelet adhesion inhibitor agents.

THROMBOLYTIC (FIBRINOLYTIC) AGENTS

The thrombolytic (fibrinolytic) agents are mentioned in **Table 6**.

Most commonly used drugs include:
- Alteplase
- Reteplase
- Anistreplase
- Urokinase
- Streptokinase.

Mechanism

- Catalyze activation plasminogen to plasmin
- Plasmin is a fibrinolytic enzyme.

Clinical Uses

Emergency thrombolysis of clot [myocardial infarction, cerebrovascular accident (emboli)].

TABLE 5: Overview of antiplatelet drugs.

Drug	Site of action	Route	T½	Metabolism	Antidote
Aspirin	COX 1–2	Oral	20 min	Hepatic	0
Dipyridamole	Adenosine	Oral	40 min	Hepatic	0
Clopidogrel	ADP	Oral	7 h	Hepatic	0
Ticlopidine	ADP	Oral	4 days	Hepatic	0
Abciximab	GP IIb/IIIa	IV	30 min	Renal	0
Eptifibatide	GP IIb/IIIa	IV	2.5 h	Renal	0
Tirofiban	GP IIb/IIIa	IV	2 h	Renal	Hemodialysis

(ADP: adenosine diphosphate; GP: glycoprotein; IV: intravenous)

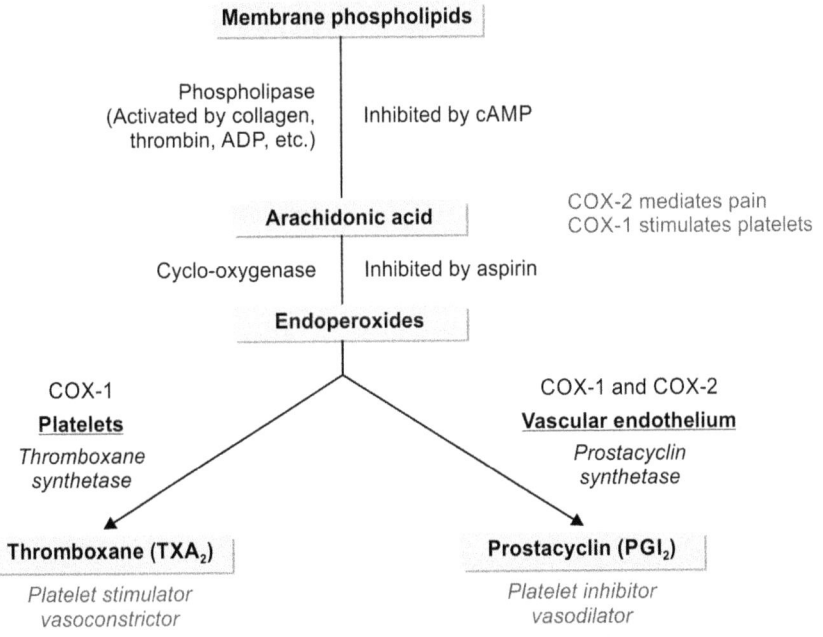

Flowchart 1: Antiplatelet drugs.

TABLE 6: Thrombolytic (fibrinolytic) agents.

First generation	Second generation	Third generation
• Streptokinase • Urokinase • Staphylokinase • Abbokinase	• Alteplase • Anistreplase • Prourokinase • Activase • Eminase	• Reteplase • Tenecteplase • Lanoteplase • Staphylokinase • Antibody-targeted PAS • Vampire bat-PA • Alfimeprase • Retavase • TNKase

Toxicity
Bleeding.

Contraindications to Fibrinolytic Therapy

Absolute
- Any history of hemorrhagic cerebrovascular event
- Any other cerebrovascular events within 1 year
- Active internal bleeding
- Known intracranial neoplasm
- Suspected aortic dissection.

Relative
- Blood pressure over 180/110 mm Hg
- Anticoagulants and INR over 2
- Prolonged cardiopulmonary resuscitation
- Prior gastrointestinal hemorrhage
- Pregnancy
- Menstruation
- Recent trauma (within 2-4 weeks)
- Major surgery within 3 weeks.

QUESTION

Q. 1. What is 4T score?

FURTHER READING

1. Horlocker TT, Vandermeuelen E, Kopp SL, Gogarten W, Leffert LR, Benzon HT. Regional Anesthesia in the Patient Receiving Antithrombotic or Thrombolytic Therapy. American Society of Regional Anesthesia and Pain Medicine Evidence-Based Guidelines, 4th edition. Reg Anesth Pain Med. 2018; 43(4):263-309.
2. Krombach JW, Dagtekin O, Kampe S. Regional anesthesia and anticoagulation. Curr Opin Anaesthesiol. 2004;17(5):427-33.
3. Oprea AD, Noto CJ, Halaszynski TM. Risk stratification, perioperative and periprocedural management of the patient receiving anticoagulant therapy. J Clin. Anesth. 2016; 34:586-99.

CHAPTER 22

Chemotherapy

Tanvi Meshram, Ankur Sharma

INTRODUCTION

The *chemotherapy* term was coined to refer to a broad range of chemicals (drugs) aimed at treating cancer by eradicating malignant cells anywhere in the body. Malignant cells are often characterized by rapid division and synthesis of deoxyribonucleic acid (DNA). Most conventional chemotherapeutic drugs exert their antineoplastic effects on cells actively undergoing division (mitosis) or DNA synthesis. Many chemotherapeutic drugs act only at specific phases of the cell cycle. Rapidly dividing normal cells of the bone marrow, gastrointestinal mucosa, skin, and hair follicles are more vulnerable to the toxic effects of chemotherapeutic drugs.

Myelosuppression is the most frequent complication that results in the temporary or permanent cessation of treatment for several chemotherapeutic agents.

CLASSIFICATION OF CHEMOTHERAPEUTICS

Chemotherapeutic drugs are classified according to their mechanism of action **(Fig. 1 and Table 1)**.

TOXIC EFFECTS OF CHEMOTHERAPY

As discussed previously, chemotherapy drugs act on various cell cycle phases and thus have

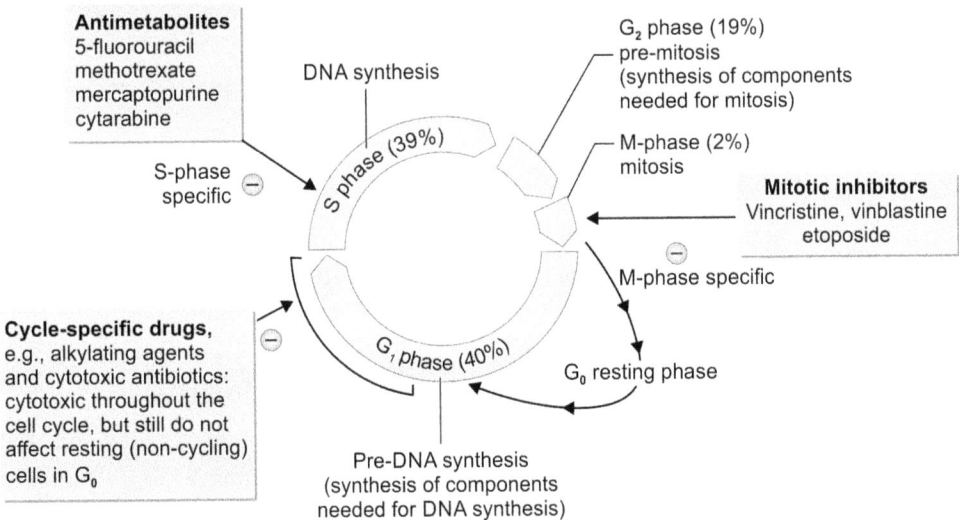

Fig. 1: Action of chemotherapeutic drugs on the cell cycle.

TABLE 1: Classification of chemotherapeutic drugs according to their mechanism of action.

Drug class	Mechanism of action	Examples
Alkylating agents	Inhibit cell function by creating covalent connections in proteins, DNA, and RNA	Cisplatin, carboplatin, chlorambucil, cyclophosphamide, ifosfamide
Antimetabolites	They either replace a metabolite that is usually integrated into DNA or RNA or compete for the catalytic site of a key enzyme	5-Fluorouracil, methotrexate, pemetrexed, mercaptopurine, gemcitabine
Antitumor antibiotics	Intercalate DNA at specific sequences, creating free radicals, which cause strand breakage	Bleomycin, anthracyclines (doxorubicin, epirubicin)
Topoisomerase inhibitors	Topoisomerase I and topoisomerase II uncoil DNA during replication	• *Topoisomerase I*—irinotecan, topotecan • *Topoisomerase II*—etoposide
Tubulin-binding drugs	Prevent the production of microtubules, which are essential during mitosis and for cell shape, intracellular transport, and axonal function	• *Vinca alkaloids*—vincristine, vinorelbine • *Taxoids*—docetaxel, paclitaxel
Signal transduction modifiers	• Hormonal treatment of cancer results in a disruption of the normal growth factor receptor interactions • Monoclonal antibodies bind to specific antigens on tumor cells and thereby modify cell proliferation • Aromatase inhibitors act by suppressing the enzyme aromatase from converting androgens into estrogen	• *Antiestrogens*—tamoxifen, toremifene, raloxifene • *Antiandrogens*—flutamide, bicalutamide, nilutamide • *Monoclonal antibodies*—rituximab, trastuzumab • *Aromatase inhibitors*—aminoglutethimide, anastrazole, letrozole • *Gonadotropin-releasing drugs*—leuprolide, buserelin • *Progestins*—megestrol acetate

(DNA: deoxyribonucleic acid; RNA: ribonucleic acid)

more significant action on rapidly multiplying malignant cells in the body. Therefore, even the rapidly multiplying normal cells of bone marrow, hair, skin, and gastric mucosa are affected, leading to myelosuppression, hair loss, and mucosal ulcers with almost all chemotherapy drugs. Nevertheless, they also act on other body systems to produce acute and long-term toxicities. Knowledge of the possible toxic effects of commonly used anticancer drugs is essential for preoperative evaluation and management of patients with a history of chemotherapy use.

Cardiovascular Toxicity

Drugs implicated: Cytotoxic antibiotics, alkylating agents, antimetabolites, 5-fluorouracil, cisplatin, interferon, interleukin-2, taxol, trastuzumab, and tamoxifen.

Mechanisms of chemotherapy-induced cardiotoxicity are:
- Direct cellular toxicity
- Effects on the coagulation system—increased thrombosis and thromboembolic event
- Arrhythmogenic effects
- Hypertensive effects
- Myocardial and pericardial inflammation resulting in myocardial dysfunction or pericardial sequels.

The anthracyclines (epirubicin, doxorubicin) are the drugs most commonly implicated in cardiotoxicity. Anthracyclines induce cardiac damage by producing free radicals, which cause myocyte apoptosis and as a result, immediate and permanent heart damage. Cardiac toxicity can manifest during as well as after the therapy and based on their appearance in relation to the time of treatment, is classified as acute, chronic, and late-onset. A decrease in ejection fraction of less than 45% is indicative of anthracycline-induced cardiotoxicity.

Acute cardiotoxicity: It may develop quickly, even after a single dosage of anthracycline treatment, presenting as nonspecific electrocardiogram (ECG) abnormalities, sinus tachycardia, arrhythmias, and heart block. Acute cardiac failure, pericarditis, and deadly pericarditis-myocarditis syndrome have also been recorded.

Chronic toxicity: It occurs within one year of treatment and progresses quickly. Cardiomyopathy is the most common type of chronic cardiotoxicity following anthracyclines. Cardiotoxicity from anthracyclines is a dose-dependent condition. The frequency of congestive heart failure caused by anthracycline-induced cardiotoxicity increases with dosage. After a dosage of 300–550 mg/m^2, there is a substantial rise in the incidence of congestive heart failure (CHF).

Late-onset cardiotoxicity: It occurs several years after receiving anthracycline therapy. Toxic effects include ventricular dysfunction, arrhythmias, conductive disturbances, and congestive heart failure.

Cyclophosphamide: It causes direct endothelium damage, resulting in hemorrhagic pericarditis or myocarditis, as well as congestive heart failure.

5-Fluorouracil: It exerts direct toxic effects on vascular endothelium, causing coronary spasm and endothelial-independent vasoconstriction, resulting in angina.

Paclitaxel and docetaxel: It can cause asymptomatic bradycardia, tachyarrhythmias, conduction disorders, and myocardial ischemia. The chronotropic effect is mediated either by histamine release or by a direct influence on the Purkinje system. The QT interval lengthening is the most significant pro-arrhythmogenic consequence of treatment.

Trastuzumab: Heart failure, and arrhythmias.

Tamoxifen: It causes alterations in cholesterol metabolism, which increases the risk of thromboembolic disease and stroke.

Pulmonary Toxicity

Drugs implicated: Cytotoxic antibiotics (e.g., bleomycin, mitomycin-C, and doxorubicin), nitrosoureas, alkylating agents, antimetabolites, plant alkaloids, biological response modifiers (e.g., GM-CSF, interleukin-2, interferon, BCG), others—taxol.

Bleomycin is most often implicated in the development of lung injury. The most frequent form of bleomycin lung injury is interstitial pneumonitis and fibrosis. Symptoms usually begin between four and ten weeks following treatment. The risk factors for bleomycin pulmonary toxicity include advanced age, a cumulative dosage >400–450 U, inadequate pulmonary reserves, radiation, uremia, and concurrent use of other anticancer medicines. Numerous mechanisms for its toxicity have been proposed, the most accepted being direct toxicity, which destroys type I pneumocytes and hyperplasia and dysplasia of type II pneumocytes and migration of fibroblasts and macrophages into the interstitium and alveoli, resulting in pulmonary fibrosis. Another mechanism suggested for bleomycin toxicity is the generation of superoxide and other free radicals, breaking nuclear DNA. The inspiration of high oxygen concentrations may accelerate the formation of these reactive radicals.

Mitomycin: It is associated with a wide variety of pulmonary syndrome, including bronchospasm during infusion, noncardiogenic pulmonary edema, acute interstitial pneumonitis, and pulmonary fibrosis.

Actinomycin: It causes pulmonary toxicity in the form of interstitial lung disease.

Busulfan: It causes pulmonary fibrosis; the mechanism remains unknown.

Cytosine arabinoside: It causes noncardiogenic pulmonary edema and pleural effusion.

Methotrexate: Noncardiogenic pulmonary edema, pulmonary fibrosis, pleurisy with acute chest pain, hypersensitivity pneumonitis has been described with its use.

Renal Toxicity

Drugs implicated: Nitrosoureas: others—bleomycin, cisplatin, cyclophosphamide, ifosfamide, methotrexate, mitomycin C, vincristine.

Cisplatin: This is the most often implicated drug. It results in coagulation necrosis of the proximal and distal renal tubular epithelial cells and collecting ducts, reducing glomerular filtration rate (GFR). It results in magnesium and potassium deficiency. A single dosage of cisplatin of 2 mg/kg or 50–75 mg/m^2 may cause nephrotoxicity, and acute renal failure can occur within 24 hours after treatment. By lowering the concentration of cisplatin in the renal tubules, adequate hydration with forced diuresis reduces the risk of renal damage.

Methotrexate: As a consequence of its intratubular precipitation, it produces acute nephrotoxicity.

Mitomycin: Chronic gradual increase in serum creatinine due to microangiopathic hemolytic anemia.

Ifosfamide: Acute tubular necrosis and renal failure.

Central Nervous System Toxicity

Chemotherapy-induced peripheral neuropathy (CIPN) is the most common neurologic complication. It develops gradually and worsens with subsequent cycles of treatment. It starts in a glove and stocking pattern and usually resolves with the withdrawal of the chemotherapy agents.

Vinca alkaloids: They are most commonly associated with neurotoxic effects. CIPN is the dose-limiting toxicity of vincristine. It may manifest itself as a disorder of the central, peripheral, or autonomic nervous systems. Peripheral neuropathies are characterized by peripheral paresthesias and a decrease in the strength of deep tendon reflexes. With treatment, the paresthesias progress proximally. Additionally, motor dysfunction and gait problems may ensue.

Taxanes: They are another class associated with CIPN. It is more commonly associated with paclitaxel than docetaxel. Single doses of paclitaxel exceeding 175 mg/m^2 predispose patients to CIPN.

Platinum compounds: Cisplatin, carboplatin, and oxaliplatin, all three are known to induce typical CIPN symptoms, with cisplatin and oxaliplatin having the highest rates. Cisplatin-induced CIPN is more often irreversible than oxaliplatin-induced CIPN. Both cisplatin and oxaliplatin have dose-limiting toxicity associated with CIPN.

Cytarabine: Irreversible cerebellar ataxia has been observed with high doses of cytarabine, and permanent neurological deficits can occur with continued treatment.

Hepatic Toxicity

Drugs implicated: Nitrosoureas; antimetabolites; cytotoxic antibiotics; others: 5-fluorouracil, vincristine, cisplatin.

Hepatotoxicity: Hepatotoxicity manifests clinically in various ways, including asymptomatic elevations in liver enzymes, overt cholestatic hepatitis, advancement to fibrosis and cirrhosis, malignant transformation, veno-occlusive disease/sinusoidal blockage, and fulminant hepatic failure.

Methotrexate: It is known to induce cirrhosis and fibrosis of the liver.

Cyclophosphamide: This has been associated with widespread hepatocellular damage.

Gastrointestinal Toxicity

Gastrointestinal toxicity is a frequent side effect of the majority of chemotherapy medicines and may manifest as nausea, vomiting, mucositis, or diarrhea. Chronic post-treatment chemotherapy-induced diarrhea and constipation have been reported in up to 49% of cancer survivors, with bouts lasting up to ten years after undergoing chemotherapy.

Hematological Toxicity

As discussed earlier, rapidly diving cells are more susceptible to chemotherapy myelosuppression is; thus, the most common side effect leading to anemia, thrombocytopenia, leucopenia and is reversible either completely or partially within 1 to 6 weeks of cessation.

QUESTION

Q. 1. Cumulative dose of various cardiotoxic chemotherapeutic agents and indications of ECHO?

FURTHER READING

1. Katzung BG. Cancer chemotherapy. Basic and Clinical Pharmacology, 14th edition. New York: McGraw-Hill Education LLC; 2017.
2. Tripathi KD. Anticancer drugs. In: Tripathi KD. Essentials of Medical Pharmacology, 8th edition. New Delhi: Jaypee Brothers Medical Publishers; 2019.

Enteral and Parenteral Nutrition

Vrinda Chauhan, Puneet Khanna

INTRODUCTION

Goals of nutrition support are to meet the energy requirements of the patients and provide adequate calories in order to correct the nutritional deficiencies, replace the ongoing losses during catabolism, support wound healing, and promote immune function.

DAILY ENERGY EXPENDITURE AND ESTIMATION OF CALORIC REQUIREMENTS

The nutrient fuels including carbohydrates, lipids, and proteins undergo oxidative metabolism to provide energy needs of the body. The heat generated during complete metabolism of a nutrient fuel equals the energy yield (in kcal/g) of that fuel **(Table 1)**.

While determining the energy needs of the critically ill patient, it is essential to consider the preadmission as well as current status of the patient including weight loss, a decline in physical performance, examination of muscle mass, and strength.

Regular reassessment thereafter includes the severity of the illness, the organ systems involved, and integrity of the gastrointestinal tract, so that the appropriate route of administration can be decided and adequate amounts of nutrients can be provided according to the individual needs of the body.

European Society for Clinical Nutrition and Metabolism (ESPEN) recommends that patients admitted to intensive care unit (ICU) >48 hours should be considered at high risk of malnutrition.

Several equations exist to estimate the resting energy requirements which are time-consuming and cumbersome, of which indirect calorimetry is considered the most accurate. It uses whole-body oxygen consumption (VO_2) and CO_2 production to measure resting energy requirements.

$$REE\ (kcal/min) = (3.6 \times VO_2) + (1.1 \times VCO_2) - 61(2)$$

A simple method to calculate the caloric requirements is using the body mass index (BMI) **(Table 2)**.

TABLE 1: Energy yield of nutrient fuels.

Fuel	Energy yield (kcal/g)
Lipid	9.1
Protein	4.0
Glucose	3.7

TABLE 2: Calorie needs based on body mass index (BMI).

BMI (kg/m²)	Energy (kcal/kg/day)
<15	35–40
15–19	30–35
20–25	20–25
26–29	15–17
29	15

Actual body weight can be used as long as the body weight is not above 125% of the ideal body weight, if it exceeds >125% then adjusted body weight is used.

$$\text{Adjusted wt (kg)} = [(\text{Actual} - \text{Ideal})] \text{ wt} \times 0.25 + \text{ideal wt}$$

Most of the daily energy requirements are provided by nonprotein calories from carbohydrates and lipids while protein intake is utilized for essential enzymatic and structural proteins **(Table 3)**.

Protein needs are calculated based on the ideal body weight (calculated by Hamwi method) **(Box 1 and Table 4)**.

In insulin-resistant critically ill patients, feeds should be initiated with calories in lower range in order to prevent hyperglycemia and infection associated with overfeeding.

TABLE 3: Basal nutritional requirements in critical illness.

Nutritional requirement	Per day (maintenance)
Water	30 mL/kg
Sodium (Na^+), chloride (Cl^-)	1–2 mmol/kg
Potassium (K^+)	0.8–1.2 mmol/kg
Calcium (Ca^{2+}), magnesium (Mg^{2+})	0.1 mmol/kg
Phosphate (PO_4^-)	0.2–0.5 mmol/kg
Energy	25 kcal/kg
Carbohydrate	2 g/kg
Protein	0.8–1.2 g/kg
Fat	1 g/kg

Note: These basal requirements may need to be increased in patients with burns and sepsis.

BOX 1: Calculation of ideal body weight.
- *Men:* 48 kg for first five feet + 2.7 kg for each inch above five feet
- *Women:* 45.4 kg for first five feet + 2.3 kg for each inch above five feet

INITIATION OF FEEDING

Enteral Nutrition

It is recommended that enteral nutrition should start within 48 hours of ICU admission, once hemodynamic stability is achieved.

There are two approaches:
1. Trophic feeding (increasing from 10–20 mL/hour, 1 kcal/mL)
2. Full feeding.

Enteral feeds can be given orally, or via nasogastric, nasojejunal, or through a surgical or endoscopic percutaneous gastrostomy. Most common route preferred is the nasogastric route. Presence of food in the bowel has a trophic influence on the bowel mucosa which preserves the integrity of the mucosa against translocation of pathogens into the portal and systemic circulation.

It also supports IgA producing immunocytes which comprise the gut-associated lymphoid tissue.

Q. When to discontinue nasogastric feed?
Ans. In patients complaining of vomiting, abdominal distention (signs of intolerance), and having high gastric residual volumes of >500 mL or who are at high risk of aspiration, enteral feeding can be provided through small bowel feeding tubes.

TABLE 4: Recommended daily protein intake for various scenarios.

Clinical condition	Protein needs (g/kg BW/day)
Normal	0.75
Critical illness	1.00–1.50
Acute renal failure (undialyzed)	0.80–1.00
Acute renal failure (dialyzed)	1.20–1.40
Peritoneal dialysis	1.30–1.50
Burn/sepsis	1.50–2.00
CVVHD	1.70–2.50

(CVVHD: continuous venovenous hemodiafiltration)

Contraindications

Absolute—complete bowel obstruction, bowel ischemia, ileus, hemodynamic instability requiring high dose vasopressors.

Composition of Feeding Formulas

Various feeding formulas with caloric densities of 1kcal/mL, 1.5 kcal/mL, and 2.0 kcal/mL are available, e.g., Osmolite, Osmolite HN, Isocal, Isocal HN, Twocal HN. Both nonprotein (85% of the caloric content) and protein calories are included in these formula feeds, with some formula feeds containing fiber, vitamins, antioxidants, and certain minerals.

Most commonly used is the formula with a caloric density of 1 kcal/mL with osmolality similar to plasma (300 mosm/L) **(Table 5)**.

Formulas with higher density (2 kcal/mL) are used in cases of severe physiological stress such as polytrauma and where volume restriction is required. These are hypertonic and may cause diarrhea.

TABLE 5: Exclusive and partial enteral nutrition.

Protein content: • Polymeric-intact proteins • Elemental (peptides) and semielemental (individual amino acids)	• Standard feeds: 35–40 g/L • High protein (HN)— 20% more proteins
Carbohydrates	40–70% of total calories
Fiber	Promotes viability of mucosa in large bowel
Lipid (omega-3 FAs-used in immune-modulating formula feeds)	30% of calories (polyunsaturated FAs from vegetable oils)
Conditionally essential nutrients	Immune modulation
Arginine	Not to be used in severe sepsis
Carnitine	Transports fatty acids for oxidation

(FAs: fatty acids; HN: hemagglutinin-neuraminidase)

Problems Associated with Tube Feedings (Flowchart 1)

- Tube occlusion
- Increased residual gastric volumes—(aspirates of >250 mL on multiple occasions or >500 mL on a single occasion, any signs of intolerance) IV metoclopramide 10 mg q6 hours for 3 days can be added (except in renal failure patients).
- *Diarrhea*—if all other causes of diarrhea are ruled out, patients can continue feeding with addition of soluble fiber to feeds or addition of loperamide 2-4 mg q6 hours (4-5 formed stools/day are normal while on tube feeds).
- *Constipation*—check for any signs of dehydration, increase free water intake, once any obstruction is ruled out, bisacodyl suppository or enema can be added.

Parenteral Nutrition

Parenteral nutrition must be initiated through a dedicated central venous catheter (CVC) or a peripherally inserted central catheter (PICC). Any contraindications to enteral feeding or complications arising due to it or where the energy requirements of the patient cannot be met via enteral route mandate initiation of parenteral nutrition **(Table 6)**.

COMPOSITION OF THE FORMULATIONS (TABLE 7)

Various preparations are available in bags containing premixed solutions containing 60% of the carbohydrates/glucose content, 40% lipid content (nonprotein calories), amino acids, electrolytes, vitamins, minerals, and trace elements.

Vitamins and trace elements are not present in parenteral preparations as they may cause instability of the preparations.

Flowchart 1: Problems associated with tube feedings.

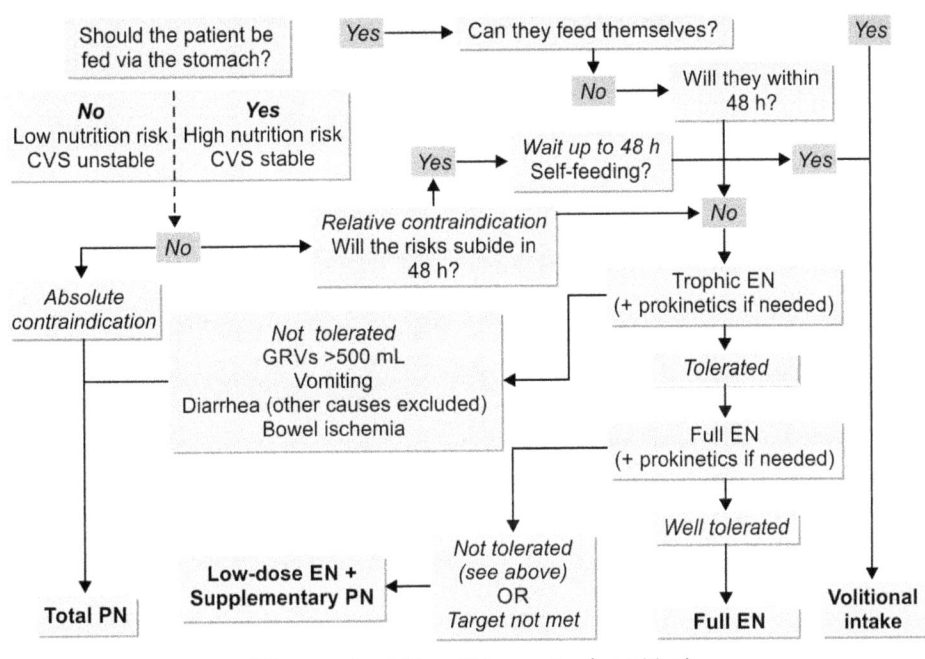

(EN: enteral nutrition; PN: parenteral nutrition)

TABLE 6: Advantages and disadvantages of enteral and parenteral nutrition.

	Advantages	Disadvantages
Enteral nutrition	• Preserves gut mucosal integrity • Less infectious complications • Less costly • Blunts hypermetabolic response	• Requires functional GI tract • Requires more time to attain target calories • Multiple contraindications
Parenteral nutrition	• Does not require functional GI tract • Full nutrition support can be given in <24 hours	• Requires CVC access • More infection related complications • Intestinal atrophy

(CVC: central venous catheter; GI: gastrointestinal tract)

TABLE 7: Composition of the formulations.

Carbohydrates	Glucose 40%, 50%, 60%, Rate <5 mg/kg/min (ESPEN)
Lipids	• Essential fatty acids, omega-3-FA, omega-6-FA • Delivered as triglycerides, Rate <1.5 mg/kg/day • Immunomodulated emulsions: Arginine, omega-3-FAs
Protein	1.3 g/kg/day (ESPEN)
Glutamine	Low protein intake (8 g/kg day) for the first 3 days and high protein intake (>0.8 g/kg/day) >3 days is suggested (PROTEINVENT study) lower 6 months mortality
Arginine	• Facilitates nitrogen transport and reduces protein catabolism • Not routinely recommended

(ESPEN: European Society for Clinical Nutrition and Metabolism; FA: fatty acids)

However, they are to be supplemented separately because of their role in modulation of immune and inflammatory response of the body.

Vitamin D_3 is recommended in critically ill patients with a severe deficiency with 25-hydroxyvitamin D plasma concentrations of <12.5 ng/mL. A single high dose of vitamin D_3 of 500,000 international units (IU) is administered within a week of admission (ESPEN recommendation).

COMPLICATIONS

They can be acute or chronic **(Table 8)**.

TABLE 8: Acute and chronic complications.

Acute	Chronic
Hyperglycemia/hypoglycemia	Liver disease
Metabolic acidosis	Metabolic bone disease
Hypophosphatemia and other electrolyte imbalance	
Hyperlipidemia	
CVC related	Infections
Extravasation and tissue necrosis	

(CVC: central venous catheter)

QUESTION

Q. 1. What is nutric score?

FURTHER READING

1. ESPEN guidelines latest.
2. Nutrition chapter in Paul Marino.

24. Minerals and Electrolytes

Puneet Khanna, Vrinda Chauhan

HYPERNATREMIA

Causes

- Loss of both sodium and water loss (water loss >sodium loss)
- Free water loss
- Retention of sodium and free water (sodium retention > free water)

Management

The management of hypernatremia is shown in **Box 1**.

Since the ongoing sodium and water losses are not considered in these equations frequent serum sodium monitoring is required.

HYPERNATREMIA WITH EUVOLEMIA

- *Central diabetes insipidus (DI):* Failure of release of antidiuretic hormone (ADH) from the posterior pituitary
- *Nephrogenic DI:* Impaired end-organ responsiveness to the action of ADH

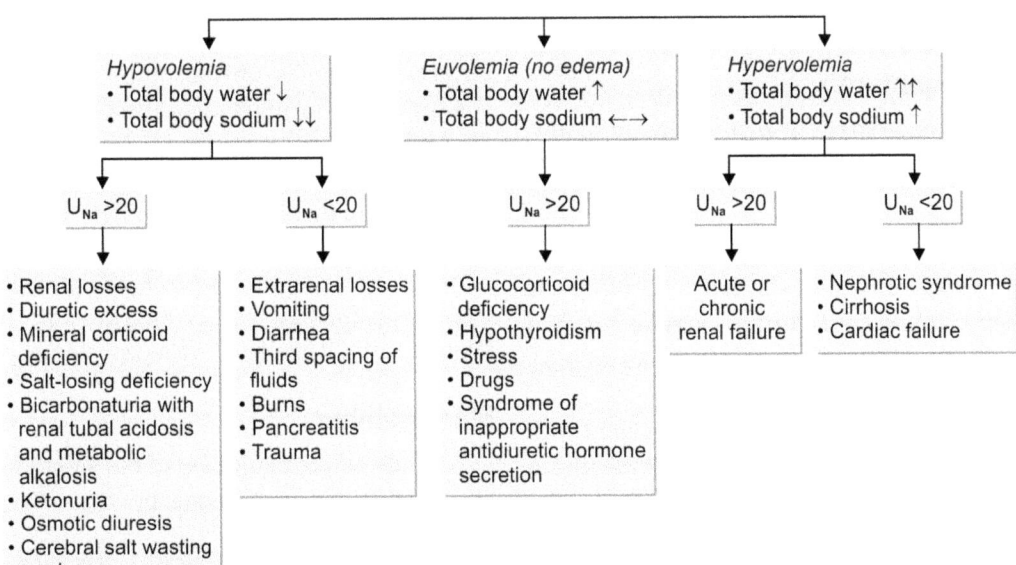

Flowchart 1: Assessment of volume status

- Hypovolemia
  - Total body water ↓
  - Total body sodium ↓↓
- Euvolemia (no edema)
  - Total body water ↑
  - Total body sodium ←→
- Hypervolemia
  - Total body water ↑↑
  - Total body sodium ↑

U_{Na} >20:
- Renal losses
- Diuretic excess
- Mineral corticoid deficiency
- Salt-losing deficiency
- Bicarbonaturia with renal tubal acidosis and metabolic alkalosis
- Ketonuria
- Osmotic diuresis
- Cerebral salt wasting syndrome

U_{Na} <20:
- Extrarenal losses
- Vomiting
- Diarrhea
- Third spacing of fluids
- Burns
- Pancreatitis
- Trauma

U_{Na} >20:
- Glucocorticoid deficiency
- Hypothyroidism
- Stress
- Drugs
- Syndrome of inappropriate antidiuretic hormone secretion

U_{Na} >20:
- Acute or chronic renal failure

U_{Na} <20:
- Nephrotic syndrome
- Cirrhosis
- Cardiac failure

Source: Jameson JL, Fauci AS, Kasper DL, Hauser SL, Longo DL, Loscalzo J. Harrison's Principles of Internal Medicine, 20th edition. New York: McGraw-Hill Education; 2015.

> **BOX 1:** Hypovolemic hypernatremia.
>
> *Volume resuscitation with hypotonic saline*
> - Any decrease in serum sodium levels leads to a decrease in extracellular fluid (ECV) which may be concerning due to the effects produced by decreased circulating volume and tissue hypoperfusion
>
> *Free water replacement*
> - Water deficit = Normal TBW − Current TBW [Normal TBW × (140/Current Serum Na)]
> - Replacement volume = Water deficit × 140/Na in IV fluid
> - Rate of sodium replacement should not exceed 0.5 mEq/L/h
> - Time required to reduce the plasma Na^+ to desired concentration at the desired rate, i.e., 0.5 mEq/L/h = Current $S.Na^+$ − Desired $S.Na^+$/0.5
> - And so the infusion rate = Replacement volume/time (Current $S.Na^+$ − Desired $S.Na^+$/0.5)

> **BOX 2:** Management of hypernatremia with euvolemia.
>
> - Diabetes insipidus (DI)—Once the diagnosis is confirmed (by fluid restriction) free water should be replaced slowly with sodium correction at ≤0.5 mEq/L/h
> - Vasopressin 2–5 units subcutaneously every 4–6 h is also used in central DI

TABLE 1: Hypervolemic hypernatremia.

Fluid management with diuresis with furosemide	1/4 normal saline can be used to partially replace the urinary losses in case of worsening hypernatremia

Management

The management of hypernatremia with euvolemia is given in **Box 2**.

■ HYPERVOLEMIC HYPERNATREMIA

Management

The management of hypervolemic hypernatremia is listed in **Table 1**.

■ HYPONATREMIA

Any value of serum sodium <135 mEq/L is hyponatremia. It is further classified as mild (130–134 mEq/L), moderate (120–130 mEq/L), and severe (<120 mEq/L).

Hyponatremia is usually associated with decreased serum osmolality unless the serum osmolality is normal or increased by the presence of other solutes which may withdraw water from the cells, e.g., glucose in the presence of insulin deficiency, mannitol, and glycine.

Pseudohyponatremia occurs in the presence of high lipid or protein concentrations.

■ HYPOTONIC HYPONATREMIA

It occurs when there is an excess of free water as compared to sodium in extracellular fluid and is usually related to the release of ADH.

In response to an increase in serum osmolality, ADH is released from posterior pituitary which causes water reabsorption in distal renal tubules. This response normally is suppressed at plasma sodium levels of <135 mEq/L.

But in conditions such as decreased BP (baroreceptor mediated) or any physiological stress there is a nonosmotic release of ADH even at plasma sodium levels of <135 mEq/L, which can further lead to aggravation of hyponatremia. It may result in encephalopathy.

Management

It depends on the acuteness of the situation and whether it is symptomatic or not.

■ HYPOVOLEMIC HYPONATREMIA

Extracellular fluid volume (ECF) volume is replaced with isotonic saline.

It occurs when there is sodium loss with excess water retention due to nonosmotic ADH release. It can occur with the use of thiazide diuretics, primary adrenal insufficiency causing renal sodium wasting due to mineralocorticoid deficiency, cerebral salt wasting.

HYPERVOLEMIC HYPONATREMIA

It mainly occurs in conditions where there is both sodium and water retention with water retention exceeding sodium retention in advanced heart failure, cirrhosis, and renal failure. The renal sodium is >20 mEq/L in renal failure and <20 mEq/L in heart failure and cirrhosis.

Treatment of the underlying cause along with fluid restriction and use of loop diuretics.

Management

The management of hyponatremia is given in **Table 2**.

POTASSIUM

It is an important intracellular ion that plays a key role in the resting membrane potential of the excitable tissue (nerves and muscles). So any disturbance in the potassium balance can lead to life-threatening cardiac arrhythmias in the perioperative period.

Flowchart 2: Syndrome of inappropriate antidiuretic hormone.

```
                          Hyponatremia
                               ↓
                    Measure serum osmolality
         ┌─────────────────────┼─────────────────────┐
         ↓                     ↓                     ↓
      Normal                  Low                 Elevated
   (280–290 mOsm/kg)      (<280 mOsm/kg)       (>290 mOsm/kg)
         ↓                     ↓                     ↓
  Pseudohyponatremia    Assess volume status   Hypertonic hyponatremia
  1. Hyperlipidemia                            1. Hyperglycemia
  2. Hyperprotinemia                           2. Hypertonic infusions
                                                  (mannitol, glycine)
         ┌─────────────────────┼─────────────────────┐
         ↓                     ↓                     ↓
   Hypervolemic            Hypovolemic            Euvolemic
   • Congestive heart failure                    • SIADH (urine osm >100 mOsm/kg)
   • Decompensated cirrhosis                     • Psychogenic polydipsia (urine osm
   • Nephrotic syndorme                            <100 mOsm/kg)
                                                  • Beer potomania
                           Check urine sodium    • Hypothyroidism
                           concentration         • Cortisol deficiency
         ↓                     ↓
   <15 mEq/L              >20 mEq/L
   (Extra-renal losses)   (Renal losses)
   1. Vomiting, diarrhea, fistulas   1. Recent diuretics (especially thiazides)
   2. Burns, sweating                2. Adrenal insufficiency
   3. Pancreatitis, peritonitis      3. Salt losing nephropathy/cerebral salt wasting
```

(SIADH: syndrome of inappropriate antidiuretic hormone)

TABLE 2: Management of hyponatremia depends on the underlying causes.

Acute hyponatremia or moderate symptomatic hyponatremia	Severe hyponatremia	Chronic asymptomatic hyponatremia
• 3% hypertonic saline is used, with an initial rate of 1 mL/kg/hour with a target of increasing sodium by 1 mEq/L/hour for the initial 3–4 hours, along with monitoring of electrolytes • Infusion rate should be adjusted sodium correction of not more >10 mEq/L/hour in first 24 hours	• Bolus of 3% hypertonic saline is given with the target of acutely increasing sodium by 2–3 mEq/L • If there is no improvement in neurological status this treatment is repeated once or twice at 10 minutes • After this treatment is continued with the target correction of not >10 mEq/L in first 24 hours	Does not need immediate correction—fluid restriction, ADH antagonists, and loop diuretics are used

The total body potassium is 50–55 mEq/kg bodyweight. Since plasma constitutes only 20% of the ECF, the potassium content of the plasma is approximately 15 mEq which is 0.4% of the total body potassium.

A total body deficit of 200–400 mEq produces a decrease in plasma level of 1 mEq/L.

A total body excess of 100–200 mEq produces a 1 mEq/L increase in plasma levels.

Hypokalemia

Serum potassium levels of <3.5 mEq/L.

TABLE 3: Causes and mechanism of hypokalemia.

GI loss	Renal loss
Vomiting	Mineralocorticoid excess
Diarrhea	Glucocorticoid excess
Fistulas	• Loop or thiazide diuretics • Renal tubular acidosis • Hypomagnesemia-causing impaired potassium reabsorption in renal tubules • Osmotic substances—glucose, urea, mannitol

(GI: gastrointestinal)

Causes (Table 3)
- *Inadequate intake:* Anorexia nervosa, alcohol, malnutrition
- *Potassium depletion:* GI loss, renal loss
- *Transcellular shift:* From extracellular to intracellular compartment—β2 agonists, insulin therapy acute alkalosis, lithium overdose.

Clinical Manifestations

Severe (<2.5 mEq/L)-severe muscle weakness; ECG abnormalities include prominent U waves, flattening and inversion of T waves, and prolongation of QT interval and arrhythmias (atrial fibrillation and ventricular extrasystoles).

Management

The management of hypokalemia is given in **Box 3**.

Hyperkalemia

Serum potassium levels >5.5 mEq/L.

Causes
- Excess intake—excess K^+ treatment, blood transfusion
- *Failure to excrete:*

BOX 3: Management of hypokalemia.
- Firstly, rule out any condition causing transcellular shifts, and treat that condition
- *Potassium replacement:* Potassium chloride (KCl) 1–2 mEq/mL preparation available in ampoules. They are highly hyperosmolar (4000 mOsm/kg) so should be always diluted
  – Standard method—20 mEq of KCl added to 100 mL saline and infused over 1 hour (maximum rate of 20 mEq/hour but doses of 40 mEq/hour may be necessary). Solutions of concentration >40 mEq/L should be given through central venous catheter
  – Continuous ECG monitoring along with electrolyte monitoring in every 1–2 hours should be done with ongoing correction
- *Refractory hypokalemia:* Consider magnesium replacement, strongly in case of refractory hypokalemia (magnesium deficiency promotes hypokalemia refractory to potassium replacement)

BOX 4: Management of hyperkalemia.
- *Antagonism of cardiac toxicity*—if S.K$^+$ > 6.5 mEq/L with ECG changes
  – Administer IV 10% Calcium gluconate 10 mL over 3 minutes and repeat after 5 minutes if necessary (onset time within a few minutes, duration 30–60 minutes)/Calcium chloride is used in case of circulatory shock
- *Intracellular potassium shift*—if S. K$^+$ levels >6.0 mEq/L
  – Administer insulin 10–20 units in 50 mL of 50% dextrose
  – (Onset within 10–2 minutes, duration 4–6 hours)
  – Nebulization with 2.5 mg salbutamol
  – Hyperventilation
  – Give NaHCO$_3$—1 mEq/kg in case S. K$^+$ levels >6.5 mEq/L
- *Increase renal excretion*—in case of moderate to severe hyperkalemia
  – IV furosemide 20–40 mg IV
  – Volume expansion with isotonic saline
  – Fludrocortisone
- *Other routes of potassium elimination*—Any sustained hyperkalemia
  – GI resin exchange
  – Sodium polystyrene sulfonate 15–30 g PO or per rectum
- In case of moderate to severe hyperkalemia with oliguria
  – Hemodialysis

- Mineralocorticoid deficiency
- Drugs causing mineralocorticoid blockade-spironolactone, ACE-1, and ARBs
- Drugs causing sodium channel blockade-amiloride, trimethoprim
- Tubulointerstitial nephritis
- Renal obstruction
- Transcellular shift—succinylcholine, insulin deficiency, acute acidosis, reperfusion of ischemic tissues.

Clinical Manifestations

Muscle weakness, paralysis, altered cardiac conduction with ECG changes as potassium levels increase
- *5.5–6.5 mEq/L:* Tall peaked T waves
- *6.5–7.5 mEq/L:* Prolonged PR interval
- *7.5 mEq/L:* Widened QRS
- *9.0 mEq/L:* Sine wave pattern, bradycardia, ventricular tachycardia, increased risk of cardiac arrest.

Management

The management of hyperkalemia is shown in **Box 4**.

CALCIUM

It is the most abundant ion in the human body. Approximately 99% is present in the bones and rest 1% in ECF. Calcium metabolism is under the control of parathyroid hormone, 1,25-OH vitamin D calcitriol and calcitonin.

It is present as three fractions in plasma:
1. Free/ionized calcium—45%
2. Bound to albumin—40%

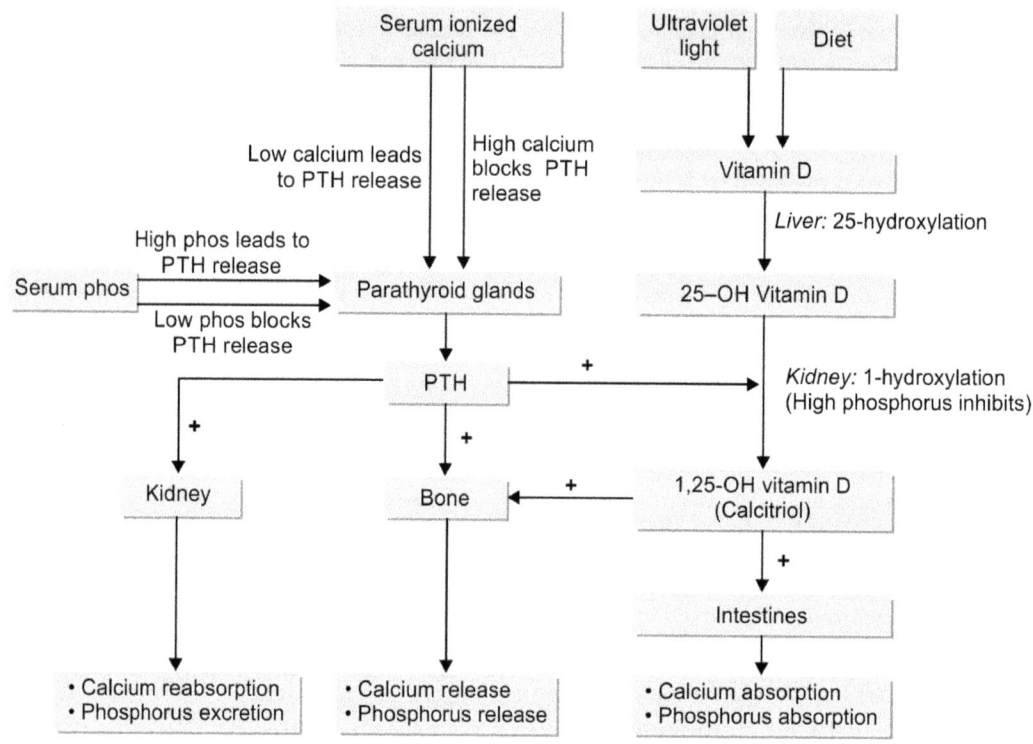

Flowchart 3: Regulation of calcium and phosphorus in the body.

(phos: phosphorus; PTH: parathyroid hormone)

3. Bound to multiple organic and inorganic anions such as sulfate, phosphate, lactate and citrate—15%

Management of Hypocalcemia

Mechanism and causes (Table 4):
- A bolus dose of 200 mg elemental calcium is given in 100 mL of isotonic saline over 10 minutes, followed by continuous infusion of 1-2 mg/kg/h for 6-12 hours (with monitoring for ionized calcium hourly for first few hours).
- Calcium should preferably be given through central vein since it is hyperosmolar. (Osmolarity of 10% calcium gluconate is 680 mOsm/L and that of calcium chloride is 2,000 mOsm/L).

Hypercalcemia

It occurs when calcium influx from GIT and/or bone outweighs the efflux from bone or excretion via the kidneys. Corrected calcium of >10.3 mg/dL or ionized calcium of >5.2 mg/dL.

Symptoms of hypercalcemia occurs at levels >12 mg/dL and are more severe with rapid elevations **(Tables 5 and 6)**.

Causes

The causes of hypercalcemia are shown in **Table 7**.

Management

The management of hypercalcemia is shown in **Box 5**.

Chapter 24: Minerals and Electrolytes

TABLE 4: Causes and mechanisms of hypocalcemia.

• Hypoparathyroidism • Pseudohypoparathyroidism • Decreased vitamin D activity	• Posthyperparathyroid/thyroid surgery • Reduced receptor response • Hyperphosphatemia/sunlight or dietary deficiency/anticonvulsants	Due to reduced regulatory hormones
• Massive transfusion • Cell lysis • Pancreatitis	Calcium chelation	
Ca prostate, breast	Increased bone deposition	
Acute respiratory alkalosis	Decreased ionic fraction	
Hypoalbuminemia	Reduced bound calcium	
Endotoxemic shock	Elevated level of procalcitonin	

TABLE 5: Symptoms of hypercalcemia.

Neuromuscular irritability	Cardiac
• Circumoral and peripheral paresthesia • Chvostek sign (facial twitching induced by tapping on the facial nerve) • Trousseau sign (forearm muscular spasm induced by inflating a pressure cuff) • Muscle cramps • Laryngospasm • Tetany • Seizure	• Impaired inotropy • Prolonged QT • Ventricular fibrillation • Heart block

TABLE 6: Manifestations of more severe hypercalcemia.

• Neurologic symptoms • Drowsiness, weakness, depression, lethargy, coma	• GI symptoms • Constipation, nausea, vomiting, anorexia, peptic ulcers	• Renal manifestations • Nephrogenic diabetes insipidus—which may further aggravate hypercalcemia through dehydration—and renal stones

TABLE 7: Causes of hypercalcemia.

Increased PTH	• Primary hyperparathyroidism • Secondary and tertiary hyperparathyroidism
Malignancy	• PTH related peptide secretion • Osteolytic metastases • Calcitriol production
• Excess vitamin D • Decreased renal excretion	• Ectopic production, excess intake • Thiazide diuretics
Increased bone turnover	Hyperthyroidism, immobilization
Increased calcium intake	Milk alkali syndrome

(PTH: parathyroid hormone)

PHOSPHORUS

Hypophosphatemia

Hypophosphatemia is a serum concentration of phosphate <2.5 mg/dL.

It causes intracellular shift (most common), increased renal excretion, reduced reabsorption from gastrointestinal tract (GIT).

Flowchart 4: Evaluation of hypercalcemia.

```
Hypercalcemia
(corrected calcium >10.3 mg/dL OR ionized calcium >5.2 mg/dL)
```

- **PTH appropriately decreased** → PTH-independent mechanism; consider checking vitamin D levels
  - **Not elevated:**
    - *PTH-related peptide:*
      - Humoral hypercalcemia of malignancy (elevated PTHrP)
    - *Bone resorption:*
      - Osteolytic malignancy
      - Paget's disease
      - Immobilization
      - Hyperthyroidism
      - Adrenal insufficiency
    - *Decreased Ca^{2+} excretion:*
      - Volume depletion
      - Thiazide diuretics
      - Milk-alkali syndrome
  - **Abnormally elevated:**
    - *Excess 25-OH:*
      - Vitamin D intoxication
    - *Excess 1,25-OH:*
      - Granulomatous disease (sarcoidosis)
      - Lymphoma
      - Calcitriol overdose
      - Acromegaly

- **PTH elevated or inappropriately normal** → Hyperparathyroid state:
  - Primary hyperparathyroidism (85% adenomas, 14% hyperplasia, 1% carcinoma) — 24 hours urine calcium >200 mg
  - Familial hypocalciuric hypercalcemia — 24 hours urine calcium <200 mg
  - Tertiary hyperparathyroidism (after renal transplantation)
  - Lithium use

(PTH: parathyroid hormone; PTHrP: parathyroid hormone-related peptide)

BOX 5: Management of hypercalcemia.

- *Isotonic saline:* 200–500 mL/h to maintain urine output of 100–150 mL/h
- *Furosemide:* 40–80 mg IV every 2 hours to maintain urine output of 100–150 mL/h
- *Calcitonin:* 4 units/kg by SC or IM every 12 hours
- *Glucocorticoids:* Oral prednisolone (20–100 mg daily) or IV hydrocortisone (200–400 mg daily) for 3–5 years
- *Bisphosphonates:* First line treatment for severe hypercalcemia takes 2 days for effect; zoledronate 4–8 mg IV over 15 minutes or pamidronate 90 mg IV over 2 hours (can be repeated in 10 hours)
- Dialysis in patients with renal failure

Causes

The causes of hypophosphatemia are shown in **Table 8**.

Mostly the hypophosphatemia is clinically silent, in most severe forms (levels <1.5 mg/dL), features may include rhabdomyolysis, leucocyte dysfunction, cardiac and respiratory failure, seizures, hypotension and coma.

Management

Intravenous phosphate replacement is given in moderate to severe hypophosphatemia only, as it may cause severe hypocalcemia.

The management of hypophosphatemia is shown in **Table 9**.

If plasma potassium is >4.0 mEq, sodium phosphate can be used, if plasma K^+ is <4 mEq—potassium phosphate can be used.

Hyperphosphatemia
Causes

The causes of hyperphosphatemia are shown in **Table 10**.

TABLE 8: Causes of hypophosphatemia.

Internal redistribution	Increased urinary excretion	Decreased intestinal absorption
• Respiratory alkalosis • Refeeding • Hormones • Sepsis • Internal redistribution Hungry bone syndrome	• Hyperparathyroidism • Disorders of vitamin D metabolism • Renal transplant • Volume expansion • Malabsorption renal tubular defects • Alcoholism • Metabolic or respiratory acidosis	• Dietary restriction • Excess antacids • Vitamin deficiency • Chronic diarrhea

TABLE 9: Management of hypophosphatemia.

Serum phosphate (mg/dL)	40–60 kg	61–80 kg	81–120 kg
<1	30 mmol	40 mmol	50 mmol
1–1.7	20 mmol	30 mmol	40 mmol
1.8–2.5	10 mmol	15 mmol	20 mmol

Sodium phosphate: PO_4 content—93 mg (3 mmol/mL), Na^+ - 4.0 mEq
Potassium phosphate: PO_4 content—93 mg (3 mmol/mL), K^+ - 4.3 mEq

TABLE 10: Causes of hyperphosphatemia.

Increased endogenous load	Increased exogenous load	Reduced urinary excretion	Pseudohyperphosphatemia
• Increased endogenous load • Tumor lysis syndrome • Rhabdomyolysis • Bowel infarction • Malignant hyperthermia • Hemolysis	• Increased exogenous load • Acidosis • IV infusion • Oral supplementation • Vitamin D intoxication	• Reduced urinary excretion • Renal failure • Hypoparathyroidism acromegaly	• Pseudohyperphosphatemia • Bisphosphonate therapy • Magnesium deficiency • Multiple myeloma • In vitro hemolysis hypertriglyceridemia

(IV: intravenous)

Management

The management of hyperphosphatemia is shown in **Box 6**.

MAGNESIUM

It is present in intracellular compartment. Over half of it is present in bone and only 0.3% fraction is present in the plasma. Total serum magnesium levels are-1.7-2.4 mg/dL out of which ionized magnesium levels are 0.8-1.1 mEq/L.

Only 67% of the magnesium (Mg) in plasma is in the ionized (active) form, and the remaining 33% is either bound to plasma proteins or chelated with divalent anions such as phosphate and sulfate.

Hypomagnesemia (Table 11)

Clinical Manifestations

It may vary depending upon associated hypokalemia/hypocalcemia or hypophosphatemia **(Table 12)**.

Magnesium Preparations

50% $MgSO_4$ solution (500 mg/mL) should be diluted to 10% (100 mg/mL), or 20% (200 mg/mL) for IV use due to high osmolarity of 4,000 mOsm/L.

Management

The management of magnesium preparations is shown in **Box 7**.

Hypermagnesemia

Usually uncommon, unless renal insufficiency is present since kidneys can excrete a large load of magnesium, so most of the cases are iatrogenic only.

Symptoms relating to different serum levels of magnesium are as follows:
- *5-7 mg/dL:* Therapeutic levels in the treatment of preeclampsia
- *5-10 mg/dL:* Impaired cardiac conduction (widened QRS, long PR), nausea
- *20-34 mg/dL:* Sedation, reduced neuromuscular transmission with

---

BOX 6: Management of hyperphosphatemia.
- Enhanced binding of phosphate in upper GIT
- Sucralfate or aluminum containing antacids
- Calcium acetate tablets in patients with hypocalcemia raises serum calcium and lowers phosphate levels
- Hemodialysis—in patients with renal failure, but rarely necessary

(GIT: gastrointestinal tract)

TABLE 11: Causes of hypomagnesemia.

• Inadequate gastrointestinal uptake (24 hours urine magnesium <2 mEq or FE Mag <2%) • Malnutrition • Prolonged vomiting or diarrhea • Intestinal fistula • Pancreatitis • Prolonged nasogastric suction • Malabsorption syndromes • Small bowel syndrome • Primary intestinal hypomagnesemia	• Increased renal losses (24 hours urine magnesium >2 mEq or Fe Mag >2%) • Chronic parenteral fluid therapy • Hypercalcemia and hypercalciuria • *Osmotic diuresis drugs:* Alcohol, loop and thiazide diuretics, aminoglycosides, cisplatin, amphotericin, cyclosporine, foscarnet • Phosphate depletion • Hungry bone syndrome • Postobstructive nephropathy • Renal transplantation • Polyuric phase of acute kidney injury • Primary hyperparathyroidism • Bartter and Gitelman syndrome

---

TABLE 12: Clinical manifestations of hypomagnesemia.

Neuromuscular	Metabolic	Cardiovascular	Musculoskeletal
• Trousseau sign • Chvostek signs • Vertigo • Seizures • Weakness	• Carbohydrate intolerance • Hyperinsulinemia • Atherosclerosis	• Wide QRS • Prolonged PR • T-wave inversion • Ventricular arrhythmias	• Osteoporosis • Osteomalacia

> **BOX 7:** Management of hypomagnesemia.
>
> - If symptomatic or ECG changes present—IV magnesium replacement is started
>   - 1–2 g MgSO$_4$ over 15 minutes followed by an infusion of 6g MgSO$_4$ in 1 L fluid over 24 hours
>   - Continuous infusion may be required for 3–7 days to replenish total body stores
>   - Magnesium levels to be assessed every 24 hours with a target to maintain levels <2.5 mEq/L
>   - Check for deep tendon reflexes, to detect developing hypermagnesemia
> - In asymptomatic cases with no ECG changes
>   - *Mild hypomagnesemia:* 240 mg PO elemental Mg^{2+} per day in divided doses
>   - *Severe hypomagnesemia:* up to 720 mg PO elemental Mg^{2+} per day in divided doses
>   - *In case of diarrhea:* 2–6 g IV MgSO$_4$ infused at 1 g/hour or less
>
> (ECG: electrocardiogram)

hypoventilation, reduced tendon reflexes, and muscle weakness

- *24–48 mg/dL:* Diffuse vasodilation with hypotension, bradycardia
- *48–72 mg/dL:* Areflexia, coma, respiratory paralysis

Management

- Hemodialysis in case of severe hypermagnesemia
- IV calcium gluconate to antagonize CVS effects (effects are transient)
- Aggressive fluid administration along with diuretics if renal function is preserved

OTHER MINERALS

Iron

The causes, effects, and treatment for the iron for the iron deficiency are shown in **Table 13**.

TABLE 13: Iron deficiency—causes, effects, and treatment.

Causes of deficiency	Effects	Treatment
• Most common cause of deficiency includes inadequate dietary intake • Increased requirements in pregnancy and blood loss • Interference with iron absorption from GIT	• Decreased iron stores • Decreased plasma concentrations of ferritin • Decreased erythrocyte content of iron	• Prophylaxis in pregnant, lactating, low birth weight infants—15–30 mg daily orally • Therapeutic dose—200 mg daily in three divided doses • Parenteral-in patients who cannot tolerate or do not respond to oral therapy • Iron dextran injection 50 mg/mL (IM/IV) • IV-A dose of 500 mg infused over 5–10 minutes
Copper	• Present in ceruloplasmin • Constituent of enzymes such as β-hydroxylase and cytochrome C oxidase • Catalyst in storage and release of iron from hemoglobin • Formation of connective tissues, hematopoiesis, and function of CNS	Copper supplements should be given in prolonged hyperalimentation

Contd...

Contd...

Causes of deficiency	Effects	Treatment
Zinc	Enzymatic cofactor required for cell growth, synthesis of nucleic acid, carbohydrates and proteins	Deficiency occurs during periods of increased requirements so should be supplemented in growing children, pregnancy, lactation, infection
Chromium	It is a cofactor complex with insulin involved in normal glucose metabolism	• Diabetes like syndrome • Peripheral neuropathy • Encephalopathy
Selenium	• Constituent of metabolically important enzymes like glutathione peroxidase in erythrocytes • Antioxidant	• Can cause cardiomyopathy
Manganese	• Concentrated in mitochondria • Influences synthesis of mucopolysaccharides, stimulates hepatic synthesis of cholesterol and fatty acids • Cofactor of various enzymes	• Unknown deficiency • Should be supplemented during prolonged hyperalimentation
Molybdenum	• Constituent of enzymes • Present in bones, liver, and kidneys	• Deficiency rare • Excess can cause gout like syndrome

(GIT: gastrointestinal tract)

FURTHER READING

1. Pandya S. Practical Guidelines on Fluid Therapy, 2nd edition.
2. Todd CA. ASPEN Fluids, Electrolytes, and Acid-base Disorders Handbook, 2nd edition.

CHAPTER 25

Intravenous Fluids

Anil Kumar, Debyani Dey, Vrinda Chauhan

INTRODUCTION

An average adult body consists of approximately 60% water, with some variation depending on the age, gender, and body composition of different tissues.

Adipose tissues contain a lesser amount of water in comparison to the other tissues, accounting for the difference in total body water among lean (75%) and obese (45%) individuals, males and females, the young and the elderly population **(Tables 1 and 2)**.

DISTRIBUTION OF FLUIDS ACROSS VARIOUS COMPARTMENTS

Laws Governing Fluid and Electrolyte Movement

Diffusion

It is the process by which the solute particles fill the available solvent volume from areas of high concentration to low concentration.

$$J = -DA\left(\frac{\Delta c}{\Delta x}\right)$$

J is the net rate of diffusion, D is the diffusion coefficient, A is the cross-sectional area available for diffusion, and $\frac{\Delta c}{\Delta x}$ is the concentration gradient.

Osmosis

The hydrostatic pressure required to resist the movement of water across a semipermeable membrane to the region of higher solute

TABLE 1: Age-related variation in total body water and ECF as per percent of body weight.

Age	TBW%	ECF%	Blood volume%
Neonate	80	45	9
6 months	70	35	
1 year	60	28	
5 years	60	25	8
Young adult (male)	60	22	7
Young adult (female)	50	20	7
Elderly	50	20	

Note: Multiply by 10 for mL/kg
(TBW: total body water; ECF: extracellular fluid)

TABLE 2: Distribution of fluids across various compartments.

Intracellular 55%	Extracellular 45%			
	Functional ECF 27.5%		Sequestrated 17.5%	
	Interstitial 20%	Intravascular 7.5%	Transcellular 2.5%	Bone and dense connective tissue 15%
	Subglycocalyx 2%	Plasma 5.5%		

concentration is osmotic pressure (depends on the number of osmotically active particles in a solution).

$$P = \frac{nRT}{V}$$

P is the osmotic pressure, n is the number of particles, R is the gas constant, R is the absolute temperature, and V is the volume.

Osmolality

Number of osmoles (each containing 6×10^{23} particles of a specific substance) present in 1 kg of solvent (used for solutions containing a different type of particles).

Normal body osmolality is 285–290 mOsm/kg.

Serum osmolality =

$$(2 \times Na) + \left(\frac{Glucose}{18}\right) + \left(\frac{Urea}{2.8}\right)$$

Osmolarity

It is the number of osmoles per liter of solution (unaffected by temperature).

Oncotic Pressure

Component of total osmotic pressure that is due to large molecular weight particles, like albumin, globulins, fibrinogen (total plasma osmotic pressure is 5545 mm Hg and Normal plasma oncotic pressure is 25–28 mm Hg).

FLUIDS

Fluids are the drugs with specific indications, given the various physiological effects they can produce on the administration of large volumes.

Fluids administered exogenously move through various barriers to distribute across various body compartments, depending on their composition.

Types of intravenous fluids can be grossly divided into:
- Crystalloids
- Colloids

Crystalloids

They are solutions of electrolytes in water that can diffuse freely from intravascular to interstitial fluid compartments.

They can further be classified according to tonicity as hypertonic, isotonic, and hypotonic or depending on the composition.

Indications

To replace free water and electrolyte and for volume expansion preoperatively or during resuscitation.

The types of crystalloids solutions are given in **Table 3**.

0.9% Sodium Chloride

- It has slightly higher osmolarity than plasma (Na⁺ 154 mEq/L vs. 140 mEq/L and Cl⁻ 154 mEq/L vs. 103 mEq/L).
- Sodium distributes freely across the ECF and is the principal determinant of extracellular volume.
- Only 25% of the infused volume remains in the intravascular compartment rest moves to the interstitial fluid compartment.
- There is a slight rise in extracellular volume due to the hypertonic nature of the fluid which causes a fluid shift from intracellular to the extracellular fluid.

Dilutional decrease in hematocrit and albumin occurs with large volumes.

Hyperchloremic metabolic acidosis (SID of 0.9% NaCl is zero which causes reduced plasma pH) and reduced renal perfusion (due to Cl⁻ mediated vasoconstriction).

Interstitial edema occurs by increased sodium load leading to increased tonicity of interstitial fluid causing sodium retention by suppressing renin-angiotensin aldosterone axis.

TABLE 3: Types of crystalloids solutions.

	Plasma	0.9% saline	Compound sodium lactate (lactate buffered solution)	Ringer's lactate (lactate buffered solution)	Ionosteril® (acetate buffered solution)	Sterofundin ISO® (acetate and malate buffered solution)	Plasma-lyte 148® (acetate and gluconate buffered solution)
Sodium (mmol/L)	136–145	154	129	130	137	145	140
Potassium (mmol/L)	3.5–5.0		5	4	4	4	5
Magnesium (mmol/L)	0.8–1.0				1.25	1	1.5
Calcium (mmol/L)	2.2–2.6		2.5	3	1.65	2.5	
Chloride (mmol/L)	98–106	154	109	109	110	127	98
Acetate (mmol/L)					36.8	24	27
Gluconate (mmol/L)							23
Lactate (mmol/L)			29	28			
Malate (mmol/L)						5	
eSID (mEq/L)	42		27	28	36.8	25.5	50
Theoretical osmolarity (mOsmol/L)	291	308	278	273	291	309	295
Actual or measured osmolality (mOsmol/kg H_2O)	287	286	256	256	270	Not stated	271
pH	7.35–7.45	4.5–7	5–7	5.0–7	6.9–7.9	5.1–5.9	4–8

So these days it is not routinely recommended in perioperative period.

Indicated in the following situations:
- As drug vehicle
- Cerebral edema

Replacement of pre-existing total body Na^+ or Cl^- deficits needs in several disorders, such as in hyponatremia, diabetic ketoacidosis, gastric outlet obstruction, etc.

Hypertonic Saline

- Available as 0.8%, 3%, 7.5% and 23.4% solutions.
- Increased tonicity draws water out of cells into the extracellular space causing

plasma volume expansion while limiting the volume infused.
- Mainly used for correction of hypoosmolar hyponatremia raised ICP.
- Concentrations >7.5% may cause endothelial damage and 11.7% NaCl may be used as a sclerosant agent (should be administered through central vein).

Ringers Solutions

Ringer lactate: These are electrically neutral solutions with decreased sodium content in order to compensate for the sodium released from the sodium lactate, and reduced chloride content to compensate for negatively charged lactate ions.

Ringer acetate: It is meant for use in patients with liver disease who are unable to metabolize lactate.

Indications: In shock-like states to correct severe hypovolemia
- Diarrhea
- Burns, sepsis
- Perioperative fluid therapy as replacement fluid
- Pediatric patients.
  No significant effect on acid-base balance.
  Calcium in ringer fluids can bind to transfused packed red blood cells (PRBCs) if the total volume infused exceeds 50% of the volume of PRBCs

Balanced Salt Solutions

These solutions have lower measured osmolality than plasma (265 mOsm/kg) and are mildly hypotonic.

Reduced anionic content is compensated by addition of buffers like lactate, gluconate, or acetate

After administration buffer is metabolized to HCO_3^- to enter the citric acid cycle, the following scenarios take place:

- Lactate undergoes hepatic oxidation or gluconeogenesis to yield HCO_3^-.
- Acetate present in trace quantities is metabolized rapidly by liver, muscle, heart to yield bicarbonate.
- Gluconate is converted to glucose to enter the citric acid cycle.
- Excretion of excess water and electrolytes is more rapid because of decreased tonicity-induced antidiuretic hormone (ADH) suppression leading to diuresis.
- pH is maintained, HCO_3^- is maintained/slightly elevated.
- Lactated solutions should be avoided in renal failure.

Dextrose Solutions

Available as D5% (50 g glucose/L), D10% (100 g glucose/L), D25% (250 g glucose/L), D50% (500 g glucose/L), DNS—50 g/1L with NaCl (154 mEq)

$$50 \text{ g glucose/L} = 170 \text{ Kcal/L}$$

These solutions are used as a source of free water and as a source of metabolic substrate that provides calories.

After administration, dextrose is taken up by the cells which leave the free water in the plasma and may cause intracellular swelling.

The osmolality of dextrose fluids is similar to that of plasma, but it becomes hypotonic as soon as the dextrose is taken up by the cells.

It causes dilution of plasma electrolytes and osmolality.

To be used with caution as it increases risk of hyponatremia

Addition of 0.9% NaCl to dextrose increases the osmolality of the plasma which may cause cellular dehydration when administered in excess.

Indications

- Correction of hypoglycemia
- Correction of hypernatremia and hyperkalemia

- As for maintenance fluids in pediatric patients and adults
- Used along with IV insulin to diabetic patients to avoid hypoglycemia.

To be avoided in the following situations:
- Conditions like cerebral edema/neurosurgical procedures
- Hypovolemia.

Colloids (Table 4)

Colloid is defined as large molecules or ultramicroscopic particles of homogenous noncrystalline substance dispersed in a second substance typically isotonic saline or a balanced crystalloid.

Molecules above 70 kDa do not pass through endothelial glycocalyx and are thus retained in the plasma leading to the plasma volume expanding effect.

They have higher colloid oncotic pressure and minimize transcapillary filtration at low capillary hydrostatic pressure.

Conditions affecting the barrier function of the glycocalyx layer or in inflammatory states where endothelial cell pore formation occurs colloid molecules may be lost from circulation or may get metabolized. So the effective half-life of colloids may vary in such situations.

Colloid osmotic pressure (COP) decides the plasma volume expanding effect of the colloid.

Normal plasma COP is 28 mm Hg (albumin being the principal determinant).

Iso-oncotic fluids have COP of 20–30 mm Hg. (COP equivalent to that of plasma), e.g., 5% albumin.

Hyperoncotic fluids have COP—>30 mm Hg (Increases plasma volume more than the infusate volume), e.g., 25% albumin.

Colloids improve blood flow by hemodilution by altering the rheology.

Disturbances in immune, coagulation, and renal systems may occur due to large doses.

Albumin

It is a type of plasma protein which constitutes 50–60% of all plasma proteins.

It is the principal determinant of COP which is near physiological (20 mm Hg) for albumin.

Heat-treated preparations of human serum albumin are available 5% and 25% in 0.9% NaCl.

5% albumin: An increase in plasma volume is 100% of the infused volume with volume effect dissipating after 6 hours and lost after 12 hours (available in 250 mL aliquot).

25% albumin: Colloid osmotic pressure (COP) is 70 mm Hg, plasma volume expansion is about 3–4 times the infused volume (due to shift of fluid from interstitial compartment—so not to be used for volume resuscitation in patients with blood loss).
- Used for hypoalbuminemia.
- Avoided in patients with renal injury and shock.

TABLE 4: Characteristics of colloids.

Fluids	Average molecular weight (kDa)	Oncotic pressure (mm Hg)	Δ Plasma volume/infusate volume	Duration of action
25% albumin	69	70	3–4	12 h
10% dextran	26	40	1–1.5	6 h
6% hetastarch	450	30	1–3	24 h
5% albumin	69	20	0.7–1.3	12 h

Hydroxyethyl Starches (Table 5)

Chemically modified polysaccharide composed of long chains of branched glucose substituted periodically by hydroxyl radicals polymers which resist enzymatic degradation.

Classified on the Basis of Molecular Weight

- High—450–480 kDa
- Medium—200 kDa
- Low—70 kDa

High molecular weight (MW) undergoes cleavage by amylase into oncotically smaller molecules exerting the osmotic effect responsible for the prolonged action.

Clearance of small molecules occurs mainly by renal excretion (size 50 kDa).

Medium-sized undergo excretion in feces and bile also.

Larger molecules resisting hydrolysis are taken up by the mononuclear phagocyte, where they may persist for several weeks causing prolonged action.

Classification on the Basis of Molar Substitution Ratio

It is the ratio of hydroxyl radical substitutions per glucose polymer (range 0–1).

Preparations with higher molar substitution ratios have prolonged activities.

Adverse Effects

- Altered coagulation with large infused volumes especially with high OH/glucose ratio (inhibition of factor VII and vWF and impaired platelet adhesiveness)
- Nephrotoxicity (especially in critically ill patients)
- Hyperamylasemia

DEXTRANS

These are highly branched polysaccharide molecules produced by bacterium *Leuconostoc mesenteroides* in a sucrose medium.

There are two available preparations:
1. 10% dextran—40
2. 6% dextran—70

   0.9% NaCl is used as diluent
   COP is 40 mm Hg
   It is 70% renally excreted in 24 hours.

Higher MW molecules are excreted into GIT or are taken up by the mononuclear phagocyte system to undergo degradation by endogenous dextrases.

Adverse Effects

- Antithrombotic effect due to red cell coating, inhibition of platelet aggregation, factor VIIIc and decrease in vWF factor
- Interference with cross-matching due to coating of RBCs
- *Anaphylactoid reactions:* Intermediate risk prevented by pretreatment with dextran (hapten inhibitor)
- Renal dysfunction.

TABLE 5: Preparations of hydroxyethyl starches.

	Concentration	MW	(OH/Glucose)
Hetastarch	6%	450 kDa	0.7
Hexastarch	6%	200 kDa	0.6
Pentastarch	6%, 10%	200 kDa	0.5
Tetrastarch	6%	130 kDa	0.4

(MW: molecular weight; OH: hydroxyl group)

GELATINS

Derived from hydrolysis of bovine collagen, with modification by succinylation or urea linkage to form polygeline.

Succinylated forms undergo conformational change due to excess negative charges yielding a larger molecule.

They have the least impact on clinically relevant hemostasis.

Calcium present in high amounts interferes with coadministration of citrated blood products in the same infusion set.

Highest incidence of severe anaphylaxis or anaphylactoid reactions.

FLUID MANAGEMENT

Routine prescription of fluid therapy is often individualized according to the body weight and nature of the surgery, gender, age, comorbidities, trauma, and anesthetic technique. Fluid management includes replacing the fasting deficits, maintenance requirements, and replacement of the losses.

Fasting deficit is calculated as—*numbers of hours of fasting × hourly maintenance requirement*. 50% of deficit thus calculated is given over first hour, 25% in 2nd hour and remaining 25% in 3rd hour.

Maintenance fluid requirement is calculated by 4-2-1 formula as:
- For 1st 10 kg = 4 mL/kg/hour
- For 10-20 kg = 4 mL/kg/hour + 2 mL/kg/hour
- For >20 kg = 4 mL/kg/hour + 2 mL/kg/hour + 1 mL/kg/hour
- Or at a low background infusion rate of 1-1.5 mL/kg/hour.

Replacement

Blood loss should be replaced with crystalloids in 1.5:1 ratio. For each mL of lost blood 1.5 mL of crystalloid should be given.

FLUID STRATEGIES

The fluid strategies are given in **Table 6**.

TABLE 6: Fluid strategies.

Liberal	Restrictive	Goal directed
• Previously used, a large volume of fluids was given to compensate for the prolonged fasting periods, bowel preparation, and ongoing losses from perspiration and urine output • Aggressive replacement of third space losses existence of which is refuted • Proven disruption of the endothelial glycocalyx by ischemia as well as hypervolemia, suggested avoiding unnecessary overloading the patients with fluids	• This strategy is often employed for special types of surgeries like lung surgery in order to avoid the risks of volume overload – This uses avoiding hypovolemia while limiting the infusion to minimum necessary. – Replacement of blood loss with colloids on a 1 mL per 1 mL basis – No replacement for 3rd space loss or urine output – Administration of vasopressors for correcting intraoperative hypotension	• This approach is a continuous dynamic process that targets physiological end points related to cardiac output or global oxygen delivery • Dynamic indices used are systolic pressure variation (SPV), pulse pressure variation (PPV), stroke volume variation (SVV), and plethysmographic variation • Use of echocardiography (TEE/TTE) in open-chest surgeries where predictive ability of dynamic indices is reduced

(TEE: transesophageal echocardiograms; TTE: transthoracic echocardiograms)

So fluid therapy should be individualized according to the needs of the patient, the rate and composition should be adjusted so as to provide adequate perfusion without overloading the patient with fluids to minimize the associated morbidity and enhance recovery.

QUESTIONS

Q. 1. Restrictive fluid therapy vs liberal fluid therapy.

Q. 2. Hydroxyethyl starch in perioperative period: Friend, foe or still unsolved issue?

Q. 3. Intravenaus fluid resuscitation rate in burns patient?

Q. 4. Balanced salt solutions vs conventional crystalloids.

FURTHER READING

1. Woodcock T. Fluid Physiology: A Handbook for Anaesthesia and Critical Care Practice.

CHAPTER 26

Anticonvulsants

Tanvi Meshram, Ankur Sharma

INTRODUCTION

The International League against Epilepsy (ILAE) defines epilepsy as a brain disease manifested by any of the following: (1) at least two unprovoked (or reflex) seizures occurring more than 24 hours apart; (2) one unprovoked (or reflex) seizure with a probability of subsequent seizures comparable to the general recurrence risk of at least 60% after two unprovoked seizures occurring over the next 10 years, and (3) epilepsy syndrome **(Flowchart 1)**.

CLASSIFICATION OF ANTIEPILEPTICS

Chemical Classification

- *Barbiturate:* Phenobarbitone, mephobarbitone
- *Hydantoins:* Phenytoin, mephenytoin, phenyl-ethyl-hydantoin, ethotoin
- *Oxazolidinediones:* Trimethadone, paramethadione
- *Phenacemide:* Phenacemide, phenyl-ethyl-acetyl urea
- *Benzodiazepines:* Nitrazepam, clonazepam

Flowchart 1: Classification of seizures according to by the International League against Epilepsy (ILAE).

Focal	Generalized	Unknown
Awareness/Impaired awareness	**Motor** • Tonic-clonic • Clonic • Tonic • Myoclonic • Myoclonic tonic-clonic • Myoclonic atonic • Atonic • Epileptic spasm	**Motor** • Tonic-clonic • Epileptic spasm
Motor onset • Automatism • Atonic • Clonic • Epileptic spasm • Hyperkinetic • Myoclonic • Tonic		**Non-motor** • Behavior arrest
Non-motor onset • Autonomic • Behavior arrest • Cognitive • Emotional • Sensory	**Non-motor (Absence)** • Typical • Atypical • Myoclonic • Eyelid myoclonia	Unclassified
Focal to bilateral tonic clonic		

TABLE 1: Anticonvulsants drugs.

Drugs	Mechanism of action	Targeted seizure	Pharmacokinetics	Dosage	Adverse effects
Carba-mazepine	Sodium channel blocker	Focal and focal-to-bilateral tonic-clonic seizures. Trigeminal neuralgia	Metabolized by the liver to an active metabolite, rapidly absorbed orally, with bioavailability 75–85%, peak levels in 4–5 hours. Protein binding 70–80%, elimination, t½: 8–24 hours	10–40 mg/kg/day in two to three divided doses	Sedation, vertigo, diplopia, nausea, vomiting, chronic diarrhea, syndrome of inappropriate antidiuretic hormone secretion. Aplastic anemia, thrombocytopenia, hepatocellular and cholestatic jaundice, oliguria, hypertension, and cardiac dysrhythmias
Lamotrigine	Sodium channel blocker	Focal seizures, generalized tonic-clonic seizures, absence seizures, other generalized seizures; bipolar depression	Metabolized by liver, Nearly complete (~90%) absorption, peak levels in 1–3 hours, protein binding—55%, t½: 8–35 hours	200–500 mg/day in two divided doses	• Tremor • Vertigo • Diplopia • Ataxia • Headache • Gastrointestinal disturbances • Stevens–Johnson syndrome
Lacosamide	Sodium channel blocker	Focal seizures	Metabolized by the liver, 40% excreted unchanged in the urine, complete absorption, peak levels in 1–2 hours protein binding <30%, t½—12–14 hours	200–400 mg/day	Dizziness, headache, nausea, and diplopia
Phenytoin, fosphenytoin	Sodium channel blocker	Focal seizures, tonic-clonic seizures	Saturable hepatic metabolism, absorption is formulation dependent, highly bound to plasma protein, no active metabolites, dose-dependent elimination, t½: 12–36 hours	15 mg/kg bolus IV	Diplopia, ataxia, gingival hyperplasia, hirsutism, neuropathy

Contd...

Contd...

Drugs	Mechanism of action	Targeted seizure	Pharmacokinetics	Dosage	Adverse effects
Valproate	Sodium and calcium ion channel blocker	Generalized tonic-clonic seizures, partial seizures, absence seizures, myoclonic seizures, other generalized seizures; migraine prophylaxis	Hepatic metabolism, Nearly complete absorption, bound to plasma proteins, t½—5–16 hours	500–3,000 mg/day in 2–4 divided doses	Anorexia, nausea, vomiting. Weight gain is common in patients treated chronically with valproic acid, fine tremors, thrombocytopenia, hepatotoxicity
Levetiracetam	It acts by engaging with synaptic vesicle protein 2A (SV2A) and altering neuron excitability	Focal seizures, generalized tonic-clonic seizures, myoclonic seizures	It is mainly eliminated via the kidneys, has a rapid onset of action, is not bound to plasma proteins, and has 6–11 hours of half-life	1,000–3,000 mg/day in two divided doses	Sedation, asthenia, anxiety, and headache
Topiramate	Sodium-ion channel blockade, enhanced GABA activity, glutamate antagonism, calcium ion channel blockade	Focal seizures, primary generalized seizures, Lennox-Gastaut syndrome; migraine prophylaxis	Renal excretion and hepatic metabolism, primarily excreted unchanged in the urine, near-complete absorption, peak levels in 2–4 hours, minimal plasma protein binding, t½–8–15 hours	500–3,000 mg/day in 2–4 divided doses	Sedation, dizziness, ataxia, nephrolithiasis
Gabapentin	It binds avidly to α2δ, a protein that serves as an auxiliary subunit of voltage-gated calcium channels	Focal seizures; neuropathic pain; postherpetic neuralgia; anxiety	Excreted unchanged in the urine, Bioavailability—50%, not bound to plasma proteins, t½–5–9 hours	10–60 mg/kg/day	• Sedation • Ataxia • Vertigo • Gastrointestinal disturbances
Pregabalin	bind avidly to α2δ, a protein that serves as an auxiliary subunit of voltage-gated calcium channels	Focal seizures; neuropathic pain; postherpetic neuralgia; anxiety, fibromyalgia	Excreted unchanged in the urine, complete absorption, not bound to plasma proteins, t½–4.5–7 hours	150–600 mg/day	• Sedation • Ataxia • Vertigo

Contd...

Contd...

Drugs	Mechanism of action	Targeted seizure	Pharmacokinetics	Dosage	Adverse effects
Tiagabine	GAT-1 GABA transporter inhibitor hence enhanced GABA activity	Focal seizures	Hepatic metabolism, complete absorption, highly protein-bound, t½—2–9 hours	32–56 mg/kg/day in two to four divided doses	Dizziness, asthenia, aphasia, tremors, mental depression
Vigabatrin	Irreversible inhibitor of GABA transaminases	Focal seizures, Infantile spasms	Excreted unchanged in the urine, not protein-bound, t½—5–8 hours	3000 mg/day in two divided doses	Permanent visual loss, anemia, somnolence, and fatigue
Phenobarbital	Potentiation of the postsynaptic actions of GABA and inhibition of excitatory actions of glutamate	Focal seizures, generalized tonic-clonic seizures, myoclonic seizures, neonatal seizures; sedation	Hepatic metabolism, 25% excreted unchanged in the urine	2–5 mg/kg/day every day or in two divided doses	Sedation, depression, hyperactivity (children)
Primidone	Sodium channel blocker-like, converted to phenobarbital	Generalized tonic-clonic seizures, partial seizures	Hepatic metabolism to active metabolites (phenobarbitone), 40% excreted unchanged in urine, complete absorption, t½—10–25 hours	500–1500 mg/day in 2–3 divided doses	Sedation, cognitive issues, ataxia, hyperactivity
Ethosuximide	Inhibit T-type calcium channels	Absence seizures	Hepatic metabolism, 25% excreted unchanged in the urine, Absorption is almost complete, unbound to plasma proteins, t½—20–60 hours	15–40 mg/kg/day in 2–3 divided doses	Nausea, vomiting, lethargy, dizziness, ataxia, photophobia
Diazepam	Potentiates GABA-mediated neuronal inhibition	Status epilepticus, sedation, anxiety, muscle relaxation (muscle spasms, spasticity), acute alcohol withdrawal	Hepatic metabolism to several active metabolites, nearly complete absorption, highly protein-bound protein, t½ of active metabolite N-desmethyldiazepam up to 100 hours		Sedation

Contd...

Contd...

Drugs	Mechanism of action	Targeted seizure	Pharmacokinetics	Dosage	Adverse effects
Clonazepam	Potentiates GABA-mediated neuronal inhibition	Absence seizures, myoclonic seizures, infantile spasms	Hepatic metabolism, near-complete absorption, highly protein-bound, t½: 12–56 hours		Sedation
Perampanel	A noncompetitive blocker of AMPA receptors	Focal and focal-to-bilateral tonic-clonic seizures, generalized tonic-clonic seizures	Hepatic metabolism, complete absorption, highly protein-bound, t½: 25–129 hours	4–6 mg/day	Dizziness, somnolence, headache, psychiatric syndromes
Retigabine	It opens KCNQ potassium channels	Focal seizures	Hepatic metabolism, Bioavailability ~60%, moderately bound to plasma proteins, t½: 7–11 hours	600–1200 mg/day	Dizziness, somnolence, confusion, blurred vision
Zonisamide	Multiple mechanisms— • Na-channel blocker • Modulation of calcium ion channels GABA-mediated neuronal inhibition	Focal seizures, generalized tonic-clonic seizures, myoclonic seizures	Hepatic metabolism, 50% excreted unchanged in the urine, moderate plasma protein binding, t½—50–70 hours	200–400 mg/day	Drowsiness, cognitive impairment, confusion, skin rashes, nephrolithiasis
Rufinamide	Na-channel blocker	Lennox-Gastaut syndrome; focal seizures	Hepatic metabolism, good bioavailability, low plasma protein binding, t½—6–10 hours	400–800 mg/days in two divided doses	Somnolence, vomiting, pyrexia, diarrhea

(GABA: gamma-aminobutyric acid; KCNQ: potassium voltage-gated channel subfamily Q member 1)

- *Iminostilbenes:* Carbamazepine
- *Miscellaneous:* Ethoxzolamide, sulthiame, sodium valproate (valproic acid).

MODE OF ACTION

- *Ion channels modulation:* Phenytoin, carbamazepine, lamotrigine, oxcarbazepine, ethosuximide, zonisamide
- *γ-amino butyric acid potentiation:* Phenobarbital, benzodiazepines, vigabatrin, tiagabine
- *Multiple action:* Sodium valproate, gabapentin, felbamate, topiramate
- *Unknown:* Levetiracetam.

PHARMACOKINETICS

All antiepileptic drugs are administered either once daily or more frequently. There is variable absorption of these drugs from the gastrointestinal tract. Protein binding varies considerably (0% for gabapentin to 90% or greater for phenytoin). They are metabolized in the liver or excreted unchanged in the urine and necessitate dose adjustment in hepatic or renal disease. The pharmacokinetics is summarized in **Table 1**.

All antiepileptic drugs, except gabapentin, levetiracetam, and vigabatrin, have been linked to pharmacokinetic drug interactions and should be anticipated in all patients receiving antiepileptics.

They increase hepatic P450 enzyme activity and may accelerate the metabolism of various drugs.

QUESTION

Q. 1. Current status of levetiracetam as an anticonvulsant.

FURTHER READING

1. Fisher RS, Acevedo C, Arzimanoglou A, Bogacz A, Cross JH, Elger CE, et al. ILAE official report: a practical clinical definition of epilepsy. Epilepsia. 2014;55(4):475-82.
2. Flood P, Rathmell JP, Urman RD. Stoelting's Pharmacology and Physiology in Anesthetic Practice; 6th edition. Philadelphia: Wolters Kluwer Health; 2021. pp. 984.
3. Katzung BG. Basic and Clinical Pharmacology, 14th edition. New York: McGraw-Hill Education; 2017. pp. 1264.
4. Sarmast ST, Abdullahi AM, Jahan N. Current Classification of seizures and epilepsies: scope, limitations, and recommendations for future action. Cureus. 2020;12(9):e10549.

SECTION 2
Anesthesia Monitoring

- **Arterial Blood Pressure Monitoring**
  Gnanasekaran Srinivasan, Kirthiha Govindaraj

- **Central Venous Cannulation Technique and Central Venous Pressure Monitoring**
  Kirthiha Govindaraj, Gnanasekaran Srinivasan

- **Pulmonary Artery Catheter Monitoring**
  Kirthiha Govindaraj, Gnanasekaran Srinivasan

- **Perioperative Cardiac Output Monitoring**
  Sayan Nath, Abhishek Singh, Puneet Khanna

- **Transcranial Doppler**
  Bhavana Kayarat, Arjun Balakrishnan, Puneet Khanna

- **Cerebral Oximetry**
  Bhavana Kayarat, Puneet Khanna

- **Electroencephalogram**
  Bhavana Kayarat, Puneet Khanna

- **Somatosensory and Motor Evoked Potentials**
  Arjun Balakrishnan, Bhavana Kayarat, Puneet Khanna

- **Bispectral Index**
  Bhavana Kayarat, Arjun Balakrishnan, Puneet Khanna

- **Entropy**
  Sudhansu Sekhar Nayak, Arjun Balakrishnan

- **Respiratory Monitoring**
  Vrinda Chauhan, Puneet Khanna, Abhishek Singh

- **Pulse Oximetry**
  Abhishek Singh

- **Capnometry and Capnography**
  Ajit Kumar, Baibhav Bhandari

- **Patterns of Neuromuscular Stimulation**
  Anju Gupta, Mitchell Gullebani

- **Nerve Stimulator**
  Anju Gupta, Manjula Sudhakar Rao

- **Temperature Monitoring**
  Tazeen Khan, Parthodeep Jha, Puneet Khanna

- **Acid–Base Status Evaluation**
  Ajit Kumar, Saurabh Chandrakar

- **Pulmonary Function Test**
  Ajit Kumar, Shivam Gupta

CHAPTER 27

Arterial Blood Pressure Monitoring

Gnanasekaran Srinivasan, Kirthiha Govindaraj

INTRODUCTION

Arterial blood pressure can be measured noninvasively by indirect cuff devices or invasively by directly cannulating certain peripheral arteries and using a pressure transducer. Arterial blood pressure is also a cardinal cardiovascular parameter similar to heart rate. It is helpful in providing crucial and timely information in many cases. Australian Incident Monitoring Study of 1993 reasserted the significance of invasive in the timely detection of hypotension over the indirect noninvasive monitoring techniques. Certain aspects are readily apparent like dicrotic notch to guide the proper timing of intra-aortic balloon counterpulsation, excessive variation in the pressure variables indicative of preload reserve, and also serves as a piece of diagnostic information regarding the changes in the patient condition. Thus, direct arterial monitoring is considered as the gold standard, providing a continual, beat-to-beat measurement of the arterial pressure, and also allows repeated sampling.

COMPONENTS OF ARTERIAL BLOOD PRESSURE MONITORING SYSTEM

The components of arterial blood pressure monitoring system includes—intra-arterial catheter itself, stopcocks for blood sampling and transducer zeroing, in-line blood sampling ports, a pressure transducer, continuous flush device, and electronic cable. Innovation to this basic system includes needleless ports and closed aspiration systems.

- *Arterial catheter kit:* Radial 20G/Femoral 18G/angiocatheter (20G for adult and older children, 22G or 24G for small children or neonates) **(Fig. 1)**.
- *3-way stopcock:* Zeroing and sampling.
- *Pressure transducer with a flushing system:* It includes flush device and transducer.
- *Flush device:* It allows continuous saline infusion at a slow rate (1–3 mL/hours) to keep the monitoring system purged and prevent the thrombus formation in the system. Dextrose-containing solutions should be avoided since flush contamination of sample blood shows erroneous measurement in blood glucose values. This device also consists of a spring-loaded valve to flush the system periodically with high pressure following

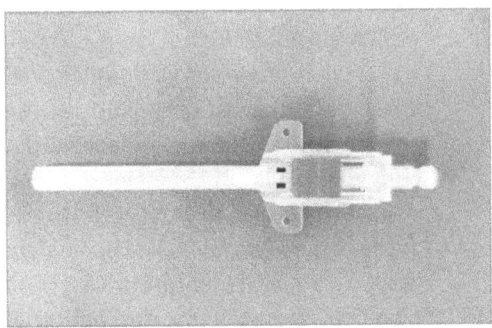

Fig. 1: Arterial cannula.

sample collection and restores the system dynamic response to the baseline.

- *Transducer set-up:* Zeroing and leveling
  - *Zeroing:* Before starting, while using the system pressure the transducer should always be zeroed, calibrated, and leveled to the appropriate position. This is done by exposure of the transducer to the atmospheric pressure and performing the zero procedure which is defined by the manufacturer of the device. Zero pressure locus should be positioned appropriately relative to the patient, and the zero reference point is the local atmospheric pressure which should be checked and rezeroed periodically. Sometimes any fault in the system can produce a significant error until the zero references is re-established.
  - *Leveling:* Appropriate level at which the zero point must be established by keeping the transducer with respect to the patient and the clinical context. Transducer zeroing and leveling are precise and different entities. Zeroing establishes the zero reference point as ambient atmospheric pressure, while the leveling aligns this reference point relative to the patient body, determining where the "0" will be. Hence, leveling is even more important when monitoring the values for which the physiological range is small, e.g., ICP. In most cases, these arterial pressure transducers should be positioned to estimate the aortic root pressure (i.e., approximately 5 cm posterior to the sternal border, however more conventional will be keeping the transducer at the midthoracic level that corresponds to the mid-left-atrial position, located halfway between the anterior sternum and the bed surface). And this reference point has to be maintained consistently throughout the monitoring period. Whereas, at a supine position, the pressures measured in both the upper limbs by either technique will be the same. But in right lateral decubitus position, arterial pressures measured from any of the radial artery will remain unaltered as long as the transducer is placed at the heart level. But the noninvasive blood pressure (NIBP) at dependent arm will be higher and the nondependent arm will be lower with respect to the arm level above and below the heart and the hydrostatic pressure differences between them **(Figs. 2A and B)**.

Special Circumstances

Sitting position in neurosurgery cases—transducer at the level of patient ear, approximating to the circle of Willis.

Lateral decubitus position: Transducer should remain fixed at the level of the heart for measuring the pressure. However, noninvasive blood pressure is higher in the dependent arm and lower in the nondependent arm **(Figs. 3A and B)**.

GENERAL PRINCIPLES

The pressure measured in the peripheral arteries varies with the pressure which is measured in the central aortic cannulation. The arterial pressure waveform becomes increasingly distorted ongoing distally, as the signal gets transmitted down the arterial system **(Fig. 4)**. The dicrotic notch disappears, systolic peak accentuates, diastolic trough attenuates and there will be a transmission delay, on moving distally. These effects are more marked

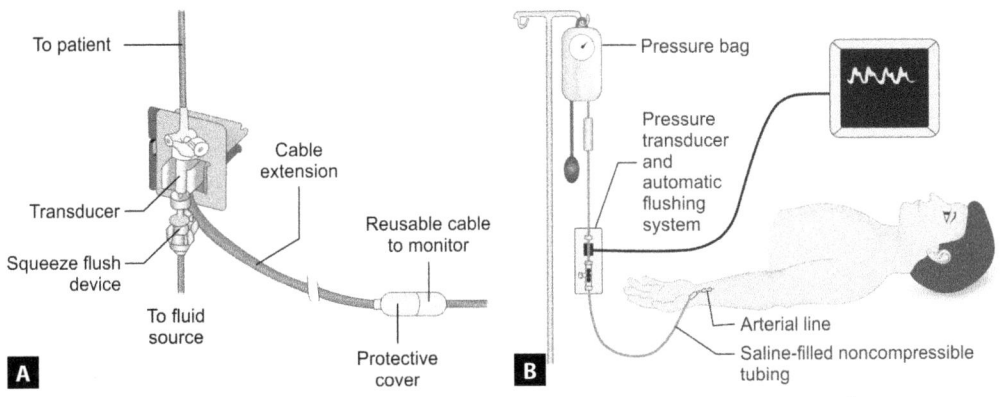

Figs. 2A and B: (A) Pressure transducer; (B) Schematic representation of arterial pressure monitoring system.

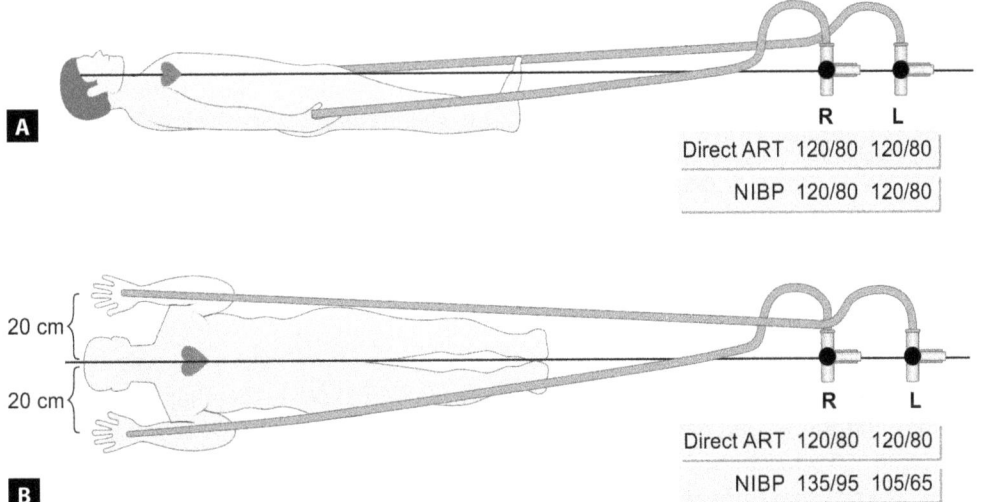

Figs. 3A and B: Demonstrates the effect of position between the direct arterial pressure (ART) and indirect noninvasive blood pressure (NIBP) measurements.

in the dorsalis pedis artery, where systolic blood pressure (SBP) will be 10–20 mm Hg higher and diastolic blood pressure (DBP) 10–20 mm Hg lower, but the mean arterial pressure (MAP) in the peripheral arteries will be similar to the central aortic pressure under normal conditions. But after the separation from cardiopulmonary bypass (CPB), the MAP measured will be lower than central aortic pressure. Additional information includes slope of the arterial upstroke correlates with the pressure derivative measured over time (dP/dt) and provides an indirect gauge of myocardial contractility. A large variation in a mechanically ventilated patient is suggestive of hypovolemia.

CHARACTERISTICS OF MONITORING SYSTEM

The displayed arterial pressure waveform is a periodic complex wave produced via Fourier analysis of a summation of multiple

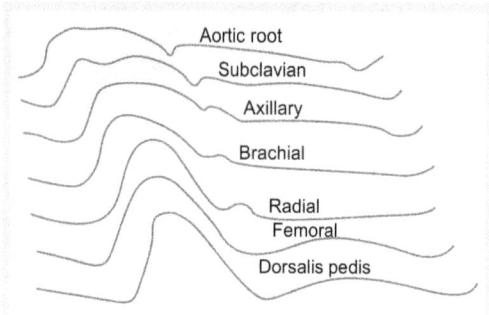

Fig. 4: Progression of the arterial waveform changes caused by propagation of forward wave and reflection of wave, observed from central monitoring through the peripheral monitoring.

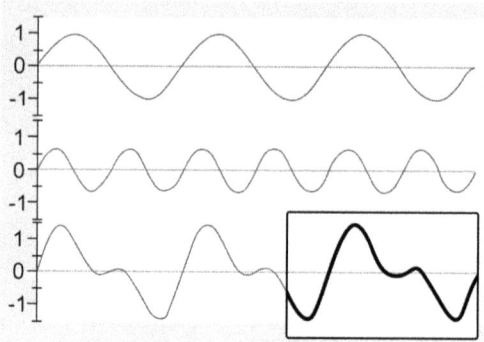

Fig. 5: Arterial pressure waveform produced by the summation of sine waves.

propagated and reflected pressure waves. The original pressure wave is characterized by its frequency, a characteristic clinically evident as the pulse rate and expressed as cycles/second (Hz).

Sine wave: The summation of sine waves producing the final complex wave has frequencies that are multiples or harmonics of the fundamental frequency (i.e., pulse rate). It is reconstructed with acceptable accuracy from only two sine waves, the fundamental frequency and the second harmonic **(Fig. 5)**. As a result, 6–10 harmonics are needed to provide arterial pressure waveforms which are distortion free. For example, patient with a pulse rate 120 beats/min (2 cycles/second or 2 Hz) requires the monitoring system dynamic response of 12–20 Hz (i.e., 6–10 waveforms × 2 Hz). Hence, the faster heart rate has greater demands on the monitoring system. This figure demonstrates that the fundamental wave added to 63% of the second harmonic wave resulting in the arterial pressure waveform **(Fig. 5)**.

The pressure monitoring system response is characterized by its natural frequency and damping. It is easily understood by snapping the end of a transducer-tubing-assembly with a finger. The waveform shows rapid oscillations both above and below the baseline, i.e., natural frequency, and then quickly returns to the straight line attributing to friction in the system, i.e., damping. *Resonance* or *ringing* of the system means the peaks and troughs seen in an arterial pressure waveform which gets amplified if there is a natural frequency in the transducer catheter assembly, which lies nearer to the underlying sine waves frequencies of the arterial pressure waveform (usually <20 Hz). It is recommended that the natural frequency of the pressure transducing system is at least 8 times higher than the frequency of the measure sine wave. This is how the arterial pressure monitoring system continues to be accurate at a higher heart rate (HR); its natural frequency should also be higher. In general, lengthy transducer tubing decreases the natural frequency of the system and amplifies the height of SBP (peak) and depth of DBP values (trough). The rigid tubing with low compliance and length of the tubing ranging from 6 inch to 5 feet has the natural frequency lessened from 34 to 7 Hz.

Damping is the propensity of certain factors like friction, compliant or soft tubing and air bubbles to absorb energy and reduce the amplitude of the peaks and troughs in the waveform. The desirable degree of damping is that which can counterbalance the distorting consequences of tubing systems of the pressure transducer with lower natural frequencies, which may not be easy to achieve. The damping of the system can be assessed by doing a rapid high-pressure flush testing of the system consisting of transducer, tubing and catheter. **(Fig. 6A)**.

Overdamping **(Fig. 6C)** causes falsely lower SBP reading and a higher DBP reading, with MAP being unaffected unless the significant distortion occurs like clot formation. *Underdamping* **(Fig. 6B)** results in opposite effects on BP recordings causing overshoot of the systolic pressure and additional small, nonphysiologic pressure waves distorting the waveform which makes difficult to distinguish the dicrotic notch, with the MAP being unaffected. Ideally damping coefficient should be 1.

The formula for calculating the natural frequency and damping coefficient are as follows:

Natural frequency: $f_n = d/8 \sqrt{3/\pi L \rho V_d}$
Damping coefficient: $\zeta = 16\eta/d^3 \sqrt{3LV_d/\pi\rho}$

d = diameter of the tubing
L = length of the tubing
ρ = fluid density
V_d = displacement of transducer fluid volume
η = fluid viscosity

INDICATIONS OF ARTERIAL CANNULATION

- Continuous, real-time monitoring of the blood pressure
- Any planned manipulation of the cardiovascular system—pharmacologic or mechanical
- Need for repeated blood sampling—electrolyte or metabolic disturbances
- Patients requiring inotropes or intra-aortic balloon counterpulsation
- Massive traumatic injury
- Patients with right heart failure, chronic obstructive pulmonary disease (COPD), pulmonary hypertension or pulmonary embolism
- Major surgical procedures involving large fluid shifts
- Failed measurement of indirect arterial blood pressure
- To obtain additional diagnostic information from the waveform
- Procedures involving deliberate hypotension or hypothermia
- Patients in any type of circulatory shock, or with multiple organ failure
- Extremely obese patients.

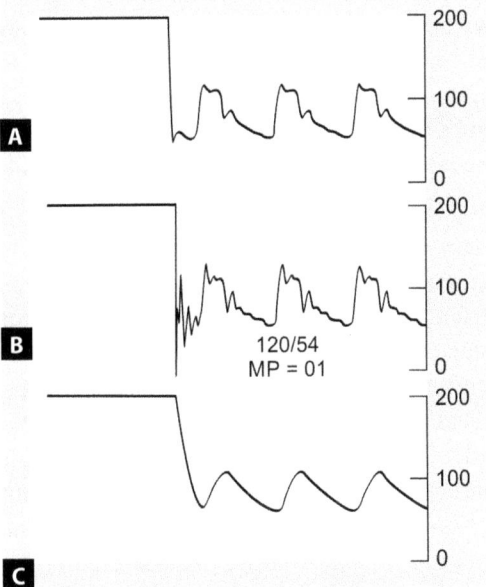

Figs. 6A to C: The Rapid high pressure flush test demonstrating the harmonic characteristics of pressure monitoring system. (A) Pressure waveform returning to baseline after a single oscillation: optimally dampened system; (B) Pressure waveform oscillates above and below the baseline several times: underdamped system; (C) Pressure waveform returning to the baseline without any oscillations: overdamped system.

CONTRAINDICATIONS OF ARTERIAL CANNULATION

- Local infection
- Coagulopathy (relative contraindications), prefer more peripheral cannulation

- Vaso-occlusive disorders such as Raynaud's syndrome or Buerger disease (thromboangiitis obliterans)—larger arteries are preferred
- Surgical considerations.

ARTERIAL CANNULATION SITES

Factors that influences the cannulation site includes the operative site, any compromise of arterial flow attributed to patient positioning or surgical manipulations, cardiopulmonary bypass and perfusion techniques, and also any prior history of ischemia or surgery on the limb to be cannulated. Monitoring arterial BP is recommended at two or more sites in complex cases requiring complex perfusion techniques or long CPB techniques. Radial arterial pressure may be supplemented by central aortic pressures obtained from axillary or femoral arteries or from the aorta itself. The advantage with central arterial tracing is the increased accuracy in patients after separation from the CPB. This monitoring usually required only for several minutes until the problem is resolved.

The sites generally chosen for arterial cannulation are as follows:

Radial and ulnar arteries: Radial artery is the most commonly cannulated artery for invasive blood pressure monitoring (IBP) monitoring, as it is easier to cannulate, readily accessible and with adequate collateral circulation. Ulnar artery supplies majority of the blood flow to the hand in 90% of the patients.

Modified Allen test: It is a simple bedside procedure, done by compressing the radial and ulnar arteries and by exercising the hand until it is pale. Then, ulnar artery is released and the time noted until the hand regains its normal color, i.e., approximately 5 seconds, however if the return of normal color of hand is delayed by >15 seconds, then cannulating the radial artery becomes controversial. In that case, another cannulation site should be chose. Plethysmography, Doppler probe and pulse oximetry has more sensitivity than the Allen test in detecting the inadequate blood supply in the collaterals.

Brachial and axillary arteries: Brachial artery measurements mirror the femoral artery measurements with lesser systolic augmentation than the radial artery tracings. It almost reflects the central aortic pressures more accurately than radial pressures with respect to the CPB. This site is not chosen most often, because if brachial artery occlusion occurs, there will be trivial or absence of collateral flow to the hand. Higher risk of thrombosis is seen in female patients with peripheral vascular disease. *Axillary artery* is cannulated near the junction of the deltoid and pectoral muscles. Left axillary artery is preferred to minimize the risk of cerebral embolization while flushing. Positioning like lateral position or adduction of arm can result in dampening of the waveform.

Femoral artery: A more reliable site for central arterial pressure monitoring after discontinuation of CPB. Recent infection prevention guidelines discourage the use of femoral cannulation. Point of entry should be distal to the inguinal ligament to prevent the risk of injuring the artery, formation of occult hematoma or even uncontrolled bleeding into pelvis or retroperitoneum. Complications include limb ischemia, pseudo aneurysm, infection, bleeding, and hematoma. It is useful in patients undergoing aortic surgery. Surgeon should be consulted before cannulating the femoral artery, because it might be useful for extracorporeal perfusion or intra-aortic balloon pump (IABP) placement.

Dorsalis pedis and posterior tibial arteries: Other less commonly used alternative sites include dorsalis pedis, posterior tibial and superficial temporal arteries, with the former two arteries being reasonable alternatives to radial artery catheterization. It resembles the radial and ulnar artery of the hand which forms the arterial arch in hand. Systolic blood pressure (SBP) is usually 10-20 mm Hg higher in the dorsalis compared to the radial or brachial arteries, and the DBP is 15-20 mm Hg lower. These arteries should be avoided in patients with significant peripheral vascular disease due to diabetes or any other etiology. Superficial temporal artery is more close to the cerebral circulation and the risk of cerebral embolization is high.

INSERTION TECHNIQUES

Direct cannulation: The wrist should be positioned in a dorsiflex position over an arm board and immobilized in a supinated position. Hyperextension needs to be avoided as it decreases the cross sectional area and also can cause damage to the median nerve by stretching. Paint the area with 4% chlorhexidine or povidone iodine and after draping, local anesthetic agent is infiltrated at the site using 25 or 27G needle. 5cc syringe with heparin flush should be kept ready for flushing if required. When the needle is entered, and once the artery is punctured, the angle between needle and skin should be reduced to 10 degrees, needle is advanced to about 1-2 mm to ensure that catheter tip lies inside the vessel, and the outer catheter is threaded off the needle. If the blood flow ceases while advancing the needle, it suggests puncture of the back wall of the vessel and in that case withdraw the needle until the blood appears and then advance. Keep the hand in normal anatomical position once the procedure is over **(Fig. 7A)**.

Transfixation: Alternatively, the artery can be transfixed by passing the needle through and through the artery at an angle of 30-45°. After the needle is withdrawn completely, the catheter is withdrawn slowly; pulsatile flow can be seen emerging from the catheter while the tip is within the arterial lumen. Depress the angle by 10-15° and now either the catheter is advanced into the artery or a guide wire is initially advanced into the lumen followed by advancing the catheter over the guide wire (modified Seldinger technique). But, direct cannulation using Seldinger technique is having increased success rate, and rarely a surgical cut down is required to place the arterial cannulation using catheter over needle assembly.

Ultrasound and Doppler-assisted techniques: Doppler assisted technique—Initially this technique is used where artery localization looks difficult, e.g., obese patient, small children, and infants. In ultrasound high frequency ultrasonic transducer (9 MHz) is used for visualization of small structures **(Figs. 7B and C)**. Both Doppler and ultrasound technique is used for difficult cannulation. It was found to be associated with increased success and fewer attempts at insertion. Procedure can be done in short axis-transverse view along with the palpation technique. Operator can choose the distance and insertion angle, depending on the depth of the target vessel. With longitudinal approach, viewing the vessel in long axis, the advancement of needle tip can be easier.

Cut down: If above measures fails, surgical cut down can be done. The target artery is cannulated under direct vision using a small incision under vision catheter over assembly is introduced.

NORMAL ARTERIAL PRESSURE WAVEFORMS

The systolic waveform immediately follows the R wave in the ECG and consists of a sharp

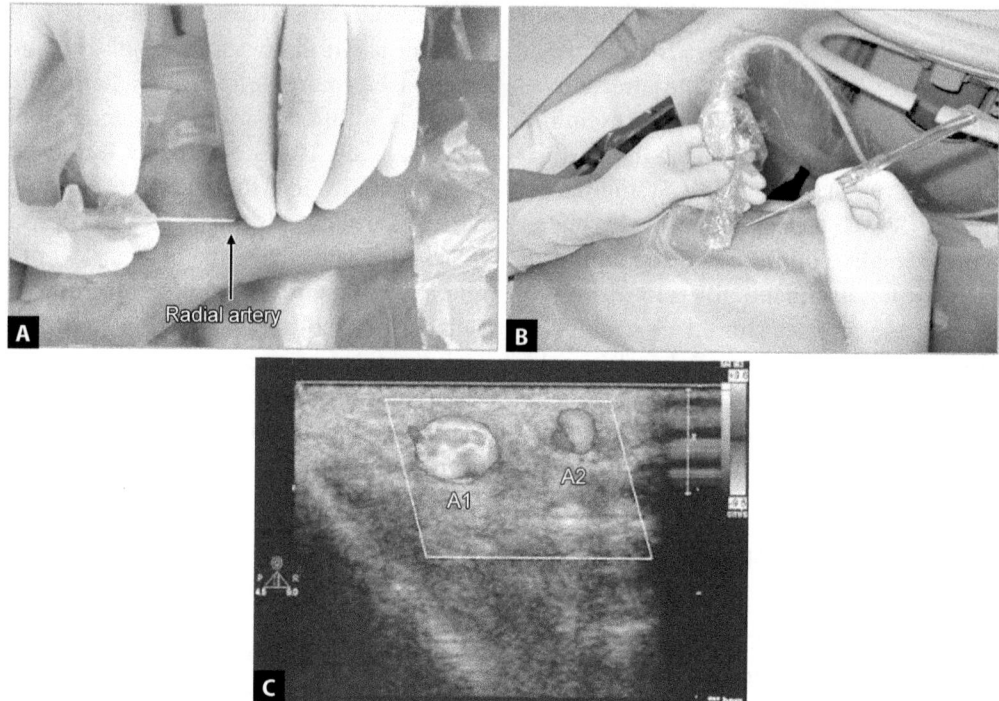

Figs. 7A to C: (A) Radial artery direct cannulation; (B) Demonstration with ultrasonic guidance; (C) Ultrasound image with color Doppler of radial artery cannulation in short axis.

pressure upstroke, peak and ensuing decline **(Fig. 8)**. A dicrotic notch interrupts the downslope and then the slope declines further after the ECG T wave and reaches its nadir at end-diastole. Systolic upstroke starts 120–180 ms after the beginning of R wave. Mean arterial pressure (MAP) describes the area beneath the arterial pressure curve which is divided by the beat period and mean value over multiple cardiac cycles; however it is dependent on device-specific algorithms. MAP is estimated as DBP plus one-third of the pulse pressure (PP), but it is valid at a slower heart rates. Arterial waveform morphology varies at different sites due to the following physical properties of the vasculature—impedance and harmonic resonance. As the pressure waveform moves from center to periphery, arterial upstroke becomes more steep, systolic peak rises, dicrotic notch appears later, diastolic wave becomes conspicuous and end diastolic pressure falls, but the MAP is only slightly increased **(Figs. 8 and 9, Table 1)**.

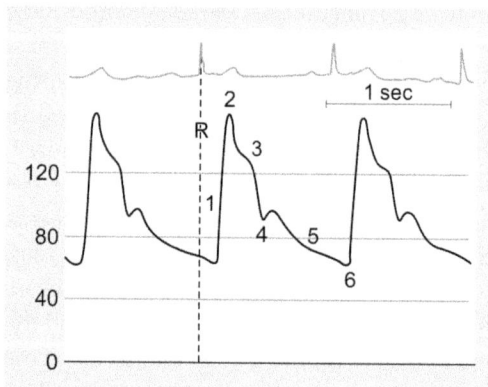

Fig. 8: Normal arterial pressure waveform with relation to the electrocardiogram 'R' wave. 1. Systolic upstroke, 2. Systolic peak, 3. Systolic decline, 4. Dicrotic notch (aortic valve closure), 5. Diastolic run-off, 6. End-diastolic pressure.

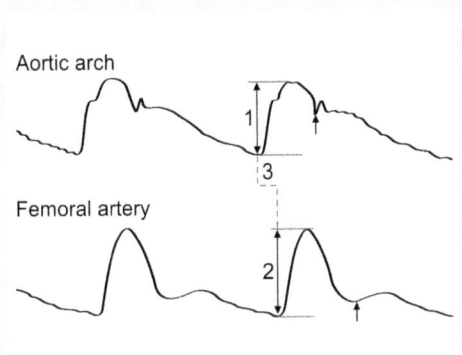

Fig. 9: Distal pulse wave amplification of the arterial pressure waveform.

ARTERIAL PRESSURE MONITORING AND WAVEFORM ANALYSIS FOR PREDICTION OF VOLUME RESPONSIVENESS

Systolic pressure variation (SPV) is the cycle of increasing and decreasing stroke volume as a result of inspiration and expiration. By the measurement of the increase and decrease in systolic pressure in relation to the end expiratory apneic baseline pressure, SPV can be subdivided into two components—inspiratory and expiratory. In mechanically

TABLE 1: Abnormal arterial pressure waveforms.

S.No.	Condition	Characteristics	Waveforms
1.	Normal arterial pressure and PAP waveform	Timing of these waveforms relative to the electrocardiographic R wave	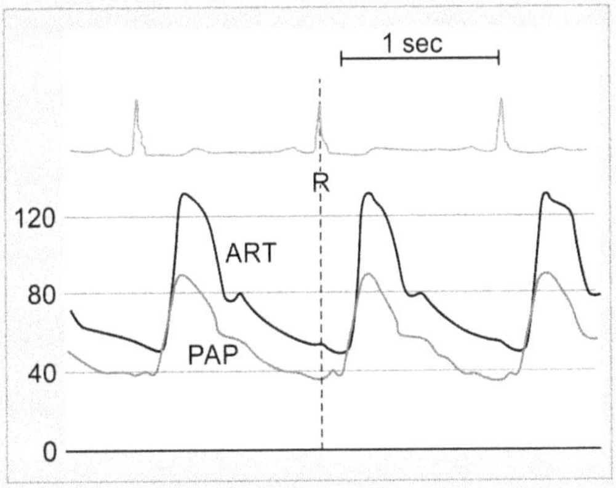
2.	Aortic stenosis	• Pulsus parvus (narrow pulse pressure) • Pulsus tardus (delayed upstroke)	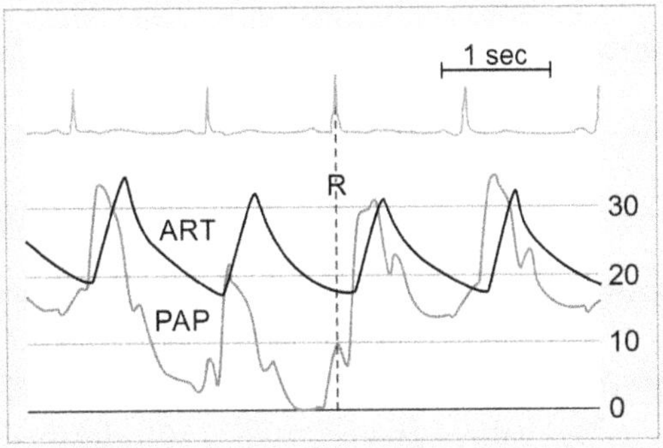

Contd...

Contd...

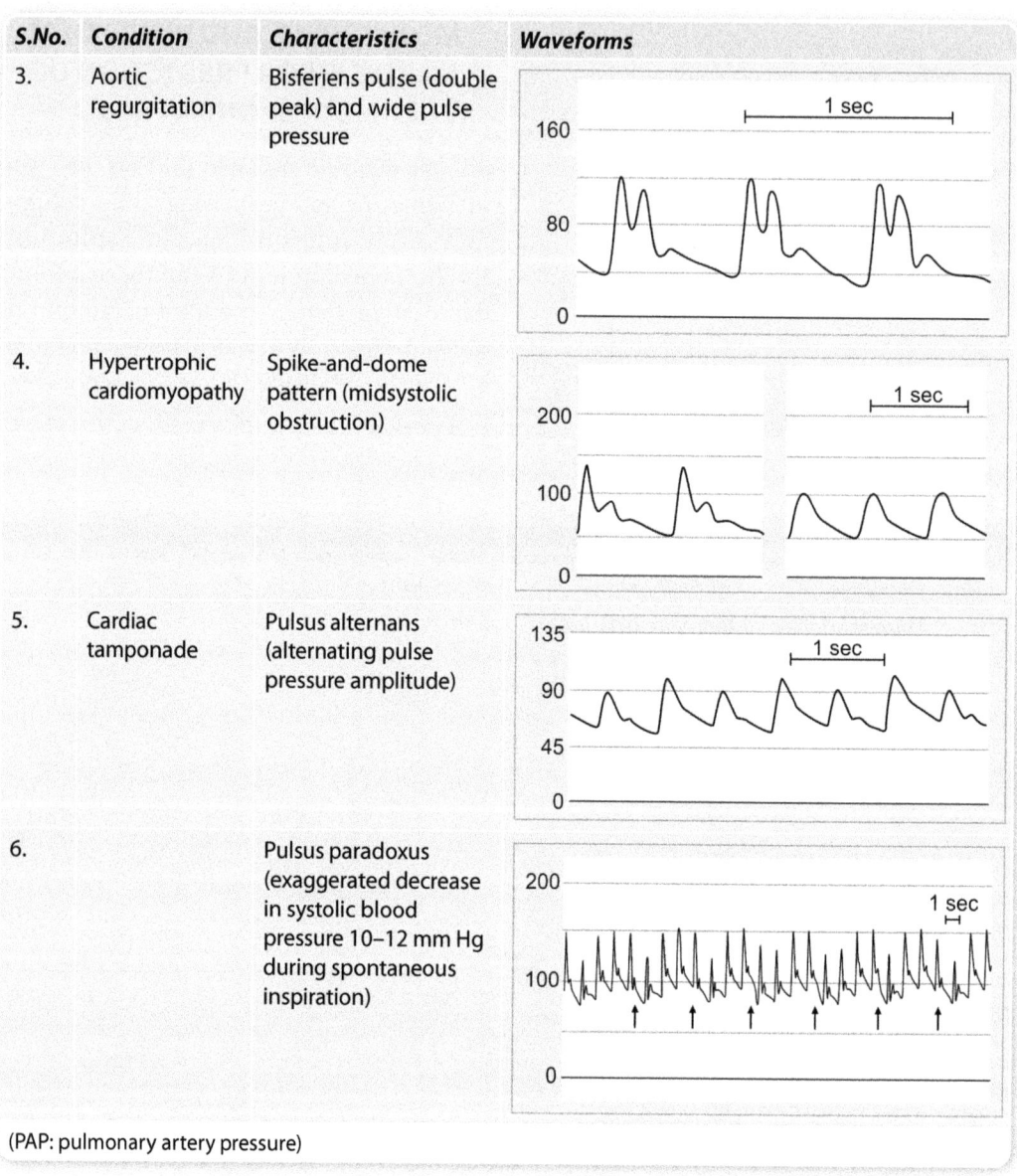

S.No.	Condition	Characteristics	Waveforms
3.	Aortic regurgitation	Bisferiens pulse (double peak) and wide pulse pressure	
4.	Hypertrophic cardiomyopathy	Spike-and-dome pattern (midsystolic obstruction)	
5.	Cardiac tamponade	Pulsus alternans (alternating pulse pressure amplitude)	
6.		Pulsus paradoxus (exaggerated decrease in systolic blood pressure 10–12 mm Hg during spontaneous inspiration)	

(PAP: pulmonary artery pressure)

ventilated patients, normal range of SPV is 7–10 mm Hg, with increases in pressure up to 2–4 mm Hg and decrease up to 5–6 mm Hg. Values greater than this indicates hypovolemia. Hence patients who manifest increased SPV during PPV may be described as having residual preload reserve or being volume responsive **(Fig. 10)**. This preload reserve depicts a physiologic state, in which the volume expansion or fluid challenge causes upward shift on the Frank-Starling Curve resulting in increase in stroke volume and rise in cardiac output as long as sustained virologic response (SVR) remains unaltered.

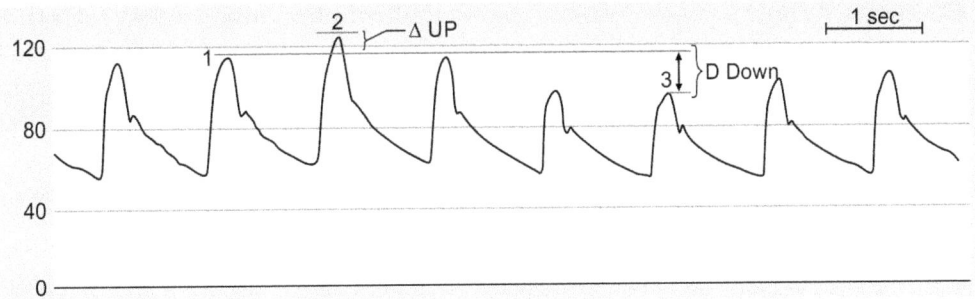

Fig. 10: Systolic pressure variation.

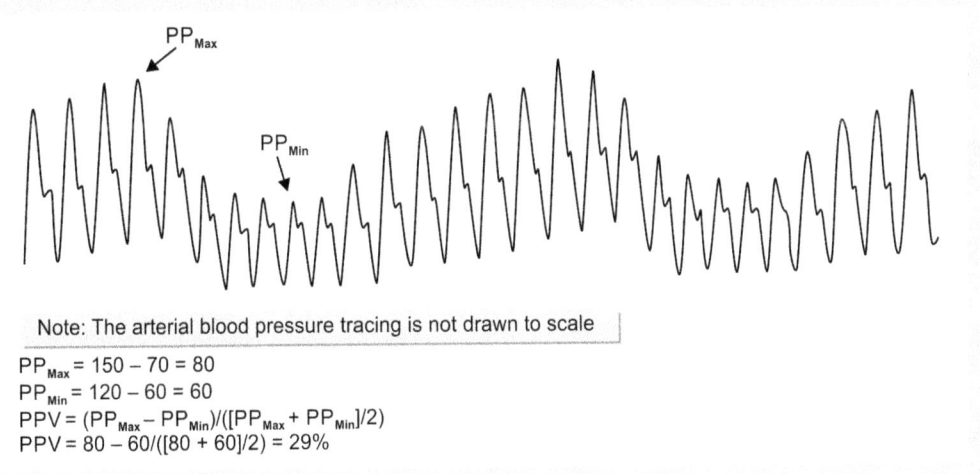

Note: The arterial blood pressure tracing is not drawn to scale

$PP_{Max} = 150 - 70 = 80$
$PP_{Min} = 120 - 60 = 60$
$PPV = (PP_{Max} - PP_{Min})/([PP_{Max} + PP_{Min}]/2)$
$PPV = 80 - 60/([80 + 60]/2) = 29\%$

Fig. 11: Pulse pressure variation.

It is a surrogate marker for left ventricular (LV) preload reserve.

Pulse pressure variation (PPV) another dynamic indicator of preload reserve, now available as standard monitoring software package. Normal PPV is <13–17%. Other sophisticated methods of pulse contour analysis allow real-time measurement of stroke volume variation as well as stroke volume variation index. When the measures exceed 10–13% and this is a positive response to volume expansion. Pulse pressure variation (PPV) shown to diverge from stroke volume variation (SVV) in the setting of the vasopressor use, in which PPV will remain low while SVV increases. It has been described that PPV >13% should receive volume expansion while those below 9% should not. PPV is significantly affected by increased intra-abdominal pressure; patient positions like prone, lateral position or steep Trendelenburg position and the use of vasopressors **(Fig. 11)**.

Less invasive alternative for assessing the preload reserve or volume responsiveness is pulse plethysmogram which is based on respiratory cycle induced variation. This transcutaneous oximetry signal of measurement is more subjected to confounding influences compared to arterial pressure waveform. Clinical studies have found that waveform analysis to be of limited utility.

COMPLICATIONS

Infection: Meta-analysis showed an incidence of arterial catheter-related bloodstream infections of 2.9/1,000 catheter days. The risk of infection was higher for the femoral site of insertion compared to radial artery insertion. Category 1A level of evidence for maintaining the sterility for all components of the pressure monitoring system using an antiseptic wipe before drawing the blood, and avoid dextrose containing flush solutions. Category 1B level of evidence was found for avoiding the femoral and axillary insertion sites. It is recommended minimum sterile precautions like a cap, mask, sterile gloves and a small fenestrated drape used during peripheral arterial insertion. Axillary and femoral artery catheter insertion requires maximal sterile barriers (category II).

Hemorrhage: Secondary to any disconnection of catheter-tubing assembly.

Arterial spasm: Temporary, resolves without intervention

Arterial thrombosis: Prolonged duration of cannulation, large catheters and small radial artery size

Embolization: Embolization of air or particulate matter that is flushed forcefully into the arterial catheter. Cerebral embolization is most likely following the axillary catheter insertion.

Hematoma: It is seen in anticoagulated patients.

Nerve damage: It occurs if the nerve and artery lies in a fibrous sheath or a limited tissue compartment. Direct nerve injury can also occur.

Pseudoaneurysm formation: Late vascular complication with progression to arteriovenous fistula

Axillary artery cannulation complications can be distal limb ischemia or limb overcirculation with limb hypoperfusion.

FURTHER READING

1. Gropper MA, Eriksson LI, Fleisher LA, Wiener-Kronish JP, Cohen NH, Leslie K (Eds). Miller's Anesthesia International Edition, 9th edition.

CHAPTER 28
Central Venous Cannulation Technique and Central Venous Pressure Monitoring

Kirthiha Govindaraj, Gnanasekaran Srinivasan

CENTRAL VENOUS CANNULATION TECHNIQUE

Introduction

Werner Forssmann, in 1929, was the first physician to introduce venous devices for central vein catheterization. Dr Sven Ivar Seldinger introduced the central venous puncture technique known as the "Seldinger technique" in the 1950s, and nowadays, it is the main method in use. Central vein cannulation (CVC) and measurement of central venous pressure (CVP) were frequently performed in hemodynamically unstable patients, in those where no peripheral access can be obtained especially in obese patients, need for frequent blood samplings, and also those patients undergoing major surgeries. It can be inserted to administer vasoactive drugs and intravenous fluids, CVP monitoring, transvenous cardiac pacing, temporary hemodialysis, pulmonary artery catheterization for cardiac monitoring, or aspiration of entrained air in those patients at risk of venous air embolism.

Site Selection

Site selection for cannulation depends on the need for the placement of a CVC catheter, the clinical scenario, the medical condition of the patient, and the expertise performing the cannulation. In patients with bleeding diathesis, it is best to choose a puncture site, where it is bleeding from the vein or adjacent artery is easily detected and controlled with local compression. And also a physician's personal experience plays a significant role in determining the safest site for cannulation **(Table 1)**.

Description of the Catheter

Central venous catheters range from single lumen to a complex combination of introducer sheaths and multilumen catheters. Most of these catheters have a fixed length. Introducer sheaths are available from size 9-11 French. This aids in introducing the pulmonary artery catheter into the circulation and can function as a large bore CVC for resuscitation. Depending on the duration of requirement, these catheters can be divided into: (1) Short-term

TABLE 1: Site selection.

Condition	Preferred site of cannulation
Bleeding diathesis	Internal or external jugular vein over subclavian vein
Severe emphysema or pneumothorax	Internal jugular vein than subclavian vein
Transvenous cardiac pacing	Right internal jugular vein
Trauma patients with a cervical collar	Femoral or subclavian vein (later is preferred if there is no risk of pneumothorax)

or temporary catheter (temporary—less than a week for perioperative usage or any acute event whereas short-term catheters—1–6 weeks) and (2) Long-term catheter (for >6 weeks usually for parenteral nutrition, antibiotics). The risk of infection is common with short-term catheters that are kept for a long period as they do not have a barrier to infection. Both are less thrombogenic **(Table 2)**.

For measuring the CVP, it is preferable to cannulate the large veins. Central venous catheters are available in various ranges of lengths, gauges, lumens, and the composition of catheter material for both adults and children. The commonly used catheter is a 7-French, 20 cm multilumen catheter with one port of 16 gauge and another two ports of 18 G each, which allows monitoring of CVP and infusion of drugs. It can be inserted using the Seldinger technique or the catheter over needle method. National Institute for Clinical Excellence (NICE) guidelines recommends the use of ultrasound for the CVC placement, particularly via IJV.

Timing of Cannulation

Decision to perform cannulation can be either before or after induction of anesthesia and it is guided by the individual patient and physician preferences.

Indications and Contraindications

Box 1 lists the indications of central venous cannulation monitoring technique whereas **Table 3** describes contraindications of the same.

BOX 1: Indications of central venous cannulation monitoring technique.

- Central venous pressure monitoring in cardiac surgical patients during cardiopulmonary bypass surgeries involving large fluid shifts or blood loss
- Administering drugs and medications in critically ill patients for vasoactive drug administration, chemotherapeutic agents, antibiotics for a prolonged period, and irritant drugs
- Aspiration of air in case of air embolism in neurological cases done in sitting position
- For fluid administration
- Unavailability of peripheral veins, e.g., obese patients
- Pulmonary artery catheterization and monitoring
- Sampling site for frequent blood sampling
- Transvenous pacing
- Major trauma

TABLE 2: Types of catheters.

Short-term or temporary catheters	Long-term catheters
• Made of polyurethane, hence the duration of cannulation is limited • Perioperative use or for any acute event • Rigid at room temperature for ease of insertion, it can cause vessel erosion if it stays for a longer time	• Made of silicone elastomer or Silastic, hence the duration can be extended • Used in patients requiring dialysis, chemotherapy • This is more flexible than polyurethane, making its insertion a little difficult

TABLE 3: Contraindications of central venous cannulation monitoring technique.

Absolute	Relative
• Superior vena cava syndrome • Pneumothorax or hemothorax on contralateral side	• Coagulopathies • Presence of newly placed pacemaker wire (4–6 weeks) • Presence of carotid disease • Diaphragmatic dysfunction • Thyromegaly • Previous neck surgery • Burns scar on the neck • Recent cannulation history at the same site • Skin infection at the puncture site • Uncooperative patient • No consent for the procedure • Application of high PEEP • Only one functioning lung

(PEEP: positive end-expiratory pressure)

Equipment (Fig. 1)

- *Nonsterile products:* Surgeon's cap and Mask with eye shield
- *Sterile products:*
  - Personal protective equipment—including gloves, gown
  - Drape
  - Gauze (4 × 4)
  - Chlorhexidine swabs or similar antiseptic agent
  - Sterile ultrasound probe cover with sterile ultrasound gel
  - Biopatch
  - "Luer locks" or catheter caps for each lumen
  - *Central venous catheter kit, which generally includes:* Central venous catheter (triple-lumen, dual-lumen, or large bore single-lumen), 18 gauge introducer needle, with a syringe, #11 blade Scalpel, Guidewire, Venodilator
  - Suture material (generally 3-0 silk suture with a straight needle or a needle driver)
  - Saline lock (number depends on the type of device)
  - 1% lidocaine, small gauge needle (25 or 27 gauge), syringe
  - Ultrasound machine with a high-frequency linear transducer.

Preparations

- Consent for the CVC procedure
- Discuss the risks, benefits, and potential complications of the procedure
- Make the equipment arranged
- Use the ultrasound machine to assess the preferable access site
- Place the patient in an anatomically advantageous position for the procedure. Trendelenburg position, contralateral rotation of the neck, and extension of the ipsilateral arm is advised for jugular catheterization. Trendelenburg position, contralateral rotation of the neck, and adduction of the ipsilateral arm are advised for subclavian catheterization. Some physicians use a cushion placed between shoulder blades to facilitate

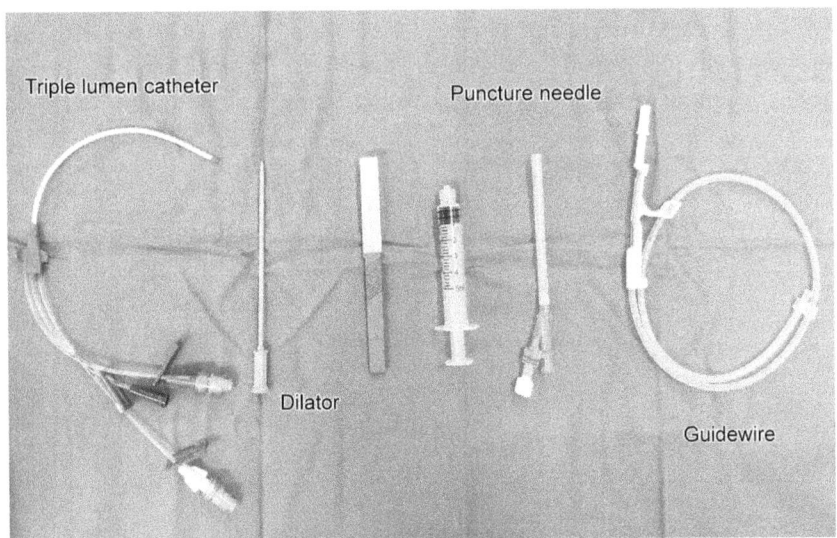

Fig. 1: Equipment of central vein cannulation (CVC).

the access. Little abduction, external rotation of the ipsilateral leg and inverse Trendelenburg position is advised for femoral vein catheterization
- Don the sterile personal protective equipment and prepare the field sterile, the probe, and then start doing the procedure
- Prepare the central venous catheter by attaching saline locks with saline flushes, and flushing all of the ports to ensure that there are no equipment issues, and remove the saline lock from the most distal port
- Assure that all equipment is within reach before initiating the procedure.

Internal Jugular Vein Cannulation

This is the most preferred method for central venous cannulation for anesthesiologists. The success rate is 90–99% and also it has a straight course to superior vena cava (SVC) with easily identifiable landmarks.

Anatomy

The picture depicts the two heads of sternocleidomastoid muscle forming the lateral boundaries, the superior border of the clavicle forming the inferior boundary. The IJV is located anterolateral to the common carotid artery, typically in the superior portion of the triangle created by the sternocleidomastoid (SCM) and the clavicle called "Sédillot's triangle". The internal jugular vein joins the subclavian vein to form the brachiocephalic vein **(Figs. 2 A and B)**. The central approach is the most commonly used, but some have argued that the posterior approach is the safest (being farthest from the lung apex and the carotid artery).

Advantages

This approach is safe in patients with emphysematous chest than the subclavian approach. It is most suitable for transvenous pacing as it is directly accessible to the right ventricle and also in patients with bleeding diathesis.

Approaches to Internal Jugular Vein Cannulation—Cannulation and its Complications

Central approach: From the apex of the sternocleidomastoid muscle. Lower risk of pneumothorax and hemothorax.

Anterior approach: From the medial border of medial head of SCM muscle approximately 5 cm above the clavicle with the needle direction towards the same side nipple. High risk of carotid puncture and hemothorax.

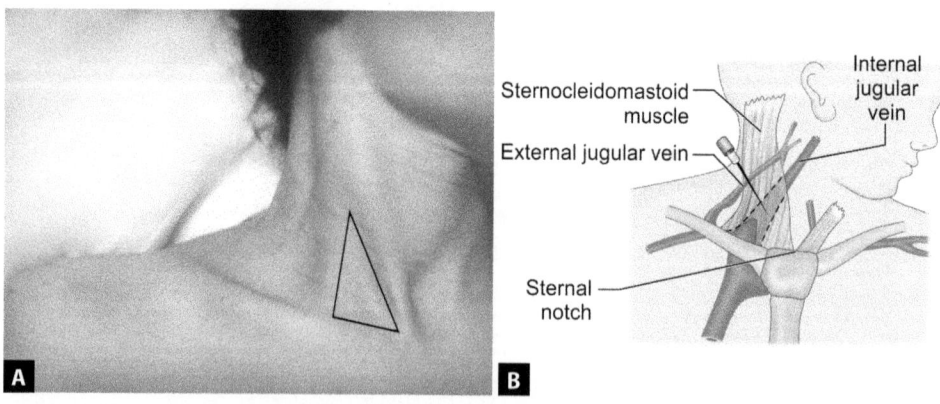

Figs. 2A and B: Anatomy of internal jugular vein cannulation. (A) Clinical image; (B) Schematic diagram.

Posterior approach: Point of intersection with a line joining the cricoid cartilage to the lateral border of clavicular of SCM. Carotid puncture risk is higher.

Supraclavicular approach: At the interscalene groove 2 cm above the clavicle, the needle is directed medially and caudally. High incidence of pneumothorax and risk of subclavian artery puncture **(Table 4)**.

Internal Jugular Vein Cannulation on the Left Side

The technique is similar to the IJV cannulation on right side with fewer anatomical differences like a high dome of pleura increasing the risk of pneumothorax, thoracic duct is close by the junction of IJV and subclavian vein leading to increased risk of duct injury. Left side vein will be smaller in caliber than right side. Carotid artery overlaps more on the vein when the head is rotated >40°. Catheter enters the brachiocephalic vein and rests on the lateral wall of SVC thus increasing the risk of vessel injury. Hence always confirm the position of tip of the catheter through fluoroscopy, X-ray, and ultrasonography.

Subclavian Vein

Most commonly used route for cannulation in patients with cervical spine injury with collars, long-term use in patients undergoing dialysis, chemotherapy, total parenteral nutrition, for emergency resuscitation, long term intravenous therapy.

Anatomy

The vein courses along the clavicle, from lateral to medial, it progresses from the lateral border of the first rib, slopes cephalad at the middle third of the clavicle, and then caudally merges with the internal jugular vein just posterior to the sternoclavicular joint. The subclavian vein lies anterior and superior to the subclavian artery. The lung is located just inferomedially to the subclavian vein, in close approximation to the lateral part of first rib **(Figs. 3A and B)**.

Technique

With head low position, arms adducted fully, roll placed between the shoulder blades, and with aseptic precautions, the skin is punctured 2-3 cm below the mid-point of the clavicle with the needle directed towards the suprasternal notch which is identified by the other hand of the operator. With a constant negative pressure aspiration, needle is advanced gently. If the vein is not punctured, the needle is withdrawn slowly and in the next attempt, needle can be moved more rostral direction by keeping the needle close to the undersurface of the clavicle and do not increase the downward angle. Once the vein is punctured, other steps will be the same as IJV cannulation.

Advantages

Patient will be comfortable as neck is free; risk of infection is less than other sites.

Complications

Pneumothorax (incidence <2%) and subclavian artery puncture (incidence is 5%). Multiple attempts can result in hematoma and pneumothorax. Bilateral side attempts should be avoided. More than 3 attempts should be discouraged.

Pinch-off syndrome: The close relationship between the clavicle and first rib may lead to crimping and intermittent positional or permanent occlusion of compressible catheters placed in this position. This complication has been referred to as the subclavian pinch-off syndrome. This problem occurs with long-term venous access catheters with an incidence of 1-5%. The resulting occlusion will render infusion and possibly

TABLE 4: Approaches to IJV cannulation and its complications.

S.No.	Steps of IJV cannulation	Rationale and problems
1.	Functioning pulse oximeter has to be applied to the patient hand	For monitoring arrhythmia and hypoxemia
2.	Rotate the patient's head to the left side and can be asked to lift the head to note the landmarks (both heads of SCM and mark the surface if required)	Aids in the visualization of landmarks
3.	Position the patient in 15° Trendelenburg position. A wedge of 6–8 cm is kept below the shoulder and the head ring can be removed	Distends IJV and decreases the risk of air embolism, which can increase congestive cardiac failure symptoms
4.	Procedure should be done under strict aseptic precautions	It is mandatory to prevent infection
5.	Under ultrasound guidance (USG) or using landmark technique, identify the vein and local infiltration given if patient is awake with 1% lignocaine to skin and subcutaneous tissues	IJV can be superficial at times, hence withdraw before giving local anesthetics
6.	Finder needle of 22 G, 3.75 cm or 1.5 inch length attached to a Luer-Lock 5 cc syringe	Use of a finder needle helps to decrease the risk of hematoma secondary to carotid puncture
7.	After reconfirming the surface anatomy, the needle is advanced in the appropriate direction facing towards the ipsilateral nipple with negative aspiration	Constant aspiration as the unit is advanced to see flashback
8.	Once the vein is located with finder needle, leave the finder needle in place, and proceed with 18G 2.5 inch in the same direction with negative aspiration until the flashback of venous blood comes and advance it by 1 mm	Finder needle can serve as a reminder for location and if it interferes with cannulation, it can be removed
9.	If blood is not aspirated freely—remove the needle, replace the syringe and aspirate, keep withdrawing until free flow is obtained, or advance it slowly into vein	• Needle could have punctured the posterior wall, hence withdraw it slowly • Patient might be hypovolemic—give fluids • Increase the Trendelenburg position or give Valsalva to make the vein prominent
10.	Confirm its placement by—lack of pulsatile flow, compare IJV and arterial samples visually or by oximetry, can compare the waveforms by attaching to the transducer	If arterial cannulation has happened, remove the needle and give pressure for 5 minutes to avoid the hematoma
11.	Pass the guidewire and once the guidewire is at 15 cm (3 marks), stabilize the wire and remove the needle, then place the dilator over the guidewire. About 1/3 to 1/2 of the length of the dilator will need to be inserted into the skin/soft tissue space. Now use USG to visualize the guidewire in a transverse and longitudinal plane	While passing the guidewire arrhythmia can happen and in that case, withdraw the guidewire little and also it indicates our tip is in the right place. Skin nick may be done to accommodate the dilator

Contd...

Contd...

S.No.	Steps of IJV cannulation	Rationale and problems
12.	Place the CVC over the guidewire after removing the dilator. Keep withdrawing the guidewire until the tip comes out of the CVC distal port, and then CVC is pushed inside. Once catheter is positioned inside the vein fully, remove the guidewire gently. Using a syringe, aspirate blood and remove air from each of the ports, and flush with sterile saline solution. "Luer Locks" may be attached to the end of each port either before or after this step	Do not blindly push the CVC inside without withdrawing and holding the guidewire tip, as it can cause dislodgement of guidewire inside the vein completely
13.	Sterile dressing done after suturing the CVC firmly in place	This prevents dislodgement and infection
14.	In addition to dynamic ultrasound guidance, there are three methods to ensure that a central venous catheter is properly in place, venous blood gas, chest X-ray, and central venous pressure from the distal port	To exclude the arterial placement of the catheter
15.	Chest X-ray should be performed in all IJV and SC CVC insertions	Both to confirm its tip placement and to verify that no complications

(CVC: central vein cannulation; IJV: internal jugular vein; SC: subcutaneous; SCM: sternocleidomastoid; USG: ultrasound guidance)

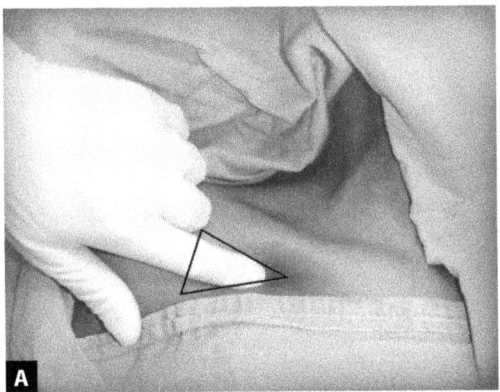
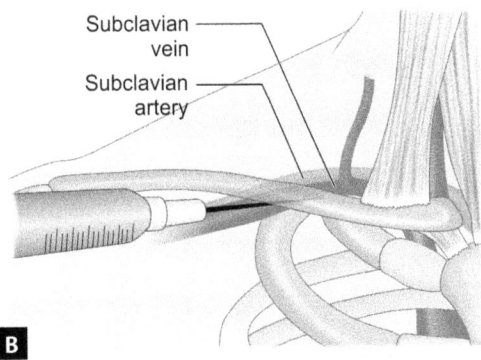

Figs. 3A and B: Anatomy of subclavian vein.

aspiration through the line will be difficult or impossible. Luminal narrowing of the catheter under the clavicle is visible on a chest X-ray and can secure the diagnosis. This radiographic sign was termed the pinch-off sign.

External Jugular Vein

The vein courses superficially across the sternocleidomastoid muscle to join the subclavian vein close to the junction of the IJV and subclavian vein. The presence of valves makes it difficult to thread the guidewire and access the central line as the vein is tortuous in the neck.

Technique

After head down position, traction to the vein is applied and 18G catheter instead of the needle is introduced and a J-tipped flexible guidewire is passed to negotiate the tortuous course. This procedure is usually easy from the left external jugular vein (EJV). Others steps are similar to IJV cannulation.

Advantages

Safe and ready venous access via angiocatheter.

Disadvantages

Risk of vessel avulsion is higher.

Femoral Vein

It is a good cannulation site when jugular veins and subclavian veins are not accessible. This occurs in patients with burns, trauma, and surgical procedures involving head and neck or upper thorax and also during cardiopulmonary resuscitation.

Anatomy

The common femoral vein is located within the femoral triangle. This region is outlined by the adductor longus medially, sartorius muscle laterally, and the inguinal ligament superiorly. Femoral vein lies medial to the femoral artery (**Fig. 4**).

Technique

Femoral artery is palpated and punctured below the inguinal ligament. Longer catheter (40–70 cm) can be inserted and positioned under electrocardiogram or fluoroscopic with its tip at the cavoatrial junction. Shorter length (15–20 cm) can be inserted with the tip at the common iliac vein.

Advantages

Usual complications like pneumothorax and neck hematoma can be avoided, but an injury to the femoral artery and nerve can occur.

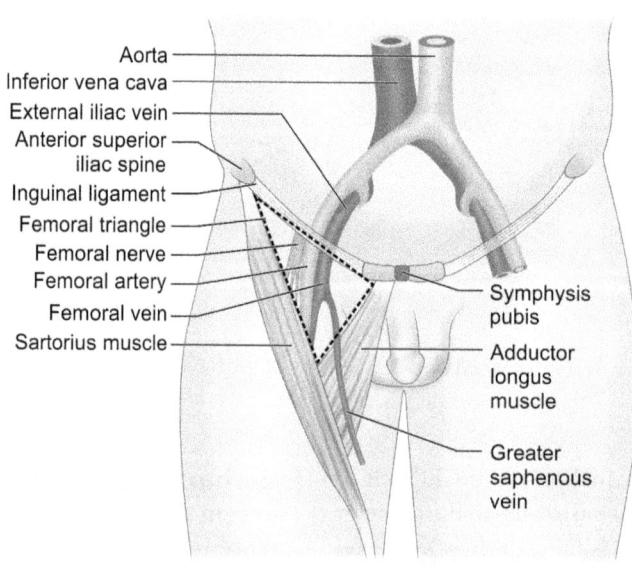

Fig. 4: Anatomy of femoral vein.

Disadvantages

Risk of infection, thromboembolic complications, vascular injury can happen which can lead to intra-abdominal, retroperitoneal hemorrhage. In children, <6 months avascular necrosis of femur, bladder injury, and gangrenous changes in the leg can also occur.

Peripherally Inserted Central Cannula

These are alternatives to CVCs with lower risk of complications. Generally, peripherally inserted central catheter (PICC) lines are inserted via the basilic and cephalic veins of the antecubital space or brachial veins. Basilic vein is preferred (largest diameter 8 mm and nontortuous) compared to cephalic vein (smaller, 6 mm diameter and also angles 90° to terminate into the axillary vein, makes catheter advancement difficult). Not advisable in patients with renal failure requiring dialysis. Polyurethane PICC lines have a higher risk of thrombosis compared to silicone. It needs to be regularly flushed 2–3 mL. Avoid using larger syringes to avoid excessive pressure and catheter rupture.

Technique

Peel away cannula technique: Intravenous access is established like a regular intravenous cannula. Stylet is removed and the catheter is inserted through the cannula. Cannula is pulled back and peeled away from the catheter.

Modified Seldinger technique: Vein is accessed through a regular hypodermic needle, a guidewire is threaded and the needle is removed leaving the guidewire in place. A nick is made in the skin beside the guidewire and an introducer sheath with a dilator is inserted over the guidewire, dilator is removed and the sheath is advanced through the introducer sheath, and then the introducer sheath is pulled back and peeled away.

Indications

Parenteral nutrition, chemotherapy, CVP monitoring, short-term infusion of vasoactive drugs.

Complications

It can produce phlebitis, thrombus formation, infection, and malposition. Increased risk of cardiac perforation or arrhythmias. Always be cautious during the placement of CVC when the PICC line is in place as there is an increased risk of shearing.

Ultrasound-guided Central Venous Cannulation

Two-dimensional (2D) ultrasound guidance helps in detecting the anatomical variations of IJV, locating the vein and it also decreases the incidence of arterial puncture.

Technique

This procedure is performed with real-time 2D 7.5–10 MHz linear probe protected by a sterile sheath. Target vessel view is obtained by holding the ultrasound probe in a non-dominant hand. The USG images of vein and artery appear as two circular black images. The compressible vein wall appearance and the anatomical location help in identifying the vein. Artery will be pulsatile. In transverse axis, both artery and vein can be visualized. But on the longitudinal axis, full length of the needle will be visible all time. After positioning the vein in the center of USG screen, vein is punctured with the 18G needle, and the guidewire is passed. After confirmation of intravenous location of the guidewire in the longitudinal view with USG, a dilator is applied and is then proceeded as described before.

Catheter Position

Confirmation of position of the catheter by radiological means done during the postoperative period. Aspiration of the dark venous blood in the multilumen catheter confirms the placement. Placing an extension line and keeping the tip at the junction of SVC and right atrium, and then look for the fluid movement with respect to the positive pressure ventilation or spontaneous ventilation also confirms the placement. Chest X-ray (CXR) after surgery confirms the tip of the catheter within the SVC and at the level of tracheal carina. Catheter tip should lie parallel to the vessel wall within the SVC, but not below the pericardial reflection of SVC as it increases the risk of pericardial tamponade and perforation. Hence tip should be positioned above the level of third rib, the tracheal carina, T4–5 interspace, division of the right main bronchus, and the azygous vein. The length of the catheter inserted to position the tip in the SVC varies according to the puncture site and it is 3–5 cm more when left IJV or EJV is chosen **(Fig. 5)**.

Few studies revealed fluoroscopically assisted measurements of guidewire length from the cutaneous puncture site to the superior vena cava-atrial junction have revealed mean distances of 16.0 cm for the right internal jugular, 18.4 cm for the right subclavian, 19.1 cm for the left internal jugular, and 21.2 cm for the left subclavian veins, respectively.

CENTRAL VENOUS PRESSURE MONITORING (TABLE 5)

Physiological Considerations for Central Venous Pressure Monitoring

Cardiac filling pressures are measured from the number of sites in the vascular system. Central venous pressure (CVP) is the least monitoring method followed by pulmonary artery and left atrial pressure monitoring. CVP is determined by the interaction of the venous return of the circulatory system and cardiac function. Isolated CVP measurement has little value.

Normal Central Venous Pressure Waveforms

Relation between waveform components and the electrocardiographic R wave is shown in **Figure 6**.

Measurement of Central Venous Pressure

Normal range of central venous pressure (CVP) is 6–8 mm Hg. It can be measured by attaching the transducer to the distal brown port. It can be measured manually at the mid-axillary line where the manometer arm or transducer is level with the phlebostatic axis, i.e., the fourth intercostals space and the mid-axillary line cross each other allowing the measurement close to the right atrium. Line up the manometer arm with the axis and ensure the bubble is zeroed by moving up and down, then turn the three-way tap off the patient and open to the manometer. Open the IV fluid to fill the manometer higher than expected CVP and turn off the fluid. Open the three-way to the patient and the fluid level inside starts falling until the gravity equals the

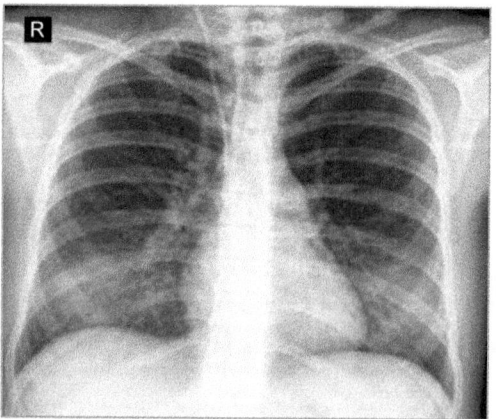

Fig. 5: Chest X-ray showing central venous cannulation.

Chapter 28: Central Venous Cannulation Technique and Central Venous Pressure Monitoring

TABLE 5: Components of central venous pressure.

Waveform component	Phase of cardiac cycle	Mechanical event
a wave	End diastole	Atrial contraction
c wave	Early systole	Isovolumetric contraction, tricuspid motion towards right atrium
v wave	Late systole	Systolic filling of atrium
h wave	Mid-to-late systole	Diastolic plateau
x descent	Mid systole	Atrial relaxation, descent of the base, systolic collapse
y descent	Early diastole	Early ventricular filling, diastolic collapse

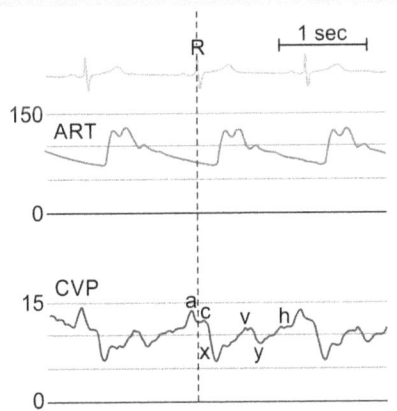

Fig. 6: Relation between individual waveforms components and the electrocardiographic R wave.

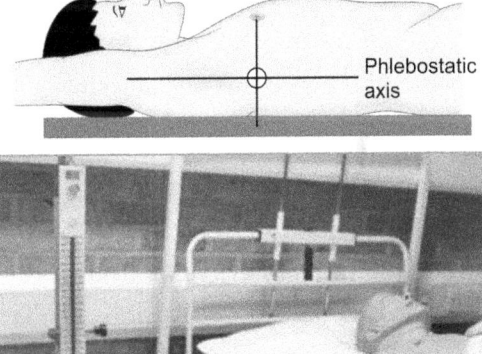

Fig. 7: Measurement of central venous pressure.

pressure in the central veins. When it stops CVP value can be read. Right IJV is the most preferred site for central venous cannulation. Static measurement is less helpful in guiding the fluid resuscitation whereas the dynamic measurements may be more informative. Preload can be assessed by dynamic changes in response to the fluid challenge (**Fig. 7**).

Relation of Central Venous Pressure with Venous Return and Cardiac Function

Central Venous Pressure and Venous Return

Venous return to the heart is determined by the gradient between the mean circulatory filling pressure (MCFP) and CVP. Normal MCFP is estimated to be between 8-10 mm Hg and CVP is 2-3 mm Hg in healthy individuals. The difference between MCFP and CVP is only 6-8 mm Hg and the small changes may be found to have profound hemodynamic consequences.

Central Venous Pressure and Cardiac Function

Central venous pressure (CVP) is affected by many cardiac conditions. Hence, assessing the CVP as a predictor of volume status or fluid responsiveness failed to demonstrate a

TABLE 6: Abnormal central venous pressure waveforms.

Condition	Characteristics
• Atrial fibrillation	• Loss of a wave, prominent c wave
• Atrioventricular dissociation	• Cannon a wave
• Tricuspid regurgitation	• Tall systolic c-v-wave, loss of x descent
• Tricuspid stenosis	• Tall a wave, attenuation of y descent
• Right ventricular ischemia	• Tall a and v waves, steep a and y descent, M or W configuration
• Pericardial constriction	• Tall a and v waves, steep a and y descent, M or W configuration
• Cardiac tamponade	• Dominant x descent, attenuated y descent
• Respiratory variation during spontaneous or positive pressure ventilation	• Measure pressures at end-expiration

relationship between the CVP and circulating blood volume.

Abnormal Central Venous Pressure Waveforms

Table 6 enlists abnormal central venous pressure waveforms.

Complications

- *Mechanical:* Vascular injury, respiratory compromise, nerve injury, arrhythmias
- *Thromboembolic:* Venous thrombosis, pulmonary thromboembolism, arterial thrombosis and embolism, catheter or guidewire embolism
- *Infectious:* Insertion site infection, catheter infection, bloodstream infection, and endocarditis
- Misinterpretation of data and misuse of equipment

FURTHER READING

1. Bannon MP, Heller SF, Rivera M. Anatomic considerations for central venous cannulation. Risk Manag Healthc Policy. 2011;4:27-39.
2. Gropper MA, Eriksson LI, Fleisher LA, Wiener-Kronish JP, Cohen NH, Leslie K. Miller's Anesthesia, 9th edition. Philadelphia: Elsevier-Health Sciences Division; 2019. p. 3112.
3. Kolikof J, Peterson K, M. Baker A. Central Venous Catheter. In: StatPearls [Internet]. Treasure Island (FL): StatPearls Publishing; 2022.
4. Laheri VV. In: Baheti DK (Ed). Understanding Anesthesia Equipment and Procedures: A Practical Approach, 1st edition. New Delhi: Jaypee Brothers Medical Publishers Pvt. Ltd; 2021.
5. Pires RC, Rodrigues N, Machado J, Cruz RP. Central venous catheterization: an updated review of historical aspects, indications, techniques, and complications. Transl Surg. 2017;2(3):66-70.

CHAPTER 29

Pulmonary Artery Catheter Monitoring

Kirthiha Govindaraj, Gnanasekaran Srinivasan

INTRODUCTION

Pulmonary artery catheter was introduced by Harold James wan and William Ganz in the 1970s. The special-purpose with its use was cardiac output monitoring, pacing, right ventricle (RV) ejection fraction monitoring, and continuous cardiac output monitoring. But still, it remains uncertain whether PAC monitoring leads to improved patient outcomes.

INDICATIONS

- Hemodynamic instability of unclear physiologic etiology
- To guide treatment in case of complicated myocardial infarction
- Cardiogenic shock, noncardiogenic pulmonary edema, acute respiratory distress syndrome (ARDS), critically ill patients on inotropes and vasopressors
- Surgeries requiring critical fluid resuscitation, e.g., liver transplant, septic shock.

CONTRAINDICATIONS

- Tricuspid or pulmonic stenosis
- RA, RV, or PA masses
- Tetralogy of Fallot (RVOT being hypersensitive, PAC may induce infundibular spasm) arrhythmias, coagulopathy, complete LBBB, WPW syndrome, and Ebstein's malformation.

CATHETER DESIGN

Pulmonary artery catheter (PAC) is a flexible, flow-directed, tipped catheter available in adult and pediatric sizes ranging from 60 to 110 cm in length, 7.0–9.0 Fr in caliber, and inflation volumes ranging from 0.5–1.5 mL. It is made up of polyvinyl chloride which softens at body temperature. It is marked at every 10 cm by thin and thick black lines to estimate the catheter tip location during the insertion. It has five lumens which vary according to the design. A Percutaneous sheath introducer and contamination shields were also provided along with the PAC. Parts include a distal lumen, proximal infusion lumen, proximal injectate lumen, balloon inflation lumen, thermistor connector lumen, additional venous infusion lumen, oximetry lumen **(Fig. 1)**.

Distal lumen: Terminates at the distal tip. It measures the pulmonary artery pressures (PAP), pulmonary capillary wedge pressure (PCWP), and blood sampling for measuring mixed venous oxygen saturation. Not used for continuous fluid or drug administration purposes.

Proximal infusion lumen: It terminates 30 cm proximal to the catheter tip and is positioned in the right atrium. It allows an infusion of solutions, central venous pressure (CVP) monitoring, and blood sampling.

Proximal injectate lumen: It terminates at 26 cm from the distal tip. This port resides

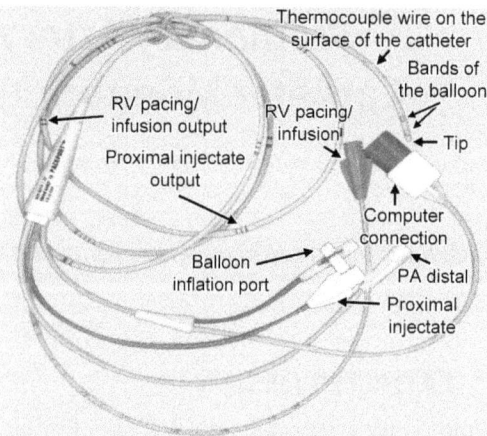

Fig. 1: Pulmonary artery catheter with its parts.

at the right atrium or vena cava. It allows RA pressure monitoring, blood sampling, or infusion of solutions.

Balloon inflation lumen: This is the third lumen that terminates within the balloon located proximal to the catheter tip, which is used to float the catheter through the cardiac chambers.

Thermistor connector lumen: It is connected by small wires to a small thermistor located 3.5–4 cm proximal to the catheter tip and used for measuring the cardiac output using the thermodilution method.

Additional venous infusion lumen: This lumen provides separate access to the right atrium and is used for continuous infusion of fluids during cardiac output measurement.

Oximetry lumen: It terminates at the distal tip and contains fiber optic bundles through which light is transmitted to the pulmonary artery and reflected to the photodetector by the hemoglobin in the blood.

INSERTION TECHNIQUE

Different pressures at different catheters positions when threading the catheter from the right. The preferred site of cannulation is the internal jugular vein (IJV) followed by the subclavian or femoral vein. The sterile sheath that covers the PAC must be secured at both ends to prevent the contamination of its outer portion of the sheath. All lumens will be flushed with the heparinized saline and the distal portion of the port is attached to the transducer. Using an 18 G needle, IJV is punctured, and a flexible guidewire is passed, the needle is removed. (Large bore introducer sheath that has a hemostasis valve at its outer end and a sidearm extension for intravenous access. Stopcock can be placed to the extension to prevent blood loss). An 8 Fr vein dilator passed over the guidewire, and the sheath remains in IJV after the dilator and guidewire, were removed. Before placing the PAC, the patency and symmetry of the balloon are tested with 1.5 mL of air from a volume-limited syringe. Start advancing the PAC to a depth of 15–20 cm and the waveform of the CVP is confirmed and the balloon is inflated. Orient the PAC curve leftwards to the sagittal plane and position the head down facilitates the passage of PAC to the tricuspid valve. When the catheter tip enters the RV, there is a rise in systolic pressure of 15–30 mm Hg with a change in diastolic blood pressure (DBP) of 0–8 mm Hg. As it passes through the pulmonic valve, a dicrotic notch appears on the waveform with a sudden increase in the diastolic pressure. PAP waveform is similar to the systemic arterial waveform but smaller and precedes slightly with PAP systolic 15–20 mm Hg and diastolic of 5–12 mm Hg. Advancing further by 3–5 cm, the tracing resembling CVP morphology is obtained, with PCWP 5–12 mm Hg. Deflate the balloon and confirm the reappearance of PAP waveforms. If it does not appear withdraw the catheter till it appears. During the catheter use, an inflation syringe will be kept attached to the gate valve to prevent the inadvertent injection of liquid into the balloon inflation lumen.

The stiffness of the catheter can be changed according to the cardiac manipulation and temperature changes that occur during the cardiopulmonary bypass. This can result in the catheter migration distally without even balloon inflation. Hence, PAC can be withdrawn 3-5 cm before the institution of CPB. Pressure monitoring lumens were kept patent by an intermittent flush of continuous infusion with heparinized saline solution. Avoid flushing the catheter, when the balloon is wedged in the pulmonary artery. **Table 1** and **Figure 2** show the pulmonary artery catheter position at a specific catheter length with characteristic waveforms.

Additional 5-10 cm from the left IJV and left external jugular vein, 15 cm from the femoral vein, and 30-35 cm from the antecubital veins need to be taken. PAOP is measured at the end-expiration when the effect of intrathoracic pressure is minimal. The tip should be within 2 cm of the cardiac silhouette on an AP chest film. The tip must lie on the west zone 3 of the lung, where the PAP and PVP exceed the alveolar pressure **(Fig. 3)**.

NORMAL PULMONARY ARTERY PRESSURES, WAVEFORMS, AND ITS INTERPRETATION

In the wedged position, a continuous static column of blood connects the PAC tip to the junction of the pulmonary veins and left atrium. Pulmonary capillary wedge pressure (PCWP) and pulmonary artery diastolic pressure (PADP) are estimates of left atrial

TABLE 1: Pulmonary artery catheter position and appropriate catheter length.

Pulmonary artery catheter position	At approximate catheter length
Right atrium	20–25 cm
Right ventricle	30–35 cm
Pulmonary artery	40–45 cm
Wedge position	45–55 cm

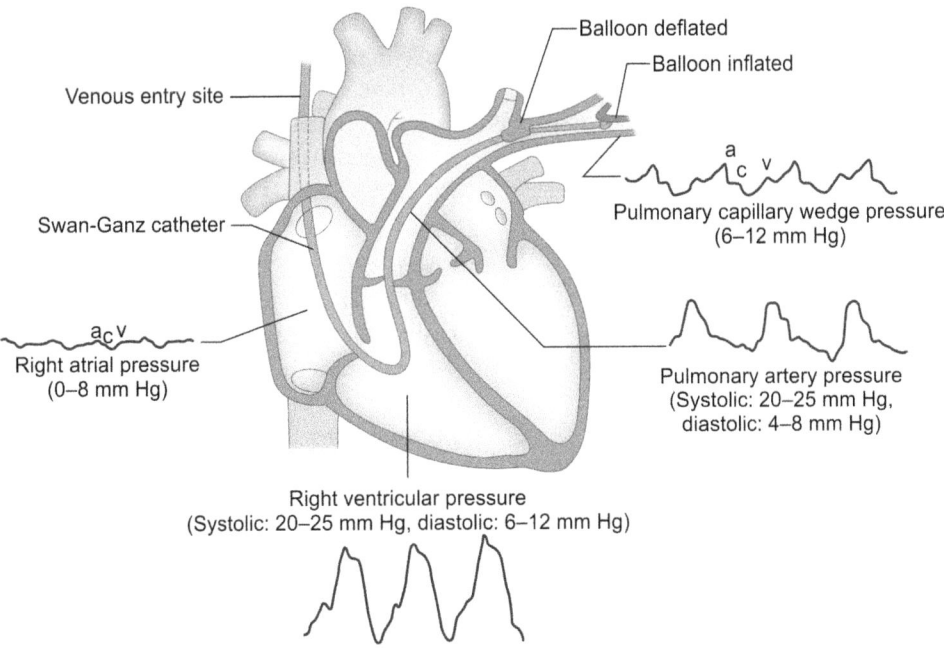

Fig. 2: Pulmonary artery catheter (PAC) catheter at specific sites with the characteristic waveforms.

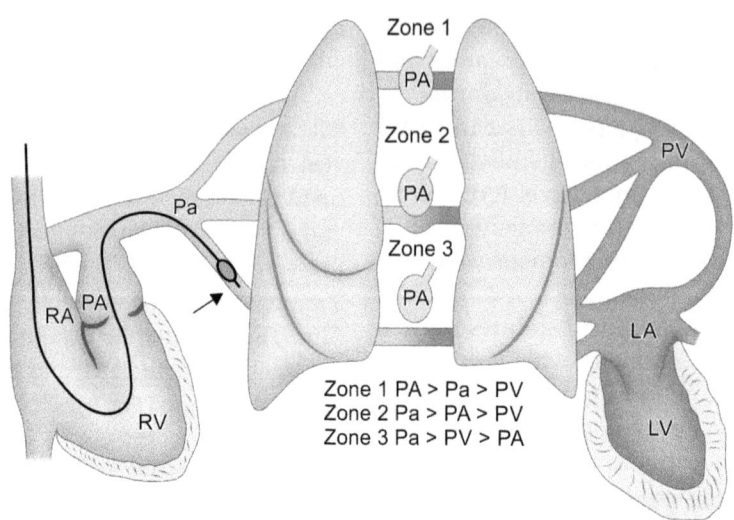

Fig. 3: The position of the pulmonary artery catheter (PAC) tip in west zone 3 of the lung indicated by the arrow.

pressure (LAP), which is a reflection of left ventricular end-diastolic pressure (LVEDP) and left ventricle (LV) preload. The factors affecting the PAP and PCWP are intrathoracic pressure, LV compliance, valvular dysfunction, etc. A properly wedged catheter with the balloon inflated does not allow the mixing of shunted venous blood with postcapillary blood so that the oxygen saturation is around 20% higher than that recorded with the balloon deflated. As the balloon-tipped PAC is floated in its proper position in the pulmonary artery, characteristic pressure waveforms are recorded according to the position of the tip of the PAC **(Table 2)**. The relationship of normal PAP and PCWP waveform with arterial pressure waveform and CVP waveform is shown in **Figure 4**.

The system is zeroed to ambient air pressure either before or after PAC insertion using the midpoint of the LA (i.e., 4th intercostal space (ICS) in the midaxillary line as the reference point). Few monitors have an automated electronic calibration after zeroing.

PAP waveform: It has a systolic phase, diastolic phase, and a dicrotic notch. Dicrotic notch: reflects the closure of the semilunar valves at the end of contraction and prior to the refilling of ventricles. Slight elevation seen at the dicrotic notch represents the transient increase in PAP.

PCWP waveform: It resembles like CVP waveform. It has a, c, v waves and x, y descents. 'a' wave may be increased in patients with high resistance to LV filling, e.g., mitral stenosis, LV failure, decreased LV compliance. Large 'v' waves seen in myocardial infarction secondary to decreased LV diastolic compliance, or mitral regurgitation secondary to ischemic papillary muscle dysfunction.

Dampened waveform: It is most commonly results from the transducer malfunction, loose connection in any part of the tubing, catheter impinging on the vessel wall, air bubbles, etc. The dampened system does not overshoot or oscillate, and there will be a delay in returning to the PAC waveform. It is usually checked with the rapid flush test where an initial horizontal straight line with high-pressure recording. After the flushing is terminated, the pressure drops immediately represented by a vertical line that plunges

TABLE 2: Position of PAC and the characteristic waveforms.

Position of PAC	Characteristics	Pressure waveforms
Superior vena cava or right atrium	CVP waveform with a, c, v waves, and low mean pressure should be observed	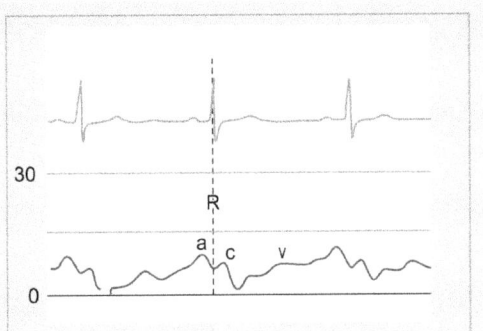
Right ventricle	Rapid systolic upstroke, wide pulse pressure, and low diastolic pressure	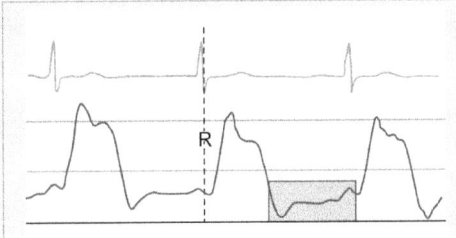
Pulmonary artery	Step up in diastolic pressure (diastolic contours) and change in waveform morphology *RV*: During diastole, it increases due to filling from the right atrium *PA*: During diastole, PAP pressure will fall due to continuous runoff flow to the lung	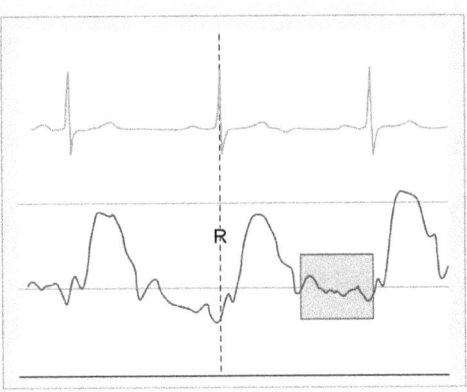
Pulmonary artery wedge pressure	Resembles the venous waveforms with the characteristic a and v waves, and x and y descents. It is also a delayed and damped representation of left atrial pressure	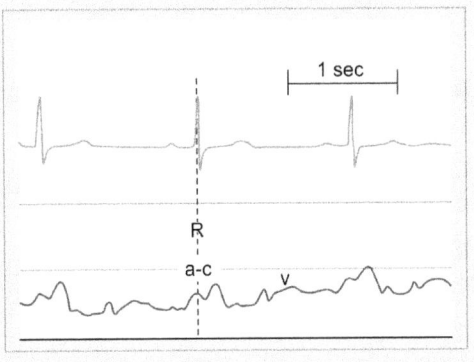

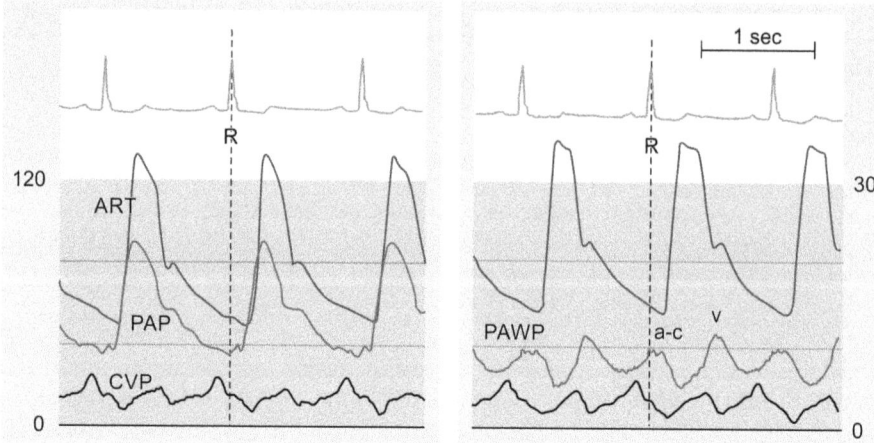

Fig. 4: Pulmonary artery pressure (PAP) and pulmonary capillary wedge pressure (PCWP) waveform in relation to arterial and central venous pressure (CVP) waveform.

below the baseline. A brief well-defined oscillation occurs followed by the return of the PA waveform.

Over wedging waveform: Over wedged pressure is devoid of pulsatility, higher than expected, and rises continuously to flush pressure. Continuous wedge trace with the balloon deflated or with minimal deflation raises the suspicion of distal catheter migration.

ABNORMAL PULMONARY ARTERY AND WEDGE PRESSURE WAVEFORMS

Artifactual pressure spikes may be distinguished from the underlying physiologic pressure waveform by the unique morphology and timing **(Table 3)**.

PHYSIOLOGIC CONSIDERATIONS FOR PULMONARY ARTERY CATHETER MONITORING: PREDICTION OF LEFT VENTRICULAR PRELOAD

- Used to estimate LV end-diastolic pressure, a surrogate measure of LV end-diastolic volume.
- PAWP provides an indirect measurement of both pulmonary venous pressure and left atrial pressure (to measure this, the catheter needs to reside, in the so-called, *West zone three of the lung*).
- PAD pressure is used as an alternative to PAWP to estimate the LV filling pressure. It also has the advantage of being available for continuous monitoring whereas PAWP is only measured intermittently.

TROUBLESHOOTING THE PULMONARY ARTERY CATHETER MONITORING

- If the RV waveform is not present after inserting up to 40 cm—coiling in the right atrium is likely
- If PAP waveform is not obtained after inserting up to 50 cm—coiling in the right ventricle has occurred
- In both scenarios, deflate the balloon, withdraw the catheter to 20 cm and the PAC floating sequence can be repeated with the additional points. As the balloon floats easily in nondependent regions as it passes through the heart into pulmonary vasculature, head down will float the

TABLE 3: Artifacts observed at different conditions and the specific waveforms.

Site and events	Artifacts observed and solution	Characteristics waveforms
• Onset of systole: Tricuspid valve closure with RV contraction and ejection with resultant excessive catheter motion	Most common artifact. Erroneously, it will show as low pressure and designated as pulmonary artery diastolic pressure—repositioning the PAC	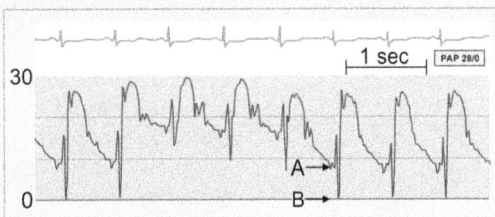 The correct value of PA-EDP is 8 mm Hg. But the monitor displays erroneously as 28/0 mm Hg
• Over-wedging: Due to distal catheter migration and eccentric balloon overinflation that forces the catheter against the vessel wall	Nonpulsatile increasing pressure-gentle catheter withdrawal to a more proximal location in the pulmonary artery	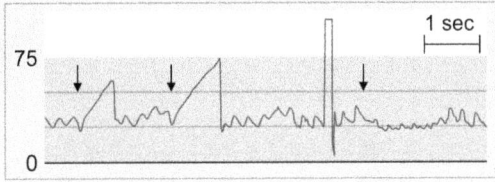 Nonpulsatile increasing pressure by occluded catheter (first two arrows). Restoring of PA and PAWP after flushing the catheter
• PAC balloon inflation and wedge measurement: Can cause migration of the catheter tip distally	The appearance of wedge pressure tracing during partial balloon inflation is suggestive of PAC location at the distal branch. Slight withdrawal of the catheter	
• Pulmonary artery and wedge pressure: Characteristic waveforms in left-sided pathology • Mitral regurgitation—distorts the systolic portion	Tall v wave (begins in early systole) in PAWP and also distorts the PAP trace—bifid appearance, causing the mean PAWP to exceed the LVEDP. It is neither a specific nor sensitive indicator of MR severity	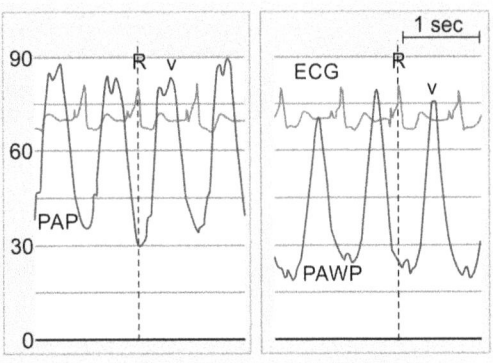 In severe mitral regurgitation, PAWP exceeds the LVEDP. LVEDP is estimated by measuring the PAWP at the time of ECG R wave, before the regurgitant v wave

Contd...

Contd...

Site and events	Artifacts observed and solution	Characteristics waveforms
• Mitral stenosis—distorts the diastolic portion	• Increased mean wedge pressure, slurred early diastolic y descent, tall end-diastolic a wave • Advanced mitral stenosis with atrial fibrillation—a wave will not present in many of these cases	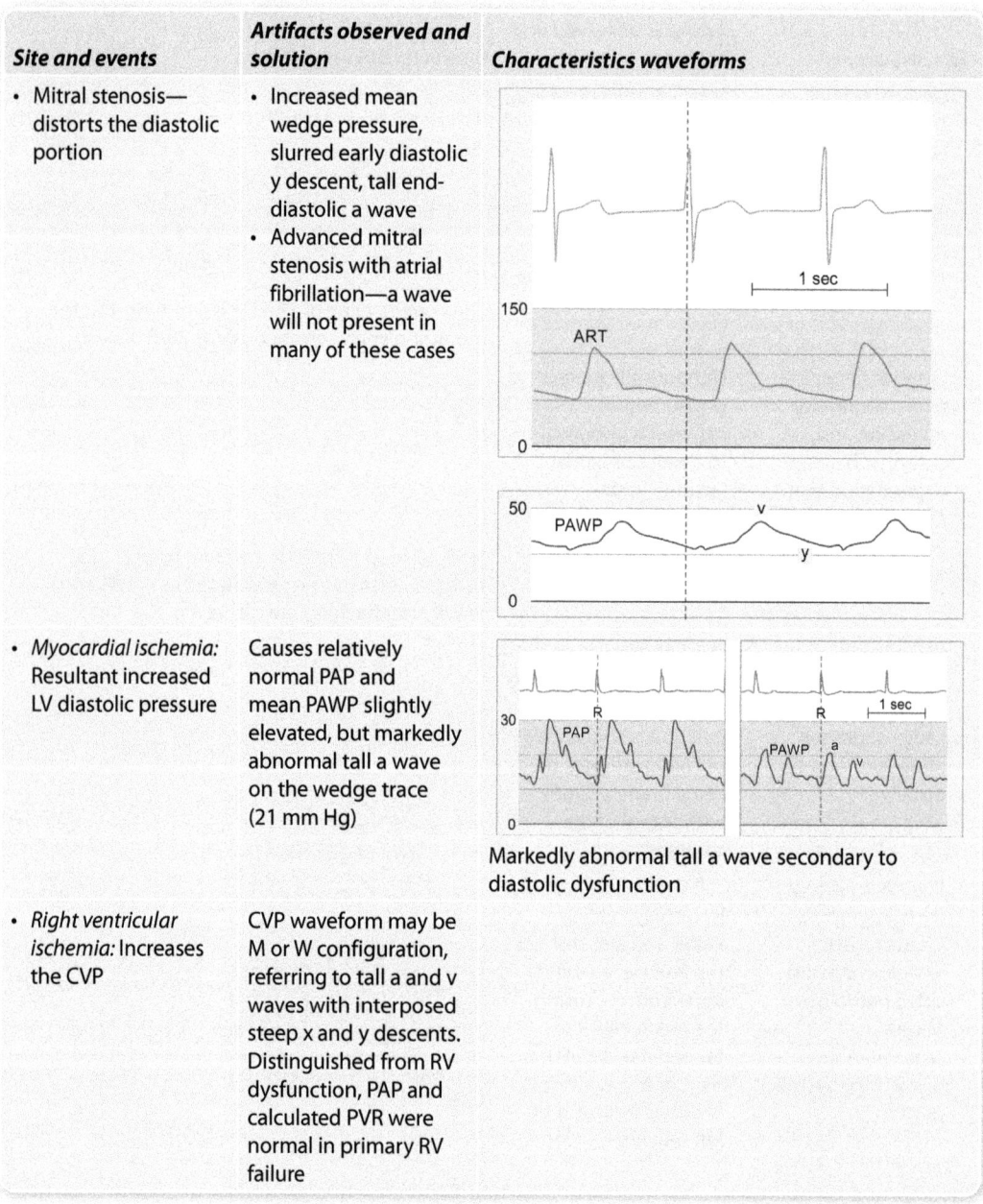
• *Myocardial ischemia:* Resultant increased LV diastolic pressure	Causes relatively normal PAP and mean PAWP slightly elevated, but markedly abnormal tall a wave on the wedge trace (21 mm Hg)	Markedly abnormal tall a wave secondary to diastolic dysfunction
• *Right ventricular ischemia:* Increases the CVP	CVP waveform may be M or W configuration, referring to tall a and v waves with interposed steep x and y descents. Distinguished from RV dysfunction, PAP and calculated PVR were normal in primary RV failure	

Contd...

Contd...

Site and events	Artifacts observed and solution	Characteristics waveforms
• RV infarction, restrictive cardiomyopathy, or pericardial constriction	Elevated mean pressures, prominent a and v waves, steep x and y descents, and a mid-diastolic plateau wave—characteristic W or M configuration in CVP trace secondary to damping effect of the pulmonary vasculature	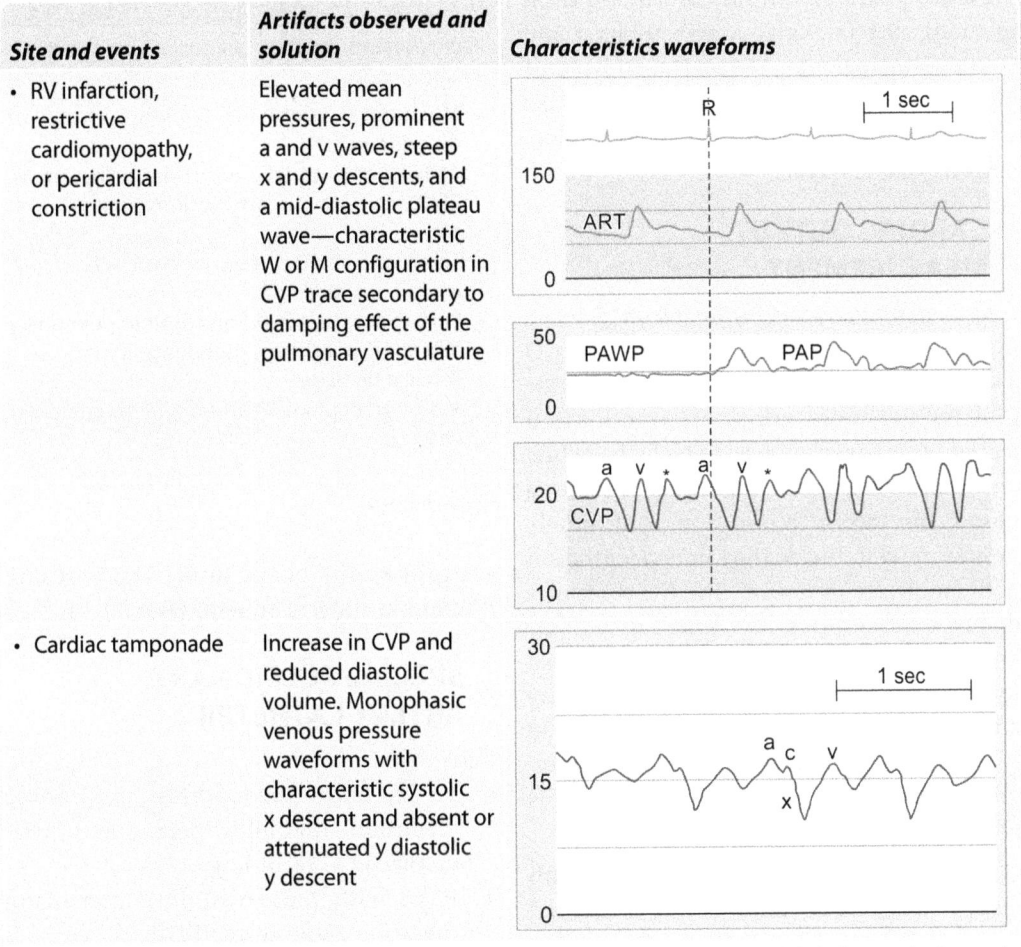
• Cardiac tamponade	Increase in CVP and reduced diastolic volume. Monophasic venous pressure waveforms with characteristic systolic x descent and absent or attenuated y diastolic y descent	

(CVP: central venous pressure; ECG: electrocardiogram; LV: left ventricle; LVEDP: left ventricular end-diastolic pressure; PA: pulmonary artery; PAC: pulmonary artery catheter; PAP: pulmonary artery pressure; PAWP: pulmonary arterial wedge pressure; RV: right ventricle)

balloon across the tricuspid valve. Further tilting the patient to the right side and placing head up encourages the floatation out of the right ventricle and also reduces the incidence of arrhythmias during the insertion. Deep inspiration during spontaneous ventilation also facilitates catheter floatation. Sometimes catheter can be floated to the proper position when stiffened by injecting 10–20 mL ice-cold solution through the distal lumen. Finally, maneuvering the PAC can also be guided by transthoracic echocardiogram (TTE) or transesophageal echocardiogram (TEE) by demonstrating its passage in the heart.

PULMONARY ARTERY CATHETER-DERIVED HEMODYNAMIC VARIABLES

Right atrial and ventricular pressures, pulmonary artery systolic and diastolic pressures,

PCWP estimates, left atrial and LV end-diastolic pressures, cardiac output (thermodilution method), mixed venous oxygen saturation, and core body temperature. Derived hemodynamic parameters were SVR, PVR, LV, and RV stroke work index, oxygen delivery and consumption, oxygen extraction ratio.

CARDIAC OUTPUT MEASUREMENT

Intermittent thermodilution technique: As many newer methods of measuring the CO are less invasive, PAC remains a valuable tool for CO monitoring. Thermodilution technique is based on the principle that when an indicator substance is added to circulating blood, the rate of blood flow is inversely proportional to the change in concentration of the indicator over time. The CO computer displays the temperature-time curve. This area under the curve is inversely proportional to the rate of blood flow in the pulmonary artery. In the absence of a shunt, this flow rate is equivalent to the average cardiac output. The modified Stewart-Hamilton equation is used to calculate the cardiac output.

Continuous thermodilution technique: With a specialized PA catheter of 10 cm thermal filament incorporated into the RV portion of the PAC approximately 15–25 cm from the catheter tip. The filament produces the low-energy heat pulses that get transmitted to the surrounding blood with the resulting temperature change. This change is measured by the Thermistor at the PAC tip. The thermodilution temperature curve is plotted and displayed value of CO every 30–60 seconds. It represents the CO measured over the last 3–6 minutes.

COMPLICATIONS

The incidence of complications from PAC monitoring varies widely, although serious

> **BOX 1:** Complications of pulmonary artery catheter monitoring.
>
> *Complications depicting pulmonary artery catheter monitoring*
>
> - Mechanical problems (kinking, knots, or dislodgement)
> - Arrhythmias (atrial, ventricular arrhythmias, RBBB, complete heart block in patients with pre-existing LBBB)
> - Thromboembolism, thrombocytopenia
> - Infection, endocarditis
> - Pulmonary artery injury and rupture, pulmonary infarction, pulmonary pseudoaneurysm
> - Valvular damage
> - Misuse of equipment and misinterpretation of data
>
> (LBBB: left bundle branch block; RBBB: right bundle branch block)

complications occur in 0.1–0.5% of PAC monitored surgical patients **(Box 1)**.

SPECIAL PULMONARY ARTERY CATHETER

It includes:
- PAC's with permanently implanted electrodes that allow pacing and intracardiac ECG recording.
- PACs with rapid response thermistor measures RVEF and RVEDV.
- PAC's with antimicrobial heparin coating are also available.

MIXED VENOUS OXIMETRY PULMONARY ARTERY CATHETER

The physiological relations described by Fick's equation forms the basis for another PAC-based monitoring technique known as continuous mixed venous oximetry. Hence the rearrangement of the equation reveals the four determinants of mixed venous hemoglobin saturation by modified Fick formula. This can be used as an indirect indicator of cardiac output. It also provides information about the balance of oxygen delivery and oxygen consumption by the body. Always remember this measurement value reflects the global, whole-body measurement.

$$S_vO_2 = S_aO_2 - \dot{V}O_2/CO \times 1.34 \times Hb$$

REMOVAL OF PULMONARY ARTERY CATHETER

Check the recent CXR film to rule out any knotting or coiling of the catheter. Make the patient position head down to prevent air embolism. The balloon needs to be deflated before its removal. The introducer sheath with the sidearm may be left at its place for IV access. Coagulation status needs to be checked before the removal of the introducer sheath. Unclip the hub of the catheter sheath, remove gently and steadily. Whenever there is resistance during the removal, suspect the attachment towards the cardiac structure.

FURTHER READING

1. Gropper MA, Eriksson LI, Fleisher LA, Wiener-Kronish JP, Cohen NH, Leslie K. Miller's Anesthesia: International Edition, 9th edition.

CHAPTER 30

Perioperative Cardiac Output Monitoring

Sayan Nath, Abhishek Singh, Puneet Khanna

INTRODUCTION

Hemodynamic monitoring has evolved leaps and bounds in last few decades owing to the increasing evidence behind its role in identifying and preventing occult hemodynamic changes which in turn transforms into improved perioperative outcomes. The invasiveness and complications associated with the use of pulmonary artery catheter (PAC) have prompted clinicians and researchers to develop less invasive and completely noninvasive techniques while PAC is still considered the gold standard but not the preferred method of hemodynamic measurements. This chapter outlines the principles of different semi-invasive and noninvasive methods of perioperative continuous cardiac output monitoring devices.

CARDIAC OUTPUT MONITORING: WHY AND WHEN?

Individual hearts fall in different parts of the slope of the Frank–Starling curve of cardiac output (CO) versus cardiac preload. Accordingly, for achieving the same cardiac output few patients will require fluid (preload optimization) while few will require inotropes (optimization of cardiac contractility) in order to achieve the maximum cardiac output in a given clinical situation. If a patient has optimized cardiac output and is still hypotensive then it is in all probability due to a decreased afterload or in other words, the shock is distributive and the patient will require vasopressors in order to maintain blood pressure.

In modern-day anesthesia practice, it is important to optimize the fluid (preload) and/or cardiac contractility in order to attain the best hemodynamic targets. Studies have shown that goal-directed fluid therapy (goal is to achieve best cardiac output) in combination with minimally invasive cardiac output monitoring (MICOM) improves perioperative outcomes. Accordingly, continuous cardiac output measurement has become the cornerstone of hemodynamic monitoring in the perioperative period for surgeries where significant hemodynamic alterations are expected owing to either the patient's preexisting cardiac disease (e.g., severe cardiomyopathies, severe valvular heart disease, recent myocardial infarction, etc.) or the invasiveness of the procedure (e.g., surgeries with a chance of major blood loss, major tumor surgeries, emergency laparotomies, etc.).

METHODS OF CONTINUOUS CARDIAC OUTPUT MEASUREMENT

There are ample novel technologies to measure cardiac output in a minimally

invasive fashion. The major principles and techniques are enumerated below:
- *Indicator dilution techniques:*
  - Thermodilution
  - Lithium dilution
  - Pulse dye densitometry
- Minimally invasive arterial waveform analysis
- Noninvasive finger blood pressure waveform analysis
- Pulse wave transit time
- Thoracic impedance
- Thoracic bioreactance
- Electrical cardiometry
- Doppler principles
- Partial CO_2 rebreathing technique (Fick principle)
- Ultrasound dilution technique.

Indicator Dilution Techniques

Transpulmonary Thermodilution

A predetermined amount of cold saline is injected into the central vein (most commonly in the superior vena cava system) which passes through the right heart, pulmonary circulation, left heart, and finally into the arterial system where the temperature drop since the injectate is measured with a thermistor tipped catheter in any of the peripheral arteries (femoral, axillary or brachial). A thermodilution curve is generated from the same by computer software and cardiac output is measured using calculations based on the Stewart–Hamilton equation much similar to the PAC (Fig. 1).

The advantage of the transpulmonary thermodilution technique is that its measurement is not affected by arrhythmias, it can be used in spontaneously breathing patients and it has an excellent correlation with pulmonary artery-based cardiac output measurement. It can also provide other important hemodynamic variables such as global end-diastolic volume (GEDV), extravascular lung water (EVLW), and

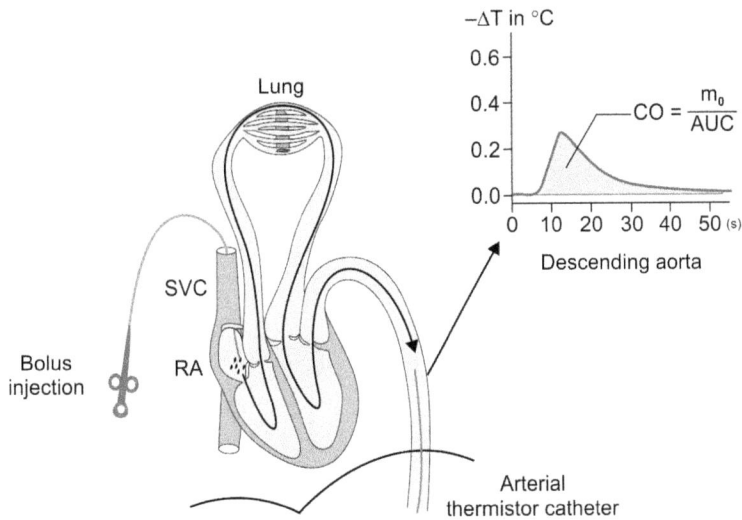

Fig. 1: Transpulmonary thermodilution technique.
(AUC: area under thermodilution curve; CO: cardiac output; m_0: [(Temperature of blood-temperature of injectate). (Amount of injectate). Constant], the value of the constant depends on the specific weight and specific temperature of blood and the injectate.

pulmonary vascular permeability index (PVPI) (**Fig. 2**).

The disadvantages are potential sources of errors such as severe valvular regurgitation, underestimation of cardiac output due to indicator recirculation from tissues, and that the method is a noncontinuous mode of cardiac output measurement.

Lithium Dilution Technique

About 0.5–2 mL bolus (0.15 mmol/mL) of lithium chloride (to a maximum cumulative dose of 20 mL) is injected through a central or a peripheral venous catheter, and lithium concentration is measured by a sensor attached to an indwelling arterial cannula. The resulting lithium plasma concentration versus time curve is used to calculate plasma flow using the Stewart-Hamilton equation. Plasma flow is converted to blood flow by dividing the value by one packed cell volume. An advantage of this system is a high signal-to-noise ratio since lithium does not naturally occur in plasma. It has a rapid redistribution time and minimal first-pass loss from circulation. Disadvantages are diminished accuracy in patients on long-term lithium treatment, concurrent administration of nondepolarizing neuromuscular blocking agents such as atracurium and rocuronium (which leads to an overestimation of cardiac output as these agents at their peak

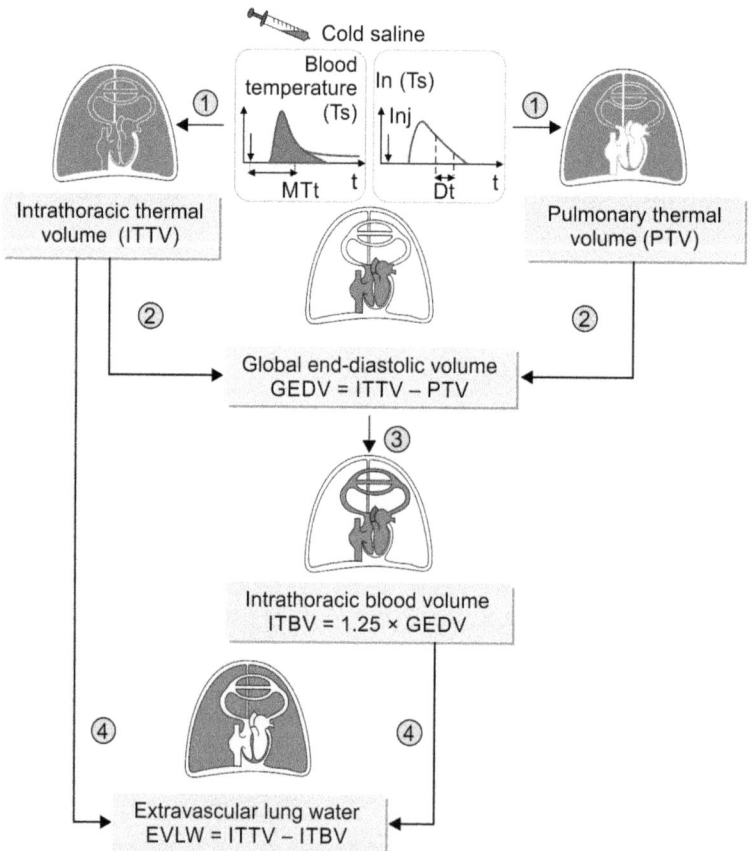

Fig. 2: Calculation of hemodynamic parameters from transpulmonary thermodilution technique.

concentration are also detected by the arterial sensor). This technique is contraindicated in patients <40 kg and during the first trimester of pregnancy.

Pulse Dye Densitometry

This method estimates the arterial concentration of a dye indocyanine green (ICG) after intravenous bolus injection. It is a completely noninvasive method. After injection of the dye in a peripheral vein, the dye passes through the pulmonary circulation and then comes into the arterial system where a fingertip or a nasal sensor detects the ICG concentration noninvasively by emitting lights at wavelengths 805 nm and 890 nm. Indocyanine green has peak optical absorption at 805 nm and insignificant at 890 mm. Absorption by oxyhemoglobin and deoxyhemoglobin is similar at 805 nm. The ratio of light absorption at 805 and 850 nm and the concentration of hemoglobin are then used to calculate the ICG concentration. Cardiac output is calculated using the area under curve (AUC) obtained from the first recirculation of ICG similar to other thermodilution techniques **(Fig. 3)**.

Arterial Waveform Analysis

Under stable circumstances,

Mean arterial pressure (MAP) ~ Stroke volume (SV) × Systemic vascular resistance (SVR)

The systemic vascular resistance depends on the vascular tone and arterial elastance. If these can be known then the arterial blood pressure trace can be used to derive cardiac output. These can be derived from population-based biometric and anthropometric data and fed into specific nomograms of the monitoring devices, or these can be derived from the arterial pressure tracing itself by analyzing its shape. Once this is known, the arterial waveform can be utilized to derive stroke volume based on the above-simplified equation **(Fig. 4)**.

A similar approach is a pulse power analysis (instead of pulse contour analysis) which assumes that the net power change in the heartbeat is a balance between the inputs of a mass of blood minus the mass that is lost to periphery during that beat. In this method, the effect of site-specific differences in arterial tone and waveforms are minimized. Since this method does not allow measurement of absolute values and tells only changes over time, it needs calibration against a standard method like lithium dilution technique. This method is utilized in the LidCO™ rapid monitoring system.

Accordingly, three types of devices are available:
1. *Noncalibrated techniques not taking into account the vascular tone:* These take into account only the aortic impedance. They do not take into account the changing vascular tone. For example, ProAQT (Getinge, Germany), and modelflow (Finapress Medical Systems, Netherlands).
2. *Noncalibrated techniques that take into account the vascular tone:* Two such devices are available. The FloTrac/Vigileo (Edwards Lifesciences, US) utilizes the arterial pressure shape (kurtosis and skewness) to derive the vascular tone and a population-based algorithm to derive

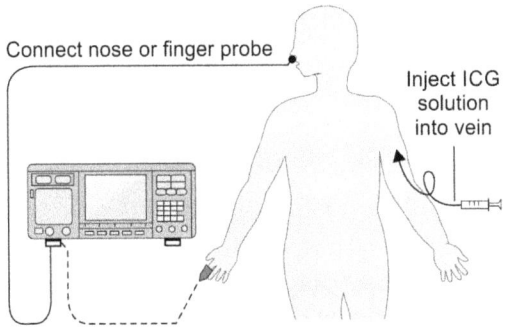

Fig. 3: Pulse dye densitometry.

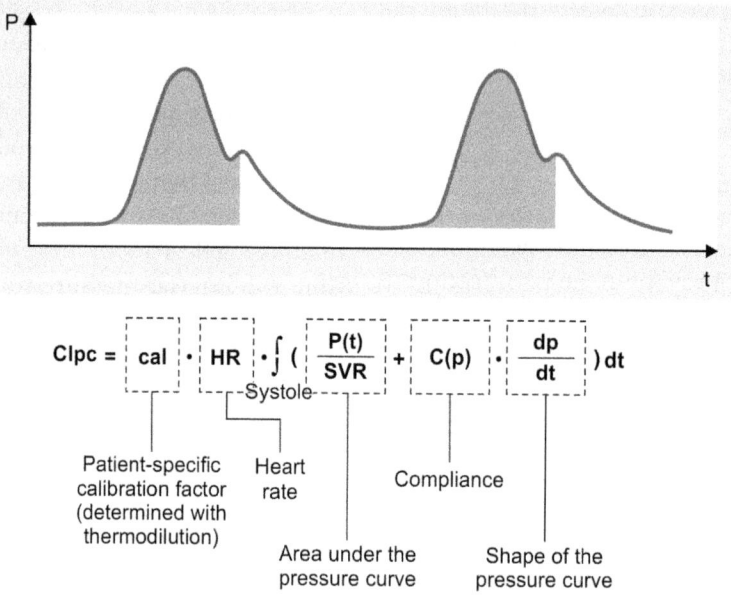

Fig. 4: Arterial waveform analysis.
(CIpc: cardiac index derived from pulse contour analysis)

aortic impedance. These are integrated into a factor c.

Cardiac output is calculated as:
Pulse rate. APsd. C,
where APsd is the standard deviation of arterial pressure over several beats. Factor c is updated every minute in the newer generations of the device.

The other device called PRAM (Vygon, Italy) uses a complex algorithm to estimate the deviation from equilibrium induced by the delivery of stroke volume from the ventricle into aorta.

3. *Calibrated techniques:* These devices do not calculate vascular tone. At a given time the calibration is performed by a standard technique like the indicator dilution method. Any subsequent change in the arterial waveform is presumed to be because of changes in SV and not the Systemic vascular resistance. This gives a continuous measure of stroke volume based on the arterial pressure waveform. For taking into account the changes in systemic vascular resistance the device has to be recalibrated at definite time intervals, at least 6–8 hourly. It might require calibration as frequently as every 15 minutes when patient is hemodynamically unstable, systemic vascular changes are changing rapidly and the patient is being resuscitated. Examples of such devices include PiCCO plus (Pulsion Medical Systems, Germany) and the EV1000/Volume View (Edwards Lifesciences, US. Both use transpulmonary thermodilution technique for calibration. The LidCO™ plus (LidCO™,UK) utilises Lithium dilution technique for calibration.

Noninvasive Finger Arterial Pressure Waveform Analysis

These methods are based on analysis of arterial blood pressure trace obtained noninvasively by measurement of finger blood pressure by inflatable cuff around the finger in other words applanation tonometry of peripheral arteries. The pulsating finger artery is clamped to a constant volume (called unloaded volume) by applying a varying counter pressure equivalent to the changing arterial pressure of the subject. The set-point of unloaded volume is determined by detecting loss of arterial pulsation in the finger using a built-in photoelectric plethysmograph (infrared light emitter and receiving light sensor) and an automated algorithm. This method is also called the volume clamp method or Penaz technique **(Fig. 5)**.

The Nexfin monitor (BMEYE, Netherlands) used an inflatable cuff around middle phalanx to trace a finger arterial pressure waveform which is then reconstructed by the software into a brachial arterial waveform. Blood pressure, heart rate, and stroke volume are obtained from this arterial waveform analysis. The cardiac output and systemic vascular resistance are derived from these parameters. The systolic pressure area of this waveform and a physiological factor for the vascular resistance (individualized for each patient) is then utilized to determine the stroke volume and cardiac output. The ClearSight® system (Edwards Lifesciences, US) is an advanced version of the Nexfin monitor (which is no longer available). It can use one cuff for up to 8 hours or two cuff systems for up to 72 hours alternating between two fingers in every 60 minutes.

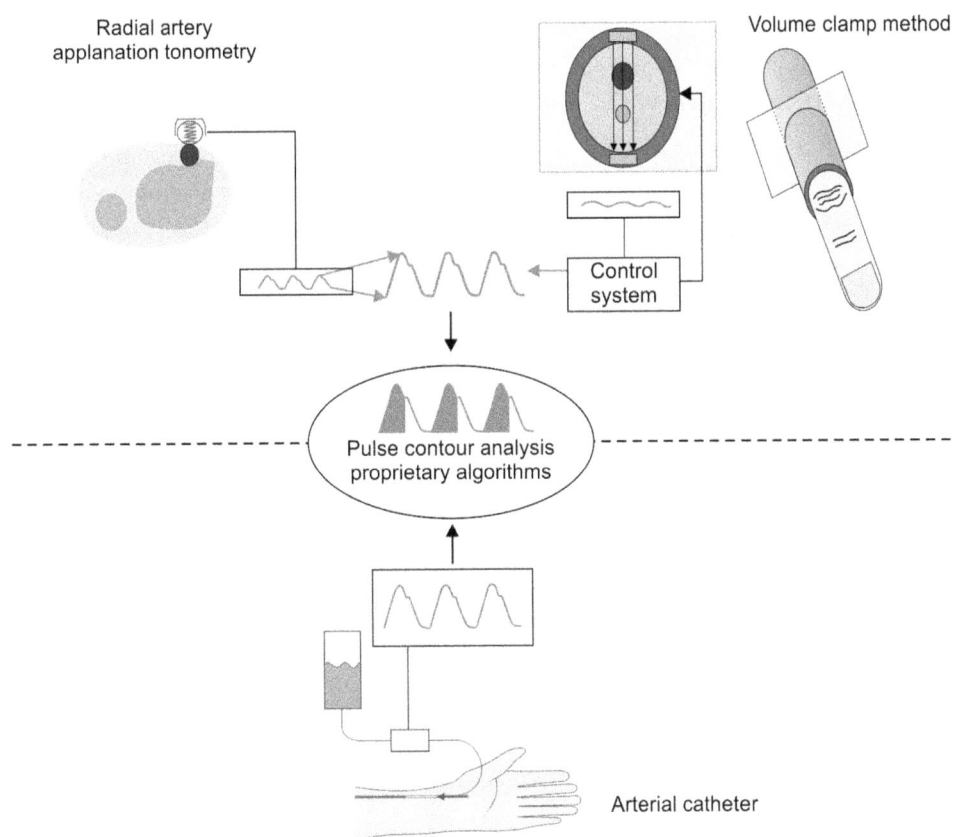

Fig. 5: Volume clamp method.

The advantages of the arterial waveform analysis systems are the minimally invasive nature of the monitoring system. They have a good correlation with PAC over wide range of circumstances. However, these systems are not accurate in extremes of hemodynamic disturbances where the vascular tone is changing rapidly such as patient on high dose vasopressors or severe septic shock.

Pulse Wave Transit Time

The esCCO (Nihon Kohden, Japan) monitoring system is a completely noninvasive technique that utilizes the pulse wave transit time (PWTT) for cardiac output measurement. Pulse wave transit time (PWTT) is the time between the time intervals between the R-wave in an electrocardiogram (ECG) to the point where the pulse wave reaches 30% of its peak amplitude. The stroke volume is inversely proportional to the PWTT.

$$esCCO = K \times (\alpha \times PWTT + \beta) \times HR$$

Where α is a fixed value that was decided experimentally by the past esCCO clinical studies. Meanwhile, constants K and β need to be individualized for each patient.

The PWTT is composed of multiple subparameters **(Fig. 6)**.

- *Preejection period (PEP):* Preejection period includes the electromechanical delay at the start of systole and isometric contraction time, with the R wave of ECG serving as the starting point.
- *T1:* The time it takes for pulse wave to travel from the aorta through the elastic arteries to the muscular arteries.
- *T2:* The time it takes for pulse wave to travel from the muscular artery to the further distal peripheral site of SpO_2 measurement.

$$PWTT = PEP + T1 + T2$$

Thoracic Bioimpedance

In this method, the stroke volume is estimated from changes in the electrical resistance of the thorax overtime when a low magnitude, and how frequency current is applied across the thorax. The patient does

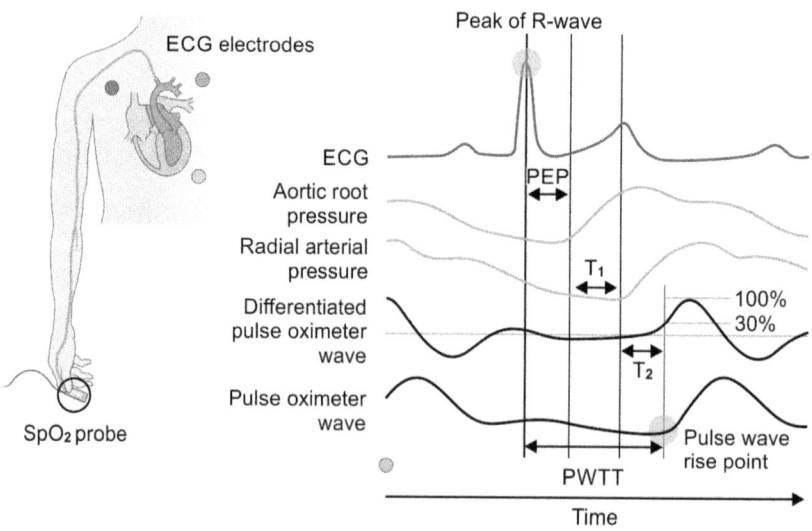

Fig. 6: Pulse wave transit time.
(ECG: electrocardiogram; PEP: pre-ejection period; PWTT: pulse wave transit time; SpO_2: oxygen saturation)

not detect the low level of current. The CO is continuously derived from electrical signals received by using skin electrodes (BioZ, CardioDynamics, San Diego, USA), shown in **Figure 7**, or electrodes mounted on the tracheal tube (ECOM TM, CONMED Corp, Utica, USA). These are used to determine the intra-beat-to-beat variations in transthoracic voltage in response to the applied high-frequency current across the thorax. The electrical current passes across the path of least resistance which is the aortic blood flow. When the left heart contracts there is a change in aortic blood volume and decrease in impedance. The amount of electrically participating tissue is estimated from the gender, height, and weight of the patient using an algorithm.

The SV is calculated using the formula:

$$SV = r \times L/Z_0^2 \times (dZ/dt)_{max} VET$$

Where r—resistivity of blood, L—mean distance between the inner electrodes (the thoracic length), ventricular ejection time (VET), $(dZ/dt)_{max}$—the absolute of the maximum value of the first derivative during systole, and Z_0—basal thoracic impedance. Ventricular ejection time is obtained from the dZ/dt versus time curve.

Though simple, this technique has multiple limitations and clinical data of its use is not robust. Change in water content in the surrounding tissue and the effect of respiration on pulmonary blood volume affects the technique. Hence it is prone to errors from pulmonary edema, effusions, and anasarca. The electrodes cannot be moved during the measurement as it measures changes in the same electrodes over time. Arrhythmias cause errors in measurement.

Thoracic Bioreactance

The bioreactance reflects the overall sum of the electrical resistance, i.e., capacitive and inductive properties of blood and biological tissues. In the NICOM Reliant system, Cheetah Medical Ltd., Maidenhead, Berkshire, UK) a high-frequency sine wave oscillating current is delivered across thorax, and the phase shift in voltage across the thorax (changes in both amplitude and direction measured in degrees) due to changes in bioreactance in response to the cyclic blood flow out of the heart are measured. It uses four electrodes two on either side of the chest and cardiac output is determined separately from each side **(Fig. 8)**. An almost linear relationship has been found between the phase shifts measured continuously and the changes in blood flow in the aorta, viz., stroke volume. This approach results in less interference from the patient movement, electrical noise, lead placement, respiratory effort, and body mass index due to a higher signal-to-noise ratio. It does not measure static impedance and also does not depend on the distance between the electrodes.

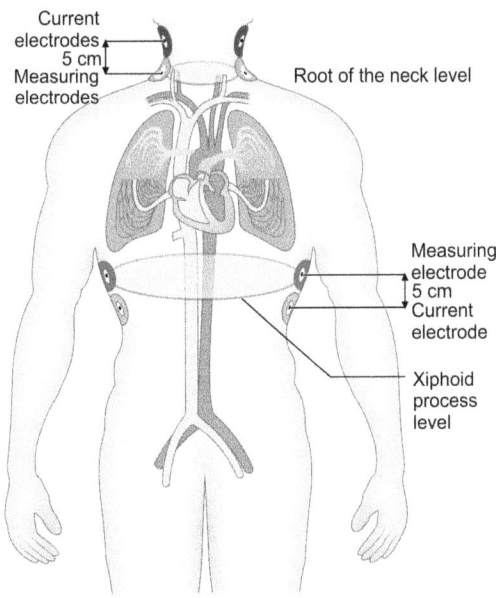

Fig. 7: Thoracic bioimpedance measurement.

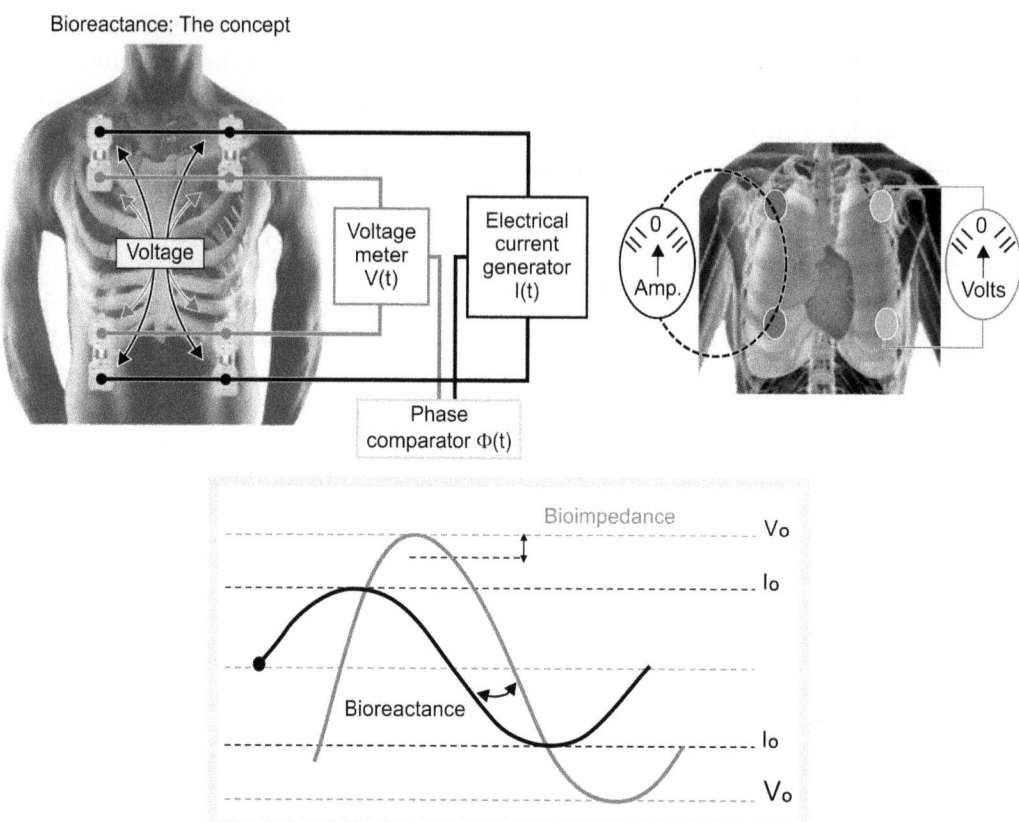

Fig. 8: Thoracic bioreactance measurement. (Amp.: ampere)

The signals are averaged over one minute period and hence can be used in arrhythmia. NICOM is not reliable when electrocautery is being used for >20 s/min. There is conflicting evidence on whether it can track CO changes due to functional challenges like fluid bolus and passive leg raise.

Electrical Cardiometry

Electrical cardiometry is a method based on the model of electrical velocimetry (EV), and noninvasively measures stroke volume (SV), cardiac output (CO), and other hemodynamic parameters through the use of 4 surface ECG electrodes. EV is based on the fact that the conductivity (inverse of impedance) of the blood in the aorta changes during the cardiac cycle. Prior to opening of the aortic valve, the red blood cells assume a random orientation (there is no blood flow in the aorta). When the electric current is applied from the outer electrodes, the current must circumference these red blood cells, therefore resulting in a higher voltage measurement, and thus, a lower conductivity. Shortly after aortic valve opening, the pulsatile blood flow forces the red blood cells (RBC) to align in parallel with the blood flow **(Fig. 9)**. When the electric current is then applied, it is able to easily pass the red blood cells in the aorta resulting in a lower voltage, and thus, a higher conductivity. The change from random orientation to the alignment of red blood cells upon opening of aortic valve

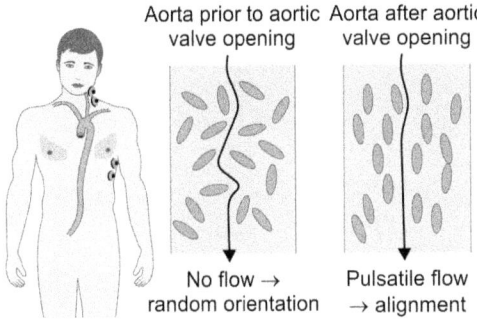

Fig. 9: Alignment of red blood cells (RBCs) before and after the opening of aortic valve.

generates a characteristic steep increase of conductivity or dZ(t) (corresponding to a steep decrease of impedance)—beat to beat.

The measured bioimpedance over time can be expressed as the superposition of three components:

$$Z(t) = Z_0 + \Delta Z_R + \Delta Z_C$$

here Z_0 is the quasi-static portion of the electrical impedance (base impedance), ΔZ_R are the changes of impedance due to the respiratory cycle, and ΔZ_C are the changes of impedance due to the cardiac cycle. ΔZ_R is considered an artifact and is therefore suppressed.

The timely measurement of ΔZ_C (dZ(t)) reveals a waveform with a shape similar to an arterial pressure waveform. The calculated first time derivative of dZ(t) is the dZ(t)/dt waveform, which contains landmarks that allow determination of left-ventricular ejection time (LVET) and peak aortic blood acceleration. The peak aortic blood acceleration occurs at the steepest slope of the dZ(t) waveform, and at the peak of the dZ(t)/dt waveform **(Fig. 10)**.

The dZ(t)/dt waveform is analyzed to determine the following landmarks **(Fig. 10)**:
- Opening of aortic valve (Point B)—begin of flow time (FT)/left-ventricular ejection time (LVET)
- Peak aortic blood acceleration (Point C, occurring in time with aortic dP/dt_{MAX})
- Closure of aortic valve (Point X)—end of flow time (FT)/left-ventricular ejection time (LVET).

The model considers the peak amplitude of dZ(t)/dt divided by the base impedance Z_0 as an index for peak aortic acceleration, and as an index of contractility of the heart, or ICON. The general equation for estimating stroke volume (SV) by means of thoracic electrical bioimpedance calculates the product of a patient's constant CP (in ml), the mean blood velocity index vFT (measured in s^{-1}) during flow time FT, and flow time (FT; measured in s):

$$SV = CP \cdot vFT \cdot FT$$

is then used to calculate the ICG concentration. Cardiac output is calculated using the area under curve (AUC) obtained from the first recirculation of vFT is derived from the measured index for peak aortic acceleration ICON. The flow time FT is corrected for heart rate. The higher the mean blood velocity during flow time, the more SV the left ventricle ejects. The volume of electrically participating tissue (V_{EPT}) is used as the patient constant (CP). The V_{EPT} is derived primarily from the body mass and hence it is important to get an accurate weight of the patient.

Doppler Principles

Doppler probes can be used to measure cardiac output.

The esophageal Doppler uses a long esophageal probe inserted orally until approximately 35–40 cm (midthoracic level in adults). It can be kept in place for 72 hours with frequent rechecking of position. It is safe to use in coagulopathic patients. Another noninvasive ultrasound probe USCOM™ (USCOM, Sydney, Australia) measures CO using a suprasternal probe.

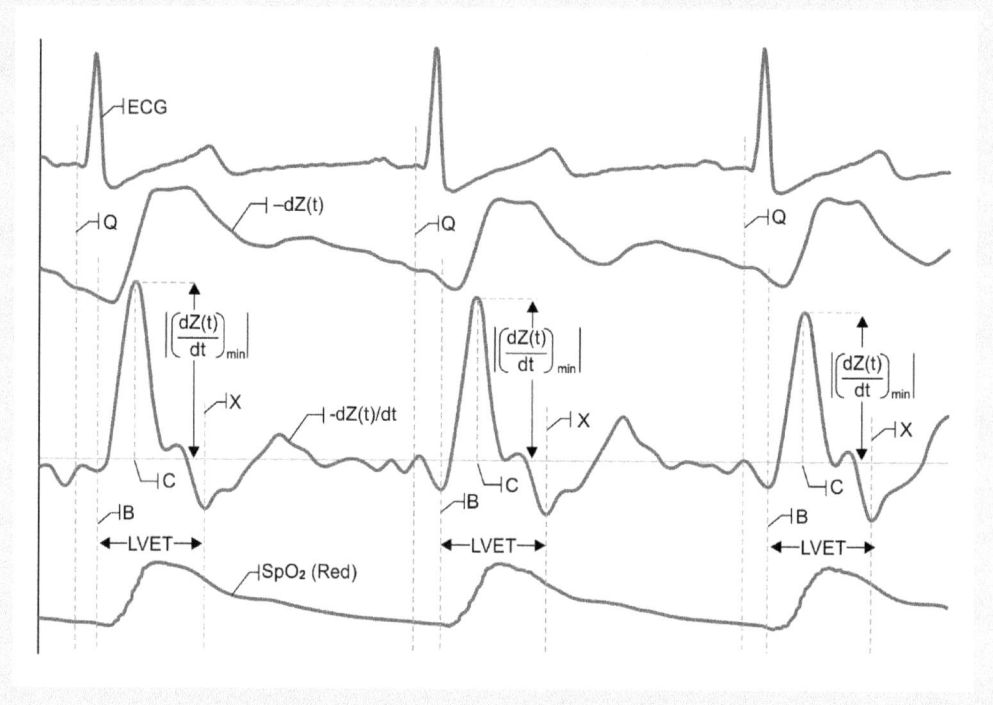

Fig. 10: Different timings during electrical cardiometry.

The ultrasound emitted by the probes is reflected by the flowing blood in aorta. The frequency shift depends on the velocity of red blood cells in the descending aorta (Doppler principle). The velocity of blood (v) is calculated using the equation:

$$v = \text{speed of sound} \times \cos\theta \times \text{transmitted frequency} \times \text{frequency shift}/2$$

(θ = angle of incidence between the beam and reflecting blood).

The stroke distance is calculated by multiplying this red cell velocity by the measured ejection time. This is called the *velocity time integral* or *VTI*. This is multiplied by the cross-sectional area (CSA), which quantifies the amount of blood that passes through at the level of Doppler interrogation (the stroke volume). Cross-sectional area is derived either by a nomogram based on age, weight, and height (Deltex monitor) or directly measured with the transducer (HemoSonic) using M-mode ultrasonography. The actual SV at the level of left ventricular outflow is then estimated by assuming that the descending aorta receives 70% of the total cardiac output. In addition to stroke volume and cardiac output the esophageal Doppler also provides a measurement of preload or volume status of the patient by measurement of corrected flow time (FTc). It is the systolic flow time corrected for the heart rate. Normal value is between 330 and 360 milliseconds. Achieving the longest possible FTc correlates well with optimal fluid status of a patient. The Doppler probe also provides peak velocity of the aortic systolic blood flow which is a measure of the contractility of heart **(Fig. 11)**.

Though the method is easy and less invasive it has multiple limitations.

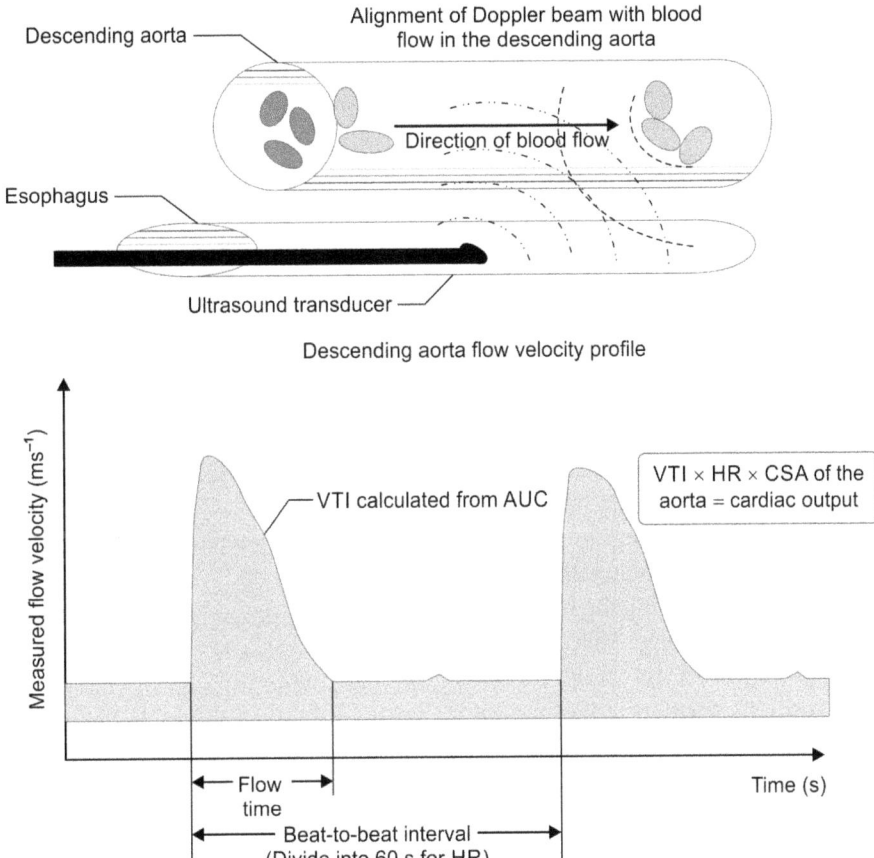

Fig. 11: Esophageal Doppler technique.

The assumption that aorta receives 70% of cardiac output might not hold true during rapidly changing hemodynamics in shock states, the aortic cross-sectional area is not fixed and the use of nomograms might produce erroneous results. The mathematical model also assumes that aorta is cylindrical with constant laminar blood flow which might not hold true in anemia, arrhythmia, and aortic valve diseases. The procedure is relatively contraindicated in esophageal varices. The device has 10% interobserver variability. The probe position is very important and any angle between the probe and the flow >20–30° will result in significant error. The device is best used for serial measurements and to measure the trends in response to therapy.

Partial CO_2 Rebreathing Technique

This technique relies on the modified Fick's principle to calculate cardiac output. The NICO™ system (Novametrix Medical Systems, Wallingford, USA) utilizes a modification of the Fick principle using carbon dioxide (CO_2) instead of oxygen to obtain CO measurements in mechanically ventilated patients. The monitor consists of a disposable rebreathing loop that is attached to the ventilator circuit, a mainstream infrared CO_2 sensor, a disposable airflow sensor, and a pulse oximeter. CO_2 production (VCO_2) is calculated as a product of CO_2 concentration and airflow during a breathing cycle, and arterial CO_2 content is derived from the end-tidal CO_2 with adjustments for the slope of CO_2 dissociation curve and the degree of dead space ventilation. The attached rebreathing loop generates a partial rebreathing state every three minutes that results in an increased end-tidal CO_2 and reduced CO_2 elimination. The difference between normal and rebreathing ratios is used to calculate cardiac output with an assumption that cardiac output does not change significantly between normal and rebreathing states. This allows the omission of the venous CO_2 content measurement which is required in the Fick's equation. Intrapulmonary shunts can affect the equation by altering the blood flow participating in gas exchange. This technique may only be applied in mechanically ventilated patients with relatively stable hemodynamics.

$$CO = [vCO_2 \text{ (normal)} - vCO_2 \text{ (rebreathing)}]/(S \times \Delta EtCO_2)$$

where S is the slope of CO_2 dissociation curve.

Ultrasound Dilution Technique

The ultrasound velocity of blood is 1,560–1,590 m/s. When blood is diluted by a bolus of isotonic saline (ultrasound velocity of saline is 1,533 m/s, i.e., lower than the blood) the ultrasound velocity of the blood also gets reduced. The changes in ultrasound velocity are sensed and measured to derive flow by using indicator dilution principle. 0.5–1 mL/kg of saline at 37°C is injected into the venous limb of an arteriovenous circuit at 6–12 mL/min for 5–6 minutes. The decrease in velocity of the blood in ultrasonogram (USG) is recorded. This requires an extracorporeal circuit prefilled with heparinized saline in

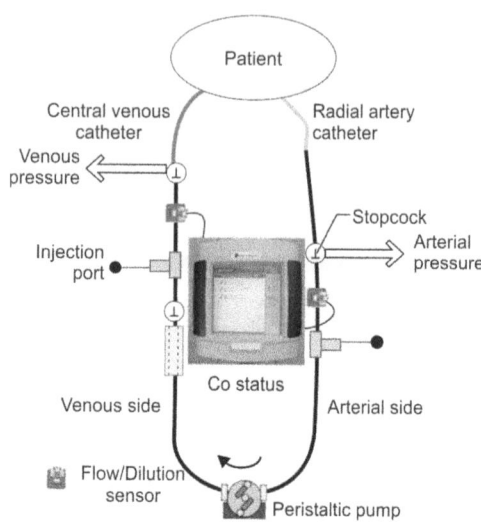

Fig. 12: Ultrasound dilution technique.

between an arterial line and a central venous catheter. It needs a peristaltic pump to circulate blood through this circuit **(Fig. 12)**. The decrease in ultrasound velocity is detected by flow sensors in the loop and a ultrasound dilution curve like thermodilution curve is obtained. The main disadvantage is the use of the heparinized extracorporeal circuit and that this method is relatively less explored and experience with this system is minimal.

QUESTIONS

Q. 1. Explain (i) Cardiac function index, (ii) Global ejection fraction.

Q. 2. Cardiac output measurement devices based upon (i) Calibrated and (ii) noncalibrated techniques.

Q. 3. Difference between bioimpedance and bioreactance.

FURTHER READING

1. Gropper MA, Eriksson LI, Fleisher LA, Wiener-Kronish JP, Cohen NH, Leslie K. Miller's Anesthesia, 9th edition.

CHAPTER 31

Transcranial Doppler

Bhavana Kayarat, Arjun Balakrishnan, Puneet Khanna

■ IDENTIFY AND INTERPRET

Aids in the noninvasive real-time assessment of cerebral blood flow (flow velocity is measured, not the adequacy of blood flow) and cerebrovascular hemodynamics.

■ PRINCIPLE (FIG. 1)

Based on the Doppler effect of sound waves:
- The perceived frequency of sound waves reflected from a moving object changes based on the direction the object is moving with respect to the source.
- Objects moving towards the probe reflect at a higher perceived frequency, and objects moving away reflect at a lower perceived frequency.
- Velocity is calculated based on the original frequency and reflected frequency.
- Calculated velocity depends on the cosine of the angle of insonation. Higher the angle (>30°) less the accuracy.
- Red blood cells (RBC) in the blood vessels act as the reflective target for the ultrasonic waves.
- Pulsed Doppler probe > graphs velocity over time.

■ CLINICAL ANATOMY (FIG. 2)

- The middle cerebral artery (MCA) → branch of the internal carotid artery (ICA), receives the majority of ICA blood flow.
- Courses laterally before bifurcating into superior and inferior segment.
- MCA does not directly take part in the circle of Willis.
- Intracranial aneurysms are commonly seen at the junction of two blood vessels.

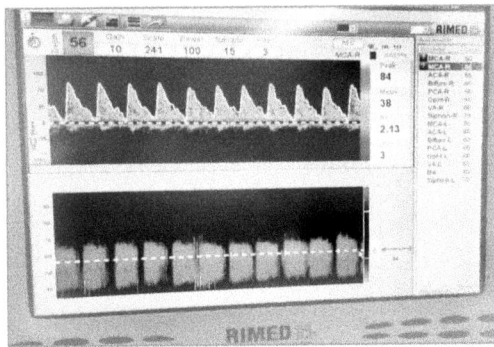

Fig. 1: Transcranial Doppler.

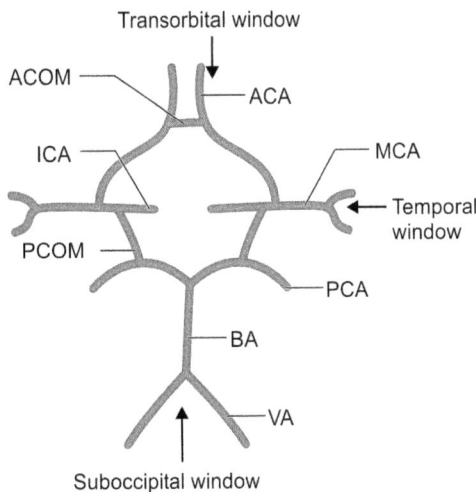

Fig. 2: Clinical anatomy.

- MCA bifurcation is a common site of intracranial aneurysms.
- Other common sites of aneurysms are the anterior communicating artery (ACOM) (most common) and posterior communicating artery (PCOM).

TECHNIQUE (TABLE 1)

- *Probe:* 2 MHz probe (waves need to penetrate the bone); scan in the supine position
- Temporal window (transtemporal) to measure middle cerebral artery (MCA) flow
- Bone thickness least
- Above the zygomatic arch, 1-2 cm anterior to tragus
- Probe is held perpendicular to skin with slight anterior angulation → insonation depth is adjusted to 45-60 mm → MCA identified by noting flow towards the probe.
- *Other approaches:* Transorbital [carotid siphon, ophthalmic artery, and also anterior cerebral artery (ACA), suboccipital (basilar and vertebral artery), and submandibular (extracranial ICA)].

INTERPRETATION
Detection of Vasospasm

- High velocity in MCA (>120 cm/s) could be due to hyperemia or vasospasm.
- Vasospasm results in the reduction of vessel caliber. The pressure head at the start of the spasmic segment is higher (Poiseuille law). This increased pressure head is responsible for the increased flow velocity seen in vasospasm.
  Lindegaard ratio = mean velocity in the MCA/mean velocity in ipsilateral extracranial ICA **(Table 2)**.

Pulsatility Index

- Pulsatility refers to ratio of peak systolic velocity (PSV) minus end-diastolic flow velocity (EDV) divided by mean flow velocity (MFV). Dimensionless and not affected by angle of insonation.
  $$PI = (PSV - EDV)/MFV$$
- Assesses flow resistance in the vessel.
- Higher the cerebrovascular resistance, higher the pulsatility index.
- Normal PI is between 0.5 and 1.0. Pulsatility index over 1.2 shows high resistance to cerebral blood flow.

TABLE 1: Techniques approaches.

Artery	Window	Mean flow velocity (MFV) (cm/s)	Depth of insonation (mm)	Direction of flow
Middle cerebral artery	Temporal	40–60	45–60	Towards
Anterior cerebral artery	Temporal	40–50	60–75	Away
ICA	Temporal	30–50	55–70	Bidirectional
Posterior cerebral artery	Temporal	30–45	60–75	Bidirectional
Basilar artery	Suboccipital	35–50	75–100	Away
Vertebral arteries	Suboccipital	30–50	50–75	Away
Carotid siphon	Transorbital	30–60	55–70	Bidirectional
Ophthalmic artery	Transorbital	10–30	30–50	Towards
Extracranial ICA	Submandibular	20–40	40–60	Away

(ICA: internal carotid artery)

TABLE 2: Detection of vasospasm.

Lindegaard ratio	Interpretation
<3	Hyperemia
3–6	Mild vasospasm
>6	Severe vasospasm

Resistive Index

The ratio of peak systolic velocity minus end-diastolic velocity to peak systolic velocity. Like PI, dimensionless and unaffected by the angle of insonation.

$$RI = (PSV - EDV)/PSV$$

Assesses flow resistance distal to the site of insonation. Normal resistive index (RI) is <0.75. Higher values indicate high resistance to cerebral blood flow.

Detection of Ischemia

A difference in flow velocities by 30% compared to the contralateral (normal) side signify reduced blood flow. Higher grades of ischemia show a reduction in MFV with PI < 1.2 followed by the absent diastolic flow.

INDICATIONS

- Detecting and monitoring cerebral vasospasm after subarachnoid hemorrhage.
- Monitoring cerebral vasomotor reactivity.
- Assessing successful thrombolysis after stroke.
- Detection of circulating cerebral microthrombi.
- Ancillary test for brain death.
- Assessment of hypoxic-ischemic encephalopathy in neonates and children.
- Noninvasive test to assess intracranial pressure. However, is less accurate than other methods.

DISADVANTAGES

- Operator dependent.
- Less sensitive than angiography for stroke.
- Difficult to insonate the distal vessels.
- Transcranial Doppler (TCD) velocities are dynamic and change with factors affecting cerebral blood flow such as hypo/hypercapnia, raised ICP, etc.
- Insonation difficult in older patients who have thicker bone.

FURTHER READING

1. Cottrell J, Patel P. Cottrell and Patel's Neoroanesthesia, 6th edition.
2. Khanna P. Ultrasound in Critical Care, Ist edition.

Cerebral Oximetry

Bhavana Kayarat, Puneet Khanna

INTRODUCTION
- It aids in noninvasive monitoring of cerebral oxygenation.
- It represents a balance between cerebral oxygen delivery and consumption.

PRINCIPLE

Beer and Lambert Laws, Near Infrared Light, and Spatial Resolution
- *Beer's law:* The intensity of transmitted light decreases exponentially as the concentration of a substance the light passes through increases.
- *Lambert's law:* The intensity of transmitted light decreases exponentially as the distance travelled by the light through a substance increase.
- Near infrared light has a wavelength of 650–940 nm and is therefore able to penetrate the skull to the underlying cerebral tissue. The absorption spectra for deoxygenated hemoglobin is 650–1,000 nm and oxygenated hemoglobin is 700–1,150 nm.
- Cerebral oximetry values are derived from venous blood and are independent of pulsatile blood flow.
- Since extracranial blood could be a potential source of error, a principle of spatial resolution is applied, i.e., by increasing the distance between the emitter and detector, the depth of tissue sampled can be increased, thus reducing interference from extracranial blood.

EQUIPMENT (FIG. 1)
- Monitor
- *Probes:* It contains fiberoptic light source (infrared range) and light detectors
- Adhesive pads attach the probes on the patient scalp
- The sensor is usually placed over the forehead on either side of the midline, few centimeters above the eyebrow, to avoid contamination by sagittal and frontal sinus.

INTERPRETATION
- *Normal value:* 60–80%
- *Adult:* 71 ± 6 %, neonate: 76 ± 8%

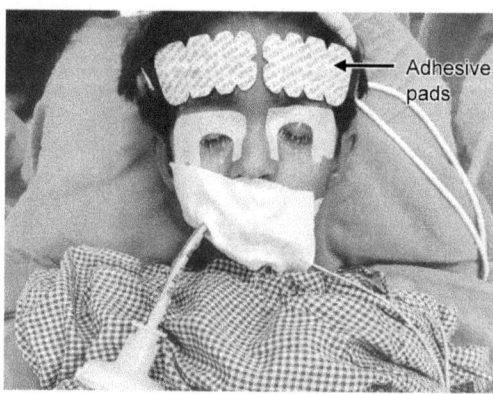

Fig. 1: Cerebral oximetry.

Flowchart 1: Approach to reduced cerebral oxygenation values.

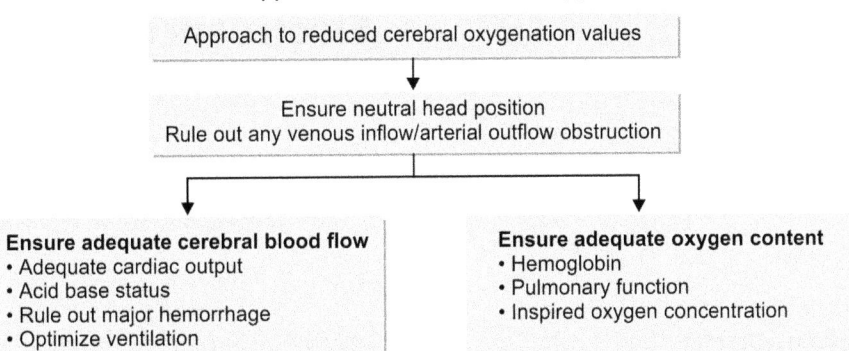

- Fall >20–25% of baseline are considered as cut off for development of cerebral ischemia

USES
- To monitor and detect the onset of cerebral ischemia, especially in surgical procedures using cardiopulmonary bypass, and carotid endarterectomy
- *Noncardiac surgery*—shoulder surgery (beach chair position) and thoracic surgery
- To detect cerebral vasospasm in subarachnoid hemorrhage
- In newborns, for early detection and prevention of periventricular leukomalacia and intraventricular hemorrhage

LIMITATIONS
- Interference from extracranial blood source (extradural hematoma) can show false low values
- Only regional cerebral oxygenation is measured (focal prefrontal cortex). Oxygenation in other areas of brain could be missed.
- Expensive-cost benefit studies still underway

FURTHER READING
1. Cottrell J, Patel P. Cottrell and Patel's Neuroanesthesia, 6th edition.

CHAPTER 33: Electroencephalogram

Bhavana Kayarat, Puneet Khanna

INTRODUCTION

Continuous noninvasive indicator of cerebral function by recording spontaneous electrical activity of the cerebral cortex.

EQUIPMENT

Electrodes are placed on the scalp in a standardized array, each scalp electrode provides continuous recording of spontaneous brain activity, i.e., 2–3 cm in diameter.

About 10–20 system of electrode placement is commonly practiced.

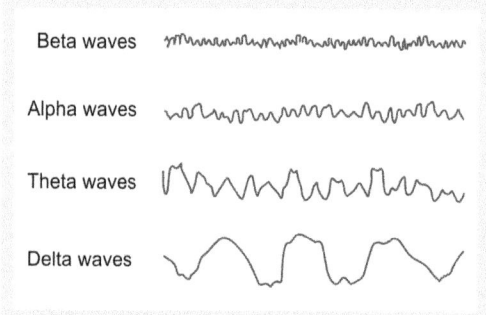

Fig. 1: Different types of waves in EEG.

Electrical activity in each electroencephalogram (EEG) channel is described in terms of amplitude and frequency **(Fig. 1)**.

INTERPRETATION

It is a plot of voltage versus time—>1–35 Hz frequency **(Tables 1 and 2)**.

USES

- To identify cerebral ischemia, i.e., during carotid cross-clamping in carotid endarterectomy and during temporary occlusion of a vessel during dissection of cerebral aneurysm
- To titrate drugs, in surgeries requiring metabolic suppression for cerebral protection
- To detect subclinical seizures
- In stereotactic EEG, implanted leads are used to localize seizure foci in patients with focal seizures, who are refractory to medical therapy
- To monitor the depth of anesthesia
- As a prognostication tool

TABLE 1: Results of plot of voltage versus time—>1–35 Hz frequency.

Waves	Frequency (Hz)	Amplitude (µV)	Characteristics
Beta (β)	>13	20	Mental activity (frontal)
Alpha (α)	8–12.5	40–100	Awake, eyes closed (occipital)
Theta (θ)	4–7.5	>50	Sedation/anesthesia/light sleep
Delta (δ)	0.5–3.5	>50	Sedation/anesthesia/deep sleep

TABLE 2: Reduction in cerebral blood flow will produce rapid characteristic changes in EEG.

Cerebral blood flow (mL/100 g/min)	EEG changes
35–70	Normal
25–35	Loss of beta frequencies
18–25	Theta range, decrease in amplitude
12–18	Delta range, decrease in amplitude
8–10	Severe amplitude loss at all frequencies
<8	Loss of activity, isoelectric EEG

(EEG: electroencephalogram)

LIMITATIONS

Surface EEG recordings do not detect ischemia in subcortical regions.

ANESTHETIC STRATEGY

- *To detect cerebral ischemia:* EEG activity to be maintained, therefore avoid excessive depth of anesthesia
- *To identify seizure focus:* Avoid inhalation agents [>0.5 minimum alveolar concentration (MAC)], benzodiazepines and propofol during the monitoring period.

FURTHER READING

1. Cottrell J, Patel P. Cottrell and Patel's Neuroanesthesia, 6th edition.

CHAPTER 34

Somatosensory and Motor Evoked Potentials

Arjun Balakrishnan, Bhavana Kayarat, Puneet Khanna

EVOKED POTENTIALS

- Records the electrical potentials produced after stimulation of specific neural tracts
- Voltage versus time graphs
- Response recorded either in the brain [somatosensory evoked potentials (SSEP)/visual evoked response (VEP)/brainstem auditory evoked potential (BAEP)] or muscle group motor evoked potentials (MEP).

Somatosensory Evoked Potentials

- Primarily checks the integrity of posterior column sensations (proprioception, fine touch).
- Stimulus is given along course of peripheral nerve.
- Commonly used nerves are median or ulnar for upper limb (UL) and tibial or peroneal for lower limb (LL).
- Conduction is measured along multiple points in the pathway to ascertain the region affected.
- Measurement sites for UL are cubital fossa, supraclavicular fossa, cervical cord, and cortex.
- Lower limb (LL) measurement sites are popliteal fossa, lumbothoracic cord, cervical cord, and cortex.

Motor Evoked Potentials

- To check the integrity of the motor pathway.
- Transcranial electrodes stimulate the motor cortex; impulse descends from the cortex, crosses the midline in lower lateral brainstem, and descends in the ipsilateral anterior funiculi of the spinal cord (corticospinal tract).
- Direct stimulation of brain and tracts can also be done using cortical or subcortical electrodes during intracranial procedures.
- Electrical activity summates in anterior horn cell and activates the alpha motor neurons.
- Alpha motor neuron activation in turn results in stimulation of neuromuscular junction resulting in a compound muscle action potential (CMAP) in 4-5% of the muscle fibers which is recorded by electrodes placed in the muscle group.
- MEPs are faster than SSEPs due to less synapses needed for signal transmission.
- MEPs are more sensitive to hypoperfusion due to greater blood flow to gray matter of anterior horn cells because of higher metabolic demands of the alpha motor neurons.
- Intracranial stimulation shows proximity of stimulating electrodes to the tracts based on strength of stimulating current.

INTERPRETATION OF EVOKED POTENTIALS (TABLE 1)

TABLE 1: Significant findings of evoked potentials.

SSEP	Fall in amplitude by 50% and increase in latency by 10%
MEP	• Fall in amplitude by 70% • Increase in latency by 10% • More stimuli are required to produce the response • Failure of signal to return to baseline • Increased strength of stimulus (>50 V) required to produce the same response

(SSEP: somatosensory evoked potentials; MEP: motor evoked potential)

ROLE OF EVOKED POTENTIALS (TABLE 2 AND FIG. 1)

- Acts as an early warning sign for procedure-related deficit.
- Allows early initiation of measures to halt/reverse change [increasing mean arterial pressure (MAP), removing screws, halt resection, etc.].
- Allows for planning extent of tumor resection during intracranial and intradural spinal cord procedures for maximum preservation of function.
- MEPs have a high negative predictive value for procedure-related deficits (>90%).

TABLE 2: Effects of various anesthetic agents on somatosensory evoked potentials and motor evoked potentials.

	Effect on SSEP		Effect on MEP
	Amplitude	Latency	
Anesthetic agents	Only at MAC 1–5		Even at 0.5 MAC
Inhalational agents			
• Isoflurane • Sevoflurane • Desflurane	Decreases	Increases	Decreases
Nitrous oxide	Decreases	Increases	Decreases
Intravenous agents			
Propofol	Decreases	–	Decreases at higher doses
Thiopentone	Decreases	Increases	Decreases
Ketamine	Increases	–	Increases
Midazolam	–	–	–
Opioids	–	–	–
Dexmedetomidine	–	–	–

(MAP: mean arterial pressure; CMAP: compound muscle action potential; MAC: minimum alveolar concentration; MEP: motor evoked potentials; SSEP: somatosensory evoked potentials)

Note:
Muscle relaxants have no effect on SSEP.
Muscle relaxants abolish CMAP, not epidural MEP.
Inhalational agents have direct depressant effects on anterior motor neurons and hence greater effect on MEPs even at low MAC values.
Intravenous agents suppress MEP responses much lesser than inhalational agents.
Decreased MAP and hypothermia can decrease the amplitude of the evoked potentials.

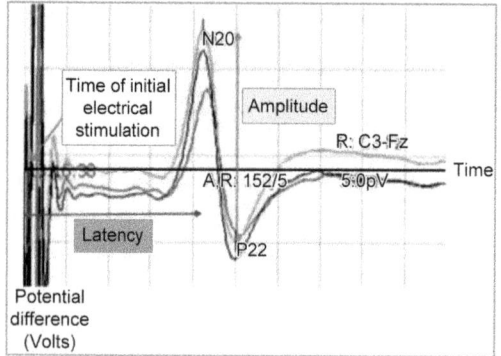

Fig. 1: Examples of an evoked response. Latency (unit: seconds) and amplitude (unit: volts) are important parameters in describing evoked potentials.

LIMITATIONS OF SOMATOSENSORY EVOKED POTENTIAL

- Artifacts, electrocautery, convection warmers, cavitron ultrasonic surgical aspirator (CUSA) can cause problems in interpretation of SSEP reading.
- Does not monitor the part of the spinal cord supplied by anterior spinal artery.
- A normal intraoperative SSEP does not rule out procedure-related neurological deficits.

LIMITATIONS OF MOTOR EVOKED POTENTIALS (FIG. 2)

- Relatively contraindicated in individuals with pacemakers, cardiac arrhythmias,

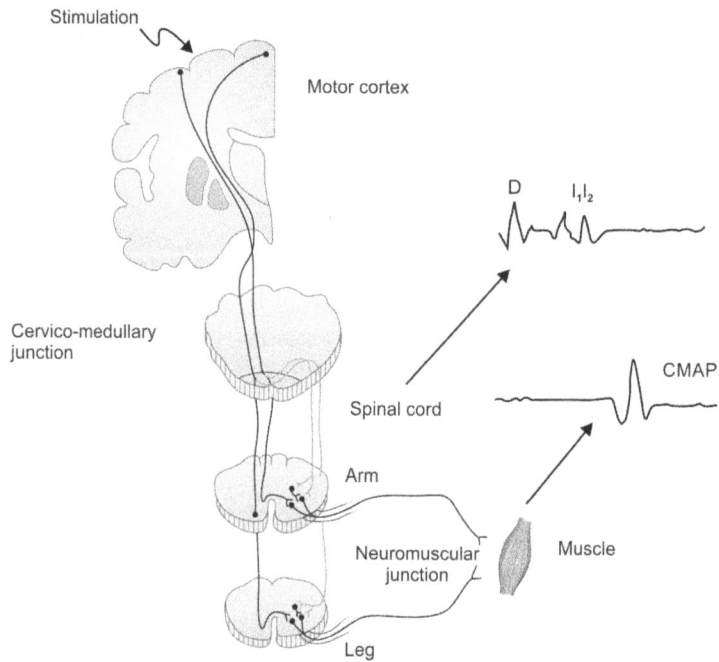

Fig. 2: Motor pathway monitored by MEP with the waveform recorded from cord level (D and I waves) and muscle level (CMAP). Stimulation of the motor cortex generates evoked potentials that propagate through the brain and spinal cord to cause a muscle contraction. The response typically is recorded near the muscle as a compound muscle action potentials (CMAP). The response can so be recorded over the spinal column as a D wave followed by a series of I waves (high-frequency repetitive discharges from the corticospinal fibers). At the spinal cord level, most motor fibers reside in the lateral corticospinal tract (gray pathway) after decussation at the brainstem level. The anterior corticospinal tract (black pathway) contians fewer motor tracts.

cochlear implants, aneurysm clips, and raised intracranial pressure.
- Positive predictive value for procedure-related deficit is low (<50%).

VISUAL EVOKED POTENTIAL
- Response recorded by stimulating retina with flashes of light.
- Response recorded in occipital cortex.
- Most sensitive of all evoked potentials to anesthetic agents.
- Does not measure clinically relevant vision.

BRAINSTEM AUDITORY EVOKED POTENTIAL
- Produced by using sound stimulus.
- Resultant potential was recorded over the course from cochlea to auditory cortex.
- Used primarily in posterior fossa surgeries, along with SSEPs and MEPs.
- Greatly affected by disorders of sound conduction (otitis media, tympanosclerosis, etc.).
- Extremely resistant to effects of anesthetic agents.

FURTHER READING
1. World Federation of Societies of Anesthesiologists. (2019) Introduction to Intraoperative Neurophysiological Monitoring for Anaesthetists. [online] Available from: https://resources.wfsahq.org/wp-content/uploads/397_english.pdf [Last accessed March, 2022].

CHAPTER 35: Bispectral Index

Bhavana Kayarat, Arjun Balakrishnan, Puneet Khanna

INTRODUCTION
- It is used to monitor the depth of sedation/anesthesia.
- Consists of processed electroencephalographic (EEG) signals based on a proprietary algorithm to obtain a numerical value between 0 and 100.
- Analysis is mainly based on three components, the EEG spectrum, bispectrum, and time spent in burst suppression measured over a specific period (time-domain).
- A value of 0 represents EEG silence and 100 represents a fully awake state. Bispectral index (BIS) values between 40 and 60 correspond to an adequate depth of general anesthesia for surgery.
- Values <40 represent a deep hypnotic state.

EQUIPMENT FOR BISPECTRAL INDEX MONITORING
- Four sensors—consist of disposable wet gel electrodes (Fig. 1).
- Cable
- Monitoring module—interfaces with anesthesia machine or monitoring system:
  - The skin on the forehead is cleaned with an alcohol swab.
  - The four electrodes are applied on the forehead and 2-5 seconds of digital pressure is applied.
  - Electromyographic activity of the frontalis muscle is measured by lead 4 (ground electrode).

The BIS view monitor displays the following:
- BIS value
- Trend of BIS values over time

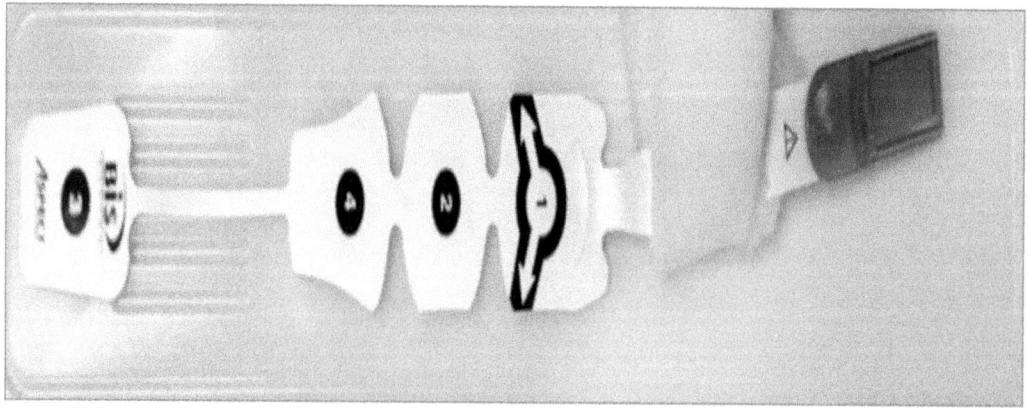

Fig. 1: Disposable adult bispectral index sensor.

- Continuous EEG graphs
- Quality and depth indicators as SQI, EMG, BSR
- Alarms and messages.

The signal-quality-index (SQI) predicts the reliability of the signal. An SQI over 50 is preferable.

The electromyographic (EMG) bar indicates muscle activity due to an increase in muscle tone or contraction.

Burst suppression ratio (BSR) is the time spent in burst suppression over normal EEG activity in the previous time domain. Value of 1.0 denotes EEG silence.

FACTORS AFFECTING BISPECTRAL INDEX VALUES

- Effect of anesthetic agents on BIS values:
  - Ketamine can elevate BIS values.
  - Etomidate can cause drug-induced myoclonus and alter BIS values.
  - Halothane can increase BIS values as compared to isoflurane or sevoflurane at equipotent minimum alveolar concentration (MAC) doses.
- Dexmedetomidine lowers BIS values without affecting ability of a patient to respond to verbal commands and therefore makes BIS unreliable during sedation with dexmedetomidine.
- *Hypothermia:* The BIS value reduces with reduction in core temperature due to reduced cerebral metabolic activity.
- *Neurological impairment:* BIS has not been validated in patients with pre-existing neurological impairment.
- *Interference from medical devices:* Electrocautery can cause artifacts and impair the ability of the BIS monitor to assess changes in the depth of anesthesia.

A BIS value is a timed average of the components analyzed by the algorithm over a 30–40 second time domain. Hence is not reliable when there are rapid changes in level of consciousness such as during induction or emergence from anesthesia.

FURTHER READING

1. Cottrell J, Patel P. Cottrell and Patel's Neuroanesthesia, 6th edition.

36. Entropy

Sudhansu Sekhar Nayak, Arjun Balakrishnan

INTRODUCTION

General anesthesia is defined as a reversible state of unconsciousness that enables the patients to undergo pain-free surgery without awareness of intraoperative events. To achieve adequate depth of anesthesia is of paramount importance during surgery. Overdosage of anesthetic agents can lead to cardiovascular instability and delayed emergence and obviously increase in costs of anesthesia. On the contrary, light plain of anesthesia can cause awareness of intraoperative events which can lead to postoperative psychological disturbances in the patients. So, measurement of the depth of anesthesia is essential for safe anesthesia practice.

Depth of anesthesia can be measured or monitored in many ways based on clinical/conventional monitoring and/or brain electrical activity monitoring. Entropy is one of the commonly used monitoring systems for assessing the depth of anesthesia. Entropy monitoring is a quantitative measurement of the depth of anesthesia. Entropy measures the irregularity or complexity or unpredictability in spontaneous brain electrical activity and facial muscular electrical activity. The Entropy Module (Datex-Ohmeda) uses a proprietary mathematical algorithm that uses electroencephalography (EEG) and frontal electromyography (FEMG) values to produce two separate entropy values to measure the depth of anesthesia.

TWO ENTROPY VALUES

1. Response entropy (RE)
2. State entropy (SE)

Response Entropy

- Response entropy scale ranges between 0 (complete cortical silence) and 100 (complete wakefulness).
- Calculated over a frequency range between 0.8 and 47 Hz.
- A rapid reacting parameter represents both EEG and FEMG signals (affected by facial muscle activation).
- Used to detect the activation of facial muscles and thus inadequate analgesia.

State Entropy

- Reflects the cortical state of the patient.
- State entropy scale ranges between 0 (complete cortical silence) and 91 (complete wakefulness).
- Calculated over the frequency range between 0.8 Hz to 32 Hz.
- The stable (slower response) parameter represents processed EEG mostly (less affected by sudden reactions to the facial muscles).
- Reflects the hypnotic effect of anesthetic agents on the brain.

Therefore, RE value is always higher or equal to SE value. Therefore, the RE-SE difference means there is a muscular activity, reflecting nociception. Motor nerve which innervates the upper facial muscles is originated from the brainstem, which is associated with the awareness centers. So, any external stimulus like pain that is perceived by patient in the upper facial region will be manifested as an EMG signal. Muscle relaxation affects EEG monitoring by causing the inhibition of frontal muscle activity.

ENTROPY CAN BE USED

- To monitor the depth of anesthesia during inhalation and intravenous induction of general anesthesia
- To predict arousal and motor responses during the maintenance phase of anesthesia.

Takamatsu et al., found that SE and RE declined significantly with rises in end-tidal sevoflurane concentration. Xing et al also found that increasing sevoflurane concentration causes a decrease in RE and SE values and without noxious stimulation, spectral entropy did not affect by neuromuscular blockade but with noxious stimulation, spectral entropy was significantly reduced by muscle relaxants and there were significant interactions in spectral entropy between NMB and sevoflurane **(Tables 1 and 2)**.

- The target value of entropy for general anesthesia is 40–60.
- If, during general anesthesia, there is an approximately 10-point difference between RE and SE, the patient is likely to move in response to external stimulation.

HOW TO USE?

Three electrodes with a disposable sensor attached to the patient's forehead. A sensor cable connects these sensors to entropy module. The module produces continuous data by interpreting the brain and facial muscular activity **(Figs. 1A and B)**.

The Entropy Module can also measure the burst suppression ratio (BSR). It is the ratio of the period of severely reduced brain activity to the total period of brain activity in EEG in one minute. Burst suppression is seen during states of severely suppressed brain activity, such as general anesthesia, hypothermia, coma, and anoxic brain injuries. The ideal value of BSR required for general anesthesia is 0%. A higher BSR is typically seen with

TABLE 1: Correlation of entropy values with different planes of anesthesia.

RE	SE	Interpretation
100	90	Awake
60	60	Low probability of recall
40	40	Clinically adequate level for most surgical operations
0–40	0–40	Deep anesthesia
0	0	Suppressed electroencephalography (EEG)

TABLE 2: The effect of neuromuscular blocking drugs (NMBDs) on entropy.

Medication	Low amount of hypnotics	High amount of hypnotics
No NMBDs	• Light anesthesia • RE > SE (high entropy)	Deep anesthesia RE ≥ SE (low entropy)
High amount NMBDs	• Risk of awareness • RE = SE (high entropy)	• Deep anesthesia • RE = SE (low entropy)

(RE: response entropy; SE: state entropy)

Section 2: Anesthesia Monitoring

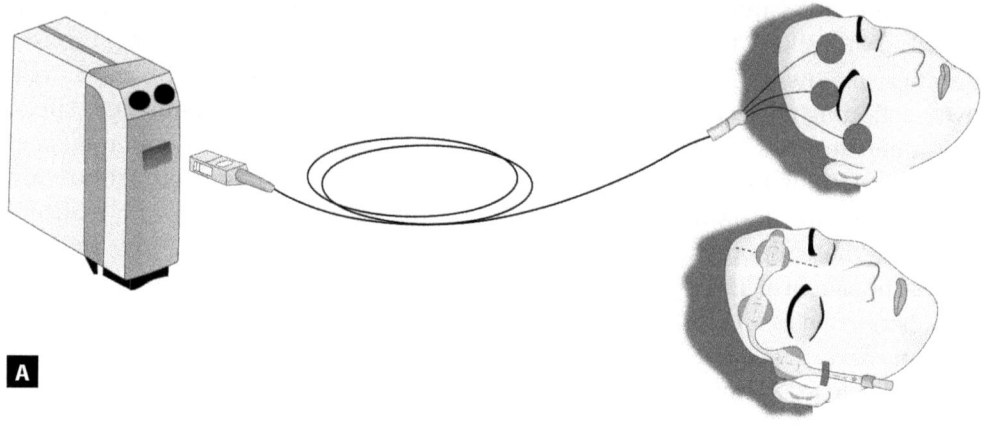

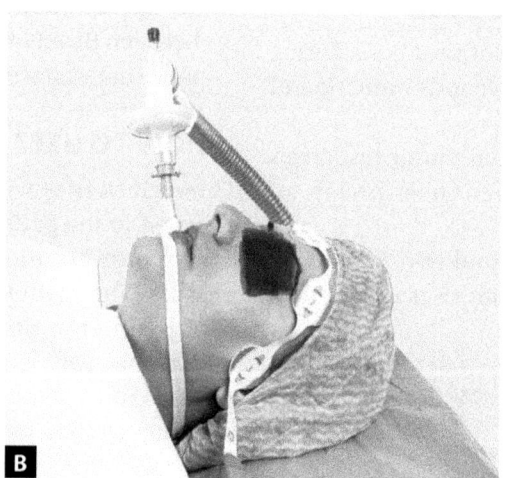

Figs. 1A and B: How to use the entropy module?

entropy values below 40 and can indicate unnecessarily deep anesthesia.

QUESTION

Q. 1. Which is better EEG/BIS/Entropy? Give reasons for advantages of each over others.

FURTHER READING

1. Takamatsu I, Ozaki M, Kazama T. Entropy indices vs the bispectral index for estimating nociception during sevoflurane anaesthesia. Br J Anaesth. 2006;96(5):620-6.
2. Xing Y, Xu D, Xu Y, Chen L, Wang H, Li S. Effects of neuromuscular blockages on entropy monitoring during sevoflurane anesthesia. Med Sci Monit. 2019;25:8610-7.

CHAPTER 37

Respiratory Monitoring

Vrinda Chauhan, Puneet Khanna, Abhishek Singh

INTRODUCTION

Respiratory monitoring refers to the continuous or periodic assessment of processes involved with the exchange of respiratory gases between the environment and the subcellular pathways where those gases are utilized and produced.

Respiratory monitoring includes assessment of the following **(Fig. 1)**:
- Transport of the gas through the conducting airways and the alveoli.

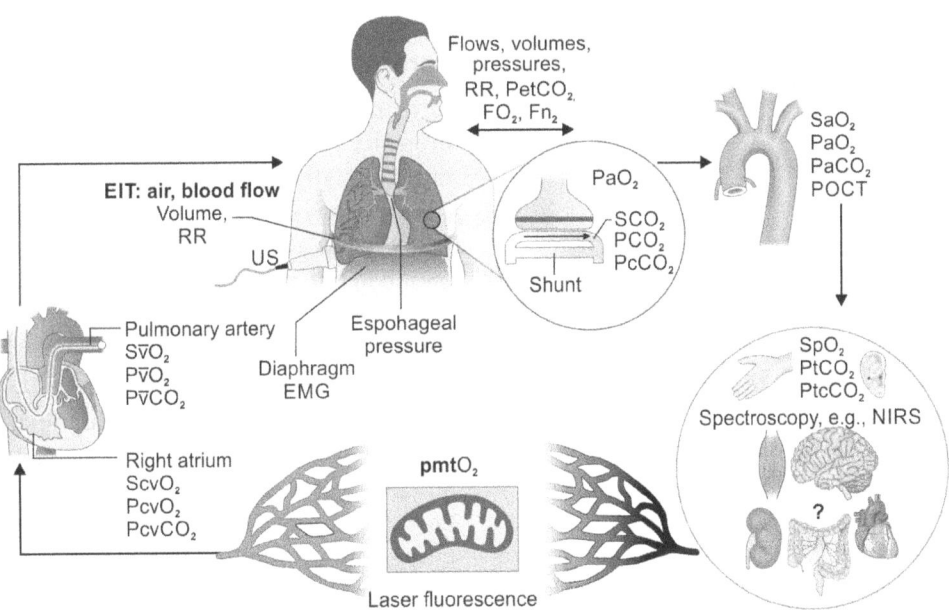

Fig. 1: Respiratory processes and measurement sites for current respiratory monitoring techniques.
(EIT: electrical impedance tomography; EMG: electromyography; NIRS: near-infrared spectroscopy; $PaCO_2$: arterial partial pressure of carbon dioxide; PaO_2: arterial partial pressure of oxygen; $PcCO_2$: cutaneous carbon dioxide; PCO_2: partial pressure of carbon dioxide; $PcvCO_2$: partial pressure of central venous carbon dioxide; $PcvO_2$: partial pressure of central venous oxygen; $PetCO_2$: partial pressure of end-tidal carbon dioxide; POCT: point-of-care testing; RR: respiratory rate; $PtcCO_2$: transcutaneously measured carbon dioxide tension; $PtCO_2$: transcutaneous partial pressure of carbon dioxide; $PvCO_2$: partial pressure of carbon dioxide in mixed venous blood; PvO_2: mixed venous oxygen tension; $P\bar{v}CO_2$: partial pressure of mixed venous carbon dioxide; $P\bar{v}O_2$: partial pressure of mixed venous oxygen; SaO_2: arterial oxygen saturation; SCO_2: supercritical carbon dioxide; $ScvO_2$: measuring continuous central venous saturation; SpO_2: peripheral oxygen saturation; SvO_2: venous oxygen saturation; $S\bar{v}O_2$: mixed venous oxygen saturation)

- Exchange of gases between alveoli and pulmonary capillary blood.
- Balance of regional ventilation and perfusion contributes to producing expired gases and arterial and mixed venous blood.
- Transport of gas between the blood and tissues through microcirculation.
- Diffusion of gas between tissues and mitochondria.
- Cellular respiration using oxygen (O_2) and carbon dioxide (CO_2) production.

PHYSICAL EXAMINATION

- It is an essential component of perioperative respiratory monitoring.
- It provides essential information for diagnosing and initiating treatment and may indicate changes in patient status requiring intervention.
- It includes inspection of the patient, and assessment of the respiratory rate which provides a measure of the breathing pattern.
- Anatomic signs often visible on inspection such as deformities of the chest wall and spine, goiter, tracheostomy scar, and tracheal deviation are all relevant to respiration.
- Functional elements include the components of inspiration and expiration diaphragmatic versus thoracic, duration, and difficulty of inspiration and expiration, paradoxical chest wall motion, use of accessory muscles, central, and peripheral cyanosis, pallor, wheezing, stridor, cough and sputum, aphonia, splinting, and clubbed fingers.
- Auscultation of the lungs for normal and abnormal breath sounds such as vesicular sounds, rhonchi, wheezes, fine and coarse crackles, inspiratory stridor, and pleural friction.

MONITORING OF INSPIRED OXYGEN CONCENTRATION

According to the American Society of Anesthesiologists (ASA) Standards for Basic Anesthesia Monitoring, 1 Standard 2.2.1 states, "during every administration of general anesthesia using an anesthesia machine, the concentration of oxygen in the patient breathing system shall be measured by an oxygen analyzer with a low oxygen concentration limit alarm in use".

Due to its highly reactive chemical nature, the presence of oxygen can be determined by various analyzers. Three types of analyzers are there—(1) paramagnetic oxygen analyzers, (2) galvanic cell analyzers, and (3) polarographic oxygen analyzers.

Paramagnetic Analyzers

Any change in sample line pressure resulting from the attraction of oxygen by switched magnetic fields can be detected. Signal changes that occur during electromagnetic switching correlate with the oxygen concentration in the sample line.

Galvanic Cell Analyzers

They measure the current produced when oxygen diffuses across a membrane and is reduced to molecular oxygen at the anode of an electrical circuit. As a result, the current flow that is produced is proportional to the partial pressure of oxygen in the fuel cell. Regular replacement of the galvanic sensor capsule and reactants is required.

Polarographic Oxygen Analyzers

- They are most commonly used. Oxygen diffuses through an oxygen-permeable polymeric membrane and the resulting current change is proportional to the number of oxygen molecules surrounding the electrode.

- Oxygen sensors on the inspired limb of the anesthesia circuit to detect and alarm in the event that hypoxic gas mixtures are delivered to the patient.
- Adequate inspiratory oxygen concentration does not guarantee adequate arterial oxygen concentration. Consequently, ASA1 Standard 2.2.2 mandates additional monitoring for blood oxygenation, including the provision of adequate lighting and exposure to assess the patient's color by direct observation.

ARTERIAL OXYGENATION MONITORING

Pulse Oximetry (Fig. 2)

- It provides a noninvasive and continuous assessment of functional arterial oxygen saturation.
- Pulsatility of arterial blood flow is required to provide an estimate of SaO_2 by differentiating light absorption by arterial blood from light absorption by other components.

Based on the Beer–Lambert law, it utilizes two techniques:
1. *Spectrophotometery:* The intensity of light transmitted through tissue is a logarithmic function of the oxygen saturation of hemoglobin (Hb) at a constant light intensity and hemoglobin concentration.
2. *Optical plethysmography:* It measures pulsatile changes in arterial blood volume at the sensor site.

Light-emitting diodes (LED) emit two wavelengths of light—(1) red 660 nm and (2) near-infrared 940 nm light.

Oxyhemoglobin absorbs more infrared light and deoxyhemoglobin absorbs more red light.

The percentage of oxyhemoglobin is determined by measuring the ratio of infrared and red light sensed by a photodetector and the ratio of absorption of red.

Functional saturation by the pulse oximetery is measured as:

$$SPO_2 = \frac{HbO_2}{HbO_2 + Hb} \times 100\%$$

Fractional saturation is measured by the co-oximeter as:

$$SaO_2 = \frac{HbO_2}{HbO_2 + Hb + COHb + MetHb} \times 100\%$$

Types of Pulse Oximetry

- *Transmission pulse oximetry:* Light beam transmitted through a vascular bed and

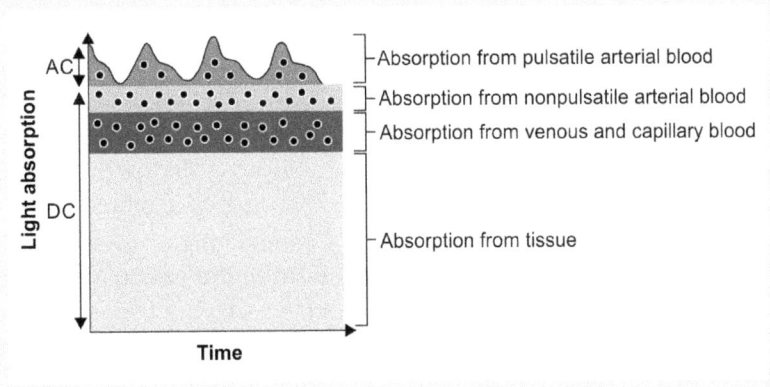

Fig. 2: Absorption of light passing through tissue is characterized by a pulsatile component alternating current (AC) and a nonpulsatile component direct current (DC).

detected on the opposite side of that bed.
- *Reflectance pulse oximetry:* Both the photodiode and LED are present on the same side and it relies on the light reflected back from the blood.
- *Co-oximetry:* Considered as gold standard, it can measure concentration of different types of hemoglobin—oxyhemoglobin, reduced hemoglobin, carboxyhemoglobin, and methemoglobin.

Limitations

Various factors can affect the accuracy and reliability of pulse oximetry such as dyshemoglobins, dyes such as methylene blue, indocyanine green, and indigo carmine, nail polish, ambient light, LED variability, and motion artifact.

These monitors do not ensure the adequacy of oxygen delivery to, or utilization by, peripheral tissues and should not be considered a replacement for arterial blood gas measurements or mixed central venous oxygen saturation when more definitive information regarding oxygen supply and utilization is required.

MONITORING OF INSPIRED AND EXPIRED CARBON DIOXIDE

Respiratory gases must be sampled continuously and measured by a rapid response device that is either attached to the breathing circuit—side stream sampling or within the breathing circuit mainstream sampling.

Carbon dioxide tension is usually measured by infrared absorption as its absorption band lies within the infrared spectrum.

Capnometry

Capnometry is the measurement and numeric representation of the CO_2 concentration during inspiration and expiration.

Capnography

Capnography is the continuous monitoring of CO_2 concentrations versus time in a gas mixture.

The size and shape of the capnogram waveform can provide additional clinical information **(Fig. 3)**.
- *Phase I:* E-A, inspiratory baseline—inspired gas devoid of CO_2.
- *Phase II:* B-C, expiratory upstroke—represents transition gas from anatomical dead space:
  - Prolonged in—partial endotracheal tube obstruction—chronic obstructive pulmonary disease (COPD), bronchospasm—upper airway obstruction.
- *Phase III:* CD, plateau phase—represents gas coming from alveoli, end of phase III at point D is end-tidal point.
- *Phase IV:* DE, inspiratory downstroke—represents patient inhalation, CO_2 levels abruptly fall to zero.
- *α angle:* Take off/elevation angle—angle between phase II and phase III.
  - Normally between 100-110°—decreased in obstructive lung disease.
  - Increased in: Airway obstruction—positive end-expiratory pressure (PEEP).
- *β angle:* Angle between phase III and descending limb of capnogram.
  - Normally around 90°—decreased in airway obstruction and PEEP and increased in rebreathing.

Capnography is the standard of care for monitoring the adequacy of ventilation in patients receiving general anesthesia. It is also now mandated for use in monitoring ventilation during procedures performed while the patient is under moderate or deep sedation.

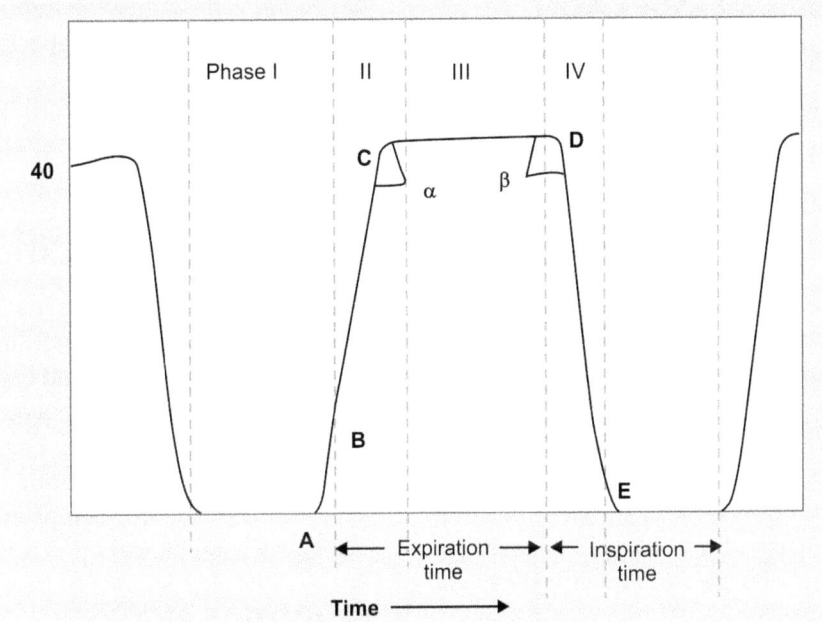

Fig. 3: Time-volume capnograph.

Limitations

- Occlusion of the sampling line with condensed water vapor during prolonged use, replacement is often required. The sampling line can be above the ventilator circuit help prevent the entry of condensed water.
- A humidifier can be used, although this will increase the response time of the capnogram.
- It is not as accurate as blood gas analysis for the assessment of the partial pressure of arterial carbon dioxide.
- In disease states characterized by increased dead space and ventilation-perfusion mismatch, single-lung ventilation, or in very low CO states, an arterial blood gas analysis is necessary for accurate determination of arterial partial pressure of carbon dioxide ($PaCO_2$).
- In infants, sidestream sampling rates can approach and even surpass the minute ventilation. Sidestream capnography systems may report erroneously low end-tidal CO_2 levels since the capnography system may be sampling gas that never actually participated in ventilation an apparently normal end-tidal carbon dioxide ($ETCO_2$) on the monitor may in fact represent inadequate ventilation, which would predispose the patient to respiratory acidemia.

VOLUME PRESSURE RELATIONSHIP (FIG. 4)

Compliance of the lungs and chest wall determines the volume-pressure relationship.

It has three components:
1. An initial increase in pressure with no significant volume change.
2. A linear increase in volume as pressure increases (the slope of which represents respiratory system compliance).
3. A further period of pressure increase with no volume increase.

DYNAMIC MEASUREMENT

It is available on most modern ventilators. A square wave inspiratory waveform constant flow and no inspiratory pause are necessary for waveform interpretation.

STATIC MEASUREMENT

- Small, incremental lung volumes are delivered with a calibrated syringe. The pressure measurement is taken under zero flow conditions.
- Measurements are more easily obtained in the relaxed, fully ventilated patient.
- The most appropriate setting for external peep is represented by a lower inflection zone to avoid gas trapping since the small airways are closed below the lower inflection zones and expiration does not reach functional residual capacity.
- Above the upper inflection zone, the lungs cannot inflate further. Therefore, the upper inflection zone represents the maximum setting for peak airway pressure.

COMPLIANCE CALCULATIONS

- Lung compliance $(L/cmH_2O) = \Delta VL/\Delta PL$ where L, is the liter above functional residual capacity (FRC), and is the slope of the linear portion of the curve.
- Total respiratory system compliance is derived from the equation: (1/total compliance) = (1/lung compliance) + (1/chest wall compliance)

BLOOD GAS ANALYSIS

A heparinized blood sample can be inserted into a blood gas machine and/or co-oximeter for measurement of gas tensions and saturations, and acid-base status **(Table 1)**.

Uses

- Identification of arterial hypoxemia and hyperoxia, hypercapnia and hypocapnia—enabling monitoring of disease progression and efficacy of treatment

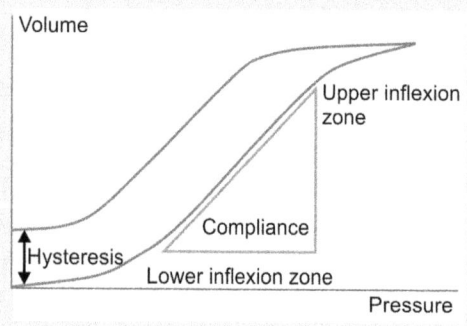

Fig. 4: Volume-pressure curve.

TABLE 1: Blood gas anomalies.

Respiratory acidosis	pH↓, PaCO$_2$↑	Excess CO$_2$ production and/or inadequate excretion, e.g., hypoventilation, excess narcotic
Respiratory alkalosis	pH↑, PaCO$_2$↓	Reduction in PCO$_2$ due to hyperventilation
Metabolic acidosis	pH↓, PaCO$_2$ → or ↓	Usually lactic, keto, renal, or tubular. Consider tissue hypoperfusion, ingestion of acids (e.g., aspirin), loss of alkali (e.g., diarrhea, renal tubular acidosis), diabetic ketoacidosis, and hyperchloremia (e.g., from excess normal saline administration)
Metabolic alkalosis	pH↑ PaCO$_2$ → or ↑	Consider excess alkali (e.g., bicarbonate or buffer infusion), loss of acid (e.g., large gastric aspirates, renal), hypokalemia, and drugs (e.g., diuretics)

(CO_2: carbon dioxide; $PaCO_2$: arterial partial pressure of carbon dioxide; PCO_2: partial pressure of carbon dioxide)

- To make appropriate changes in ventilatory parameters
- pH, PaCO$_2$, and base deficit or bicarbonate values can be used for diagnosis of acidosis and alkalosis, whether it is respiratory or metabolic in origin, and whether any compensation has occurred.
- Co-oximeter can be used for accurate estimation of hemoglobin oxygen saturation and also the total Hb level.
- The more sophisticated co-oximeters permit the measurement of the fraction of methemoglobinemia (MetHb), carboxyhemoglobin (COHb), deoxyhemoglobin (deoxyHb), and fetal Hb.
- Measurement of mixed venous oxygen saturation—for calculation of oxygen consumption and monitoring of oxygen supply—demand balance.

FURTHER READING

1. Dorsch JA. Understanding Anesthesia Equipment.
2. Gropper MA, Eriksson LI, Fleisher LA, Wiener-Kronish JP, Cohen NH, Leslie K. Miller's Anesthesia, 9th edition.

38
Pulse Oximetry

Abhishek Singh

INTRODUCTION

Pulse oximetry is one of the major advancements in patient monitoring. It has the unique advantage of providing information regarding cardiorespiratory function of the patient continuously without involving sophisticated instruments noninvasively. Pulse oximetry has now become the standard of care for patients in operation theatre (OT), emergency, recovery room, and intensive care unit (ICU).

PHYSICS OF PULSE OXIMETRY

Oxyhemoglobin concentration in the blood is measured on the physical principle of Lambert-Beer law. Fractional oximetry (SaO_2) is the measurement of arterial oxygen saturation. It is calculated as:

$$SaO_2 = HbO_2/\text{total hemoglobin}$$
HbO_2 - oxygenated hemoglobin

Total hemoglobin = HbO_2 + deoxyhemoglobin (HHb) + methemoglobin (metHB) + carboxyhemoglobin (COHb)

Functional oximetry is the measurement of oxygen saturation by a pulse oximeter.

It is calculated as:

$$SpO_2 = HbO_2/HbO_2 + HHb$$

The physical basis of pulse oximetry is that oxy and reduced hemoglobin absorbs more light at a different wavelength **(Fig. 1)**.

Oxyhemoglobin (HbO_2) absorbs more light in the infrared range (850–1000 nm) while deoxygenated hemoglobin (HHb) absorbs more light in the red band (600–750 nm). Various pulse oximeters consist of two light-emitting diodes which emit light at a different wavelength **(Figs. 2 and 3)**. One is in the red band (660 nm) while the other is in the infrared band (940 nm). After placing the probe on the patient, the light at different wavelength which is emitted by LED passes through the intervening medium consisting of blood and tissue and is detected by the sensors present on the probe. The light emitted by the LED is detected by the probe which helps inaccurate estimation of the peak and trough of each pulse waveform. During diastole (pressure trough), the emitted light is absorbed by arterial, venous, and capillary blood along with intervening tissue. During systole (pressure peak) extra light is absorbed in both the bands by an additional amount of arterial blood which constitutes the *pulse volume*. Pulse oximeters remove the pulsatile component from the blood volume signal and calculate the red/infrared ratio. The ratio obtained is compared with the algorithm based on a nomogram which is derived from studies of healthy volunteers and is used to calculate the SpO_2 value of a patient.

How much accurate are pulse oximeters?
Pulse oximeters are generally found to be accurate in the range of 70 to 100%. For values

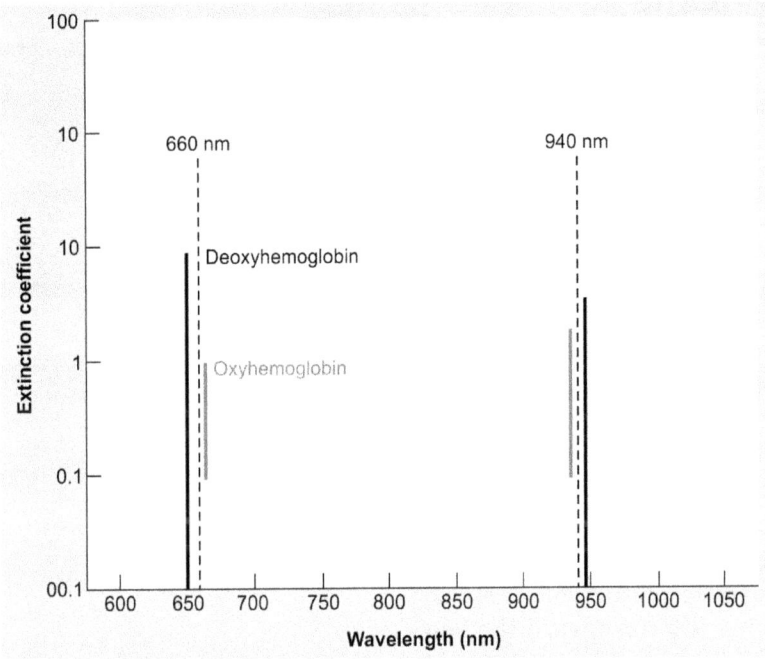

Fig. 1: Principle of pulse oximetry.

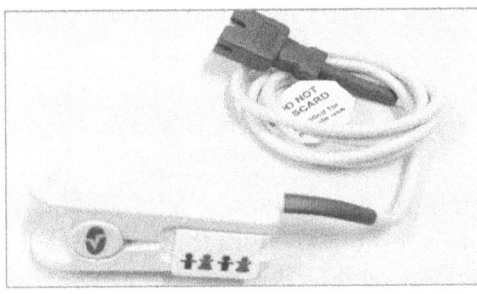

Fig. 2: Adult pulse oximeter probe.

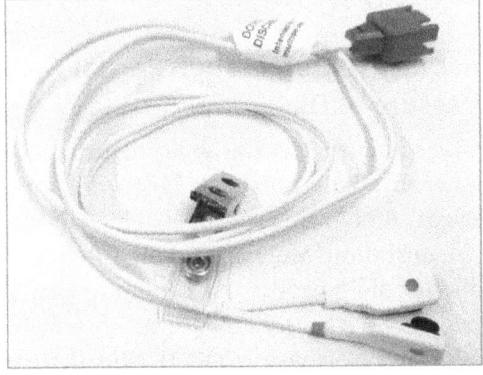

Fig. 3: Pediatric pulse oximeter probe.

less than 70%, there are certain limitations. First, since pulse oximeters have been calibrated using data from healthy volunteers, it is unethical that saturation below 70% will be allowed for healthy volunteers. Any saturation below this value would be an extrapolated one and hence inaccurate. Second, the absorption spectrum of reduced hemoglobin is maximal steep at 600 nm and any deflection of light emitted by LED can introduce significant measurement error into the system.

RESPONSE TIME

Most pulse oximeters take 5–8 seconds for displaying the value. It also depends upon probe location and perfusion state of the body. Desaturation response times range from 40 to 70 seconds for toe probes, 7 to 20 seconds for ear probes, and 19 to 35 seconds for finger probes.

LIMITATIONS OF PULSE OXIMETERS

Dyshemoglobinemia

A conventional pulse oximeter can measure only HbO_2 and HHb as they use only two wavelengths of light. Therefore, the presence of methemoglobin or carboxyhemoglobin can interfere with pulse oximetry measurement by causing interference in the absorption of light in the red and infrared region. The presence of COHb in the blood is interpreted as 90% of HbO_2 and 10% of HHb by a pulse oximeter. Thus, in presence of a high blood level as in the case of a fire accident or cigarette smoking, the pulse oximeter will give an erroneous high reading. The presence of methemoglobin is also known to affect pulse oximeter reading. Methemoglobin is formed when the heme iron is oxidized from the ferrous (Fe^{2+}) to the ferric (Fe^{3+}) state. It absorbs red and infrared light in an equal amount resulting in red/infrared ratio of 1. This ratio of 1 corresponds to a saturation of 85% on the calibration curve. Therefore, with an increase in MetHb concentration, saturation approaches 85% regardless of oxyhemoglobin level. The recent advances in pulse oximetry, some of which use >7 wavelengths (Rainbow SET Technology, Masimo Corp., Irvine, CA) which allow an approximate measure of levels of COHb and MetHb **(Fig. 4)**. Some new pulse oximeters can measure total hemoglobin either continuously or as a spot-check device **(Fig. 5)**.

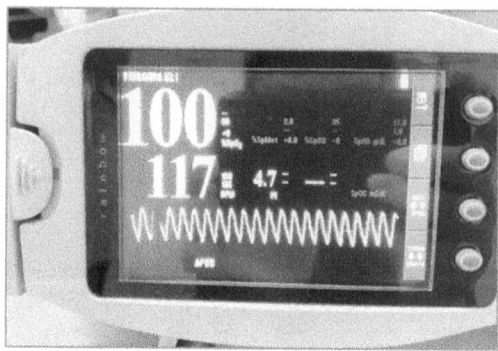

Fig. 4: Masimo pulse oximeter showing SpO_2, %SpMet, and %SpCO.

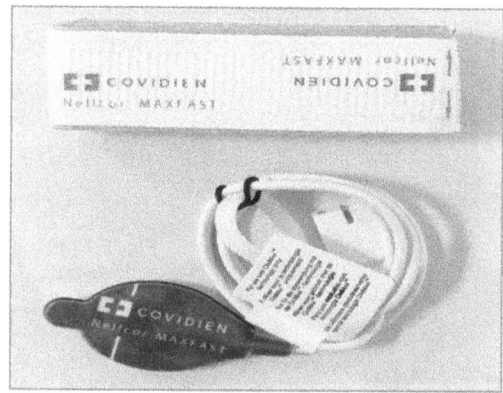

Fig. 5: Covidien forehead probe for use in low-amplitude state.

Low-amplitude States

Pulse oximeters need a pulsatile waveform to calculate blood oxygen saturation. Hence, under the condition of absent or low amplitude pulse such as cardiac arrest, cardiac bypass, hypovolemia, hypothermia, blood pressure cuff inflation, or tourniquet application may show a false reading or may not show any value. In such scenarios, earlobes, and forehead probes can be used for monitoring as they are least sensitive to decreased pulse amplitude.

Inability to Detect High Partial Pressure of Oxygen

Pulse oximeters lack the ability to distinguish between a safe and high level of arterial oxygen. Prolonged exposures of high oxygen concentration are harmful in premature infants who have the risk of retinopathy as well as in patients with chronic obstructive pulmonary disease (COPD) who depend upon the hypoxic drive for respiration.

Therefore, pulse oximeters should be used with caution under such conditions.

Delay in Detecting Hypoxic Events

Generally, the pulse oximeters have a good response time but it is still possible that there may occur a significant delay between the development of arterial hypoxia and a change in pulse oximeter reading. Sensor location plays an important role in displaying the response of pulse oximeter during hypoxia. A centrally placed sensor display results quickly while the response time will increase in cases of poor perfusion to the site being monitored. Peripheral nerve block reduces the response time while vasoconstriction, hypothermia, venous obstruction, etc., increases the response time of pulse oximeter.

Poor Performance during Arrhythmias

Irregular heart rhythms may result in abnormal performance. Pulse oximetry is extremely unreliable in the presence of rapid atrial fibrillation.

Dyes and Pigments

Various dyes produce variable changes in pulse oximeter reading. Injection of Methylene blue, indocyanine, and indigo carmine produce a decrease in SpO_2 readings for a variable time while the elevated concentration of bilirubin has no effect on the accuracy of pulse oximeter. Sometimes obtaining pulse oximeter reading may not be possible in deeply pigmented patients as led light from the emitter may not reach sensor due to heavy pigmentation.

Ambient Light

Pulse oximeters may give false readings due to interference of light coming from surgical lamps, fiberoptic lamps, fluorescent lights, and other lightning sources used in ICU or OT.

Motion Artifact

Motion artifact results in erroneous interpretation of oxygen saturation. *Repetitive motion artifact* results in a pulse oximeter to display local venous saturation. The susceptibility of pulse oximeter to motion artifacts also depends on its signal processing algorithm.

Nail Polish

Nail polish interferes with pulse oximeter functioning. It usually results in low SpO_2 reading but its effect also depends on color and number of layers of nail polish. Therefore, the best solution is to remove the nail polish or use another site for monitoring.

Electrocautery

Wide spectrum radiofrequency emission from electrocautery affects the pulse oximeter probe resulting in decreased SpO_2 reading. Some latest manufacturers have taken care of this problem by properly shielding the sensors and cable of pulse oximeter apparatus.

Discrepancies in Readings from Different Monitors

Different brands of pulse oximeters may show different readings on the same patient at the same time. It is mainly due to the different calibration methods that are used by different monitors.

OTHER USES OF PULSE OXIMETER

Waveform generated by a pulse oximeter, called *plethysmograph*, can provide the most valuable information about patient volume status. Some pulse oximeters also provide

TABLE 1: Limitations of pulse oximetry.	
Limitations	Conditions
Low reading	Venous pulsation such as severe right-sided heart failure, and severe tricuspid regurgitation
False hypoxemia	Elevated arterial oxygen tension level
Inadequate signal	• Dark skin • Anemia • Intravenous dye • Nail polish • Low perfusion states • Bright external light
Unreliable reading	• Dyshemoglobinemia • Methemoglobin • Carboxyhemoglobin

measurements of perfusion in a digit which is useful to assess change in sympathetic tone after a regional block or as an intraoperative clue of successful surgical sympathectomy **(Table 1)**.

COMPLICATIONS OF PULSE OXIMETRY

They are generally minor and consist of mild skin erosion, blistering, and rarely skin necrosis.

QUESTIONS

Q. 1. What is (i) Perfusion index, (ii) Peripheral perfusion index, (iii) Oxygen reserve index?

Q. 2. Explain the advantages and mechanism of percutaneous oxygen measurement. What is oxygen challenge test?

Q. 3. What is SvO_2 and $ScvO_2$?

Q. 4. What is venoarterial carbon dioxide composition?

Q. 5. What is capillary refill time and its values?

FURTHER READING

1. Dorsch JA, Dorsch SE. Understanding Anesthesia Equipment, 5th edition. Philadelphia: Lippincot Williams & Wilkins; 2012.

CHAPTER 39

Capnometry and Capnography

Ajit Kumar, Baibhav Bhandari

INTRODUCTION

The most abundant gas produced by a human body is carbon dioxide (CO_2). Breathing is primarily driven by it. Capnography is nothing but monitoring exhaled CO_2 noninvasively. The changes in the elimination of CO_2 from the lungs are indicated as well as an indirect measure of tissue production of CO_2 and its delivery to the lungs.

Luft in 1943 introduced the first infrared CO_2 measuring and recording apparatus. The earlier version of CO_2 monitors was very bulky and unreliable and they were only used for research purposes. Thanks to the recent development in technology, that made capnometer smaller, inexpensive, and reliable.

Adverse events on operation theatre as well as outside theatre which can range from esophageal intubation, disconnected circuit can be prevented to a great extent with capnometer and thus preventing major anesthesia accidents and thereby reducing financial liabilities.

- *Capnometry:* Measurement and display of CO_2 concentrations on a digital or analog indicator.
- *Capnometer:* It displays the readings.
- *Capnography:* It is a graphical record of CO_2 concentration.
- *Capnograph:* It is a machine that generates the waveform.
- *Capnogram:* It is the actual waveform.

There are five physical methods to measure CO_2 concentration namely—(1) infrared, (2) spectography with molecular correlation, (3) Raman's spectrography, (4) mass spectrography, and (5) photo-acoustic spectrography.

Infrared spectrographs are the most popular used technique for monitoring CO_2. The capnometers utilizing this method is compact and cheap as compared to other spectrographs.

CAPNOGRAPHY

It works on the principle of Beer and Lambert law and when it is applied to infrared waves; it says "amount of infrared rays absorbed is proportional to the concentration of the infrared absorbing substance". Different gases absorb infrared waves of different wavelengths. Carbon dioxide maximally absorbs infrared waves with a wavelength of 4.25 nm. By using this principle, infrared source emitting wavelength of 4.25 nm is utilized. Absorbed infrared waves are directly proportional to the amount of CO_2 present **(Fig. 1)**.

For an infrared spectrograph to be CO_2 specific it is so designed to emit infrared waves having a wavelength of 4.25 μm (wavelength which is maximally absorbed by CO_2).

Factors Affecting Infrared Spectrography

- Ambient atmospheric pressure
- N_2O
- O_2

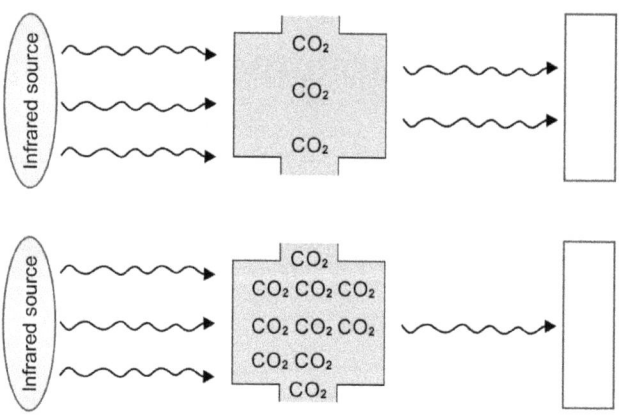

Fig. 1: Capnography.

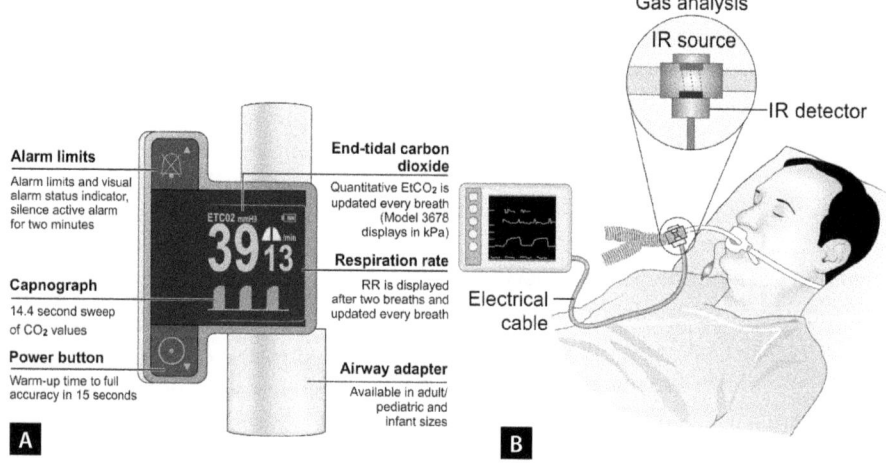

Figs. 2A and B: Mainstream capnograph.

- Water vapor
- Inhalational anesthetic agents
- Response time.

MAINSTREAM CAPNOGRAPH

Conventional capnograph consists of sample line which is directly connected between endotracheal tube (ETT) and airway. Nowadays the CO_2 is measured straightaway in the airway itself whereas previously the gas has to be sampled away from the airway where it was tested for CO_2. This recent innovation has resulted in more crisper waveforms and has decreased the delay time significantly.

The mainstream capnograph has to be kept somewhat warm above than the body temperatures to prevent water vapor formation which can result in faulty CO_2 measurements. In addition to lesser response time they are light weight, has negligible moving parts and are compact which makes them all the more attractive as compared to side stream capnographs **(Figs. 2A and B)**.

SIDESTREAM CAPNOGRAPHS

As the name suggests CO_2 sensor is situated away from the airway and a small sampling unit connects airway (via T-piece connected to ETT or mask) and sensor, and a suction pump drives the gas towards sensor which contains aesthetic gases and thus these gases have to be recycled to breathing circuit or redirected to scavenging systems. These capnographs can be used for measuring CO_2 in nonintubated patients **(Fig. 3)**.

Based upon whether CO_2 is plotted against volume or time, capnograph can still be divided into volumetric capnography or time capnography.

VOLUMETRIC CAPNOGRAPHY

If the expired CO_2 is plotted against lung volume then it is known as volumetric capnography **(Fig. 4)**. It is helpful in the breath by breath estimation of alveolar dead space (Vd). Newer ventilators namely Hamilton-T1, Dräger Evita XL, and Maquet Servo-I, have inbuilt volumetric sensors which helps in the estimation of Vd as well as mixed expired CO_2 pressures ($PECO_2$).

- *Phase I:* Carbon dioxide free gas which includes anatomical dead space as well as apparatus dead space.
- *Phase II:* Mixing of dead space and alveolar gas results in S-shaped rise.
- *Phase III:* The rising PCO_2 on this phase results in a positive slope and the alveolar plateau is indicative of alveolar gas which is rich in CO_2.

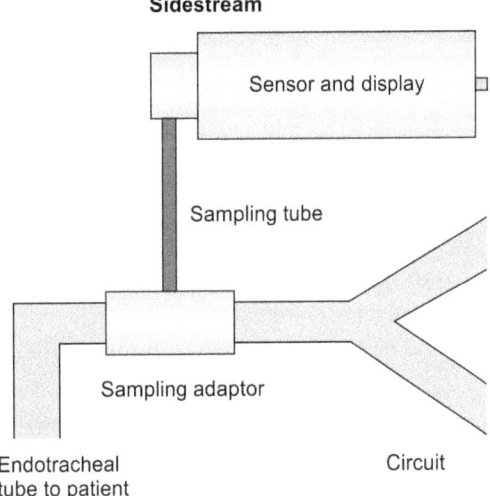

Fig. 3: Sidestream capnograph.

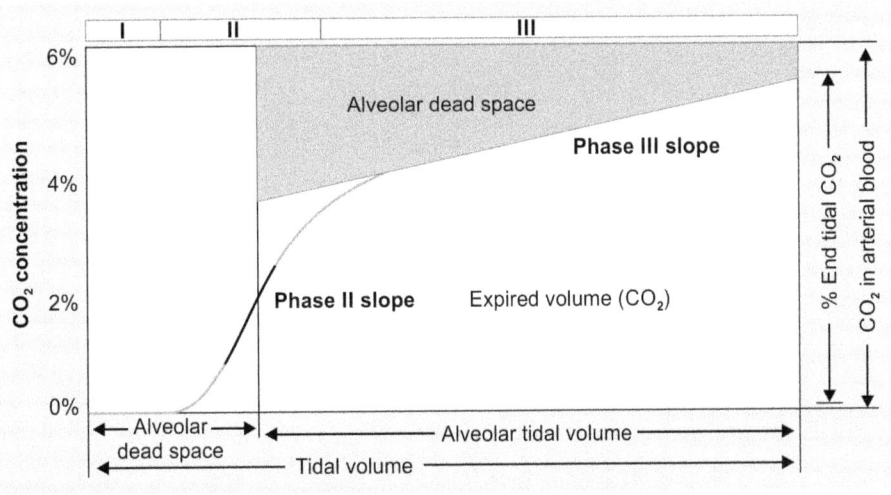

Fig. 4: Volumetric capnography.

TIME CAPNOGRAM

Carbon dioxide when plotted against time is known as a time capnogram which consists of an expiratory segment and inspiratory segment and two angles namely alpha and beta.

Expiratory Segment

The expiratory segment mainly consists of three phases: namely I, II, III. Occasionally, phase IV which is marked by terminal upswing after the end of phase III may occur (Fig. 5).

- *Phase 0:* It represents carbon dioxide from the start of inspiration to start of expiration and on the graph it is represented by descending limb and early part of horizontal baseline. Once phase III is over, which represents inspiratory phase when fresh gas which is essential. Free carbon dioxide is inhaled and thus CO_2 concentration falls all the way to zero. The later half of horizontal baseline is phase I of expiratory segment.
- *Phase I:* It represents anatomical and apparatus dead space.
- *Phase II:* It represents a mixture of anatomical and alveolar dead space. It is marked by a rapid S-shaped ascent of the capnogram.
- *Phase III:* It represents CO_2 rich gas from alveoli which forms a plateau with a positive slope indicating a gradual rise of partial pressure of carbon dioxide (PCO_2). The positive slope thus formed is due to the following:

Consistent Discharge of CO_2 into the Alveoli

As alveoli become progressively smaller and smaller towards the end of expiration which leads to a steady increase in alveolar PCO_2 concentration and thus rising positive incline of phase III is formed with expiration.

Difference in Ventilation and Perfusion Ratio Ventilation to Perfusion

Dependent areas of the lung have lower ventilation to perfusion (V/Q) ratio as compared to nondependent areas of the lungs. These low V/Q areas representing the under ventilated region of lungs have relatively

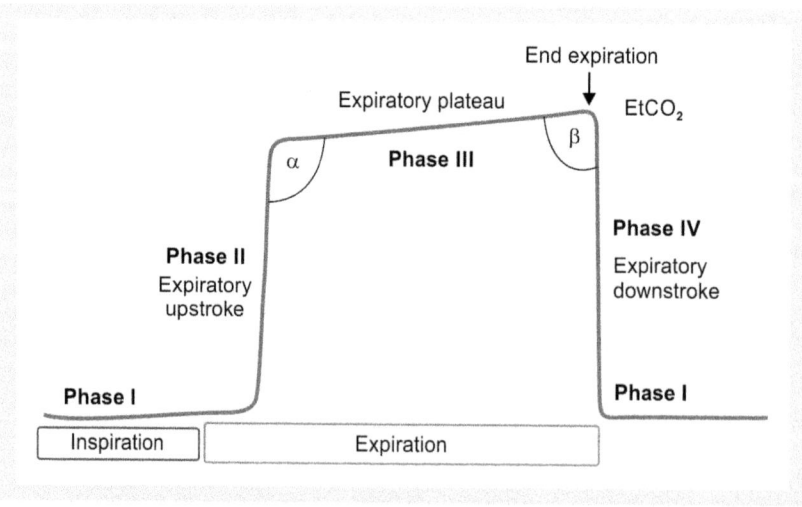

Fig. 5: The expiratory segment.

higher PCO_2 as compared to areas with a higher V/Q ratio or over ventilated region. The emptying of regions having a lower V/Q ratio is delayed which is responsible for the rising slope of phase III.

Inspiratory Segment

Phase 0

Phase 0 represents carbon dioxide from the start of inspiration to start of expiration and on the graph it is represented by descending limb and early part of horizontal baseline.

Once phase III is over, which represents inspiratory phase when fresh gas which is essential. The free CO_2 is inhaled and thus CO_2 concentration falls to zero. The later half of horizontal baseline is phase I of expiratory segment.

Alfa angle: Phase II and phase III forms an alfa angle which indirectly indicates V/Q status of the lungs.

Beta angle: Phase III and descending limb forms Beta angle which is around 9°. An increase in beta angle can be seen during rebreathing and also when there is prolongation of response time of the capnometer as compared to respiratory cycle time.

A normal capnogram is indicative of healthy lungs **(Fig. 6)**. If there is some physiological or pathological abnormality in lung mechanics is reflected by the change in shape of capnogram.

Other possible causes: Foreign body in the airway, occlusion of the breathing circuit.

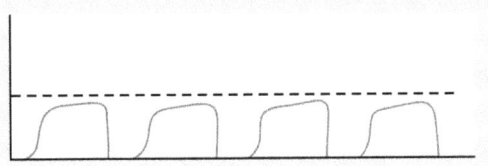

Fig. 6: Normal capnogram.

Other possible reasons: Increase in metabolic rate, hyperthermia, rebreathing, and faulty expiratory valve.

CLINICAL APPLICATIONS (FIGS. 7 TO 11)

- Patient end-tidal carbon dioxide ($PetCO_2$) acts as surrogate estimate of $PaCO_2$

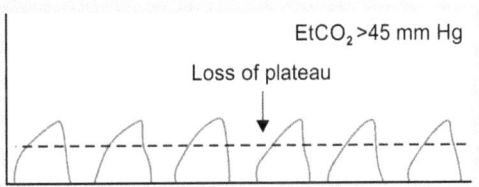

Fig. 7: Bronchospasm/asthma.

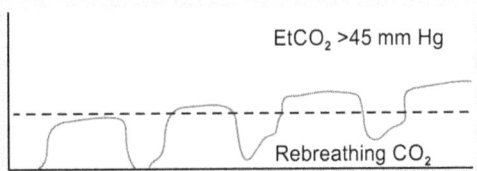

Fig. 8: Increasing CO_2 (hypoventilation).

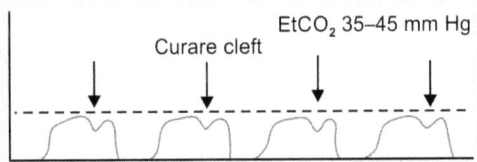

Fig. 9: Curare cleft.

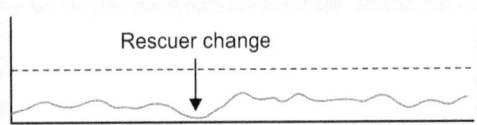

Fig. 10: Cardiac arrest.

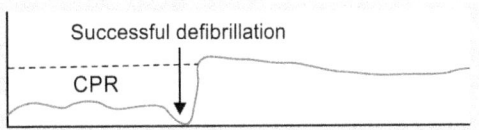

Fig. 11: Return of spontaneous circulation.

- Adequacy of spontaneous respiration
- Fresh gas flow rates (FGF) in rebreathing systems can be adjusted based on capnograms
- Integrity of anesthetic apparatus
- Accidental esophageal intubation
- Blind nasal intubation
- Proper placements of double lumen-tubes
- Hypermetabolic states
- Detection of pulmonary embolism
- Detection of Venous CO_2 embolism
- Determining adequacy of cardiopulmonary resuscitation.

CONCLUSION

Capnography has taken a significant position in the anesthetists' armamentarium to increment patient safety in the operation theatre as well as in the postoperative monitoring and emergency unit.

These technological advancements in patient monitoring has resulted in improved patient outcomes and reduced the occurrence of major intraoperative accidents and resultant legal suit following it.

Further research work should focus on minimizing issues related with CO_2 sampling in capnometers and at the same time increasing its accuracy, and also making capnometers more pocket friendly. While anesthetists have valued the worth of capnography somewhat recently, doctors in different specialties will see the value in its worth later on, as various research has proactively shown the use of capnography outside the realm of anesthesia.

FURTHER READING

1. Capnocheck.com
2. Davey A, Diba A. Ward's Anaesthetic Equipment, 5th edition.

40: Patterns of Neuromuscular Stimulation

Anju Gupta, Mitchell Gullebani

INTRODUCTION

Clinical criteria alone cannot serve as an optimal guide to the degree of neuromuscular blockade. Residual neuromuscular blockade may persist postoperatively and thus objective monitoring of the degree of the block during and after anesthesia may negate complications such as airway obstruction, hypoxemia, aspiration pneumonia, need for tracheal intubation culminating longer stay in the postanesthesia care unit.

PRINCIPLE OF PERIPHERAL NERVE STIMULATION

The neuromuscular function is evaluated by applying a supramaximal stimulus to a peripheral motor nerve and then measuring the associated response.

The reaction of a single muscle fiber to a stimulus follows an *all or none pattern*. The electrical stimulus must be at least 20–25% above that necessary for a maximal response.

The nerve chosen must fulfill the following criteria:
- It must have a motor element.
- It must be closer to the skin.
- Contraction in the muscle or muscle group supplied by the nerve must be visible or attainable for evoke response monitoring.

ESSENTIAL FEATURES OF THE NERVE STIMULATOR

- The current applied should be of sufficient magnitude and duration, e.g., 0.1–0.3 ms.
- It should be battery operated.
- It should deliver a constant current of 80 mA, rather than only deliver constant voltage.
- Adequacy of electrical contact should be displayed on the monitor screen.
- E-pulse stimulus—monophasic, square wave type—no longer than 0.3 ms.
- Polarity of the electrode needs to be indicated.
- Capable of delivering a variety of patterns of stimulation (single twitch, train of four, double burst, and post-tetanic count).
- A built-in time constant system to facilitate post-tetanic count—the tetanic stimulus should last for 5 seconds followed by 3 seconds later a first post-tetanic stimulus.

PATTERNS OF NERVE STIMULATION

Single Twitch Stimulation

A single supramaximal electrical stimulus is applied to a peripheral motor nerve at frequencies ranging from 1–0.1 Hz for a period of 0.2 ms, at regular intervals and the evoked response is observed.

Most Common Application

Onset of neuromuscular blockade where a single twitch of 1 Hz is applied (1 twitch every second) to assess the level at which supramaximal stimulus is obtained.

Limitation

A control twitch needs to be measured before administering a neuromuscular blocking agent.

Figure 1 clearly depicts that besides the time factor, no difference exists in the strength of evoked responses between the two blocks.

Train-of-four Stimulation

Introduced by Ali and associates during the early 1970. Four supramaximal stimuli of 2 Hz are given every 0.5 seconds. Each set (train) of stimuli is usually repeated every 10 seconds and the response provides the basis for evaluation.

Train-of-four Stimulation Ratio

Dividing the amplitude of the fourth response to the first response provides the ratio.

In the control response (before administration of muscle relaxant), the four responses are the same. The ratio of 1.

Application (Fig. 2)

- In nondepolarizing blockade, the *fade response* is seen; hence the degree of block can be ascertained by the train-of-four (TOF) response.
- No fade is seen in depolarizing block. If fade is seen, then it signifies phase 2 block.
- Monitoring recovery from neuromuscular blockade. Train-of-four ratio of 0.7 or greater generally means adequate reversal (**Fig. 2**).

Fade is the gradual decrease in twitch height first of T4, T3, T2, and finally T1 once a neuromuscular blocking agent is given.

Reversal from block T1 reappears first, then T2, T3, and finally T4.

Disadvantage

Less useful for monitoring depolarizing neuromuscular block as each twitch is decreased equally in size.

Tetanic Stimulation (Fig. 3)

Delivery of rapid electrical stimuli (3,050, 100 Hz). The most commonly used is 50 Hz for 5 seconds.

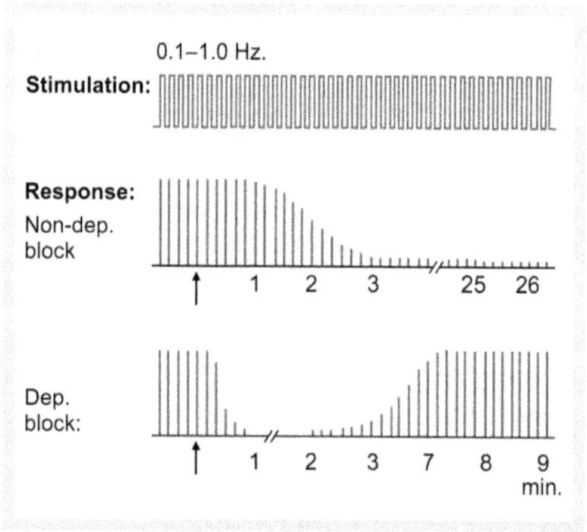

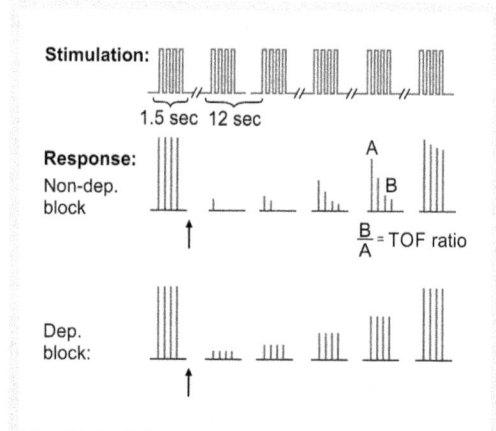

Fig. 1: Pattern of electrical nerve stimulation and evoked muscle responses to single twitch nerve stimulation (0.1–1 Hz) after injection of nondepolarizing (Non-dep) and depolarizing (Dep) neuromuscular blocking drugs.

Fig. 2: Pattern of electrical nerve stimulation and evoked response to TOF nerve stimulation before and after administration of nondepolarizing (Non-dep) and depolarizing (Dep) neuromuscular blocking agents.

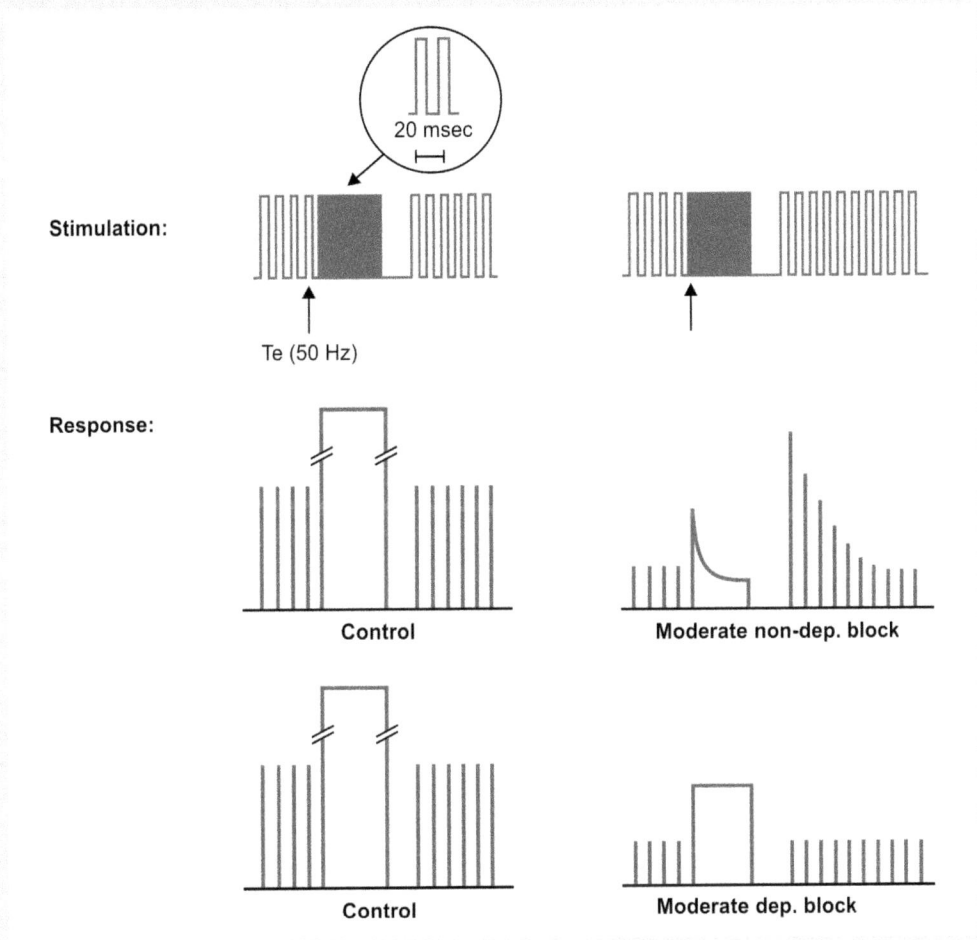

Fig. 3: Tetanic stimulation of 50 Hz for 5 seconds and post-tetanic twitch of 1 Hz is applied. (dep.: depolarizing; non-dep.: nondepolarizing)

Evaluation

- Response to a depolarizing block is sustained.
- Response to a nondepolarizing block and phase 2 block is not sustained but fades.
- Evaluate residual neuromuscular blockade.

Explanation

It is a presynaptic event with large amounts of acetylcholine being released from the nerve terminal during the tetanic stimulus into the synaptic cleft. In the presence of nondepolarizing neuromuscular blocking agents, the competitive block at the presynaptic level reduces the amount of acetylcholine being mobilized and released, contributing to fade.

Role in the Present-day

A little place in everyday anesthesia and is extremely painful.

Fade response and post-tetanic facilitation in the moderate nondepolarizing neuromuscular block.

During depolarizing block, the tetanic response is well sustained, and no post-tetanic facilitation occurs.

Post-tetanic Count Stimulation

Technique

Evaluation of intense neuromuscular blockade can be done by applying tetanic stimulation of 50 Hz for 5 seconds and observing the post-tetanic response to a single twitch given at 1 Hz starting 3 seconds after the end of stimulation.

Response

During the intense neuromuscular blockade, there is no response to either tetanic or post-tetanic stimulation. In the early stages of recovery, the first response to post-tetanic twitch stimulation occurs, even before the first response to TOF stimulation reappears. This is called *post-tetanic facilitation.*

Role in Anesthesia

- Assessment of the degree of neuromuscular blockade when there is no response to either a single twitch or TOF nerve stimulation.
- Profound neuromuscular blockade is required, for example, retinal surgery where any movement could be devastating.

Point to Note

If two post-tetanic counts are administered in quick succession, the degree of the neuromuscular block will be underestimated. It is recommended not to repeat it for a period of 6 minutes.

The *intense block* in **Figure 4** shows no response to TOF, TE, and PTS. However, in *the deep block and surgical block*, the post-tetanic facilitation is present and in the surgical block, it further gets intensified with appearance to first response of TOF.

Double Burst Stimulation

Technique

Two short bursts of 50 Hz tetanic stimulation separated by 750 ms. The duration of each square wave impulse in the burst is 0.2 ms, although the number of impulses may vary. Most commonly three impulses in two tetanic bursts are used.

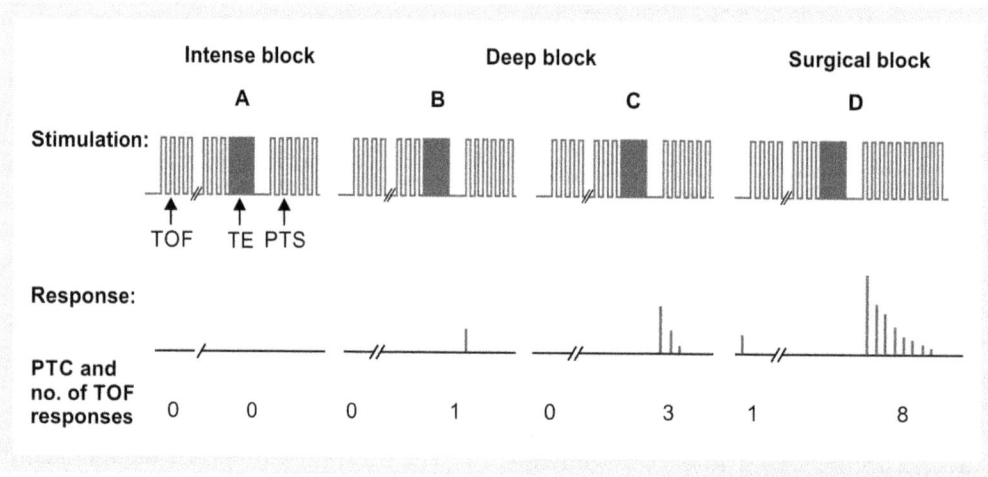

Fig. 4: Patterns of nerve stimulation and evoked response during TOF, 50 Hz tetanic stimulation for 5 seconds, and 1 Hz PTS during different levels of nondepolarizing neuromuscular block.

Response

- In a nonparalyzed person, two separate muscle contractions of equal intensity will occur.
- In partially paralyzed with nondepolarizing drugs, the response to the second burst is reduced/faded.
- Double burst stimulation (DBS) ratio—response of the second burst to the first burst. Similar to the TOF ratio but tactile evaluation of the former has been considered to be more accurate than the latter.

Role in Anesthesia

Detection of a small amount of residual block during recovery and immediately after surgery.

Figure 5 is depicting DBS response to stimulation, before administration of neuromuscular blocking drugs and during recovery from nondepolarizing block.

TYPES OF PERIPHERAL NERVE STIMULATION

- Electric—most commonly used
- Magnetic

Magnetic Stimulation

Advantages of Magnetic Stimulation

- Less painful
- Does not require physical contact with the body.

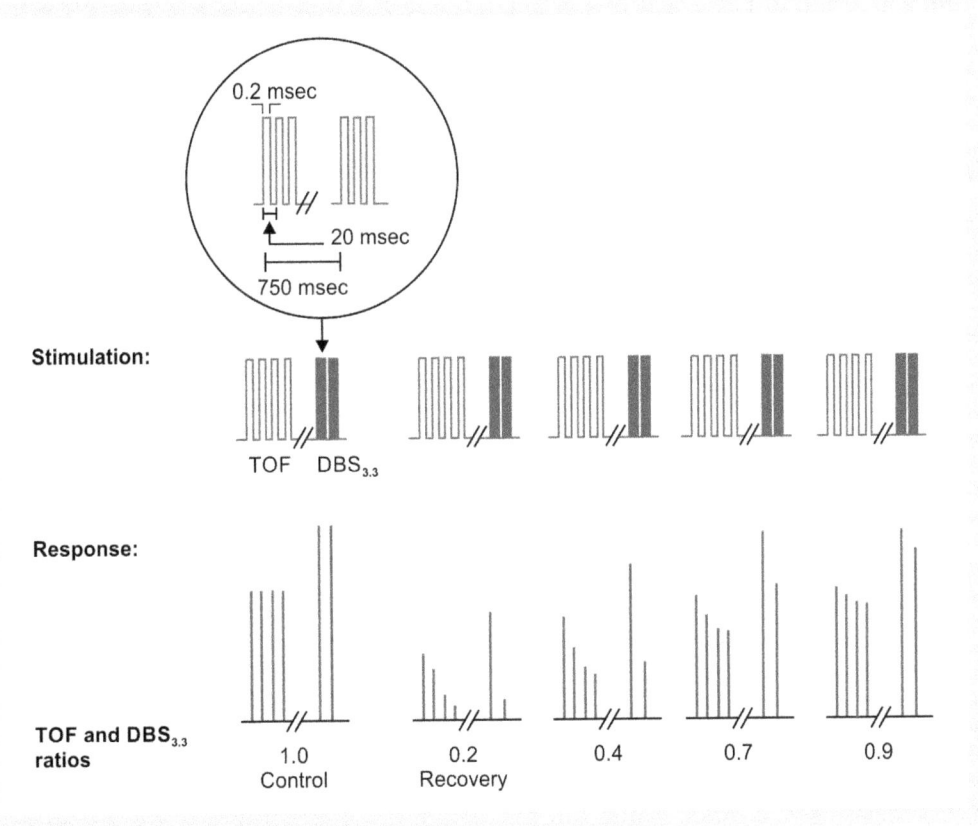

Fig. 5: Deep brain stimulation (DBS) showing the response to stimulation, before administration of neuromuscular blocking drugs and during recovery from nondepolarizing block.

Disadvantages of Magnetic Stimulation
- Bulky and heavy
- Cannot be used for TOF stimulation
- Difficult to achieve supramaximal stimulation.

STIMULATING ELECTRODES
- Surface—most commonly used
- Needle

Points of Care
- The actual conducting area should be small 7-11 mm in diameter
- The skin should always be cleaned properly
- When supramaximal stimulus cannot be obtained with surface electrodes, needle electrodes should be used
- The needle electrodes should be placed subcutaneously but never in a nerve.

Sites of Nerve Stimulation
- Ulnar nerve—most commonly used. Muscle—adductor pollicis
- Median nerve
- Posterior tibial nerve
- Common Peroneal nerve
- Facial nerve.

Points to Note
- The diaphragm is the *most resistant* of all the muscles for both depolarizing and nondepolarizing blocks. Requires nearly twice as much relaxant as the adductor pollicis for an identical blockade.
- *Onset time* is shorter for the diaphragm (central muscle) compared with the adductor pollicis owing to its good blood supply.
- *Recovery time* is also faster for the diaphragm compared with other peripheral muscles.
- Most sensitive are the abdominal muscles, the orbicularis oculi, the peripheral muscles of the limb, and the upper airway muscles.
- During recovery, if the adductor pollicis (relatively sensitive muscle) has recovered, it can be assumed that no residual neuromuscular blockade exists in the diaphragm.

Which Nerve to Stimulate and When?
One can stimulate the nerve by going through the following:
- *Induction of anesthesia:* Orbicularis oculi as it is more like a central muscle.
- *Maintenance of anesthesia:* Orbicularis oculi will reflect the diaphragm more closely as the adductor pollicis is a more sensitive peripheral muscle.
- *Reversal of anesthesia:* Peripheral muscle monitoring like adductor pollicis is best.

RECORDING OF EVOKED RESPONSES
Assessment of neuromuscular response by tactile and visual means is difficult. Quantitative and numerical display of the evoked responses is desirable. Commonly employed methods are given in **Table 1**.

NEUROMUSCULAR MONITORING
Clinical Significance of Neuromuscular Monitoring
- Onset of neuromuscular block and assessment of the intubating condition (**Table 2**).
- Maintenance of block during surgery.
- Reversal of neuromuscular blockade.

Conditions Where Neuromuscular Monitoring is Essential
- Prolonged infusion of long-acting neuromuscular blocking agents.

Chapter 40: Patterns of Neuromuscular Stimulation

TABLE 1: Techniques for quantitative neuromuscular monitoring.

Method	Principle	Technique
Mechanomyography	Force-displacement transducer by *isometric* muscle contraction	The thumb is stabilized by placing a fixed tension, then evoked response is measured as change in tension develops MC muscle—Adductor P
Electromyography	Compound action potential is produced by stimulation of a peripheral nerve	Stimulating electrodes are placed over the ulnar nerve (muscle belly, tendinous insertion of muscle and third as a third site distant to muscle) MC nerve—ulnar and median nerve
Acceleromyography	Force equals mass times acceleration. Piezoelectric ceramic wafers with electrodes on both sides are used. On stimulation the transducer produces a voltage proportional to its acceleration and voltage is displayed as twitch	Adductor pollicis is most commonly used for this too. This is a nonisometric measurement hence less stringent requirements for immobilization of arm and preload is not necessary
Piezoelectric neuromuscular monitor	Stretching of a piezoelectric film in response to nerve stimulation generates a voltage that is proportional to the amount of stretching	Adductor pollicis is used for this too
Phonomyography	Low-frequency sound waves produced by muscle contraction is recorded by special microphones	Many muscles besides adductor pollicis like the diaphragm, larynx, and eye muscles are employed. The advantage is it is easy to use

TABLE 2: Nondepolarizing neuromuscular block and TOF/PTC relation.

TOF count	Neuromuscular blockade	PTC value
>1	Onset of block	
0	Intense block	0
0	Deep block	>1
1–3	Moderate block	
Measurable	Recovery phase	

(PTC: phenylthiocarbamide; TOF: train-of-four)

- Prolonged surgery and anesthesia
- Adequate reversal is of paramount importance, for example, severe respiratory disease and morbid obesity
- Severe liver or renal dysfunction
- Neuromuscular disorders such as Myasthenia Gravis and Eaton-Lambert syndrome.

Shortcomings of Neuromuscular Monitoring

- Neuromuscular response may appear normal despite the occupancy of receptors by neuromuscular blocking agents.
- Genetic variability in evoked responses can result in weakness even in TOF ratio of 0.8–0.9.
- Values for adequate recovery do not correlate with the adequacy of airway protection.

- Evoked responses may be hampered by skin impedance owing to perioperative hypothermia.

CONCLUSION

Neuromuscular monitoring should always be employed in all cases when neuromuscular blocking agents are given. Clinical tests are highly uncertain in assessing adequacy and reversal from neuromuscular block. Quantitative methods for measuring block depth like mechanomyography and acceleromyography are preferred.

FURTHER READING

1. American Society of Anesthesiologists. Standards and Guidelines and Related Resources [online]. Schaumburg, IL: American Society of Anesthesiologists; 2014.
2. Checketts MR, Alladi R, Ferguson K, Gemmell L, Handy JM, Klein AA, et al. Recommendations for standards of monitoring during anaesthesia and recovery 2015: Association of Anaesthetists of Great Britain and Ireland. 2016;71(1):85-93.
3. Difficult Airway Society Extubation Guidelines Group, Popat M, Mitchell V, Dravid R, Patel A, Swampillai C, et al. Difficult Airway Society Guidelines for the management of tracheal extubation. Anesthesia. 2012;67(3):318-40.
4. Dorsch JA, Dorsch SE. Understanding Anesthesia Equipment, 4th edition. Philadelphia: Lippincott Williams & Wilkins; 1999.
5. Durga P, Mantha S. Monitoring of neuromuscular junction. Indian J Anaesth. 2002;46(4):279-88.
6. Miller R, Eriksson L, Fleisher L, Wiener-Kronish J, Young W. Miller's Anesthesia, 7th edition. Philadelphia: Churchill Livingstone; 2009.

CHAPTER 41

Nerve Stimulator

Anju Gupta, Manjula Sudhakar Rao

ESSENTIAL FEATURES OF THE NERVE STIMULATOR

- The current applied should be of sufficient magnitude and duration (0.2 ms)
- It should deliver a constant current of 80 mA
- It should be battery powered
- Adequacy of electrical contact should be displayed on the monitor screen
- A monophasic impulse with a rectangular waveform no longer than 0.3 ms is to be delivered
- The polarity of the electrodes needs to be indicated
- Should be capable of delivering a variety of patterns of stimulation (single twitch, train of four, double burst, and post-tetanic count)
- A built-in time constant to facilitate post-tetanic count.

SITES OF NERVE STIMULATION (FIG. 1)

- The nerve chosen must have a motor element
- It must be close to the skin
- The contraction in the muscle/muscle group supplied by the nerve must be visible or accessible for evoked response monitoring.

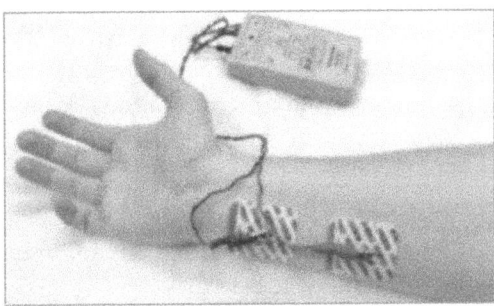

Fig. 1: Nerve stimulator.

COMMON NERVE–MUSCLE UNITS USED

- Ulnar nerve-adductor pollicis muscle
- Facial nerve-orbicularis oculi/corrugator supercilii
- Tibial nerve-flexor hallucis brevis
- Common peroneal nerve-extensor hallucis longus
- Median nerve-abductor pollicis.

Which nerve–muscle unit to stimulate when?

Facial nerve-corrugator supercilii muscle for optimal intubation condition (diaphragm and abdominal wall muscle paralysis).

Ulnar nerve-adductor pollicis is the better choice for pharyngeal muscle recovery. Onset and recovery time is shorter for the diaphragm when compared with an adductor pollicis owing to its better blood supply.

THE STIMULATING ELECTRODE

Surface Electrode
- The actual conducting area should be small (7–11 mm in diameter)
- The skin should be cleaned properly
- It has to be placed at a site to ensure the stimulation of the target nerve.
- The negative electrode should be placed distally.
- Ag/AgCl electrodes/special neuromuscular monitoring electrodes can be used.
- Skin temperature should be maintained at >32° to avoid the hypothermia-related increase in skin impedance.

Needle Electrodes
- When supramaximal stimulus cannot be used with surface electrode.
- It should be placed subcutaneously.
- Should never be placed in a nerve.

Stimulating a peripheral nerve with an electrical impulse results in a muscular response following the "all or none" principle. For clinical application of neuromuscular monitoring, a supramaximal stimulus, i.e., 15–20% above the level of maximal response is used. This is to ensure that factors like variability in skin impedance do not have a significant influence on the muscular response and quality of measurement.

TYPES OF QUANTITATIVE MONITORS

Whenever a neuromuscular blocker is administered, the neuromuscular function must be monitored by observing evoked muscle response to peripheral nerve stimulation. Objective monitoring (a TOF ratio ≥ 0.9) ensures a near-total recovery from neuromuscular blockade. Various types of nerve stimulators have been summarized in **Table 1**.

Mechanomyography (Fig. 2)
It was considered the gold standard method of neuromuscular monitoring, which measures the force of isometric muscle contraction using a force transducer. The ulnar nerve is commonly stimulated and the force of contraction of the adductor pollicis is measured. This requires the use of a preload which is 200–300 g resting tension applied to the thumb.

Drawbacks

The setup of the system, the sophisticated calibration process, the sensitivity to temperature changes, and the requirement of a stable baseline have made them unsuitable for routine clinical use. This method has become obsolete in clinical settings and is only used for research purposes.

Electromyography (Fig. 3)
This measures the compound muscle action potential on stimulation of the nerve. The force of muscle contraction is measured based on the amplitude of the compound muscle action potential (CMAPs), which is directly proportionate to the number of muscle fibers activated.

Advantages
- Good correlation with mechanomyography (MMG)
- Applicable to several nerve-muscle units
- Does not require hand immobilization/use of preload
- Increasing adoption of robotic surgery creates a special use case for electromyography (EMG) devices
- Calibration is simpler and faster compared to acceleromyograph/MMG
- Temperature changes effects to a lesser extent
- More reliable for use in daily practice.

TABLE 1: Various nerve stimulators.

Modality	Principle	Pros	Cons	Monitoring site	Current availability
MMG	Directly measures isometric muscle contraction force	Measures muscle force directly. The "reference" modality	Cumbersome and time-consuming setup. Not suitable for clinical practice	• Ulnar nerve—adductor pollicis muscle • Posterior tibial nerve—flexor hallucis brevis muscle	Commercially not available
EMG	Measures compound muscle action potentials evoked by neurostimulation	• Many muscles can be examined • Does not require freely moving limbs • Easy and fast setup and short calibration	Possible interference from other electrical equipment (electrocautery). Currently available in modular form only	• Ulnar nerve—adductor pollicis, abductor digiti minimi, and first dorsal interosseous muscles • Posterior tibial nerve—flexor hallucis brevis muscle • Phrenic nerve—diaphragm	E-NMT (GE Datex-Ohmeda NMT, Waukesha, WI, USA)
AMG	Measures the acceleration of the thumb or any freely moving muscle. The acceleration is directly proportional to the force according to Newton's second law	• Current NMB management guidelines are based on AMG measurements • Most widely used technique	Requires the use of hand adapter, fixation of arm and fingers, free movement of the thumb, normalization of recovery TOF ratios	• Ulnar nerve—adductor pollicis muscle • Facial nerve—orbicularis oculi, corrugator supercilii muscles • Tibial nerve—flexor hallucis brevis muscle	• Infinity Trident NMT SmartPod (Dräger, Lübeck, Germany) • IntelliVue NMT (Philips, Amsterdam, the Netherlands) • TOF-Scan (IDMed, Marseille, France) • Stimpod NMS450 (Xavant Technology, Pretoria, South Africa)
KMG	Measures the distortion of a piezoelectric film sensor. The level of distortion is proportional to the force of thumb contraction	Easy to apply	Available only in modular form	Ulnar nerve—adductor pollicis muscle	M-NMT (GE Datex-Ohmeda NMT, Waukesha, WI, USA)

Contd...

Contd...

Modality	Principle	Pros	Cons	Monitoring site	Current availability
PMG	Measures the emitted low-frequency sound of sliding muscle fibers	Many muscles can be examined	• Relatively expensive microphones • Commercially not available	• Ulnar nerve—adductor pollicis, abductor digiti minimi, and first dorsal interosseous muscles • Facial nerve—orbicularis oculi, corrugator supercilii muscles • Posterior tibial nerve—flexor hallucis brevis muscle • Recurrent laryngeal nerve—posterior cricoarytenoid and lateral arytenoid muscles	Implemented in an anesthesia robot system (McSleepy) but commercially unavailable at the moment
CMG	Measures the pressure change in an air-filled balloon due to the hand muscle's contraction in response to ulnar nerve stimulation	Seemed to be a reliable technique	Commercially not available.	Ulnar nerve—all hand muscles innervated by the ulnar nerve	Not available
Cuff pressure modality	Measures the pressure change in a modified noninvasive blood pressure cuff due to upper arm muscle's contraction evoked by brachial plexus stimulation	Easy to apply	Needs further validation	Brachial plexus—muscles of the upper arm	TOF-Cuff (RGB Medical, Madrid)

(AMG: acceleromyography; CMG: compressomyography; EMG: electromyography; KMG: kinemyography; MMG: mechanomyography; PMG: phonomyography)

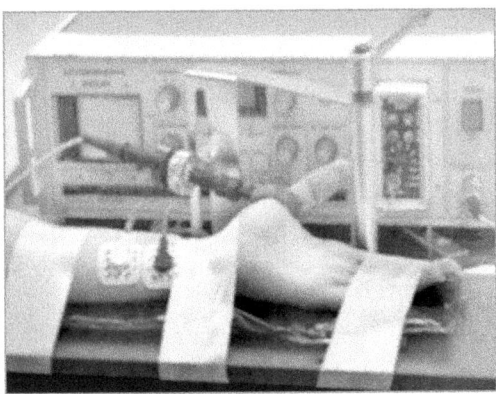

Fig. 2: Mechanomyography (MMG).

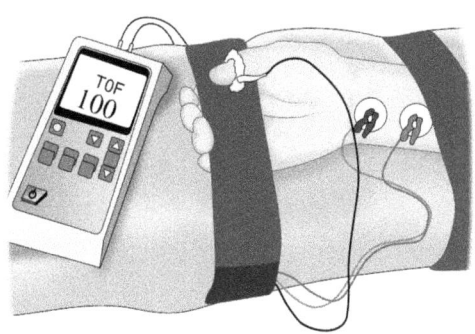

Fig. 4: Acceleromyography (AMG).

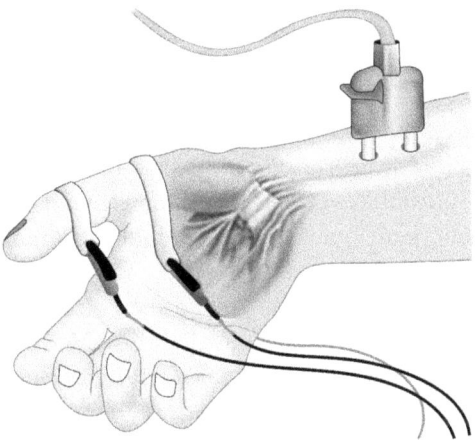

Fig. 3: Electromyography (EMG).

Drawbacks

Susceptible to direct muscle stimulation and interference from surgical cautery.

Currently, there is only one EMG-based monitor available that is incorporated into the anesthesia workstation (GE Datex-Ohmeda NMP, Waukesha, WI, USA). The portable EMG-based monitor Tetragraph is under clinical trial.

Acceleromyography (Fig. 4)

It was developed by Viby-Mogensen et al. in 1988. Over years it has become the most popular monitoring technique. The newer versions are most widely used in a clinical setting. (Portable TOF-Watch series), it measures the acceleration of the thumb using a piezoelectric transducer placed at the thumb tip when the ulnar nerve is stimulated. The force of contraction of adductor pollicis muscle is calculated by using the formula $F = MA$. Other sites like—corrugator supercilii, orbicularis oculi, great toe, and trapezius were used. But not recommended for routine monitoring in view of a high level of uncertainty. The user must ensure the thumb returns to the same position by fixing the forearm and fingers to eliminate the motion artifact.

The recently introduced portable acceleromyography (AMG) monitors are *Stimpod NMS 450* (South Africa) and **TOF-Scan** (France) they have a modified three-dimensional (3D) piezoelectric transducer that senses the motion of thumb in all directions. Hence improving the precision of AMG technology **(Fig. 5)**.

TOF-Watch

Acceleration of the thumb is measured only in one direction that is perpendicular to the face of the monitor **(Fig. 6)**.

Drawbacks

- The thumb needs to be stabilized using a preload device

Section 2: Anesthesia Monitoring

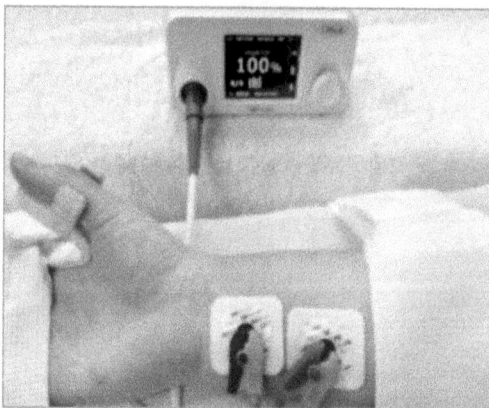

Fig. 5: TOF-Scan.

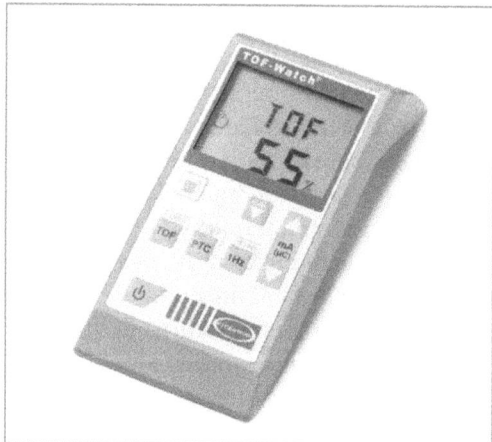

Fig. 6: TOF-Watch.

- Overestimation of TOF ratio for which the baseline value has to be normalized.
- Baseline TOFR = 1.25, adequate recovery (0.9) = 1.25 × 0.9 = 1.125
- Staircase effect—repeated indirect stimulation may enhance the evoked mechanical response of the muscle **(Fig. 7)**.

TOF Watch SX

Fixes issues with overestimated TOFR.

When the staircase occurs, the monitor displays T4/T2 rather than T4/T1. If this ratio is more than 1, the monitor will limit the display to 100%.

Kinemyography

It can be considered as a variant of AMG. It uses piezoelectric film embedded in a flexible molded strip. The electrical signal is directly proportional to the extent of bending of the probe kept between the thumb and index finger in response to ulnar nerve stimulation. The technique was introduced in 1994. Currently, the device available is M-NMT integrated neuromuscular transmission module (GE-Datex-Ohmeda) kinemyography (KMG) is less susceptible to reverse fade phenomenon compared to AMG.

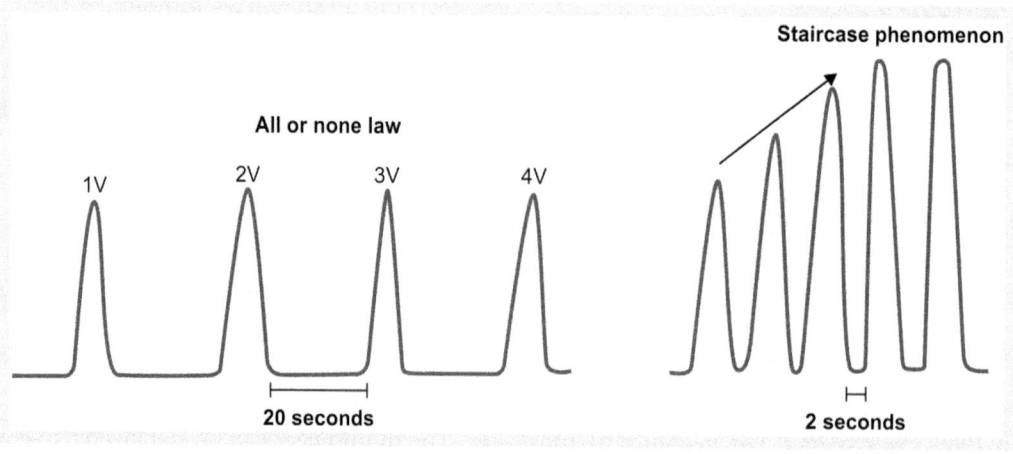

Fig. 7: All or none law and staircase phenomenon.

Compressomyography

An air-filled balloon is placed in the palm of the patient with fingers closed and secured around the balloon with a flexible strap. The force of contraction of hand muscles is transmitted to the balloon via two plastic strips which ensure even distribution of force and uniform deformation of the spherical balloon with each hand contraction. A pressure transducer is connected to the balloon and a pressure monitoring unit.

Advantages

Free of pre-relaxation reverse fade phenomenon allowing faster and easier calibration.

It has a low bias regarding T1% and TOFR when compared to MMG. It is not available for clinical use as of now.

Phonomyography

The lateral movement of muscle fibers produces low-frequency sound. This can be detected by using special microphones. These microphone systems are easy to set up and correlate well with MMG data. It can be applied to any superficial muscle (laryngeal and corrugator supercilii muscles). It is not commercially available at present. However, it is available as a part of a closed-loop anesthesia management system.

Cuff Pressure Modality (TOF Cuff) (Fig. 8)

It relies on specifically designed noninvasive blood pressure (NIBP) monitors that detect pressure changes due to muscle contraction.

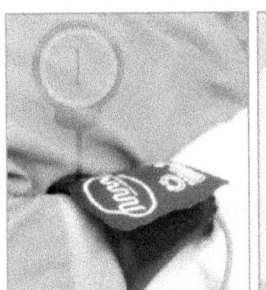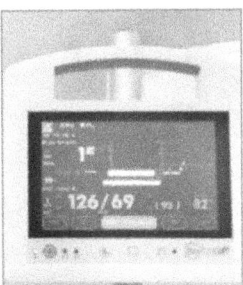

Fig. 8: Cuff pressure modality (TOF cuff).

Stimulating electrodes are integrated into the inner surface of the BP cuff. Further clinical investigations are needed to prove the reliability of this new monitoring modality.

FURTHER READING

1. Bowdle A, Bussey L, Michaelsen K, Jelacic S, Nair B, Togashi K, et al. A comparison of a prototype electromyograph vs. a mechanomyograph and an acceleromyograph for assessment of neuromuscular blockade. Anaesthesia. 2020;75(2):187-95.
2. Checketts MR, Alladi R, Ferguson K, Gemmell L, Handy JM, Klein AA, et al. Recommendations for standards of monitoring during anaesthesia and recovery 2015: Association of Anaesthetists of Great Britain and Ireland. Anaesthesia. 2016;71(1): 85-93.
3. Claudius C, Fuchs-Buder T. Neuromuscular monitoring. In: Gropper MA (Ed). Miller's Anesthesia, 9th edition. Philadelphia: Elsevier; 2020. pp. 1354-72.
4. Iwasaki H, Nemes R, Brull SJ, Renew JR. Quantitative neuromuscular monitoring: current devices, new technological advances, and use in clinical practice. Curr Anesthesiol Rep. 2018 (8):134-44.
5. Murphy GS. Neuromuscular monitoring in the perioperative period. Anesth Analg. 2018;126(2):464-8.

CHAPTER 42: Temperature Monitoring

Tazeen Khan, Parthodeep Jha, Puneet Khanna

INTRODUCTION

Body temperature is a vital sign indicating proper physiological functioning and thus needs to be carefully monitored. Maintenance of normothermia is a primary function of the autonomic nervous system in warm-blooded animals. In humans, core body temperature is maintained between a narrow range of 36.5–37.5°C through behavioral and physiological responses. Body temperature varies significantly from the core to the periphery, higher at the core due to highly perfused central tissues and lesser at the periphery due to heat dissipation. The variation ranges between 2 and 4°C.

PHYSIOLOGY

Maintenance of normothermia is through a physiological system consisting of peripheral and central thermoreceptors, an integrating control center, and an efferent response system that enables a compensatory action. Afferent thermal inputs are provided by the cold and warm receptors that are either central or peripheral. The main control mechanism is via the hypothalamus which determines the mean body temperature by integrating various thermal signals and comparing the mean body temperature to a predetermined set-point temperature. In humans, the efferent response to maintain normothermia is via behavioral and physiological responses. The physiological response involves

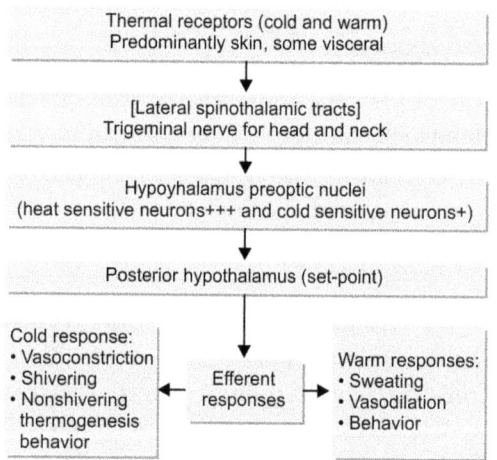

Flowchart 1: Control of thermoregulation.

vasodilation and sweating when heat loss is indicated whereas vasoconstriction, shivering, and nonshivering thermogenesis when increased heat production is indicated. In conscious individuals, behavioral modification is much more significant than autonomic response. In cases of excessive cold, impulses pass from the hypothalamus to the cerebral cortex resulting in a sensation of cold and increased motor activity, moving to warmer surroundings, and increasing clothing or coverage **(Flowchart 1)**.

EFFECT OF ANESTHESIA ON THERMOREGULATION

Both general and regional anesthesia obtunds normal temperature control mechanisms. General anesthesia causes an impairment

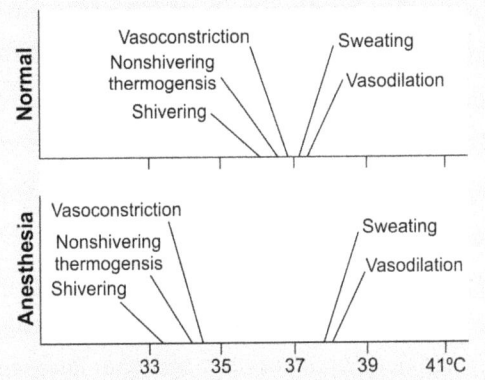

Fig. 1: Activation of thermoregulatory effector responses is triggered at specific temperatures for a given individual (threshold temperature).
Note: Under general anesthesia, the threshold temperatures for activation of cold responses (including vasoconstriction and shivering) are "decreased", whereas those for activation of warm responses (including sweating and vasodilation) are "increased". Thus, the narrow range of temperature between the vasoconstriction and sweating thresholds (normally ~0.4°C) is widened during general anesthesia to ~4.0°C.

characterized by a decrease in threshold towards response to cold whereas an increase in threshold towards response to heat. All general anesthetic agents impair thermoregulation to a certain extent and thus close monitoring is required for any procedure under general anesthesia lasting for >30 minutes **(Fig. 1)**.

Neuraxial anesthesia both epidural and spinal anesthesia decreases the vasoconstriction and shivering thresholds to a significant extent but lesser than general anesthesia.

Sedation and regional blocks do not cause significant impairment of the thermoregulatory mechanism.

MEASUREMENT OF TEMPERATURE

Temperature is the degree of "hotness" of a substance and reflects its potential for heat

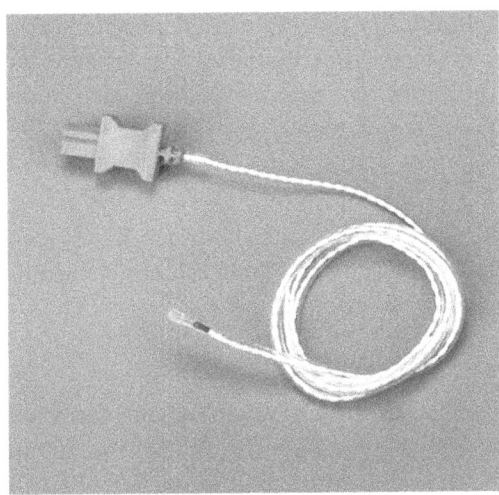

Fig. 2: Nasopharyngeal temperature probe.

transfer. The standard international (SI) unit of temperature measurement is Kelvin (K). It is based on the triple point of water, which is the temperature at a specific pressure at which water exists in all three phases of solid, liquid, and vapor (273.16 K or 0.01°C at a pressure of 0.006 atm). A change in temperature of 1 K is equivalent to a change in temperature of 1°C.

SITES FOR MONITORING

Core temperature monitoring sites can be:
- Pulmonary artery
- Distal esophagus
- Nasopharynx **(Fig. 2)**
- Tympanic membrane.

Possibly the best single estimate of core temperature is the pulmonary artery, although rarely available.

Near the core, temperatures can be obtained by oral and axillary both reliably used in patients recovering from anesthesia. Bladder and rectal temperatures are less reliable sources as both sites are poorly perfused and thus cannot give accurate readings.

Skin is also a site for near-core temperature monitoring. The heat from the skin is mostly dissipated by radiation and convection. Skin surfaces are lower than the core temperature. The core to forehead temperature also varies amongst individuals.

TYPES OF THERMOMETERS

Temperature measurement can be divided into nonelectrical, electrical, and infrared-based methods.

Nonelectrical Methods

- *Liquid expansion thermometer (mercury and alcohol-based):* These are based on the volumetric expansion of a liquid with increasing temperature; cheap and easy to use. However, they are slow and the glass thermometers can break and mercury is now classified as a hazardous substance.
- *Gas expansion thermometers:* They are based on the volumetric expansion of gas with temperature and the associated pressure changes that ensue due to this volume expansion. They can be used outdoors in harsh environments, are cheap, and robust but has poor accuracy and needs frequent calibration.
- *A bimetallic strip dial thermometer:* It has a coil consisting of two different metals with different expansion coefficients. As the temperature increases, these metals expand by different amounts causing the coil to tighten and move a pointer over the temperature scale. Used outdoors in harsh environments. Cheap, robust, and gives continuous measurements but has poor accuracy and requires recalibration.
- *A chemical thermometer:* It consists of a strip of small cells that melts over a range of temperatures to produce temperature-dependent color changes. Nowadays reusable liquid crystal form is available. These types have a fast response time, are disposable, and have no risk of glass breakage. However, are not very accurate at low-temperature differences.

Electrical Methods

- *A thermocouple:* It consists of two different metals such as copper and constantan (an alloy of copper and nickel) joined to form two separate junctions. One junction is kept at constant temperature and known as the *reference junction* while the other junction acts as the temperature-measuring probe **(Fig. 3)**. When there is a temperature difference across these two junctions, a small voltage is produced. This voltage is proportional to the temperature difference across the junctions and is measured using a galvanometer. This phenomenon is known as the Seebeck effect. They have a rapid response time, accurate to within 0.1°C. However, has a low voltage and needs frequent voltage amplification.
- *Resistance thermometer (platinum wire resistance thermometer):* A linear relationship between temperature and electrical resistance of a wire (such as

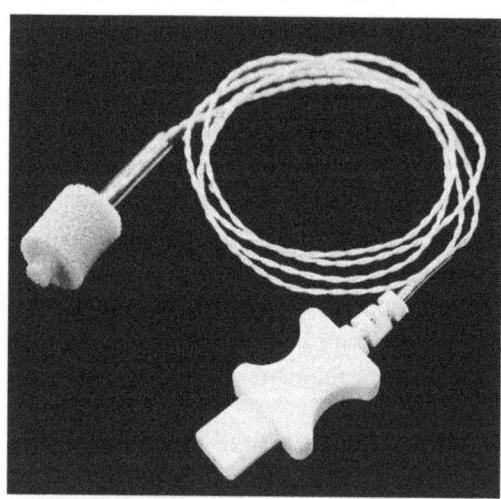

Fig. 3: Skin temperature probe.

platinum, copper, or nickel) such that as temperature increases, the resistance within a platinum wire increases in a predictable manner. These are extremely accurate but have a slow response time and are bulky.
- *Thermistor semiconductors:* They are composed of heavy metal oxide (nickel, iron, or manganese) and display a negative exponential relationship between electrical resistance and temperature. Used clinically in pulmonary artery catheters to measure core temperature. They have a rapid response time, accurate, small, and cheap. However can undergo hysteresis, aging, and variability within a batch.

Infrared
- *Infrared tympanic membrane thermometers* are based on the principle that all objects emit electromagnetic radiation which is dependent on the temperature of that object. Tympanic membrane thermometers receive infrared radiation from the tympanic membrane, which is close to the brain and therefore represents core body temperature **(Fig. 4)**.

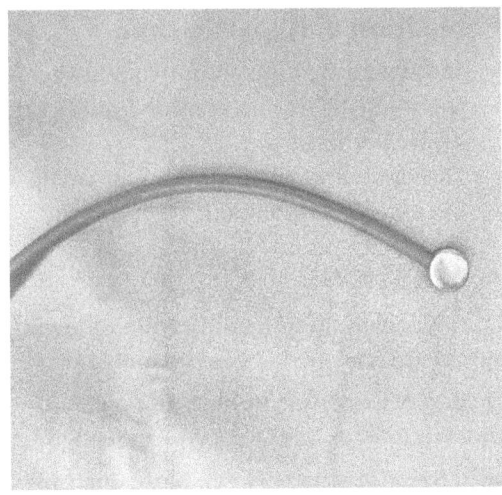

Fig. 4: Tympanic membrane temperature probe.

- Primarily based on two sensors the pyroelectric sensor and the thermopile sensor.
  1. The pyroelectric sensor contains crystals that alter their polarization depending on the temperature.
  2. The thermopile sensor is made up of numerous thermocouples connected in series and allows continuous measurements to be made. They are noninvasive with rapid response time.

■ CAUSES OF HYPOTHERMIA
Hypothermia during general anesthesia results mainly due to impaired thermoregulation and exposure to a cold environment **(Table 1)**.

Prevention of Hypothermia
- Preoperative warming.
- Airway heating and humidification-using low flow rates and semi-open circuits heat and humidity loss via evaporation is minimized.
- Warm intravenous fluids—the only method that provides directs core warming. Fluids can only be heated up to body temperature.
  - Heat loss also occurs between warmer and patient.
  - Also depends on the rate of fluid being transfused and the type of fluid.
  - Red blood cells (RBCs) are stored at 4°C and hence transfusion at a fast rate results in a drop in core temperature.
  - Fluid warmers are recommended in all intraoperative infusions ≥500 mL in adults.
- Cutaneous warming—heat is primarily lost through the skin via radiation, convection, and evaporation.
  - Increasing room temperature is an effective means of minimizing heat loss.

TABLE 1: Causes of hypothermia.

Causes of hypothermia	Mechanism
OT environment	• Exposure of body surface • Cold irrigation fluid • Skin preparation
Cold intravenous fluids	• 1 U RBC can decrease body temperature by 25–35°C • Cold crystalloids

Anesthesia	• Impaired thermoregulatory mechanisms
	• Muscle relaxants
	• Reduction in metabolic rate:
	  – Intravenous sedatives/hypnotics such as dexmedetomidine/clonidine, propofol, and some opioids increase the sweating threshold
	  – Regional anesthesia causes vasodilatation and impaired shivering below the level of block

Surgical technique	• Exposure of body cavity • Duration of surgery

- Passive insulation is the easiest method of cutaneous warming.
- Cotton blankets and surgical drapes all contribute. The layer of air still trapped beneath the layer provides the insulation.
- Appropriate airflow changes with at least four air changes with fresh air component, unidirectional and downward on the OT table.
- Postoperative warming—radiant heaters and forced air blankets are most commonly used.

CAUSES OF HYPERTHERMIA

Hyperthermia occurs when the core temperature exceeds normal values. Passive hyperthermia occurs due to excessive patient heating with inadequate core temperature monitoring. It is a common occurrence in infants and children as sweating is less effective under general anesthesia. Fever develops because the endogenous pyrogens interfere with the set point of the thermoregulatory system.

Causes range from a mismatched blood transfusion, to allergic reactions. Malignant hyperthermia can be caused by all inhalational anesthetics except nitrous oxide. Succinylcholine is also another cause. Characterized by rapidly increasing temperature >38.8°C and end-tidal carbon dioxide ($EtCO_2$) along with other criteria. Dantrolene is the antidote used.

Prevention of Hyperthermia

- Intraoperative temperature monitoring is the mainstay for preventing both hypo- and hyperthermia.
- Discontinuing active warming and removing excessive insulation.

QUESTIONS

Q. 1. Mechanism of hypothermia following spinal anesthesia and general anesthesia.

Q. 2. Prewarming before general anesthesia: Good or bad?

Q. 3. Relationship between perfusion index and central temperature.

Q. 4. What is noninversive body temperature (SpO$_2$ ON).

Q. 5. Bair Hugger: Potential side effects.

FURTHER READING

1. Barkha B, Bindra A, Rath G. Temperature management under general anesthesia: compulsion or option. J Anaesthesiol Clin Pharmacol. 2017;33(3):306-16.
2. Buggy DJ, Crossley AWA. Thermoregulation, mild perioperative hypothermia and postanaesthetic shivering. Br J Anaesth. 2000;84:615-28.
3. Sessler DI, Nolt RJ. Perioperative temperature monitoring: reply. Anesthesiology. 2021;135(1):190.

CHAPTER 43

Acid–Base Status Evaluation

Ajit Kumar, Saurabh Chandrakar

INTRODUCTION

Extreme changes in acid–base (pH <7.0 or >7.7) can be life-threatening. Such severe abnormalities can cause organ dysfunction—seizures, cerebral edema, decreased myocardial contractility, pulmonary vasoconstriction, and systemic vasodilatation. *Acidemia* is associated with an increased adrenergic tone and can be *arrhythmogenic*. The clinically acceptable range (beyond which therapy is mandatory) is not the same as "normal physiological" values **(Tables 1 and 2)**.

In evaluating the acid–base disorder, the first step is the *clinical assessment* **(Flowchart 1)**, which includes a detailed history, clinical examination, medication, and surgery details, and status of chronic disorders. The second step is to *collect data* and *correlate* it clinically. An arterial blood gas (ABG) documents, specifies the problem (oxygenation failure, ventilatory failure, or a metabolic problem), and quantitates the severity of the *derangement*. Simultaneously, if possible, collect laboratory parameters such as albumin, phosphorus, urea, and creatinine. We should interpret data accordingly whenever a peripheral venous blood gas (PVBG) or central venous blood gas analysis is used for assessment. We can use the Henderson-Hasselbalch equation for internal consistency to ensure that the variables (pH, PaCO$_2$, and HCO$_3^-$) are consistent.

$$pH = 6.1 + \log_{10}\left(\frac{[HCO_3^-]}{0.0307 \times PCO_2}\right),$$

The third step is to rule out any *existing chronic acid–base disorders*. Any baseline blood gas or laboratory data work as a guiding tool for patients with chronic respiratory acidosis **(Table 3)**. The fourth step is to determine if the primary issue is *acidemia* or *alkalemia*. While the standard value for the arterial pH may be between 7.35 and 7.45, multiple acid–base disturbances may still be present in a patient with a pH in this range. Therefore, it is essential to evaluate the pH, PaCO$_2$, and serum HCO$_3$ for every patient. The fifth step is to determine the primary disorder present, then examine for appropriate compensation and identify any secondary acid–base disorders present **(Table 4)**.

TABLE 1: Physiological and clinically acceptable acid–base parameters.

Parameter	2 SD normal	Clinically acceptable
pH	7.35–7.45	7.30–7.50
PCO$_2$	35–45 mm Hg	30–50 mm Hg
PaO$_2$ (on 21% oxygen)	97 mm Hg	>70 mm Hg
PO$_2$ (on ventilator)		60–90 mm Hg
HCO$_3$ (mEq/L)		24–28

(SD: standard deviation)

Chapter 43: Acid–Base Status Evaluation

TABLE 2: Definition of terms.

pH	The negative logarithm of the H⁺ ion activity
Acid	An H⁺ ion donor
Base	An H⁺ ion acceptor
Acidosis	An abnormal process that tends to lower the arterial pH
Alkalosis	An abnormal process that tends to increase the arterial pH
Acidemia	Blood pH lower than the acceptable range
Alkalemia	Blood pH higher than the acceptable range
Actual base excess (ABE)	Amount of strong acid/base required to be added to a liter of blood/ECF in vitro at 37°C to return the pH to normal (7.40) with the carbon dioxide held at a normal level (40 mm Hg) and with the hemoglobin fully saturated and temperature at 37°C
Standard base excess (SBE)	Base excess when the hemoglobin value is taken as 5 g%—a value it would have if the Hb were diluted in the entire ECF. The SBE gives a more accurate picture of what is happening in vivo
Standard HCO_3	It would represent the bicarbonate value if the $PaCO_2$ were 40 mm Hg with a hemoglobin oxygen saturation of 100% at a temperature of 37°C. The logic being that if the respiratory component were to be eliminated by making the $PaCO_2$ = 40 mm Hg, the resulting bicarbonate value would represent the metabolic component

Flowchart 1: Algorithm for acid–base evaluation.

Clinical evaluation
(History, physical examination, medication, chronic illness, surgery)
↓
Collect data and correlate clinically
(ABG/ peripheral vs. central VBG/laboratory parameters/confounders/internal consistancy)
↓
Identify patient's baseline acid–base status
(Rule out chronic respiratory acidosis)
↓
Identify acidemia or alkalemia
(Serum pH)

(ABG: arterial blood gas; VBG: venous blood gas)

TABLE 3: Primary (simple) acid–base disorder.

Respiratory acidosis	Elevated $PaCO_2$ as the initial change
Respiratory alkalosis	Reduced $PaCO_2$ as the initial change
Metabolic acidosis	Reduced HCO_3 as the initial change
Metabolic alkalosis	Elevated HCO_3 as the initial change

POTENTIAL PRACTICAL PROBLEMS WITH BLOOD GAS

- In a hypotensive patient, forceful aspiration of blood from the artery may create a negative pressure adequate to pull the dissolved oxygen in the sample into a gas bubble in the syringe. If this bubble is then expelled, the measured PaO_2 will be falsely low.
- If the sample is kept at room temperature for >20 minutes, the $PaCO_2$ will rise (with a resultant fall in pH) due to the metabolism of cells in the blood. The same can happen faster with high white cell or platelet counts.

TABLE 4: Different approaches to acid–base disorder.

	Classical approach		*Strong ion approach*
The Boston (American) approach using "expected limits of compensation"	The Copenhagen (European) approach using base excess: separating the respiratory and nonrespiratory components of HCO_3 utilizing the concept of base excess		Stewart approach

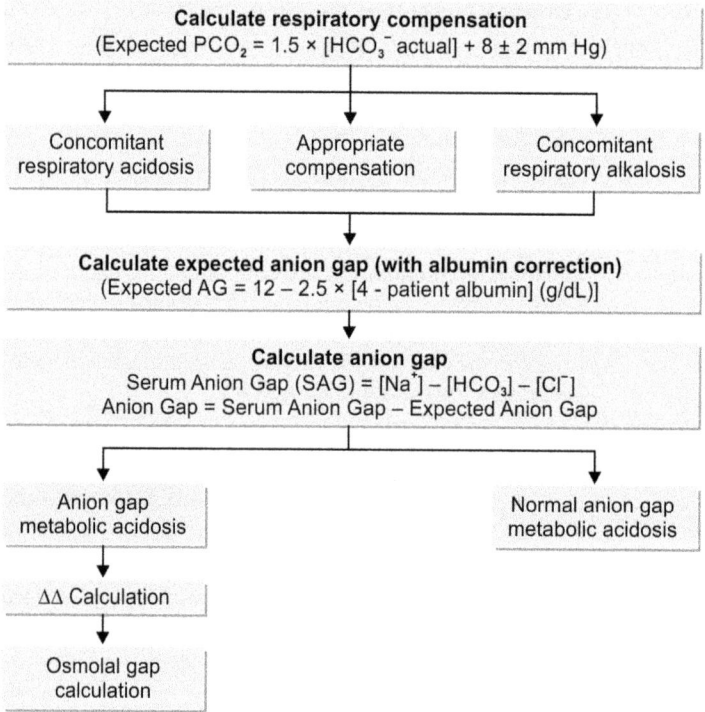

Flowchart 2: Algorithm for metabolic acidosis evaluation.

- A plastic (not glass) syringe allows a high $PaO_2/PaCO_2$ to diffuse out, and the measured levels will then be below.
- The effect of an air bubble will depend on the actual value of the PaO_2 and $PaCO_2$ in blood. The partial pressure of oxygen in the air is about 150 mm Hg, and carbon dioxide is almost zero. The values in the sample will tend to equilibrate to these values in the presence of an air bubble in the syringe—an actual PaO_2 of less than 150 mm Hg will tend to rise, but an actual PaO_2 value >150 mm Hg will tend to fall. The $PaCO_2$ will tend to fall.

CLASSICAL APPROACH

Respiratory abnormalities are due to an increase or decrease in carbon dioxide. Still, the nonrespiratory (also called *metabolic*) abnormalities can be due to multiple causes—renal (retention of hydrogen ions, loss of bicarbonate), tissue (hydrogen ion production), or gut-related (loss of hydrogen ion or bicarbonate) problems.

- *Metabolic Acidosis (Flowchart 2)*
  The first step in evaluating metabolic acidosis is to assess for an adequate compensation (starts in minutes and

completes in 24 hours) by Winter's formula.

Expected $PCO_2 = 1.5 \times [HCO_3^- \text{ actual}] + 8 \pm 2$ mm Hg

Respiratory compensation will be appropriate if it falls in the expected range. If expected PCO_2 falls below range, *concomitant respiratory alkalosis* is present, and if higher, it will be termed as *concomitant respiratory acidosis*. The next step is to calculate the anion gap to look for anion gap acidosis.

- *Anion Gap*

  The anion "gap" is a misnomer and should be more accurately termed the "unmeasured anions." It exists because not all electrolytes are measured and is calculated as:

  $$AG = (Na + K) - (Cl + HCO_3)$$

  It has a value of 16 + 4 mEq/L. The anion gap is the difference between the unmeasured cations and unmeasured anions. The total unmeasured cations is 6.5 mEq/L and the total unmeasured anions is 23 mEq/L thus giving the anion gap as 16.5 mEq/L (Range = 10–18 mEq/L). In reality, there is no gap as the body is electroneutral and the equation is:

  $$Na^+ + K^+ + Ca^{2+} + Mg^+ + Protein^+ = Cl^- + HCO_3^- + Protein^- + HPO_4^{2-}/HPO_4^- + SO_4^{2-} + OA^-$$

- An increase in the anion gap (>18 mEq/L) can occur with:
  - Increase in unmeasured anions—ketoacidosis (alcohol, starvation, diabetes), lactic acidosis, renal failure, some poisons.
  - Decrease in cations and not in the equation (these will cause a compensatory increase in the cations which are in the equation)—hypocalcemia, hypomagnesemia.
- A decreased or even negative anion gap (<10 mEq/L) can occur with:
  - Decrease in unmeasured anions—hypoalbuminemia.
  - Spurious hyperchloremia—false increase in measured chloride due to an increased serum bromide (from consumption of cough medication) can occur because the bromide interferes with the automated analyzers measuring chloride and gives a false hyperchloremia.
  - Increase in unmeasured cations and not in the equation (these will cause a compensatory decrease in the cations which are in the equation)—hypercalcemia, hypermagnesemia, lithium, increased [immunoglobulin (IgG)] (a cationic protein).
- It is important to note that a high anion gap acidosis can be masked by a process tending to lower the anion gap. These are:
  - Low serum albumin—for every 1 g% reduction in serum albumin below 4 g%, the anion gap drops by 2.5–3.0 mEq/L

    Expected AG = 12 − 2.5 × [4 − patient albumin] (g/dL)
  - Increase in unmeasured cations
  - Normal renal function—a normal kidney can excrete the excess organic anions and replace them with chloride, thus reducing the anion gap.
- IgA is anionic, but IgA myelomas usually have a variable (standard or high) anion gap.
  - *Gap-Gap or Delta-Delta Ratio ($\Delta\Delta$)*
    In patients having anion gap acidosis, the next step is to evaluate for the presence of *concomitant nonanion gap acidosis* or *metabolic alkalosis*.

This is evaluated by *gap-gap or delta-delta ratio* (ΔΔ):

ΔΔ = (Measured AG − Normal anion Gap)/(24 − Measured HCO$_3^-$)

The interpretation of ΔΔ the ratio is as per **Table 5**.

- *Osmolal Gap*
  In patients with metabolic acidosis, the osmolar gap can rule out the presence of ingested toxins/alcohols. Initially, serum osmolality will be calculated as:

  Calculated serum osmolality (mOsm/kg)
  = 2 × [Na$^+$] + [glucose]/18 + [BUN]/2.8
  + [ethanol]/3.8 + [methanol]/3.2
  + [isopropyl alcohol]/6.0 + [ethylene glycol]/6.2 + [acetone]/5.8
  + [β-hydroxyl butyrate] + [lactate],

  where units are serum osmolality: (mOsm/kg), sodium in mmol/L, glucose in mg/dL, BUN in mg/dL, alcohol in mg/dL, β-hydroxybutyrate, and lactate in mmol/L.

  Osmolal gap will be calculated as:

  Osmolal gap = (measured − calculated) serum osmolality

  Normal range of osmolal gap: −10 to +10 mOsm/kg. Positive serum osmolal gap will be considered if the difference is more than + 10 mOsm/kg.

  Interpretation of osmolal gap is as per **Table 6**.

- *Nonanion Gap Metabolic Acidosis*
  Gastrointestinal losses of bicarbonate, acid ingestion or infusion and renal tubular acidosis (RTA) are common etiologies for nonanion gap acidosis. History, clinical correlation, and urine studies (urine pH, urine anion or osmolal gap, presence of kidney stones) and serum potassium can help differentiate the cause of underlying nonanion gap acidosis.
  - *NAGMA with low serum potassium:*
    - Gastrointestinal loss—diarrhea, pancreaticoduodenal fistula, urinary, intestinal diversion
    - Renal—type 1 RTA (distal), type 2 RTA (proximal)
    - Medications/exposures—carbonic anhydrase inhibitors, toluene
  - *NAGMA with high or normal serum potassium:*
    - *Gastrointestinal loss:* Elevated ileostomy output
    - *Renal:* Type 4 RTA or CKD
    - *Medications:* NSAIDs; antibiotics (trimethoprim, pentamidine); heparin; ACE Inhibitors, ARBs, aldosterone antagonists (spironolactone); acid administration (TPN)
  - *Respiratory acidosis* (**Flowchart 3**).

TABLE 5: Delta-delta ratio and acid–base status.

ΔΔ Ratio	Acid–base status
<0.4	Nonanion gap metabolic acidosis
0.4–0.9	Both anion gap and nonanion gap metabolic acidosis
1.0–2.0	Anion gap acidosis
>2.0	Anion gap acidosis and metabolic alkalosis

TABLE 6: Clinical scenarios with elevated serum osmolal gap and metabolic acidosis.

Increased osmolal gap and anion gap	Increased osmolal gap and normal anion gap
• Alcoholic ketoacidosis • Diabetic ketoacidosis • Salicylate poisoning • Chronic kidney diseases • Organic alcohols (methanol, ethylene glycol, propylene glycol, diethylene glycol)	• Mannitol, glycerol • Acetone • Isopropyl alcohol • Hyper-triglyceridemia • Hyperproteinemia

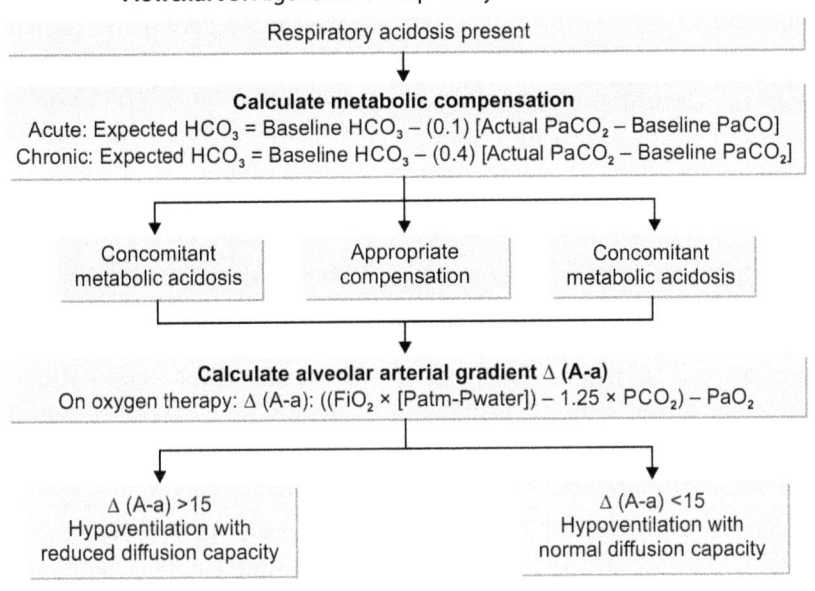

Flowchart 3: Algorithm for respiratory acidosis evaluation.

Once respiratory acidosis is diagnosed, the first step is to assess history, clinical condition, baseline carbon dioxide, and bicarbonate status to check for acute versus chronic acidosis nature and whether the compensation is appropriate or not. If baseline status is not available, then bicarbonate of 24 mEq/L and carbon dioxide of 40 mm Hg will be used. The following equations will be used depending on the underlying nature of the disease.

For acute respiratory acidosis:

Expected HCO_3 = Baseline HCO_3 + (0.1) [Actual $PaCO_2$ - Baseline $PaCO_2$]

For chronic respiratory acidosis:

Expected HCO_3 = Baseline HCO_3 + (0.4) [Actual $PaCO_2$ - Baseline $PaCO_2$]

If the actual bicarbonate value is higher than expected, concomitant metabolic alkalosis is present, however, if bicarbonate value is lower than anticipated, concomitant metabolic acidosis is present. If the bicarbonate value is in the expected range, compensation is appropriate.

After assessing for compensation, calculate the *alveolar-arterial gradient* (A-a) using *gas equation*. However, the A-a gradient is affected by many variables like age, left to right shunt, dead space ventilation, and hypoventilation, so it should be interpreted carefully.

Potential causes of respiratory acidosis are:

- Neuromuscular and central nervous system—head trauma, vascular (ischemic/hemorrhagic stroke), drugs (opioids, other sedatives), neuromuscular (myasthenia gravis, Guillain-Barré syndrome or variants), myxedema, multiple sclerosis.
- Pulmonary—central sleep apnea, airway obstruction, aspiration, laryngospasm/bronchospasm, chronic obstructive pulmonary disease (COPD), status asthmaticus, interstitial lung disease, pulmonary embolism/fat embolism, esophageal intubation, hypoventilation/air trapping on mechanical ventilation,

pneumonia, acute respiratory distress syndrome (ARDS).
- *Respiratory Alkalosis (Flowchart 4)*

Similar to the algorithm of respiratory acidosis, the first step is to determine history, clinical condition, baseline carbon dioxide, and bicarbonate status to check for acute versus chronic respiratory alkalosis nature and compensation is appropriate or not. If baseline status is not available, then bicarbonate of 24 mEq/L and carbon dioxide of 40 mm Hg will be used. The following equations will be used depending on the underlying nature of the disease:

For acute respiratory alkalosis:

Expected HCO_3 = Baseline HCO_3^- (0.2) [Actual $PaCO_2$ − Baseline $PaCO_2$]

For chronic respiratory alkalosis:

Expected HCO_3 = Baseline HCO_3^- (0.4) [Actual $PaCO_2$ − Baseline $PaCO_2$]

After evaluating respiratory alkalosis, the next step is to calculate the A-a gradient, to understand underlying clinical pathology.

Causes of respiratory alkalosis are:
- *Neural:* Anxiety, pain, psychosis, fever, trauma, stroke, sepsis, hypoxemia, central nervous system (CNS) stimulation due to cerebral edema, drugs (catecholamines, doxapram).
- *Pulmonary:* Pneumonia, asthma, pulmonary emboli, interstitial lung disease, pulmonary edema, high altitude.
- *Miscellaneous:* Pregnancy, cirrhosis, heatstroke, secondary to metabolic alkalosis, Mechanical ventilation, drugs (nicotine, progesterone, xanthines, salicylates).
- *Metabolic Alkalosis (Flowchart 5)*

The first step in the evaluation of metabolic alkalosis is to look for appropriate respiratory compensation. The following equation will be used:

(Expected PCO_2 = Baseline PCO_2 − 0.7 × [HCO_3^- actual − HCO_3^- baseline]

Once the evaluation of adequate compensation is done, the next step is to re-examine the patient (to look for cystic fibrosis, exogenous

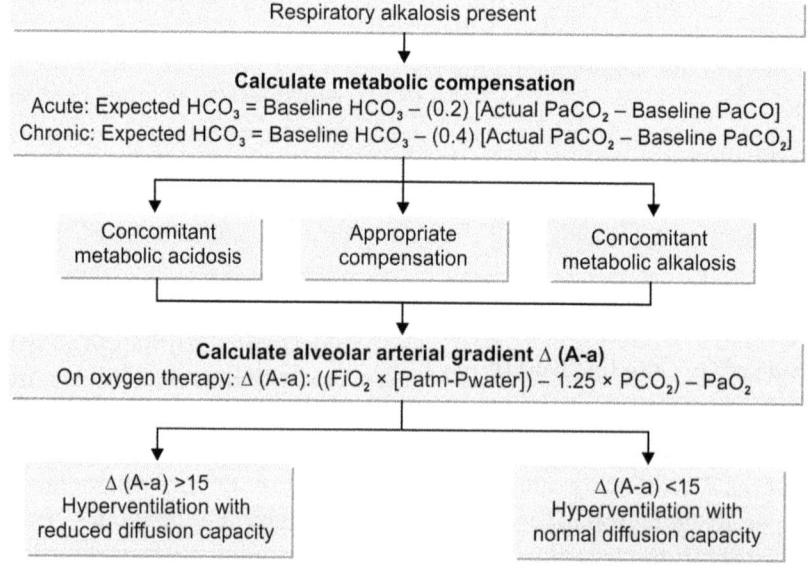

Flowchart 4: Algorithm for respiratory alkalosis evaluation.

Flowchart 5: Algorithm for metabolic alkalosis evaluation.

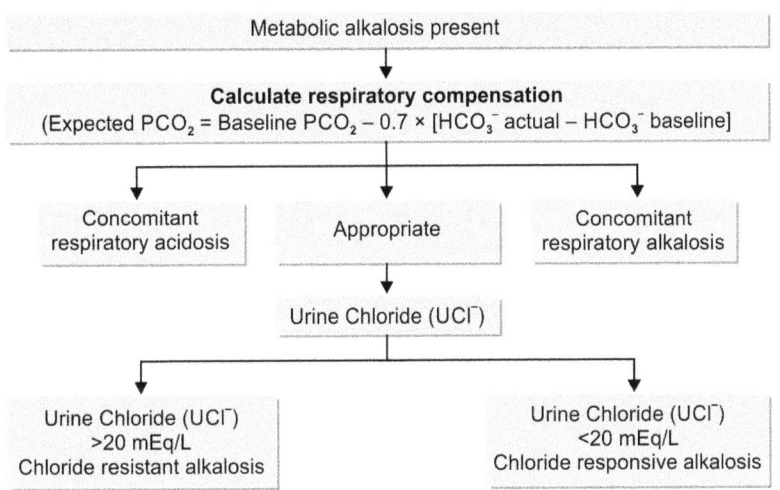

alkali administration, hypercalcemia, use of β-lactam antibiotics presence of hypertension or features suggestive of hyperaldosteronism) followed by urinary chloride level. Urine potassium, plasma renin, and aldosterone levels may be required **(Table 7)**.

Sustained metabolic alkalosis occurs if there are two conditions:
1. A mechanism to increase extracellular fluid (ECF) bicarbonate
    a. Net gain of HCO_3
        i. Loss of gastric HCl - vomiting
        ii. Administration of absorbable alkali
        iii. Increased renal production of HCO_3.
            - Hyper mineralocorticoidism
            - Increased Na delivery to the distal nephron.
    b. Contraction of ECF volume by concentrating the bicarbonate in a smaller ECF volume.

This is known as "contraction alkalosis" and occurs when a rapid decrease in ECF volume. The bicarbonate concentration rises (if the ECF loss does not include a bicarbonate loss as well). Although the $PaCO_2$ also grows, the increased carbon dioxide will be removed by ventilation. As a result, the bicarbonate/carbonic acid ratio changes, and a contraction alkalosis results.

2. An increase in the renal threshold for HCO_3 loss (increased reabsorption), thus preventing extra HCO_3 excretion (as the kidney has an enormous capacity to excrete HCO_3):
    a. Reduced ECF volume.
    b. K^+ depletion.

Metabolic alkalosis can thus occur in those with low ECF volume and those with average or increased ECF volume. The urinary chloride can be used to differentiate between these two scenarios. A low urinary chloride is seen in those with a depleted ECF, while a normal or increased chloride is seen in those with normal or high ECF. The urinary sodium is less reliable in this situation because the renal threshold for bicarbonate may be exceeded, and sodium can spill into the urine as the accompanying cation along with the bicarbonate.

- *Mixed disorder*

    Examples of mixed disorders:
    - Metabolic acidosis + metabolic alkalosis

TABLE 7: Causes of metabolic alkalosis.	
Urine Chloride <20 mEq/L (chloride responsive causes)	Urine Chloride >20 mEq/L (chloride-resistant causes)

• Loss of gastric acid (hyperemesis, high nasogastric output)
• Recent diuretic use
• Post-hypercapnia
• Villous adenoma
• Congenital chloridorrhea
• Chronic laxative abuse
• Cystic fibrosis
	• Urine potassium <30 mEq/L:
	  – Hypokalemia or Hypomagnesemia
	  – Laxative abuse
	• Urine potassium variable:
	  – Diuretics
	  – Bartter Syndrome
	  – Gitelman Syndrome
	• Hypertension, urine potassium usually >30 mEq/L, elevated plasma renin:
	  – Renal artery stenosis
	  – Renin secreting tumor
	  – Renovascular disease
	• Hypertension, urine potassium usually >30 mEq/L, low plasma renin, low plasma aldosterone:
	  – Cushing syndrome/exogenous minerlocorticosteroid
	  – 11-hydroxylase or 17-hydroxylase or 11 β-hydroxysteroid dehydrogenase deficiency
	  – Liddle syndrome
	  – Licorice toxicity
	• Low plasma renin, high plosmo aldosterone:
	  – Primary hyperaldosteronism
	  – Adrenal adenoma
	  – 3. Bilateral adrenal hyperplasia

- Renal failure and vomiting
- Vomiting and hypotension (lactic acidosis)
- Metabolic acidosis + respiratory acidosis
  - Cardiac arrest
  - Severe pulmonary edema
  - Drug ingestion with CNS depression
- Metabolic acidosis + respiratory alkalosis
  - Septic shock
  - Salicylate overdose
- Metabolic alkalosis + respiratory acidosis
  - Chronic diuretic (furosemide) use in chronic lung disease
- Metabolic alkalosis + respiratory alkalosis
  - This is a rare combination and can occur in patients on ventilators who are hyperventilated (e.g., for cerebral edema) and given diuretics or nasogastric suction.
- Mixed acute and chronic respiratory acidosis
  - Patients with chronic respiratory failure with acute decompensation.

- *Base Excess*

Base Excess (BE) is defined as the amount of strong acid/base required to be added to a liter of blood/ECF in vitro at 37°C to return the pH to normal (7.40) with the carbon dioxide held at standard level (40 mm Hg) and with the hemoglobin fully saturated and temperature at 37°C. The normal reference value for standard base excess is 0 mmol/L, and the normal range is −3-3 mmol/L, with increasingly negative values indicating metabolic acidosis and positive values indicating metabolic alkalosis.

The significance of base excess/deficit is that it performs the following:
- Evaluates the entire buffering system, not just bicarbonate
- The total ECF base deficit/excess is estimated
- The metabolic component of a mixed acid–base disorder is quantified.

Base excess can be calculated by Van Slyke equation:

$$BE = [[HCO_3] - 24.4 + (2.3 \times [Hb] + 7.7) \times (pH - 7.4)] \times (1 - 0.023 \times [Hb]).$$

When applied in vivo, there was an inaccuracy in extrapolating it to clinical scenarios because the calculation involved the hemoglobin value in whole blood. In reality, the entire ECF volume buffers pH, not just intravascular fluid (blood). The equation was modified to hemoglobin of 5 g%, to give Standard Base Excess (SBE). Actual Base Excess (ABE) is the BE in blood with a standard hemoglobin value. SBE gives a more accurate picture of what is happening in vivo.

However, it cannot determine which the primary is and which the secondary dysfunction is—that needs a clinical evaluation. It provides no means to differentiate between anion gap and nonanion gap causes of metabolic acidosis.

THE STEWART STRONG ION DIFFERENCE: AN ALTERNATE APPROACH

The Stewart approach (Dr Peter Stewart formulated the principles on which this approach is based) emphasizes the application of the "principle of electroneutrality" and "principle of conservation of mass."

The three independent variables which determine the H^+ concentration of the human body in the Stewart approach are:
1. The Strong Ion Difference (SID)
2. $PaCO_2$
3. Weak acids.

The Strong Ion Difference

In plasma, there is an excess of strong cations over strong anions. The difference is made up of weak anions. This difference (gap) between the sum of strong cations and strong anions is known as the strong ion difference (SID). In healthy humans, this value is between 40 mEq/L and 42 mEq/L.

As SID increases (either because strong cations increase or strong anions decrease), the weak cation (H^+) dissociates less to maintain electroneutrality, and hence pH rises (alkalosis). The reverse (acidosis) occurs when the SID falls (when strong cations decrease or strong anions increase). Therefore, decreases in the strong ion difference (such as those occurring in hyperchloremia, hyperlactatemia, and ketonemia) lead to increases in dissociation of water (to maintain electroneutrality) and a fall in the pH. The opposite happens if the strong ion difference increases.

The SID can be obtained in two ways; in health, both are nearly equal and are valid estimates of SID:

Apparent SID (SIDa) = difference of the "strongs" (indirect calculation)

Based on the principles of electroneutrality and conservation of mass, the strong ion difference represents the net balance between positive strong ions (cations) and negative strong ions (anions) according to the following formula (all concentrations in mEq/L):

(Na + K + Ca + Mg) − (Cl + lactate)

More accurately,

$$[SID]a = (Na + K + Mg + Ca) - (Cl + lactate + urate) \text{ - all in mEq/L}$$

This equation, however, does not take into account the weak acids present in the blood; therefore, this is called the apparent strong ion difference (SIDa).

Effective SID (SIDe) = adding the "weaks" (direct measurement and addition)
$$HCO_3^- + A^-$$

More accurately,

[SID]e = mEq/L due to PCO_2, protein and phosphate (all corrected for pH) = A + B + C

$A = 1000 \times 2.46 \times [10^{-11} \times (PCO_2 \text{ in mm Hg})] / (10^{-1} \times pH)$

$B = [\text{albumin in g\%}] \times [(0.123 \times pH) - 0.631]$

$C = PO_4 \text{ in mmol/L} \times ([0.309 \times pH] - 0.469)$

SIDe is the same as the buffer base in the classical approach to acid–base analysis.

Strong Ion Gap

In critically ill patients, both lactate and unmeasured ions are likely to increase. Unmeasured anions, measured by the strong ion gap (SIG), represent the "gap" between apparent and effective strong ion differences.

Strong Ion Gap (SIG) = [SID]a - [SID]e

The Strong Ion Gap is similar to the serum anion gap and incorporates measurements of anions and cations present at low concentrations.

Interpretation

The normal values for both [SID]a and [SID]e are about 40 mEq/L. The normal SIG = 0.

If the gap is >0, then there is an increase in unmeasured anions. SIG reflects the contribution of unidentified anions to SID.

The value is positive when unmeasured strong anions > unmeasured strong cations—the usual scenario is due to accumulation of lactate (sepsis), acetoacetate (diabetic ketoacidosis), or sulfate/phosphate (renal failure).

The value is negative in the reverse scenarios (theoretically possible but clinically unusual).

From a practical point of view, a positive SIG may be considered equivalent to the strong unmeasured anion, and in one review, the term "Strong Ion Gap" has been replaced by a new term - net unmeasured ions (NUI).

SIG/NUI = unmeasured anions minus unmeasured cations.

The equation is similar to the Classical Anion Gap but the difference is as follows:

Classical Anion Gap = $(Na + K) - (HCO_3 + Cl)$
Strong Ion Gap (NUI) = $(Na + K + Ca + Mg) - (A^- + HCO_3^- + Cl + lactate + urate)$

The difference is that the SIG has a smaller unmeasured list as compared to the classical AG. Hence the value of SIG is almost zero while the value of the classical anion gap is 8–12 mEq/L. It is essential to be aware that strong ion gap (SIG) is not the same as anion gap (AG).

Carbon Dioxide

The level of PCO_2 is affected by the production rate and alveolar ventilation. $PaCO_2$ influences the acid–base status via the hydration reaction. A rise in $PaCO_2$ results in compensation by the body by altering another independent determinant of pH—the SID.

Weak Acids: A_{tot} (Total Concentration of Weak Acids)

The total concentration of nonvolatile weak acids in any compartment is termed A_{tot}. The degree of dissociation is related to temperature and pH. Changes in the total value of this component usually do not occur acutely. The independent effect of A_{tot} (total concentration of weak acids) depends on absolute levels and dissociation equilibria.

- The total levels of these depend on their production, loss, and volume of distribution and are not determined by the acid–base status. A reduction in serum albumin or phosphate results in metabolic alkalosis, while an increase in serum phosphorous leads to metabolic acidosis.
- The amount of dissociation of these affects the acid–base status. Its concentration has a direct influence on the final concentration of H^+ for a given SID and $PaCO_2$. An increase in these anions will result in more dissociation of H^+ from water (causing acidosis) to maintain electroneutrality and a reduction will cause reduced H^+ ionization (resulting in alkalosis).

The A_{tot} does not vary with pH and is, therefore, an independent variable. An increase of A_{tot} causes metabolic acidosis, while reduction of A_{tot} causes metabolic alkalosis.

The normal A_{tot} is 17.2 mmol/L. In plasma, it consists of albumin, globulin, and phosphate in 73%, 22%, and 5%, respectively, while in erythrocytes (whole blood), it consists primarily of Hemoglobin. A reasonably accurate way to estimate A^- in plasma is to use the following formula:

$$A_{tot} = 0.25 \times \text{albumin (g/L)} + 0.09 \times \text{globulin (g/L)} + 2 \text{ (phosphate in mmol/L)}.$$

EFFECT OF CHANGES IN ALBUMIN

Albumin behaves as a weak acid, and thus hypoalbuminemia has an alkalinizing effect. A loss of weak acid secondary to hypoalbuminemia leads to a renal-mediated increase in chloride so that the SID decreases without any changes in H^+ and HCO_3^-. The renal response to chronic hypoproteinemia is to retain chloride, and the chloride concentration increases by 1.4 mmol/L for every 1 g% reduction in total protein. It has also been shown that hypoalbuminemia is also strongly associated with low serum sodium, and correction of the hypoalbuminemia with albumin infusion results in a significant increase in serum sodium without significant change in urine osmolality. Hence the change in serum sodium associated with hypoalbuminemia is due to a shift in the distribution of sodium between plasma and interstitial fluid resulting from the Gibbs-Donnan effect. Therefore, hyponatremia in a hypoalbuminemia person does not necessarily indicate fluid overload or water excess. Consequently, in a patient with hypoalbuminemia, if serum sodium rises, the strong anions, Cl and XA (XA stands for unidentified strong anions), will increase to preserve electroneutrality.

However, hypoalbuminemia does not necessarily lead to a clinically significant disorder of acid–base balance. Critically ill patients are often hypoalbuminemia but are not always alkalemia. Their SID is reduced. This can be considered a physiological response to a decreased level of nonvolatile weak acids.

UNDERSTANDING AN ACID–BASE DISORDER BASED ON THE STEWART APPROACH

In a dynamic multi-compartmental physiological system, a change in $[H^+]$ secondary to a change in one independent variable is compensated for by a complementary change in another. For example, an increased CO_2 increase $[H^+]$ (respiratory acidosis) is compensated by a decrease in Cl^- and a resultant increase in SID. Conversely, a decrease in SID due to a metabolic derangement (metabolic acidosis) is compensated by hyperventilation and decreased CO_2. In a nutshell, the $[H^+]$ and $[HCO_3^-]$ reflect the influence of SID and $PaCO_2$ for a given A_{tot}. However, the compensatory response to a change in A_{tot} (loss of weak acid) is unclear. Intuitively, hypoventilation (resulting in hypercarbia) would be expected in those with alkalosis due to hypoproteinemia. The empirical data on this is not consistent as both hypercarbia and hyperventilation have been reported in hypoproteinemia. In other studies, it has been observed that hypoproteinemia is compensated for by an increase in Cl^-, such that SID decreases. Some have stated that there is no unique compensatory mechanism for the alkalosis associated with hypoproteinemia.

A decrease in SID produces metabolic acidosis. The reduction in SID produces an electrochemical force which increases free H^+ concentration. A decrease in SID can occur due to the generation of organic anions (ketones, lactate), the addition of exogenous anions (excess chloride administration as normal saline, poisoning, or drugs), or the loss of cations (diarrhea, renal tubular acidosis). Excess administration of normal saline causes metabolic acidosis not by diluting HCO_3 but by decreasing the SID. Although normal saline contains an equal number of anions (chloride) and cations (sodium), the plasma does not. Thus, when large amounts of sodium chloride are added, the effect will be proportionately more on total body chloride than on total body sodium, causing a reduction in SID. Similarly, if hydrochloric acid is added to plasma, the chloride concentration increases with a resultant decrease in the SID. This results in more "acidity" and a drop in bicarbonate concentration.

Metabolic alkalosis occurs as a result of a large SID due to loss of anions over cations (vomiting, diuresis) or the administration of cations over anions (transfusion of a large volume of bank blood).

A summary of the classification of metabolic acidosis/alkalosis as per the Stewart approach is mentioned in the following:

- Metabolic Acidosis: Low Sid
  - Low SIG: Renal tubular acidosis, TPN, saline infusions, diarrhea, pancreatic loss, rapid response team (RRT) using solutions with low lactate and high chloride.
  - High SIG: Keto-, lactic-acidosis, salicylate, formic acid, methanol poisoning.
- Metabolic Alkalosis: High Sid
  - Low albumin states: Cirrhosis, nephrotic syndrome.
  - Chloride loss: Vomiting, loop diuretics, hyperaldosteronism, Bartter syndrome, Liddle Syndrome.
  - Na load with a weak base: Sodium acetate, citrate, lactate.

Using the Stewart Method at the Bedside

Stewart's method is based on physicochemical principles, diminishes the importance of bicarbonate, and acknowledges other factors controlling pH. However, one of the valid criticisms of the Stewart approach has been that its calculations are too complex for bedside use. The solution has been one of two approaches–to use a computer (calculator available online) or to use a simplified approach. One such is the base excess partitioning approach (Fencl–Stewart approach).

The base excess is partitioned into three components:
1. Component due to SID
2. Component due to albumin
3. Component due to unmeasured anions (UMA) may be strong anions such as

sulfate, acetate, lactate, or weak acids such as phosphate.

Base Excess = (SID component) + (Albumin component) + (UMA component)

Base Excess = [(Na − Cl) − 38] + [0.25 (40 − serum albumin)] + [minus UMA]

An increase in strong anions (chloride, UMA) has an acidifying effect = decreases base excess (increases base deficit). Decrease in albumin has an alkalinizing effect = increases base excess (decreases base deficit). The algebraic signs in the above equation are therefore vital. A decreasing chloride (relative to Na) or decreasing albumin (relative to normal) has alkalinizing effects.

CONCLUSION

Arterial blood gas is close to an ideal point of care test which document, specify, and quantitate the severity of an abnormality. Interpretation of ABG with clinical correlation can help the physician in the treatment of critically ill patients. All three schools (Copenhagen, Boston, and Stewart) can be reconciled and are merely descriptions of the same processes from three different vantage points and should be used appropriately.

QUESTION

Q. 1. Role of ABG for assessment of severity in COVID.

FURTHER READING

1. Berend K, J de Vries AP, Gans ROB. Physiological approach to assessment of acid-base disturbances. N Engl J Med. 2014;371(15):1434-45.
2. Feldman M, Soni N, Dickson B. Influence of hypoalbuminemia or hyperalbuminemia on the serum anion gap. J Lab Clin Med. 2005;146(6):317-20.
3. John G, Subramani K, Peter J V, Pichamuthu K, Chacko B. Essentials of Critical Care, 2nd edition. Vellore: Christian Medical College; 2011.
4. Kellum JA. Disorders of acid-base balance. Crit Care Med. 2007;35(11):2630-6.
5. Kimura S, Shabsigh M, Morimatsu H. Traditional approach versus Stewart approach for acid-base disorders: inconsistent evidence. SAGE Open Med. 2018;6:2050312118801255.
6. Krasowski MD, Wilcoxon RM, Miron J. A retrospective analysis of glycol and toxic alcohol ingestion: utility of anion and osmolal gaps. BMC Clin Pathol. 2012;12:1.
7. Kraut JA, Madias NE. Differential diagnosis of nongap metabolic acidosis: value of a systematic approach. Clin J Am Soc Nephrol. 2012;7(4):671-9.
8. Kraut JA, Xing SX. Approach to the evaluation of a patient with an increased serum osmolal gap and high-anion-gap metabolic acidosis. Am J Kidney Dis. 2011;58(3):480-4.
9. Laski ME, Sabatini S. Metabolic alkalosis, bedside and bench. Semin Nephrol. 2006;26(6):404-21.
10. McNamara J, Worthley LI. Acid-base balance: part II. Pathophysiology. Crit Care Resusc. 2001;3(3):188-201.
11. Morgan TJ, Clark C, Endre ZH. Accuracy of base excess-an in vitro evaluation of the Van Slyke equation. Crit Care Med. 2000;28(8):2932-6.
12. Rastegar A. Use of the DeltaAG/DeltaHCO$_3^-$ ratio in the diagnosis of mixed acid-base disorders. J Am Soc Nephrol. 2007;18(9):2429-31.
13. Sood P, Paul G, Puri S. Interpretation of arterial blood gas. Indian J Crit Care Med. 2010;14(2):57-64.
14. Stewart PA. Independent and dependent variables of acid-base control. Respir Physiol. 1978;33(1):9-26.

CHAPTER 44

Pulmonary Function Test

Ajit Kumar, Shivam Gupta, Revant Babu Chala

INTRODUCTION

Pulmonary function testing is an important investigation in managing patients with suspected or diagnosed pulmonary diseases. A wide range of important information regarding small airways, pulmonary parenchyma, and the size and integrity of the pulmonary capillary bed can be availed by it. They help in establishing diagnosis by identifying different patterns of abnormalities in various pulmonary diseases. Though there is not any single test available that can completely provide details about every aspect of lung function. Therefore, a combination of different tests is generally performed to come to a clinical conclusion regarding the disease. There are various tests available for determining pulmonary function, which can be divided into different categories, based on the aspect of pulmonary function they measure **(Table 1)**.

SPIROMETRY (FIG. 1)

The spirometry test is commonly used for the evaluation of airway function. It is easy to perform, comparatively economical, and has a standardized algorithm for interpretation. It measures lung function by measuring different volumes in the lung against time. All volumes (tidal volume, inspiratory reserve volume, expiratory reserve volume) and capacities (vital capacity, inspiratory capacity) can be measured except residual volume, functional residual capacity, and total lung capacity. Maximum air is inhaled and exhaled by the patient for as long and as quickly as possible during this procedure.

Indications

- To identify the disease in patients with signs and symptoms of cough, wheeze dyspnea, crepitations, and abnormal chest X-ray findings.
- In patients with known lung diseases (obstructive pulmonary disease, interstitial fibrosis, pulmonary vascular disease) to monitor the progression of disease and treatment response.
- To monitor for respiratory complications in systemic diseases such as connective tissue disorder and neuromuscular disorders.
- During pre-anesthetic check-up for patients undergoing cardiothoracic/Abdominal surgery or lung resection.
- In occupational settings to evaluate patients at risk of pulmonary diseases.
- Postlung transplant to assess for acute rejection, infection, and obliterative bronchiolitis.

Contraindications

- Recent abdominothoracic surgeries
- Pregnancy

TABLE 1: Tests and parameters for determining pulmonary function.

Pulmonary function	Test	Parameters measured
A. Airway function	• Spirometry • Forced vital capacity maneuver (FVC) • Maximal voluntary ventilation (MVV) • Maximal inspiratory/expiratory pressures (MIP/MEP) • Airway resistance (raw) and compliance (CL)	• VC, ERV, IC • FVC, FEV_1, FEF, PEF, MEFV curves
B. Lung volumes and ventilation	• Functional residual capacity (FRC) • Total lung capacity (TLC), residual volume (RV), RV/TLC ratio • Minute ventilation, alveolar ventilation, and dead space • Distribution of ventilation	• Open-circuit (N2 washout) Closed-circuit/rebreathing (He dilution) • Thoracic gas volume (VTG) • Multiple-breath N2 • He equilibration • Single-breath techniques
C. DLCO tests	• Single-breath (breath holding) • Steady-state	
D. Blood gases and gas exchange tests	• Blood gas analysis and blood oximetry • Pulse oximetry • Capnography	Shunt studies
E. Cardiopulmonary exercise tests		

(ERV: expiratory reserve volume; FEF: forced expiratory flow; FEV1: forced expiratory volume in 1 second; FVC: forced vital capacity; IC: inspiratory capacity; IC: inspiratory capacity; MEFV: maximum expiratory flow-volume curve; DLCO: diffusing capacity of the lungs for CO_2; VC: vital capacit)

- Severely breathless patients
- Myocardial infarction within the last month
- Unstable angina
- Recent eye surgery
- Pneumothorax
- Bronchopleural fistula
- Ruptured tympanic membrane
- Abdominothoracic aneurysms
- Critically ill.

General Considerations

Spirometry can be performed in a sitting or standing position, but a sitting position is preferred to prevent the risk of fall and injury in the event of sympathetic attacks. Patients are advised not to wear tight clothing, avoid heavy meals two hours before and avoid smoking 1 hour before the test.

A wide range of apparatus is available to perform spirometers ranging from handheld

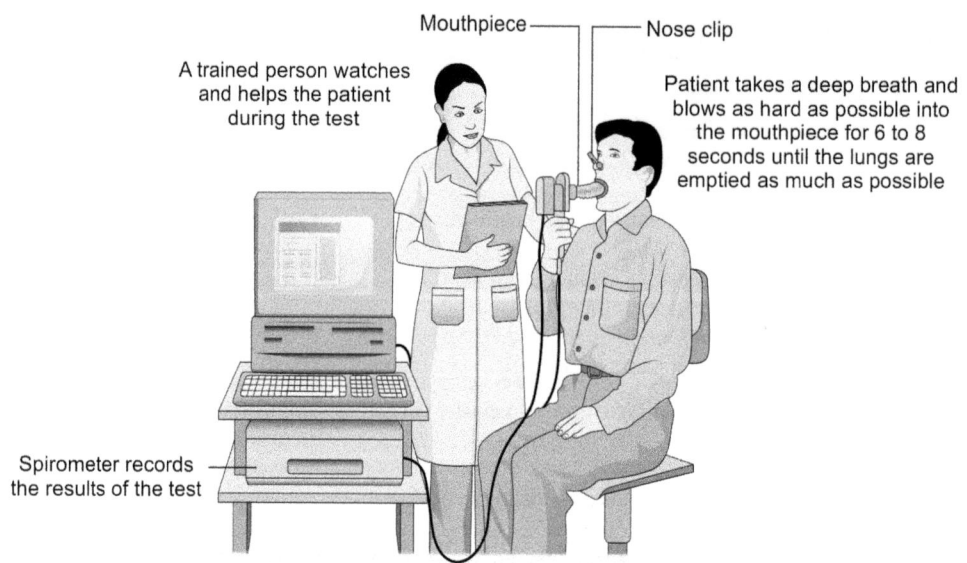

Fig. 1: Spirometry.

manual devices to completely automated large devices. American thoracic and European respiratory societies have laid some minimum technical specifications to obtain valid results. These mainly focus on precision, accuracy, and resolution. Spirometers can be of two broad categories, one with volume displacement principle and the other with flow sensing principle.

While performing the test, the patient should be constantly motivated to obtain the best possible effort by the patient. Initially, gentle breath is taken via the mouthpiece of the spirometer to give us the tidal volume. Then maximal inspiration at end-tidal exhalation followed by forced expiration which determines the forced vital capacity. Postbronchodilator assessment can also be performed to characterize the airflow limitation. Spirometry helps in the measurement of static and dynamic lung volumes.

STATIC LUNG VOLUMES AND CAPACITIES (FIG. 2)

Static lung volume indicates the volume measured when there is no movement of air

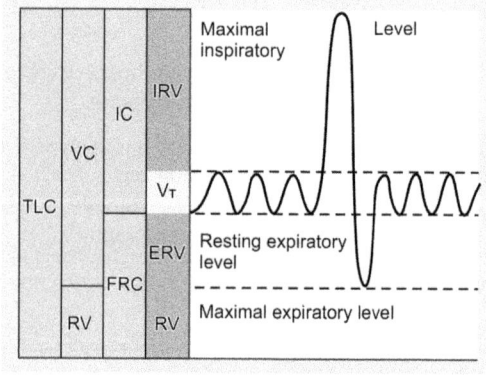

Fig. 2: Lung volumes and capacities.

in or out of the lung. These emphasize on elastic properties of the lung and the chest wall. Static lung volumes which include RV can be measured by alternate techniques such as gas dilution, nitrogen washout, and body plethysmography.

- Lung volume: These are measured directly with the help of a spirometer or by gas dilution technique.
  - Tidal volume (V_T): Normal = 500 mL
    The volume of air inspired or expired every breath while the subject is breathing normally.

- Inspiratory reserve volume (IRV): Normal = 2,500 mL
  The volume of air which can be inspired above tidal volume.
- Expiratory reserve volume (ERV): Normal = 1,500 mL
  Expiration of additional volume of air following tidal volume exhalation.
- Residual volume (RV): Volume of air that remains in the lungs after maximum expiration.
■ Lung capacities: It is derived by adding two or more lung volumes.
  - Functional residual capacity (FRC): Normal = 3,000 mL
    ◆ FRC = RV + ERV
  - Vital capacity (VC): Normal = 4,500 mL
    ◆ VC = ERV + VT + IRV
  - Inspiratory capacity (IC): Normal = 3000 mL
    ◆ IC = VT + IRV
  - Total lung capacity (TLC): Normal = 6,000 mL
    ◆ TLC = RV + ERV + V_T + IRV

DYNAMIC LUNG VOLUMES (FIG. 3)

As the name indicates, some of these volumes are measured while the individual is inhaling or exhaling. Patient inspires fully followed by forced expiration resulting in expiratory volume—*time curve*. This helps in understanding the caliber and integrity of the airways. It measures forced expiratory volume in 1 second (FEV_1), forced vital capacity maneuver (FVC), the ratio of FEV_1/FVC is calculated, peak expiratory flow rate (PEFR), expiratory flow-volume curves, and flow-volume loops (F-V loop).

- FEV_1: After a maximum inspiration volume of air which is forcefully expired in the 1 second.
- FVC: After a maximum inspiration total volume of air that is forcefully expired.

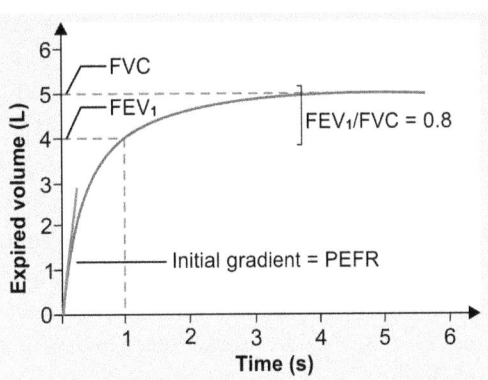

Fig. 3: Dynamic lung volumes.

- *PEFR:* Forced spirometry trace can help in knowing the PEFR. As we know that flow is nothing but volume per unit time. Therefore, the gradient of the spirometry curve represents flow. Hence the peak flow is nothing but the initial gradient of the volume time curve.
  This helps in understanding obstructive and restrictive diseases.

OBSTRUCTIVE LUNG DISEASES

If the forced spirometry is compared with the predicted values of obstructive lung disease such as asthma, chronic obstructive pulmonary disease (COPD) can be identified. Forced expiratory volume in 1 second (FEV_1) <80% of predicted and the ratio of FEV_1/FVC <0.7 is required to diagnose obstructive diseases.

- Mild obstructive lung disease → FEV_1 50–79% predicted
- Moderate obstructive lung disease → FEV_1 30–49% predicted
- Severe obstructive lung disease → FEV_1 <30% predicted.

Asthma and COPD are two common obstructive airway diseases. These can be differentiated based on history and if the airway obstruction is reversible or not. Improvement in FEV_1 of 400 mL postbronchodilator administration represents significant airway reversibility implying disease as asthma.

RESTRICTIVE LUNG DISEASE

Restrictive lung diseases can be diagnosed with forced spirometry if the FEV_1 <80% predicted, FVC <80% predicted, and the ratio of FEV_1/FVC >0.7 predicted. This ratio can be normal or even high in restrictive diseases. High FEV_1 is because of a decrease in the lung compliance.

EXPIRATORY FLOW-VOLUME CURVE

The expiratory flow-volume curve can be obtained by plotting flow against expired volume. *Flow* is plotted on the vertical axis and *volume* on the horizontal axis. Initially while expiring forcefully there is a rapid rise in flow which reaches maximum up to PEFR. This part of the curve is effort-dependent. Following this, there is an effort independent steady fall in flow rate till all air is expired reaching up to the residual volume.

OBSTRUCTIVE DISEASE

Obstruction in the small airway causes resistance to the airflow which reduces expiratory flow rate. Peak expiratory flow rate (PEFR) is reduced, which can be seen in the first part (effort-dependent part) of the curve. The second part (effort independent part) of the curve shows a change from linear to concave. This concavity is related to the severity of the disease. Residual volume is increased in obstructive airway diseases because of air trapping.

RESTRICTIVE DISEASE

There will be a significant reduction in TLC. PEFR can be decreased because of respiratory muscle weakness. The second part of the

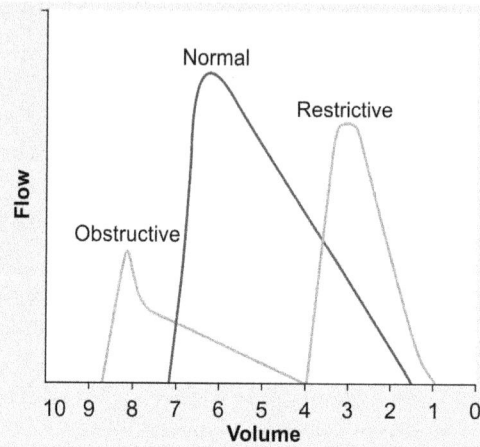

Fig. 4: Flow–volume curves on absolute lung volumes.

curve remains linear because there is no dynamic compression in pure restrictive lung disease.

FLOW-VOLUME LOOP (FIGS. 4 AND 5)

It consists of an inspiratory flow-volume curve along with an expiratory flow-volume curve making a loop. An inspiratory portion of the loop gives additional information about the disease. Flow volume loops help to identify the location of the airway obstruction. By convention expiratory flow is in an upward position and the inspiratory flow is downwards. With the patient at TLC, maximum exhalation begins till the volume in the lung reaches RV. Maximal deflection on the flow axis shows *peak expiratory* (PEF) and *peak inspiratory flow* (PIF). Abnormalities of the small and large airways can be identified by changes in the maximal flow rate.

OBSTRUCTIVE LUNG DISEASE (FIG. 5)

The inspiratory part of the curve is usually unaffected in small airway obstructive diseases. Effort independent part of the curve shows concavity or scooped out

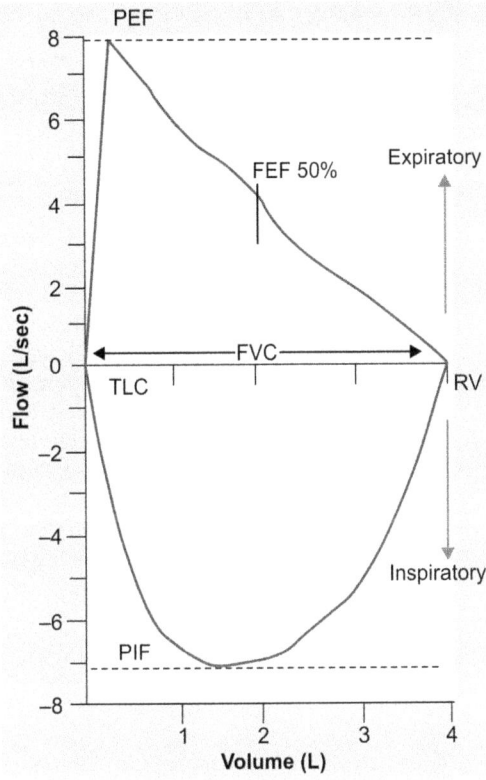

Fig. 5: Flow/volume loops.

pattern rather than linear appearance. This is because the expiratory part of this F-V loop is determined by the elastic recoil and small airway resistance, which is abnormal in obstructive diseases such as emphysema, bronchitis, or asthma. PEFR is reduced and an increase in residual volume is seen because of air trapping.

RESTRICTIVE LUNG DISEASE

Restrictive lung diseases may show linear decreases in flow versus volume with normal or greater than normal peak flows. There will be a normal appearance of the effort-independent portion of the curve and a significantly reduced vital capacity. Depending on the severity of the disease, the TLC is substantially lower whilst the residual volume is proportionally less reduced. Reduced flows are primarily caused by the decreased cross-sectional area of the small airways at low lung volumes. flow-volume loop here appears rightward-shifted with a substantially reduced FRC.

Variable Extrathoracic Airway Obstruction (Fig. 6)

"Variable" here refers to flow limitation in both expiration and inspiration and level above the sixth tracheal is the extrathoracic region and below it is the intrathoracic region. In variable extrathoracic obstruction expiratory flow is usually normal but the inspiratory flow is diminished. In the inspiratory phase of respiration, there will be a diminution of airway pressure (paw) in the trachea to a subatmospheric level that causes obstructing lesions to be pulled inwards, resulting in a reduced inspiratory flow. This leads to flattening of the inspiratory flow-volume curve. In the expiratory phase, the obstructing lesion is pushed outward because of a positive paw. Due to this, the expiratory flow is not affected. A common example for this is vocal cord dysfunction, in which there will be paradoxical closure of the vocal cords during inspiration resulting in a truncated inspiratory flow.

Variable Intrathoracic Airway Obstruction (Fig. 6)

During inspiration, intrathoracic pressure is negative which pulls the airways apart. Therefore, if there is an intrathoracic airway obstruction that gets opened up and inspiratory flow is unaffected. However, during forced expiration, positive intrathoracic pressure causes dynamic airway compression along

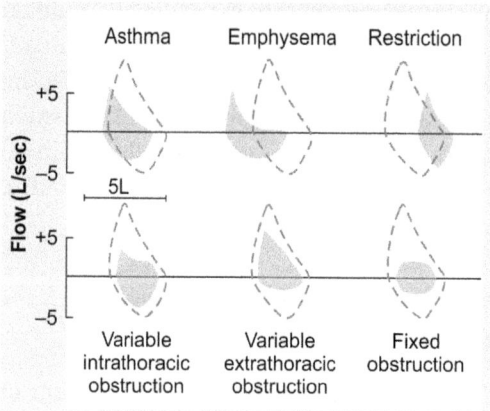

Fig. 6: Obstructions.

with obstructing lesion resulting in flattening of the expiratory flow-volume curve of the F-V loop.

Fixed Upper Airway Obstruction (Fig. 6)

In fixed airway obstruction, airway narrowing is unchanged during both inspiration and expiration. There will be a flattening of both the inspiratory and expiratory flow-volume curves, because of reduction in peak expiratory and inspiratory flows, while the lung volumes will remain unchanged. This kind of pattern is seen in cases of tracheal stenosis, foreign body, etc.

FURTHER READING

1. Altalag A, Road J, Wilcox P, Aboulhosn K. Pulmonary Function Tests in Clinical Practice, 2nd edition. UK: Springer, Cham; 2019.
2. Bhavna G, Lalit G. Pulmonary function tests-relevance to anesthesiologists. Anaesth Critic Care Med J. 2018;3(1):000131.
3. Chambers D, Huang C, Matthews G. Basic Physiology for Anaesthetists, 2nd edition. UK: Cambridge University Press; 2019.
4. Graham BL, Steenbruggen I, Miller MR, Barjaktarevic IZ, Cooper BG, Hall GL, et al. Standardization of spirometry 2019 update. An Official American Thoracic Society and European Respiratory Society Technical Statement. Am J Respir Crit Care Med. 2019; 200(8):e70-88.
5. Jindal SK. Textbook of Pulmonary and Critical Care Medicine, 2nd edition. New Delhi: Jaypee Brothers Medical Publishers (P) Ltd; 2017.
6. Johnson JD, Theurer WM. A stepwise approach to the interpretation of pulmonary function tests. Am Fam Physician. 2014;89(5): 359-66.
7. Mottram Carl D. Indications for Pulmonary Function Testing. Ruppel's Manual of Pulmonary Function Testing, 11th edition. Philadelphia: Mosby; 2016.
8. Ntima NO, Lumb AB. Physiology and conduct of pulmonary function tests. BJA Educ. 2019;19(6):198-204.
9. Ntima NO, Lumb AB. Pulmonary function tests in anaesthetic practice. BJA Educ. 2019; 19(7):206-11.

SECTION 3
Anesthesia Instruments

- **Medical Gas Cylinders**
  Ranjitha N, Puneet Khanna
- **Gas Pipeline**
  Abhishek Singh
- **Suction Apparatus**
  Ranjitha N, Puneet Khanna
- **Anesthesia Machine**
  Richa Saroa, Sanjeev Palta, Swati Jindal, Rajni Kalia
- **Vaporizers**
  Richa Saroa, Sanjeev Palta, Tenzin Nyima, Arun A Bevoor
- **Breathing Circuits**
  Richa Saroa, Sanjeev Palta, Deepika Gupta, Chaitra TS
- **Manual Resuscitators**
  Ajeet Kumar, Kunal Singh, Chandni Sinha
- **Humidification Equipment**
  Chandni Sinha, Abhinav Prakash, Pratik Singh
- **Circle System**
  Abhyuday Kumar, Chandni Sinha, Ajeet Kumar
- **Face Masks and Airways**
  Prachi Agrawal, Amit Kohli
- **Supraglottic Airway Devices**
  Deepak Kumar, Abhijit Kumar, Amit Kohli
- **Laryngoscopes**
  Anisha Singh, Abhijit Kumar
- **Endotracheal Tube**
  Rahil Singh, Nishant Sood
- **Lung Isolation Devices**
  Ayushi Mahajan, Amit Kohli
- **Devices for Difficult Airway Management**
  Ridhima Sharma, Ripon Choudhary
- **Gas Monitoring Equipment**
  Abhishek Singh
- **Spinal and Epidural Needles**
  Richa Saroa, Sanjeev Palta, Umang Sharma, Amitesh Chugh
- **Patient-controlled Analgesia Pumps**
  Richa Saroa, Sanjeev Palta, Puja Saxena, Parul Sood
- **Cleaning and Sterilization**
  Chandni Sinha, Abhinav Prakash, Ajeet Kumar

45

Medical Gas Cylinders

Ranjitha N, Puneet Khanna

Q. 1. How are cylinders constructed?
Ans. Earlier cylinders were generally made of low-carbon steel. But now they are made of aluminum, molybdenum steel, and chrome. These modern cylinders are stronger and have thinner walls, hence light in weight. Gas cylinders available in the magnetic resonance imaging (MRI) suite are made of aluminum. The wall thickness of aluminum cylinder and steel cylinder is 6 mm and 3 mm respectively.

Q. 2. What are the parts of the medical gas cylinder?
Ans. The cylinder consists of the body, shoulder, and neck. The base may be flat or concave. The upper part of the body is curved which is called as the *shoulder*. The neck is represented by the top end which ends into a tapered screw thread that is linked with a valve. The thread is generally sealed with a material which is called *Woods metal* - It is an alloy of bismuth, lead, tin and cadmium as it has the property of melting when the cylinder is exposed to intense heat. This safety feature allows the gas to escape from the cylinder, thereby, reducing the risk of explosion.

Q. 3. Mention the various safety features incorporated in medical gas cylinders?
Ans.
- Pin index safety system
- Color coding of gas cylinders—labeling of cylinder contents and symbol of the gas
- Woods metal for ceiling valve
- Pressure relief valve.

Q. 4. What is cylinder valve and its importance?
Ans. Medical gas cylinders are filled and discharged with the help of a valve shown in **Figure 1** which is fitted to the neck. They are made of brass or bronze. They are one of the most important parts of the cylinder which helps in connecting it to the yoke assembly on the anesthesia machine. The valve consists of a stem which helps in opening or closing of cylinder through rotational movement. There is a hand wheel for turning the valve system. The conical depression on the opposite present on the opposite side should not be

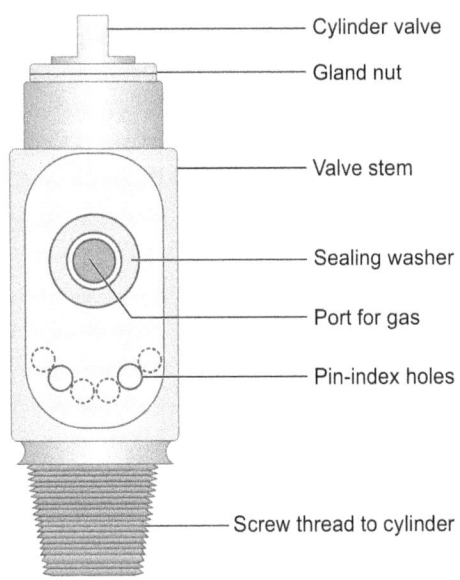

Fig. 1: Cylinder valve.

misunderstood as a port. Its function is to receive the retaining screw present on the yoke assembly.

Q. 5. What are the different types of valves?
Ans. There are two types of valves which are named—(1) packed valve and (2) diaphragm valve. The most commonly used is packed valve. The stem in the packed valve is sealed with a resilient packing like Teflon which helps in preventing the leaks around the thread. It is also called as a direct-acting valve since turning the stem causes the seat to turn. This valve can withstand high pressures. It needs 2–3 full turns to open the valve.

In the diaphragm valve, upper and lower stem is separated by the diaphragm. The lower stem participates in gas movement through the valve. These valves are less susceptible to leaks. They need only ½–¾ turns to open fully.

Q. 6. What are pressure relief devices and their importance?
Ans. Pressure relief device is part of a cylinder valve which helps to inventing the cylinder content to the atmosphere whenever the pressure in the cylinder rises above a dangerous level due to overfilling or high temperature. They are of different types such as frangible disk, fusible plug, or a combination of the two. These relief valves consist of springs that are designed in such a way that they will reclose and prevent the content of the cylinder from getting emptied when the set pressure inside the cylinder has been restored.

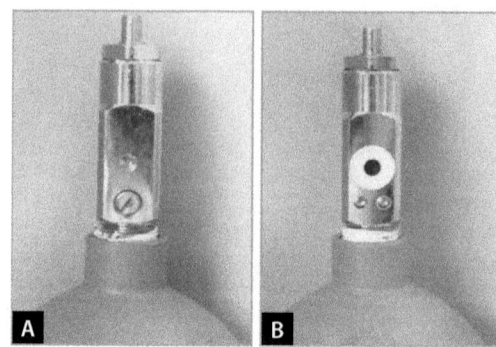

Figs. 2A and B: Pin index safety system.

Q. 7. Describe the pin index safety system and its importance.
Ans. Small cylinders (size E or less) have a safety feature of pin index **(Figs. 2A and B)**. These cylinders are used in the back of anesthesia machine which are connected through yoke assembly. This system has a unique configuration of holes and pins which match precisely to eliminate wrong connection of cylinders and thereby prevent delivery of wrong gas to patients. This system is also used by the supplier to fill correct gas in the cylinder.

FURTHER READING

1. Dorsch, JA, Dorsch SE. Understanding Anesthesia Equipment, 5th edition. Philadelphia: Lippincot Williams & Wilkins; 2012.
2. Srivastava U. Anaesthesia gas supply: gas cylinders. Indian J Anaesth. 2013;57(5):500-6.

CHAPTER 46

Gas Pipeline

Abhishek Singh

INTRODUCTION

Production of anesthetic gas, its storage, and delivery is a complex process. One should be aware of such a system so that the delivery of such gases is safe and economical. The gases commonly used in anesthesia and intensive care are oxygen, medical air, nitrous oxide, carbon dioxide, Entonox, and heliox. Medical vacuum, though, it is not a gas, but it is an important part of medical gas supply system. Medical gases such as oxygen and air can be supplied in bulk but gases such as nitrous oxide, medical air, and Entonox can be supplied from a cylinder manifold. These gases are then delivered through pipelines to the wall outlets.

Piped medical gas and vacuum consist of system, where gases from a central supply are delivered to different areas of the hospital. The pipeline system is made of high-quality deoxidizes, nonarsenic, phosphorus-containing copper alloy which stops the degradation of gases flowing through it and it also has *bacteriostatic properties*. Copper to copper fitting along with silver solder brazing alloy in the pipeline system reduces its corrosion. The size of the pipeline system depends upon the amount of gas flowing through them. Pipes with a 42 mm diameter are usually used at the manifold end of the system while smaller 15 mm pipes ultimately end as gas outlets. These gas outlets are labeled with gas names, are color-coded, and have self-sealing sockets. These self-sealing sockets shut down automatically which helps in servicing individual units without shutting a larger part of the system.

An anesthesia machine is connected to the outlet with the help of flexible color-coded hoses. These hoses consist of a Schrader probe at one end and a gas-specific threaded connector at other end. The gas-specific Schrader valve utilizes a collar indexing system that has a unique diameter that fits into the matching recess of specific gas at the terminal outlet. An anesthesia machine is connected to the hoses with the help of a unique connector which is mainly configured in the form of a *nut* and *probe*. The nut consists of the same diameter and thread for all gas services, but it can be connected to the anesthesia machine only when the probe is correctly attached. This assembly is called a *noninterchangeable screw-threaded connection* in the UK and a diameter indexed safety system in the US.

Isolation of pipeline connection is done with the help of isolating valves, which are positioned at the strategic location in various clinical areas of the hospital. These are called *area valve service unit (AVSU)*. They function as an isolating mechanism for delivery of gas to a particular clinical area for maintenance, fire, or any other emergency.

PROBLEMS WITH PIPELINE SYSTEM

Some of the most common problems encountered with the pipeline system are damage during installation, theft, fire, low pressure, human error, obstruction, leak, kinking, and contamination.

SAFETY MANEUVERS FOR PIPELINE SYSTEM

All clinical establishments should have reserve cylinders in case of failure of primary supply. A low-pressure alarm senses the failure of gas supply. Cross-connection is checked by a single hose test while misconnection by *tug tests*. Worn and damaged hoses increase the risk of fire if they carry gases under high pressure from a primary source such as anesthesia machines and ventilators. Heavy wear and tear increases the risk of rupture, especially in oxygen hoses used with transport devices. Therefore, all medical hoses should be checked and replaced at regular intervals in order to avoid any incident **(Table 1)**.

There should also be proper upkeep and maintenance of the system which can be done by the following:
- By following standard operating procedures.
- By maintaining a logbook.
- By doing regular maintenance of the equipment.
- By doing a leak test of the pipeline at a regular interval.
- Round-the-clock manning by trained workers.

TABLE 1: Modalities of pipeline testing.

Test	Process
Initial press test	Pipeline system is subjected to 1.5 times of its working pressure to detect a leak in the system
Standing press test	Pipeline system is subjected to 20% of higher working pressure for 24 hours
Blowdown	Oil-free dry nitrogen is used to clear the pipelines
Piping purge	Each gas outlet is purged to extent that there is no discoloration of white cloth held over the outlet
Cross-connection test	Gas systems are checked one by one using an oxygen analyzer
Final tie in test	Vacuum pipelines are tested using an ultrasound leak detector

- Regular training of manifold workers.
- Mock drills of pipeline failure, fire, and explosion should be regularly conducted.

FURTHER READING

1. Das S, Chattopadhyay S, Bose P. The anaesthesia gas supply system. Indian J Anaesth. 2013;57(5):489-99.
2. Sarangi S, Babbar S, Taneja D. Safety of the medical gas pipeline system. J Anaesthesiol Clin Pharmacol. 2018;34(1):99-102.

CHAPTER 47

Suction Apparatus

Ranjitha N, Puneet Khanna

Q. 1. What are the components of the suction apparatus (Fig. 1)?

Ans.
- Vacuum source
- Energy source
- Filter
- Collection vessel.

Q. 2. How much energy source/pressure is appropriate for suctioning?

Ans.
- The negative pressure for suction through a soft catheter or Ryle's tube should be 70–150 mm Hg (9.3–20 kPa).
- For infants, the negative pressure should be not >60–80 mm Hg (8–10 kPa).
- Maximum energy for suction through an endotracheal tube (ET) should be 60 kPa.

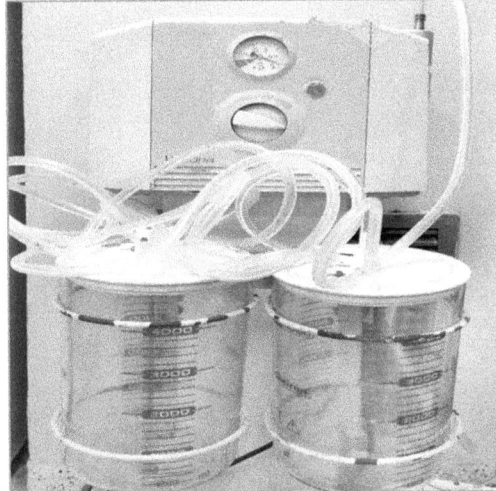

Fig. 1: Suction apparatus.

- The source of energy is a pipeline or electrically driven.

Q. 3. Describe the working principle of the vacuum source.

Ans.
- It works on the *venturi principle*.
- Subatmospheric or negative pressure is generated through the motor.
- Pump types may be either *piston pump* or *venturi pump* that works on simple bellows mechanism.

Q. 4. Mention the uses of filters in suction apparatus.

Ans.
- Filters are used between the collection vessel and the vacuum source to remove any particulate matter that could damage the source.
- Should remain dry and must be replaced regularly.

Collection vessel:
- It stores the aspirate that can be disposed.
- It consists of a rigid outer transparent container with volume markings on the sides.
- Suction tubing must be of suitable length with a detectable rigid suction handpiece.

Q. 5. What are the factors that determine the efficiency of the suction apparatus?

Ans.
- Degree of vacuum → negative atmospheric pressure

- Internal resistance of suction apparatus
- The viscosity of the matter being suctioned.

Q. 6. What are the uses of suction apparatus?
Ans. The uses of suction apparatus are given as follows:
- Used for removing secretions from the oropharynx.
- For suctioning of gastric contents through Ryle's tube.
- Suctions blood and other fluids from the surgical field.

Q. 7. What is the rationale between suction before extubation?
Ans. Prior to extubation, the secretions in the oral cavity and pharynx has to be expelled. Also there is a practice of extubating the patient with suction in the oral cavity to remove any secretions that may have passed through the trachea after deflation of the endotracheal tube cuff.

QUESTIONS

Q. 1. What is slow suction device? Where and why it is used?

Q. 2. What is VAP care cone system?

FURTHER READING

1. Davey A, Diba A. Ward's Anaesthetic Equipment 5th edition.

CHAPTER 48

Anesthesia Machine

Richa Saroa, Sanjeev Palta, Swati Jindal, Rajni Kalia

Q. 1. Who invented anesthesia machine?
Ans. Henry Edmund Gaskin (HEG) Boyle invented Boyle's machine in 1917.

Q. 2. What do you mean by BOC?
Ans. British Oxygen Company (BOC). It is the name in respect of Boyle.

Q. 3. Before Boyle's machine, what was used?
Ans. In 1912, James Taylor Gwathmey invented the Gwathmey machine. Later during First World War (1914-1918), Geoffrey Marshall developed a machine based on the Gwathmey machine.

Q. 4. What is anesthesia workstation?
Ans. To ensure patient safety, there have been many updates on the basic performance of an anesthetic workstation. The term "workstation" was introduced by American Society for Testing and Materials (ASTM) standard F1850-00 in distinction to "anesthesia (or gas) machine." The anesthesia workstation was referred to a technique utilized for the administration of anesthesia to patients consisting of the anesthesia gas supply device, target controlled inhaled anesthesia, facility for total intravenous anesthesia, breathing system, anesthetic gas scavenging system, anesthesia ventilator suitable from neonates to adults, and modular monitoring devices and monitoring recording systems and patient protection devices.

Q. 5. How has anesthesia machine modified from basic to advanced form?
Ans. The technological advancements have made the anesthesia workstations as a full-fledged anesthesia delivery as well as monitoring console though the basic concepts integral to the delivery of the anesthetic agents and operational mechanisms remain the same. Modern machines are amalgamation of complexity with incorporation of numerous devices like pneumatic gas appliance, ventilators with advanced mechanical ventilation modes, automated peripheral nerve and depth of anesthesia monitoring, monitoring for airway gas analysis, pulse oximeter and automated invasive and non-blood pressure, flow indicators, or virtual flowmeters displayed on an electronic panel. The gas flow-control needle valves have been replaced with the electronic flow controllers. The mechanical compressed gas gauges have been replaced by the digital pressure gauges in newer anesthesia workstations.

Q. 6. What are the functions of an anesthesia machine?
Ans. The function of the anesthesia machine still remains to maintain a physiological state in an anesthetized patient by ensuring the supply of compressed gases from either pipeline or cylinder and deliver a gas mixture at a constant flow rate with calibrated

composition to the central gas outlet and thereby to the patient through a breathing circuit. The relation between pressure and flow is governed by the Ohm's law that states that flow is directly proportional to the pressure and inversely proportional to the resistance of the breathing circuit. While the older machines worked on the principle of pneumatics and were pressure driven, the newer workstations are electrically driven and need the master switch to activate both the electric and pneumatic systems.

$$Flow = Pressure/Resistance$$

Q. 7. Enumerate the three pressure systems of basic anesthesia machine.
Ans.
- The high pressure system (comprising cylinder manifold/cylinder, hanger yoke assembly, pressure regulator first pressure reducing valve) (700–2,200 psig)
- The intermediate pressure system (40–55 psig)
- The low pressure system (12–16 psig).

Q. 8. Under normal conditions, from where does the anesthesia machine receive gases?
Ans. Usually the gas supply is drawn from pipeline system though an E type cylinder is always attached to the workstation to deal with any exigency or failure of the pipeline supply. Large H type cylinder with a pressure regulator is usually employed at remote places where pipeline supply is unavailable or at remote locations.

Q. 9. Describe briefly the high pressure system.
Ans. The high pressure system constitutes the part of machine that receives gases at high cylinder pressure (750 psig for nitrous oxide, 2,200 psig for oxygen) and reduces it to more constant intermediate pressure.

The parts of high pressure systems include:
- The hanger yoke assembly
- The yoke block
- The cylinder pressure gauge
- The pressure regulator.

Q. 10. Describe the parts of high pressure system in detail.
Ans.
- The hanger yoke assembly aligns the cylinder, ensures tight seal to avoid leak and warrants unidirectional flow of gas into the machine. The body has the principle framework and supporting structure. Retaining screw (retaining bar, clamping device) is used to tighten the cylinder to the yoke. Nipple allows the flow of gas to enter into machine. Index pins that are located below the nipple prevent attachment of the wrong cylinder. A neoprene washer that is surrounded by a metal ring named as Bodok seal (Bonded disk) imparts airtight seal between the cylinder and yoke. There should be no combustible material in seal as change in pressure will lead to changes in temperature creating a potential for fire. A filter (100 µm) that is mostly installed between the cylinder and the reducing valve, allows the removal of the particulate matter. The workstations usually have provision of at two yoke assembly for oxygen and single assembly for nitrous oxide administration.
- *The pin index safety system:* This system is employed for cylinder size A through E for attachment to the machine into the yoke assembly. To prevent the attachment of wrong cylinder into the yoke assembly, two pins projecting from the inner surface of the yoke fit into two corresponding holes in the cylinder head that is tailored to specific cylinder. The seven holes are

positioned on the circumference of a circle of 9/16 inch radius that is centered in the port. The pins are 4 mm in diameter and 6 mm long except for pin 7 that is thicker than the rest. Two pins are assigned for each gas, one on either side of midline. There are at least two hanger yokes one for oxygen and one for nitrous cylinder on the back of anesthesia workstation. The pin index for commonly used anesthesia gases is mentioned in **Table 1 (Figs. 1A to C)**.

- *Bourdon's pressure gauge:* It measures the pressure of the pipeline or cylinders. The hollow metal tube inside the gauge is curved as part of a circle that is further connected to the pressure line that has a clock like mechanism. This flexible tube straightens on exposure to gas pressure and this movement is transmitted to the indicator needle through a gearing mechanism. In most modern machines, the pressure gauges are placed on the front panel of the machine that allows a continuous check on the pipeline/cylinder pressure. To withstand the high pressure, face of pressure gauge is made of a special heavy glass window and the escape/release mechanism is provided through the back in case of sudden increase in pressure **(Figs. 2A and B)**.

Pressure gauges are designed such that they are easily read, color coded, labeled to indicate the gas, and symbolized to indicate the cylinder or pipeline pressures being displayed.

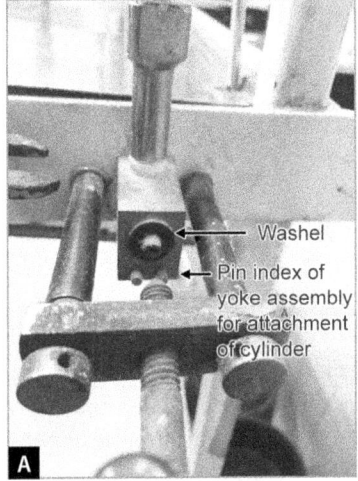

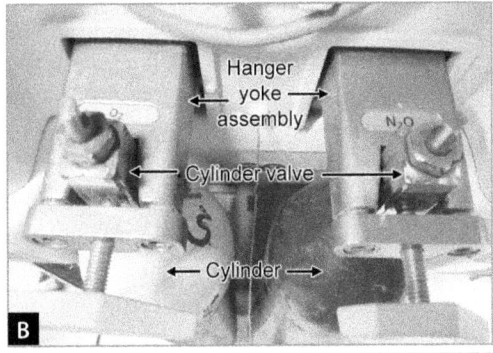

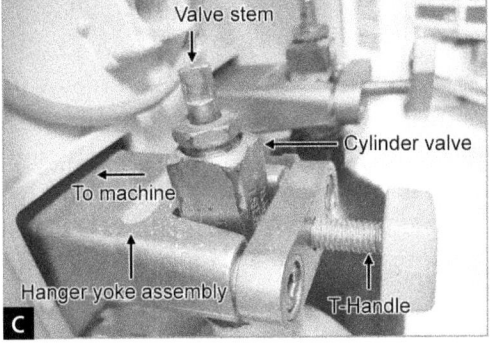

Figs. 1A to C: Parts of high pressure system.

TABLE 1: Pin index safety system.

Gas	Index pins
Oxygen	2, 5
Nitrous oxide	3, 5
Cyclopropane	3, 6
O_2:CO_2 (CO_2 <7.5%)	2, 6
O_2:CO_2 (CO_2 >7.5%)	1, 6
O_2:He (He >80.5%)	4, 6
O_2:He (He <80.5%)	2, 4
Air	1, 5
Nitrogen	1, 4
N_2O-O_2	7

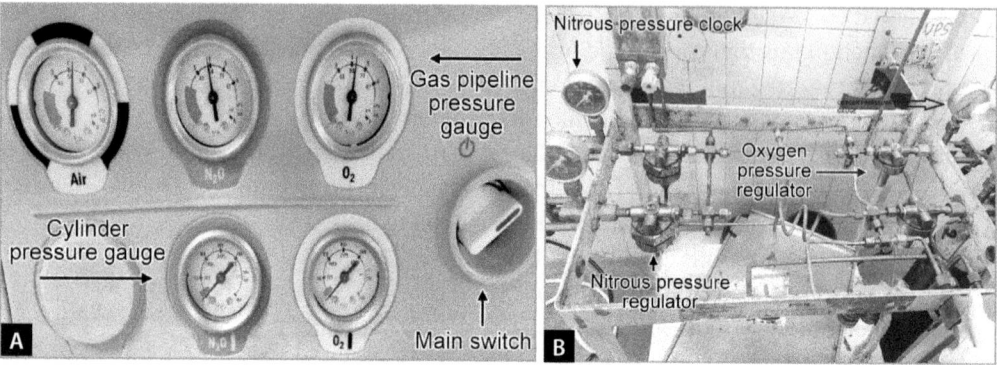

Figs. 2A and B: Bourdon's pressure gauge.

- Pressure regulator (pressure reducing device, reduction valves) primarily performs a function of reducing the high and variable pressure to maintain a constant pressure of gases flowing through the workstation. The uninterrupted flow at constant pressure eliminates the need for frequent adjustment through the flowmeter and thus contributes toward patient safety by preventing chances of building up high pressures in the machine. The standards of safety deem it necessary to have a reducing valve/device for each gas being supplied to the workstation. The reduced pressure thus provides patient safety and eliminates the chance of dangerous high pressure build up in machine. The regulator reduces oxygen pressure in cylinder from 2,200 psig to 45–60 psig and nitrous pressure from 750 to 45–60 psig.

By physics, pressure = force/area, therefore higher pressure exerted on a small area may be balanced by a low pressure acting on a large area (large diaphragm in the regulator). This principle is used in reducing pressures as cylinder contents empty. To ensure constant flow at reduced pressure, a set of high force springs are added in the regulator.

Q. 11. How is the proper working pressure of cylinders checked in premachine checkup?

Ans. Presence of two oxygen hanger yokes and placement of the cylinder gauge may complicate precheck process. In anesthesia machines with a single yoke hanger assembly, the gauge usually indicates the pressure in the cylinder by virtue of its presence upstream to the check valve. The gauge tends to indicate the pressure when cylinder is opened and indicates the same of zero if the cylinder is closed. However, in machines where two hanger yoke assemblies are present, the cylinder is usually placed downstream to the check valve and therefore always displays a higher pressure even if the cylinder is closed. The only way to ensure an adequate pressure in such scenario is by closing the oxygen cylinder and disconnecting the pipeline supply. Subsequently, the oxygen flow is turned and oxygen cylinder is opened that displays the true pressure in the cylinder after opening. The pipeline is connected after checking the cylinder pressure the second cylinder in the same way **(Fig. 3)**.

Q. 12. What is the function of a yoke plug?

Ans. The yoke assembly that is not in use may allow leak of small amount of gas that can be minimized by either attaching a full cylinder

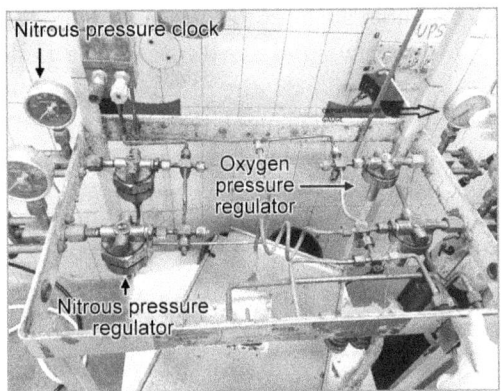

Fig. 3: Cylinder pressure test machine.

or a yoke plug also known as dummy cylinder block or plug. The yoke plug is usually a block of metal or material and has an inbuilt conical depression to make room for the retaining screw and a hollow area that fits onto the nipple. While the yoke plug prevents the escape of gases, it also prevents damage to the yoke by keeping the nipple free from dust. In the absence of yoke plug, the gas leakage may be up to 15 mL/min that can result in the delivery of hypoxic mixtures, especially in the older machines.

Q. 13. What is the pressure of gases at which anesthesia machine works?

Ans. While oxygen is stored as gas in the cylinders and follows the Boyle's law (pressure × volume = constant), nitrous oxide is stored as a liquid that converts to vapor and therefore gives a constant pressure till the entire liquid is converted to the vapor form.

The working pressure of anesthesia machine is primarily derived from primary intermediate system comprising the pipeline source of all gases usually has a working pressure of 40–55 psig (that is 5 psig higher than the reduced pressure from cylinder). Second stage pressure regulator or a flow restrictor is located between the pipeline and rest of the machine that controls the pipeline pressure surges.

The oxygen cylinder pressure varies from 1,800 to 2,200 psi which is regulated to approximately 45 psi upon its entry to the machine. A full nitrous oxide cylinder pressure is regulated from 750 psi to approximately 45 psig in the intermediate system. Air cylinder pressures are similar to oxygen. The cylinder pressure is regulated below the pipeline pressure to reduce the emptying of cylinders, if they are accidentally left open with preferential usage from the pipeline itself.

Q. 14. Enumerate components of intermediate system.

Ans.
- Pipeline inlet connections
- Oxygen fail-safe system
- Oxygen flush
- Second stage pressure regulator (reduced to 26 psi for N_2O and 14 psi for oxygen)
- Pipeline pressure gauges
- Ventilator power outlets
- Flowmeter-needle valves.

Q. 15. Describe salient features of each component of intermediate system.

Ans.
- Each pipeline that is usually made up of copper and is a reinforced, flexible, and color-coded gas line. Usually, the oxygen pipeline has an outer diameter of 0.05 inch and that of other medical gases is 3/8 inch. The display of the name and direction of the flow of gas is mandatory and all the pipelines must be identified in all the rooms and the floors to which is being supplied. The pipeline terminal toward the wall has gas-specific Schrader connection. The other machine end of the pipeline has noninterchangeable screw thread (NIST) connection or diameter index safety system (DISS) system that provide noninterchangeable connection

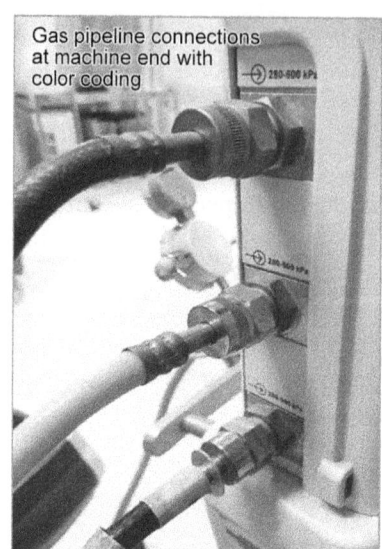

Fig. 4: Component of intermediate system.

for the medical gases. The pipelines of different gases (oxygen, nitrous oxide, and air) have different diameters. Gas enters the machine passes through filter and a one-way check valve, which prevents backward flow if there is pipeline disconnection or cylinder is in use. The pipeline gas pressure is measured by a pressure gauge that is upstream to the pipeline check valve **(Fig. 4)**.

- Second stage regulators are present in some machines (Datex-Ohmeda) before flowmeters and oxygen flush. It reduces the oxygen pressure further to approximately 14 psig for oxygen and 26 psig for nitrous oxide in case of pressure fluctuations in the intermediate system. This ensures lower pressure at oxygen flush, minimize pressure fluctuations to flowmeter and hence maintain constant flow and decrease war tear of needle valves of the flowmeter. In other machines, the oxygen failure protection device (OFPD) is incorporated as a failsafe valve for all the medical gases. While with second regulators, the oxygen is delivered at a constant pressure till pressure is more than the 40 psig, the pressures may fall proportionally for all the gases in OFPD system if supplying pressure reduction occurs. This may contribute to a lower flow rate at the central gas outlet and can cause rebreathing.
- Oxygen flush receives oxygen from pipeline inlet or oxygen cylinder. It delivers oxygen through common gas outlet (CGO) at rate of 35–70 L/minute with a pressure of 45–60 psig. This part receives direct oxygen supply from oxygen pressure regulator that is directed to the CGO. When in use, despite vaporizer and nitrous oxide being on, bypassing the rotameters and back bar, pure oxygen will be delivered at the patient end. In older machines with locking mechanism, accidental and unobserved use of oxygen flush could cause barotrauma owing to fresh gas flow through the circuit at rate of 1 L/minute. In modern machines, flush is in a recess to prevent accidental activation and there is no locking mechanism.
- The flowmeter assembly measures, controls the flow of individual gases that are being delivered at the CGO. It consists of series of needle valves that regulate the flow and flowmeter subassembly.
  • Flow control (needle) valve also known as needle or pin valve, fine adjustment valve or flow adjustment valve. They are located at the base of the associated flowmeter tube and control the flow of gas through the flowmeters by mechanical adjustment.

Components of flow control valve consist of control knob, stem, and seat. The control knob is usually made up of brass within built screws that extend into the base of the flowmeter through a body ending into a needle. The flow control valve for each gas is color and touch coded. The oxygen flow control valve is the largest, white, protruding, and octagonal knob with widely spaced flutes. The flow control valve for nitrous knob is smaller, blue in color with narrow flutes. With the valve closed, the pin fits into the seat of metal allowing no gas to flow. The gas flow occurs after the stem is turned counterclockwise that creates an opening between the pin and the seat.

Q. 16. Explain in detail about the oxygen pressure fail safe system.

Ans. Various safety features have been incorporated into anesthesia machine to prevent delivery of hypoxic mixture to the patient.

Master and slave mechanism: This mechanism primarily is safety mechanism where nitrous oxide cannot flow through the machine in the absence of oxygen flow. The oxygen pressure regulator works as primary regulator and the nitrous oxide pressure regulator allows the gas to flow through only if the oxygen pressure is adequate. This mechanism prevents the delivery of the hypoxic mixture to the patient in case of failure of oxygen supply that used to be witnessed in older machines. Since the flow of nitrous oxide is dependent upon the flow of oxygen through the oxygen pressure valve, this is commonly referred to as slave and master mechanism denoting the nitrous and oxygen regulators respectively.

There are two types of oxygen failure safety devices:
1. Fail safe valves (a) pressure sensor shut-off valves and (b) OFPD.
2. Oxygen ration proportioning systems.

Fail safe valves were earlier present in older machines where supply of gases was from cylinders and inspired oxygen concentration could not be measured. Fail safe device would ensure a set concentration of oxygen at the CGO even during reduced oxygen pressures. However, it was fraught with hazard of delivery of hypoxic mixture to the patient in case the oxygen cylinder emptied and went unnoticed in the absence of alarm systems.

In older GE Datex-Ohmeda machines, the presence of pressure sensors shutoff valves ensured the complete cut-off of nitrous oxide supply, in case the oxygen pressures fell below 25 psig.

Oxygen failure protection device synchronously decreases the flows of other gases when oxygen supply pressure falls below 12 ± 4 psig.

Fail safe mechanism is actually a misnomer as it does not ensure adequate oxygen flow and only senses the pressure in the oxygen pipeline. It is unable to detect any other gas that may accidently be present in the oxygen pipeline. Fail safe systems thus do not prevent hypoxic mixtures which is the function of hypoxic guards.

Proportioning systems: Newer machines are equipped with proportionating systems to ensure minimum FiO_2 that is delivered at all the times.

In Datex-Ohmeda, Link-25 proportion-limiting control device consists of a stainless steel chain that links nitrous oxide and oxygen flow control valves, ensuring the delivered oxygen concentration never inadvertently falls below 25%. When oxygen flow decrease, the gear engages both control knobs simultaneously. So when nitrous oxide flow control valve turns two revolutions; oxygen flow control valve turns one revolution. This mechanical system is supported by pneumatic system whereby both the flowmeters operate at different pressures due to different settings in the second stage pressure regulator. A second stage pressure regulator reduces the pressure at the nitrous oxide flow control valve to 26 psig and at the oxygen flow control valve to 14 psig. So the final flow ratio is 3:1.

Oxygen ratio monitor controller (ORMC): In newer Drager machines, this shuts off N_2O when oxygen pressure is <10 psi.

Oxygen supply failure alarm: Reduced oxygen pressure results in audible and visual alarms. It usually works through a pressurized canister filled with oxygen that produces whistle-like sound on when oxygen flows through it. Fall in oxygen pressure induces a reverse stream of oxygen that leads to activation of sound and gives an alarm indicating low oxygen pressure. The alarm is usually activated when the oxygen pressure are below 30 psig.

The stream of oxygen passing through the whistle produces a sound when machine is turned on. If oxygen pressure falls below a certain value, this canister will empty and direct a reverse stream of oxygen through the whistle. The alarm is usually activated in 5 seconds when oxygen supply pressure decreases to 30 psig at 60 decibels at one meter. Restoration of the oxygen supply will switch off the alarm.

Limitations of oxygen safety failure device:
- They prevent the hypoxic mixture delivery that may be secondary to various causes as disconnected oxygen, low oxygen pipeline pressure, and depletion of oxygen cylinders. However, accidental turning off of the oxygen flow control valve may lead to delivery of hypoxic gases.
- The devices are not foolproof in equipment related (leaks) or operator related errors (closed or partially closed oxygen flow control valve) that occur downstream.
- They do not guard against hypoxia secondary to pipeline or cylinder crossovers

Q. 17. Write short note on oxygen analyzer.
Ans. An oxygen analyzer is a device that measures the percentage of oxygen by paramagnetic method or by a fuel cell. For the proper functioning of oxygen analyzer, these should be calibrated at regular intervals at room air (21%). Despite the incorporation of oxygen failure safety measures in anesthesia machine, the best method to detect and prevent delivery of hypoxic mixture to the CGO/patient is installation of oxygen analyzer in inspiratory limb of circuit.

Q. 18. Enumerate components of low pressure system.
Ans.
- Flowmeter subassembly
- Vaporizers mounted on back bar
- Vaporizer
- Pressure relief valve
- Common gas outlet.

Q. 19. Describe each component of low pressure system in detail.
Ans. The back bar is a gaseous pathway on which the flowmeter block and vaporizers are mounted. After the vaporizer is attached and turned on gas flow is diverted through the vaporizer that delivers the required concentration of anesthetic vapor in the gaseous mixture flowing through the back bar to the CGO.

Flowmeter subassembly: Conventionally, nondigital anesthetic flowmeter is a rotameter. A rotameter is a constant pressure, variable orifice device that consist of tapered tubes (Thorpe's tubes) through which gas flows. The indicator also known as bobbin or float, a stop at the top of tube and the scale to indicate the flow are integral to the designing of a flowmeter. The rotameter has tapered glass which narrows at the bottom and is made gas tight because of neoprene washers (O rings) at both ends of the flowmeter.

Each rotameter is calibrated for the specific gas at 20°C at ambient pressure of 760 mm Hg. Therefore, if the flow tube breaks, the entire rotameter assembly including the float should be replaced. The gap between the walls of the rotameter and the bobbin is also known as the annular space. At low flows the annular space is comparatively small, the flow through the tube is similar to a hole that is laminar and depends upon the viscosity (Hagen–Poiseuille law). Since viscosity is independent of barometric pressure; therefore, the readings at low flows are accurate. At higher flows, the annular space widens, therefore, the flow is turbulent, similar to that through an orifice and is dependent on the density of the gases (Reynold's number). As different gases have different density and viscosity, the rotameters are calibrated for a specific gas at atmospheric pressure and temperature (accurate within ± 2–2.5%) and cannot be used interchangeably. At high altitude, density decreases and the flowmeter under-reads at higher flow. In a hyperbaric chamber, it over-reads at higher flows. Most machines have rotameters for oxygen, nitrous, and air.

Flowmeter tubes are tapered with bore of the tube increasing from bottom to the top and are made up of borosilicate glass Pyrex. The tubes may be either single-tapered or double-tapered tubes the former being utilized for both low-flow and high-flow anesthesia delivery systems separately and the latter in case there is a single tube for a delivery of anesthetic gas mixture. The lower portion of the double tapered flow usually has finer calibrations to measure low flows and the upper tubing depicts a coarse taper for higher flows rates. Flow is read from the top of the float. If there is sphere instead of bobbin, then flow rate is taken from the equator of the sphere. Some anesthetic machines have a pair of tubes for each gas: one to be used for low flows and the other for higher flows. As the pair is arranged in series, the second tube indicates total flow. The tubes have an antistatic coating on their inner and outer surfaces. This prevents bobbin from sticking to the tube wall.

Indicator also variously known as rotameter, bobbin, or float is made up of aluminum and comprises an upper rim that is wider as compared to the body of the float. The upper rim has grooves cut at an angle along the surface, known as flutes, that contribute to the rotatory movement of the same with the flow of gas through the tubes that are visible by a fluorescent marker on the center of the indicator. The indicator moves within the flowmeter tube and rotatory movement of the same as the gas flows through the flowmeter denotes accurate readings through the same. The float rotates at point where gravity and pressure of upward gas flow are equal. Occasionally, the flowmeter may get stuck to the sides of the tubes mostly due to development of static electricity, particularly in dry atmospheres or presence of dirt or grease. While the effects of static electricity may be minimized by the use of antistatic agent such as croxtine (BOC) sprays, the cleaning requires dismantling the entire assembly. A rotating flow should be ensured during anesthesia machine check as a nonrotating flow may lead to erroneous flows and contribute to either hypoxia or barotrauma.

Scale is usually marked either directly or toward the right side of the tube. The gradations corresponding to increments in flow rate are nearer at the top of the scale secondary to wider annular space than those at the bottom of the tube.

Rotameter flow scales glows in the dark owing to a fluorescent background that one

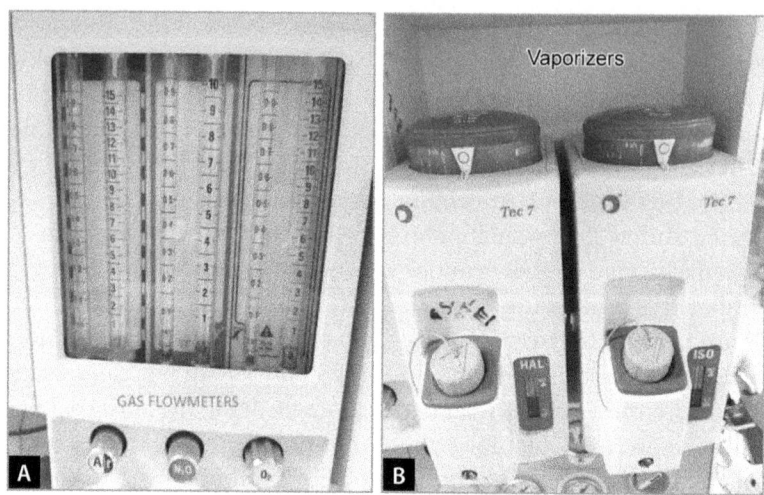

Figs. 5A and B: Gas flowmeters and vaporizers.

of safety features inducted for easy identification in dim/no light. By rule of thumb, oxygen is always downstream so as to avoid any hypoxic mixture being administered to the patient in case of damage to other rotameter tubes **(Figs. 5A and B)**.

Common gas outlet receives gases ± mixed with inhalational agent from the vaporizer. Breathing circuit is connected to the CGO, either directly or by a shifting to an in-built closed circle system. A 22-mm male and 15-mm female connection provides an airtight seal between the anesthetic machine and the breathing circuit toward the patient. Pressure relief valves downstream to the vaporizer ensure the direction of flow of gas through the anesthetic machine. A check valve that is present downstream of vaporizer bank to prevent back pressure changes being transmitted to the vaporizer particularly when oxygen flush is activated **(Fig. 6)**.

Q. 20. Describe salient features in an anesthesia machine which ensures patient safety.
Ans. It has been seen that major anesthetic mishaps due to machine have been due to lack of familiarity with equipment and precheck failures (75%) and only 24% were actually due to equipment failure.

Salient features of the anesthetic machine that enhance patient safety and make mishaps rare are:
- Two oxygen supplies
- Color-coded and labeled cylinders
- Color-coded pressure gauges
- Schrader connector at the wall, specific to each gas
- Color-coded tubing for each gas
- Color-coded cylinders for each gas
- Noninterchangeable screw thread system to prevent incorrect pipeline attachment
- Pin index system to ensure incorrect cylinder attachment
- One-way valves to prevent the retrograde flow when gases enter the machine
- Rotameter design with specified features:
  - O_2 flow control valve being color coded and a different size, shape, and texture
  - O_2 flow control valve downstream in the rotameter block
  - Link mechanism between oxygen and nitrous/antihypoxia device between O_2 and N_2O (or electronic equivalent)
  - Oxygen being always downstream and thus last gas to enter the mixed gas flow

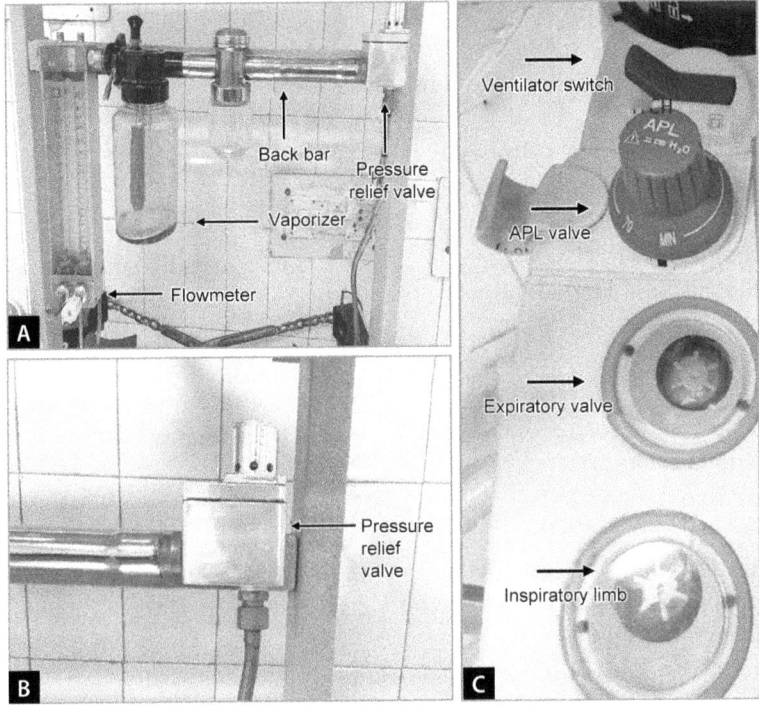

Fig. 6: Valves.

- Antistatic coating in rotameters to prevent sticking of the float
- Rotation of float that provides visual confirmation of flow
- Emergency O_2 flush that bypasses the back bar
- Oxygen concentration analyzer or monitor
- Alarm for failure of oxygen supply
- Ventilator disconnection alarm
- Preuse machine checks
- Vaporizers have several safety features:
  - Color-coded vaporizer and vapor bottles for each agent
  - Unique key-filling devices calibrated for specific agent
  - Anti-spill mechanism that allows a tilt up to 180°
  - Selectatec or Interlock systems that prevents the use of more than one vaporizer at a time
  - An agent-level indicator to indicate the total agent in the vaporizer.

Q. 21. What are the steps for the preanesthesia checkout procedure?

Ans.

- Verify that auxiliary oxygen cylinder and self-inflating manual ventilation device are available in the near vicinity and functioning of the same should be performed.
- Ensure that the suction pressure is adequate to clear the airway that can be assessed by occluding the suction tube orifice with the underside of thumb and ascertain if it can be supported at height corresponding to the waist.
- Confirm backup AC power and availability of backup battery prior to delivery of anesthesia.
- Confirm the proper functioning of the appropriate monitoring supplies prior to each anesthetic procedure. Appropriate audible or visual alarms to indicate

problems with patient oxygenation, ventilation, circulation, and temperature should be intact and reset to default values.
- Confirm that the oxygen cylinder is at least half with pressure of at least 1,000 psig to ensure acceptable amount of backup oxygen.
- Confirm that displayed piped gas pressure is ≥50 psig.
- Establish that the vaporizers are appropriately filled and filler ports are tight enough to prevent unrecognized leakage. Also confirm that vaporizers are not at a tilt or lifted from their mounts.
- Ensure that gas supply lines are leak proof between the flowmeter and the CGO.
- Scavenging system function needs to be verified before anesthesia.
- Calibration/verify calibration of oxygen monitor and check low oxygen alarm by deliberately reducing FiO_2 and confirming the alarm generation with the same. Oxygen sensor calibration should occur at least once per day.
- Carbon dioxide absorbent must be checked and replaced if exhausted before anesthesia delivery.
- Breathing system leak test is mandatory to perform before using the same.
- Confirm that gas flows properly through breathing circuit during both inspiration and expiration.
- Always document completion of the checkout procedures.
- Confirm ventilator settings and evaluate readiness to deliver anesthesia care.

QUESTIONS

Q. 1. Role of artificial intelligence in anesthesia machinery.

Q. 2. MRI compatible anesthesia machine.

Q. 3. Patient safety and low flow anesthesia. Disadvantages.

Q. 4. How to convert anesthesia machine into ICU ventilator?

Q. 5. Anesthesia information management system? (Charting)

Q. 6. What is fuzzy logic control theory in clinical anesthesia?

Q. 7. Target control inhalation anesthesia.

Q. 8. Waste anesthetic cases collection and consequences.

Q. 9. Fine hazards in an anesthesia machine. Measures adapted to prevent it.

Q. 10. Anesthesia related CO exposure. Methods to prevent it.

FURTHER READING

1. Davey A, Diba A. Ward's Anaesthetic Equipment, 5th edition. Amsterdam: Elsevier Saunders; 2005.
2. Dorsh JA, Dorsch SE. Understanding Anesthesia Equipment, 5th edition. Philadelphia, PA: Lippincott Williams and Wilkins; 2008.

CHAPTER 49

Vaporizers

Richa Saroa, Sanjeev Palta, Tenzin Nyima, Arun A Bevoor

■ RELATED PHYSICS

- *Vapor:* Vapor is a gaseous state of a substance that exists below its critical temperature.
- *Gas:* Gas is a material that exists in a gaseous state above its critical temperature.
- *Critical temperature:* The temperature above which, no matter how much pressure is applied, a gaseous substance cannot be condensed into a liquid.
- *Saturated vapor pressure (SVP):* When the liquid and its vapor are in equilibrium in a closed container at a constant temperature, the pressure that is exerted by the vapor molecules is the SVP. Saturated vapor pressure remains unaffected by ambient pressure. Temperature and liquid are the two determining factors. SVP determines the volatility of the agent (higher SVP, higher volatility).
- *Boiling point:* It is the temperature of a liquid at which its vapor pressure is equal to atmospheric pressure.
- *Partial pressure:* It is the pressure exerted by an individual gas in a mixture of gases. Partial pressure depends on the temperature of the agent.

$$P_{total} = P_1 + P_2 + P_3 + P_4$$

- *Volume percent:* It is the proportion of individual gas in a gas mixture that is expressed in percentage.

  V/V% = partial pressure/total pressure

- *Minimum alveolar concentration (MAC):* MAC value of inhalation agent is the MAC in vol% of end-tidal alveolar gas at 760 mm Hg (1 atm) that causes a lack of responses to painful stimulation in 50% of patients.
- *Specific heat:* The specific heat is the amount of energy required to increase the temperature of 1 g of substance by 1°C.
- *Latent heat of vaporization:* It is the amount of energy in joules or calories required to change 1 g of liquid into vapor at a constant temperature.
- *Thermal conductivity:* It is the measurement of the rate at which heat passes through a substance. To achieve thermostabilization, a vaporizer of high thermal conductivity metal is required.

■ QUESTIONS AND ANSWERS

Q. 1. What is a vaporizer?
Ans. A vaporizer converts liquid anesthetic into vapor and delivers a safe dose of vapor to the fresh gas flow or the breathing circuit.

Q. 2. What is the purpose of a vaporizer?
Ans. Due to its highly volatile nature and potency, inhalational agents have higher saturated vapor pressures at clinically relevant temperatures therefore if they are allowed to vaporize freely it can lead to overdose. Hence, vaporizers are required to provide a calibrated concentration of these agents to the patients.

Q. 3. Classify vaporizers according to Dorsch and Dorsch's classification of vaporizers.

Ans. The classification of vaporizers is as follows:
- *Based on the method of vaporization*:
  - Flow over type
    - *With wicks:* Temperature compensation (TEC), Epstein Macintosh Oxford (EMO), Oxford Miniature Vaporizer (OMV)
    - *Without wicks:* Goldman bottle
  - *Bubble through:* Copper kettle
  - *Flow over or bubble through:* Ether bottle
  - *Injection:* Desflurane
- *Based on the regulation of output concentration:*
  - *Variable bypass:* Ether bottle, TEC
  - *Measured flow:* Copper kettle
- *Based on temperature compensation:*
  - *Thermocompensated:* TEC 4,5,7
  - *Nonthermocompensated:* Goldman
  - *Thermobuffered:* EMO
  - *Electronic:* TEC 6, Aladin Cassette
- *Based on agent specificity:*
  - *Agent specific:* TEC
  - *Multiagent:* Goldman bottle
- *Based on resistance:*
  - *Plenum (High resistance):* TEC
  - *Draw over (Low resistance):* Goldman bottle, EMO
- *Based on the location of the vaporizer:*
  - *In-circuit (VIC):* EMO, Goldman bottle
  - *Out of circuit (VOC):* TEC.

Q. 4. Enumerate various materials used in the construction of the vaporizers according to their thermal conductivity.

Ans. Copper > aluminum [magnetic resonance imaging (MRI) compatible] > brass > steel >> glass

Q. 5. Enumerate properties of an ideal vaporizer.

Ans. Properties of an ideal vaporizer are as follows:
- Economical and safe to use
- Resistant to corrosion and solvent
- Leakproof
- Lightweight for easy transport and durable
- Unaffected by variable fresh gas flows, pressures, temperature
- Can be adjusted to a vaporizer interlock system.

Q. 6. How to calculate the quantity of liquid agent which a vaporizer uses per hour?

Ans. It can be calculated in two ways:
1. *Avogadro's hypothesis:* According to Avogadro law, at constant temperature and pressure, equal volumes of all gases will contain the same number of molecules. (1 mole of gas = 22.4 L at 1 atm and 0°C)

   For example, the molecular weight of sevoflurane is 200 g/mol

   1 mol of sevoflurane = 200 g

   According to Avogadro's hypothesis, 1 mole of a substance = 22.4 L of gas

   Therefore 22.4 L of sevoflurane weighs 200 g

   Hence density of sevoflurane vapor = M/V (mass/volume) = 200 g/22.4 L = 8.92 g/L, therefore 1 g = 1L/8.92 g = 1,000/8.9 mL of vapor.

   Density of sevoflurane liquid is 1.5 g/mL, therefore 1 g = 1/1.5 mL of liquid

   1/1.5 mL of liquid = 1,000/8.9 mL of vapor
   1 mL of liquid = 1,000/8.9 × 1.5 = 168 mL vapor

   Hence for most commonly used agents, 1 mL of liquid yields 200 mL of vapors.

   Therefore amount of vapors used per minute = Fibroblast growth factor (FGF) × time × concentration setting.

   For example, FGF = 3 L, time = 60 minutes, concentration setting = 1.5%

= 5,000 × 60 × 1.5/100 = 2700 mL of sevoflurane vapor
= 2,700/168 = 16 mL of liquid sevoflurane will be used.
- *Ehrenworth and Eisenkraft formula:* mL of liquid used per hour = 3 × FGF (L/min) × dial concentration setting (v/v%)

Q. 7. Discuss the vaporizers on the basis of method of regulating their output.

Ans.

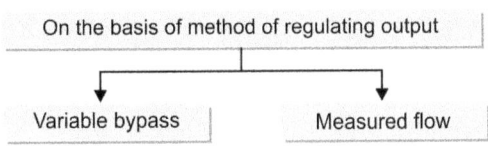

- *Variable bypass vaporizer:* It consists of a vaporizing chamber and a bypass chamber. Total fresh gas flow received from the machine splits into two, a very small amount passes through the vaporizing chamber, and the remaining passes through the bypass chamber.

  This ratio of the carrier gas flows through the vaporizing chamber and bypass chamber is a *splitting ratio* (**Fig. 1**).
  Splitting ratio = vaporizer flow/total flow – vaporizer flow

- *Measured flow vaporizer:* In this method, only a measured amount of gas is used to pick up an anesthetic agent. For this vaporizer output and the carrier gases are dialed separately. A measured amount of carrier gas is directed through the flow meter and to the vaporizer circuit control valve. The saturated vapors are redirected to the vaporizer control valve from where it mixes with fresh gas flow and delivers to the patient.

Q. 8. Calculate the splitting ratio of FGF in sevoflurane vaporizer when FGF is set at 5 L/min and the concentration dial is set at 2% at 20°C and 1 atmospheric pressure.

Ans. Known—SVP of sevoflurane at 20°C is 157 mm Hg

At 760 mm Hg (1 atm) sevoflurane vapor is 157/760 = 21% of total volume ---------(1)

Therefore FGF in vaporizing chamber will be 100 – 21 = 79%

Since concentration dial is set at 2%, for 5,000 mL of FGF sevoflurane consumed will be 2/100 × 5,000 = 100 mL

From (1), we know that sevoflurane forms 21 % of total volume, which is 100 mL in this case

Therefore, FGF in vaporizing chamber will be 100/21 × 79 = 376 mL

Hence FGF in bypass chamber will be 5,000 – 376 = 4,623 mL

Splitting ratio = FGF in bypass chamber/ FGF in vaporizing chamber
= 4,623/376
= 12.29: 1

Splitting ratios for various concentration dial settings are tabulated in **Table 1**.

Q. 9. Enumerate differences between plenum and draw over vaporizers.

Ans. The differences between plenum and draw over vaporizers are mentioned in **Table 2**.

Q. 10. Enumerate characteristic features of vaporizers outside the circuit (VOC) and vaporizers inside the circuit (VIC).

Ans. The characteristic features of vaporizers outside the circuit (VOC) and vaporizers inside the circuit (VIC) are mentioned in **Table 3**.

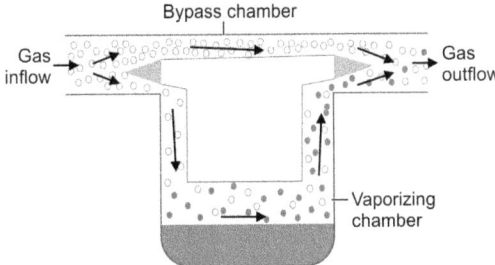

Fig. 1: Variable bypass vaporizer.

TABLE 1: Splitting ratios for various concentrations dial settings.

Concentration dial setting (v/v%)	Halothane	Isoflurane	Sevoflurane
1	46:1	45:1	25:1
2	23:1	22:1	12:1
3	15:1	14:1	8:1

TABLE 2: Differences between plenum and draw over vaporizers.

Plenum (air-filled space in a structure)/pressure vaporization chamber	Draw over
A pressurized source of FGF is required	Depends on the patient's inspiratory efforts or negative pressure at the outlet of the vaporizer
Unidirectional flow	Bidirectional flow
Not affected by the respiratory cycle	Affected by patient's minute ventilation and respiratory pattern
Flow rates depend on the flow meter settings	Flow rates vary as per peak inspiratory pressures up to 60 L/min
Operator dependent	Patient dependent
Accurate (0–15 L/min)	Inaccurate
Used only for VOC	Can be used for both (VIC and VOC)

(FGF: fresh gas flow; VIC: vaporizer inside the circuit; VOC: vaporizers outside the circuit)

TABLE 3: Characteristic features of VOC and VIC.

	VOC	VIC
Position	Between flow meters and common gas outlet or between the common gas outlet and breathing system	In the circle system, i.e., in the inspiratory limb or the expiratory limb
Resistance	Can work in both low or high resistance because it can overcome by the positive pressure of fresh gases	Requires low resistance to function
Output concentration	Lower than dialed concentration and is independent of minute ventilation	Higher than the set dialed concentration because of recirculating gases vapor and is dependent on minute ventilation
Condensation	No condensation because expired gas does not pass through the vaporizer	Condensation can occur
Care	No cleaning or washing is required as it is not exposed to expired gases from the patient	Requires frequent cleaning and washing
Examples	TEC vaporizers	Goldman, EMO

(EMO: Epstein Macintosh Oxford; TEC: temperature compensation; VIC: vaporizer inside the circuit; VOC: vaporizers outside the circuit)

Q. 11. Describe various factors causing variations in vaporizer's functioning.

Ans. Various factors causing variations in vaporizers functioning are as follows:
- Temperature
- Backpressure changes
- Flow rate
- Liquid levels
- Additives and composition of agents
- Carrier gases
- Altitude variation.

Q. 12. Explain backpressure changes in vaporizers in tabulated form.

Ans.

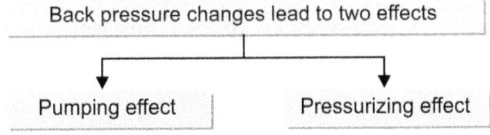

The back pressure's two effects are elaborated in **Table 4**.

Q. 13. Discuss different temperature compensation methods in vaporizers.

Ans.
- *Electrically heated:* TEC 6 desflurane.
- *Thermobuffering or thermocompensation:* TEC vaporizers bimetallic strips act as heat sink and lead them to thermocompensation, whereas in thermobuffering water bath compensates, e.g., in Boyle's bottle.

Q. 14. Explain the effect of altitude on vaporizers.

Ans. As already discussed saturated vapor pressure does not change with a change in ambient pressure and vaporizers are calibrated at sea level (1 atm). The partial pressure of the vapor does not change much with increasing altitude; therefore vaporizers do not need much calibration. The exception is TEC 6 vaporizers, which are pressurized to 2 atm hence, need higher dial settings to achieve the same effect.

Q. 15. List the safety features of a vaporizer.

Ans.
- Color-coded (both colored bottle collar and adapter)
- Agent specific
- Interlock system
- Low-filling port.

Q. 16. Enumerate various hazards associated with vaporizers.

Ans.
- Incorrect concentration, low or high
- Wrong agent delivery
- Tipping—entry of liquid agent into bypass chamber can lead to the delivery of high concentration to patients
- Overfilling
- Leaks can lead to operation theater pollution.

TABLE 4: Two effects of back pressure.

	Pumping effect	Pressurizing effect
Mechanism	During inspiration, pressure in the anesthetic circuit and vapor chamber increases leading to an increase in the saturated vapor into the inlet path. While during expiration, the pressure falls hence these saturated vapor enter the bypass chamber and result in increased output	When carrier gas is compressed in the vaporizing chamber, the number of molecules as such does not increase resulting in dilution of the anesthetic agent and hence a decrease in the output
Flows	Low flows	High flows
Output	Increased vapor output	Decreased vapor output
Significance	More significant	Less significant

Q. 17. Tabulate the physical properties of different inhaled anesthetic agents?

Ans. The physical properties of different inhaled anesthetic agents are mentioned in Table 5.

Q. 18. Describe TEC 7 vaporizer.

Ans. TEC 7 vaporizer is plenum type, variable bypass; flow over with wick, temperature compensated, out of circuit, concentration calibrated, and agent-specific.
- *Capacity:* 300 mL
- *Color coding:*
  - Halothane—red
  - Isoflurane—purple
  - Sevoflurane—yellow
  - Enflurane—orange

In a variable bypass vaporizer, the fresh gas is split into two streams. One stream flows into bypass chamber and the other stream flows into vaporizing chamber where it is saturated with the vapor of the liquid anesthetic agent. Finally, both streams mix together and deliver fresh gas with a diluted anesthetic agent into the breathing circuit. The ratio in which fresh gas is split into two chambers is called the *splitting ratio*.

WORKING MECHANISM

- *Plenum vaporizers with thermocompensation:* The concentration dial setting in the vaporizer determines the splitting ratio. This variable bypass regulates the concentration of the anesthetic agent. The fresh gas in vaporizing chamber flows over wicks and baffles to maximize the surface area of vaporization. The automatic devices ensure the steady vaporizer output by thermocompensation in different OR temperatures. The FGF which is split at the vaporizer inlet is combined at the vaporizer outlet to give the final concentration of inhaled anesthetic which is the ratio of the inhaled anesthetic to the total gas flow. These vaporizers are agent-specific as they are calibrated for specific gas and are used to deliver sevoflurane, isoflurane, and halothane.
  - Examples:
    - TEC 5 and TEC 7 vaporisers® (GE)
    - Vapor 2000® series (Dragger)
    - Sigma Delta® (Penlon)
- *Plenum vaporizers with electronic control:* They are functionally similar to a conventional vaporizer with bypass chamber and vaporizing chamber. A single electronic control system is designed in an anesthetic workstation to deliver different volatile anesthetics. It consists of two parts: (1) an electronic control system that is integrated with an anesthesia workstation and (2) the portable cassettes which are filled with a volatile anesthetic agent. The central processing unit (CPU) receives inputs from concentration dial, pressure sensor, temperature sensor, and flow meters. Using these data CPU precisely delivers desired vapor concentration by regulating in and out of fresh gas flow.

TABLE 5: Physical properties of different inhaled anesthetic agents.

Parameter	Enflurane	Halothane	Isoflurane	Sevoflurane	Desflurane
SVP at 20°C (mm Hg)	175	243	238	160	669
MAC at 1 atm (v/v%)	1.68	0.75	1.2	1.9	6.0
Boiling point at 1 atm (°C)	56.5	50.2	48.5	58.5	22.8

(MAC: minimum alveolar concentration; SVP: saturated vapor pressure)

- *Examples:* Aladin and Aladin2 Cassette vaporizers (GE/Datex-Ohmeda)

Q. 19. Why TEC 7 vaporizer is not appropriate for desflurane delivery?
Ans. Conventional TEC 7 vaporizer cannot be used for desflurane for the following three reasons:
1. *High SVP:* Desflurane has a high saturated vapor pressure of 669 mm Hg at 20°C which is considerably higher when compared to other volatile anesthetic agents. The fresh gas in vaporizing chamber carries a large amount of desflurane vapor which needs a very high bypass chamber flow rate for dilution. For example, to produce a 1% desflurane effect 73 L/min of bypass chamber flow is required.
2. *High MAC:* Desflurane has a higher MAC compared to other volatile anesthetic agents. To produce such a high MAC more amount of desflurane is consumed over a period of time leading to cooling of the vaporizer and a reduction in output. This wide range of temperatures needs an external heat source for compensation and cannot be compensated by the temperature compensating mechanisms available in the conventional vaporizers.
3. *Low boiling point:* Boiling temperature of desflurane is low, i.e., 22.8°C at 1 atm. Thus desflurane boils at normal room or OT temperature making its output uncontrollable in variable bypass type of vaporizer.

Q. 20. Describe TEC 6 vaporizer used for desflurane delivery.
Ans. TEC 6 is an electrically heated, pressurized vaporizer specially designed for the delivery of desflurane. Its internal design and mode of operation are different from conventional variable bypass vaporizers.

TEC 6 is plenum type and gas-vapor blende, saturated vapor generator, injection type, electrically supplied heat, specific to desflurane, out of circuit **(Fig. 2)**.

Capacity: 390 mL

It has a concentration dial which is calibrated with graduation of 1% from 1 to 10% and 2% from 10 to 18%. This concentration dial will be in standby mode during warm-up. At front, it has an agent level indicator and 5 light emitting diode (LED) lights (operational, no output, low agent, warm-up, alarm battery low). Operational LED shows amber for warm-up, green for operative, and red for no output.

WORKING PRINCIPLE

The vaporizer has two independent circuits (one for vapor and other for fresh gas flow) placed in a parallel position. The fresh gas passes through a fixed restrictor (R_1) and vapor passes through a concentration control valve (R_2) which is controlled by the operator. Both fresh gas and vapor join at the vaporizer outlet.

The desflurane sump is electrically heated to 39°C to produce vapor of approximately 1,300 mm Hg. When concentration dial is on, it opens shut-off valve. Pressure-regulating valve regulates background gas pressure. The differential pressure transducer senses a difference in the pressure exerted by fresh gas and vapor and relays it to control electronic system. The control electronic system adjusts the pressure regulating valve so that pressure in the vapor circuit and fresh gas circuit becomes equal. This tuning of pressure regulating valve occurs if there is a change in fresh gas flow rate or concentration dial setting.

Q. 21. Discuss the Aladin Cassette vaporizer.
Ans. Aladin Cassette is plenum type, variable bypass; flow over with wick, electronically temperature compensated, out of circuit, injection type, color-coded, and agent-specific.

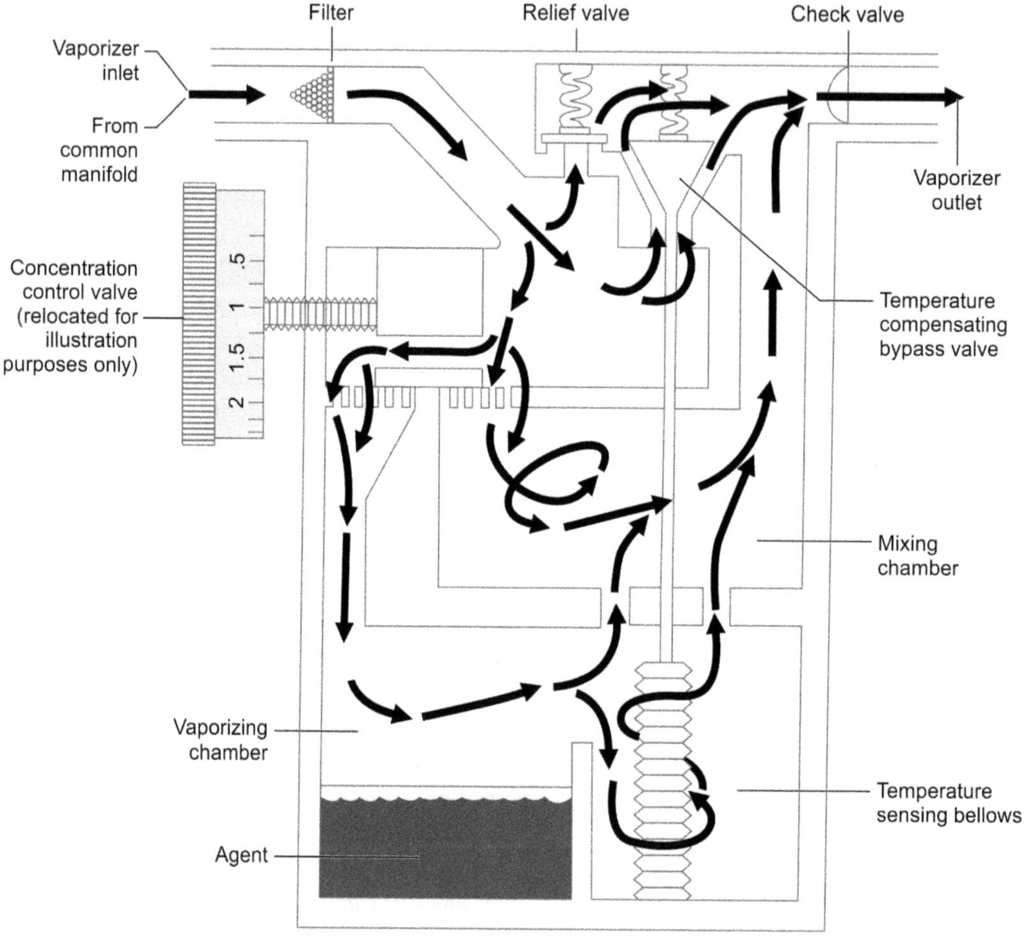

Fig. 2: Schematic diagram of TEC 6 vaporizer.

Capacity: 250 mL

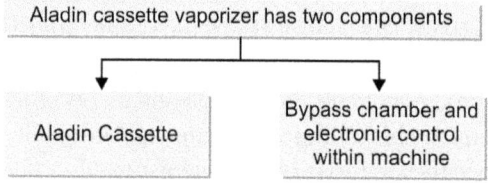

Aladin cassette vaporizer has two components

- Aladin Cassette
- Bypass chamber and electronic control within machine

ALADIN CASSETTE

Parts of Cassette are as follows:

- *Front:*
  - Filling port
  - Prismatic slide glass
  - Handle with lock
  - Handle release
  - Magnetic sensors
  - Temperature sensors
- *Back:*
  - Inflow port
  - Outflow port
  - Temperature sensor.

WORKING PRINCIPLE

As the bypass chamber is inside the anesthesia machine, only vaporizing chamber gas flows into the cassette. The resistor in the bypass controls the gas flows through the cassette which in turn is controlled by temperature and pressure sensors along with flowmeters and dialed agent concentration in contrast to conventional vaporizers which are mechanically controlled.

It also works with desflurane.

Q. 22. What are the advantages of Aladin Cassette over other vaporizers?
Ans.
- Lightweight
- Works at low fresh gas flows and over a wide range of ambient temperatures
- Provide minimum oxygen centration, hence preventing hypoxic mixture delivery to the patient
- Audible alarm if the level of agent falls below 10%
- Electronic control
- Low maintenance.

Q. 23. Enumerate different filling systems with examples.
Ans.
- Draw over vaporizers: Goldman, Boyle's
- Screw fill: Plenum vaporizers
- Key fill system
- Easy fill system: TEC 7
- Quik fill
- Saf-T-Fil: TEC 6.

FURTHER READING

1. Davey A, Diba A. Ward's Anesthetic Equipment, 5th edition.
2. Dorsch JA, Dorsch SE. Understanding Anesthesia Equipment, 5th edition.

CHAPTER 50

Breathing Circuits

Richa Saroa, Sanjeev Palta, Deepika Gupta, Chaitra TS

Q. 1. What is a breathing circuit and who invented it?

Ans. A breathing circuit constitutes an assembly that helps connect the patient's airway with an anesthesia machine or ventilator and creates an artificial atmosphere to deliver the mixture of gases to the patient and remove out the exhaled gases. Gas flow occurs at respiratory pressures and controlled composition of gaseous mixture is dispensed.

The breathing circuits were first described by Sir William Wellesley Mapleson who explained five breathing circuits: A, B, C, D, and E in 1954. A 6th circuit "The Jackson Rees (JR) modification" of Ayre's T-piece; (F) was later described in 1975 by Willis, Pender, and Mapleson.

Q. 2. What is the purpose of the breathing systems?

Ans. The purpose of the breathing systems is:
- Oxygen delivery to the patient
- Deliver inhalational anesthetic agent
- Remove carbon dioxide (CO_2)
- Provide a method for assisted or controlled ventilation
- Provide ports for the sampling of gaseous mixture and pressure as well flow and volume monitoring.

Q. 3. What are the basic requirements desired of a breathing system?

Ans. The breathing ideally should be able to cater to the following requirements:

- Certain characteristics that should be definitely catered to, include:
  - Deliver gases from the machine to the alveoli in the same concentration as set by the anesthesiologist in the shortest possible time.
  - It should eliminate CO_2 effectively and prevent rebreathing.
  - It should possess minimal apparatus dead space.
  - It should have low resistance.
- The desirable factors include:
  - The circuit is lightweight and inexpensive
  - Regulation of temperature and humidity of the gaseous mixtures
  - Circuit accounts for the economy of the anesthetic gases
  - Efficient for both spontaneous and controlled ventilation
  - Efficient at low fresh gas flow and hence minimize wastage of gases
  - Suitable for both adults and children
  - Provision to reduce theater pollution.

Q. 4. What are the general principles for working of breathing systems?

Ans. The working of a breathing system involves the basics of principles of physics as integral to anesthesia as discussed here.
- *Resistance:* While gas passes through a tube, the pressure at the distal end is lower than that at the proximal end.

A drop in pressure is an indirect measure of resistance required to overcome the movement to be overcome as the gas moves. Resistance varies with volume of gas passing through per unit of time. Hence flow rate is important when talking about resistance.

- *Flow rate* is either laminar or turbulent depending upon the Reynolt's number.
  - *Laminar flow:* Flow is smooth and orderly and particles move parallel to the walls of the tube with flow being faster in the center secondary to less friction.

    The Hagen–Poiseuille law applies in a laminar flow that is as follows:

    $$\Delta P = (L \times v \times V)/r^4$$

    Where "r" is the radius of the tube, "ΔP" is the pressure gradient across the tube, "v" is the viscosity of the gas, "L" is the length, and "V" is the flow rate. Resistance is directly proportional to the flow rate during laminar flow.
  - *Turbulent flow:* The flow lines are no longer parallel and the particles move across or opposite the general direction of flow. Flow rate is same across the entire length of the tube. As with laminar flow, the factors responsible for the pressure drop along the tube are similar for turbulent flow. However, gas density becomes more important than viscosity.

    $$P = (L \times V^2 \times K)/r^5$$

    In this equation, "K" is a constant that includes such factors as gravity, friction, gas density, and viscosity. Resistance is proportional to the square of the flow rate with turbulent flow.
- *Significance of resistance:* Resistance imposes a strain on the patient and thus affects the work of breathing. Changes in resistance can be depicted by flow-volume loops.
  - *Compliance:* It is the ratio of change in volume to the change in pressure. It is a measure of distensibility. It can be measured by pressure-volume loop.
  - *Rebreathing:* It essentially refers to inhaling the previously expired gas. Rebreathing may be partial or complete and may or may not be associated with raised CO_2 concentration.

Q. 5. What are the components/arrangement of Mapelson's breathing circuits?

Ans. There are five components of Mapelson's breathing circuits that include:

1. *The breathing tubes:* usually large bore, corrugated, preferably clear and lightweight. May be made of plastic or rubber.
2. *Adjustable pressure limiting (APL) valve:* It is a one-way adjustable spring-loaded valve and that helps the exhaled gases to exit and pops up in case the pressure exceeds the maximum limits.
3. *Reservoir bag:* Most distensible part of the circuit and acts as a reservoir for the fresh gas flow. Used to deliver assisted or controlled breaths to the patient. It is made up of plastic or rubber. The capacity of the reservoir bag is usually 2 L for adults though 1 L is available for pediatric use. The JR circuit has a reservoir bag of 500 mL.
4. *Fresh gas flow (FGF) end:* It is connected to the oxygen delivery source (anesthesia workstation, machine, or cylinder via flow meter).
5. *The patient end* is fitted to a face mask or endotracheal tube via a 15 mm connector.

Section 3: Anesthesia Instruments

Q. 6. How do you classify and identify Mapelson's breathing circuits?

Ans. They are called flow control breathing circuits. They are classified into A, B, C, D, and E. Later on circuit type F was added. They all potentially allow rebreathing and are called semiclosed or semiopen circuits. These systems are therefore defined in terms of fresh gas flow (FGF) needed to maintain unchanged partial pressure of carbon dioxide ($PaCO_2$) in face of unchanged ventilation.

Q. 7. Describe Mapelson's A system in detail.

Ans. Mapleson A is also called the *Magill's system*. The APL valve is situated at the patient end and the reservoir bag and the fresh gas inlet is situated at the opposite machine end. There is a corrugated tubing of 110 cm in length in between the two ends **(Fig. 1)**.

Technique of use: APL valve is kept fully open in a spontaneously breathing patient and exhaled gases are vented out through the APL valve. While during controlled ventilation the APL valve is partially closed, and sufficient pressure is generated with each positive pressure ventilation that initiates an inspiratory cycle with the APL valve popping up.

Q. 8. What is the modified Mapelson's A circuit and what are its advantages and disadvantages?

Ans. Modified Mapelson circuit is called the *Lack's system* **(Fig. 2)**. Here the expiratory and inspiratory limbs are separate.

- It may be available as:
  - *Coaxial tube system*—expiratory limb is concentrically outside the Inspiratory outer limb.
  - *Parallel tube system*—both the expiratory and inspiratory limbs runs parallel to each other.
- *Advantages:* It facilitates the scavenging of gases and avoids theater pollution.
- *Disadvantages:* It increases the work of breathing.

Q. 9. Describe the functional analysis of Mapelson's A and its checking before use.

Ans.
- *Spontaneous breathing:* During inspiration fresh gas flows from the FGF inlet and reservoir bag flows towards the patient and during expiration FGF moves towards the bag and fills it. The expired gas consisting of alveolar gas and dead space gas also moves towards the bag and fills it. When the reservoir bag is filled the APL valve opens and releases the gas into the atmosphere.

If FGF is more than minute ventilation (70–100 mL/kg/min, i.e., 5–6 L/min) the alveolar and dead space gas which was filled in the bag during expiratory pause will escape through the APL valve but if the FGF is less than the minute ventilation the rebreathing will occur.

System is maximum efficient when the FGF is equal to minute ventilation as the

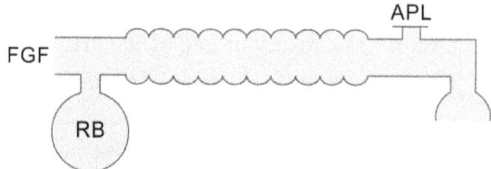

Fig. 1: Mapelson's A circuit.
(APL: adjustable pressure limiting; FGF: fresh gas flow; RB: reservoir bag)

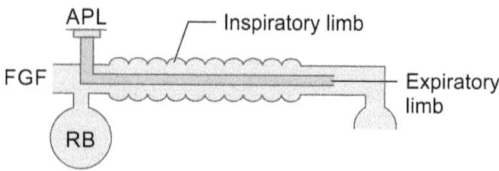

Fig. 2: Lack's system.
(APL: adjustable pressure limiting; FGF: fresh gas flow; RB: reservoir bag)

maximum alveolar gas is vented out and dead space gas which was not used in the previous breath is rebreathed and used in the next breath.
- *Controlled breathing:* The APL is partially closed. During inspiration, patient receives FGF and part of it is ventilated out by the APL valve. During expiration fresh gas flows into the bag along with the expired gas gets accumulated and leads to rebreathing. Controlled ventilation should be avoided with this circuit and only be practiced in presence of end tidal carbon dioxide ($EtCO_2$) monitoring.
- *Checking:* Occlude the patient end and close the APL valve and then pressurize the system by connecting to the O_2 inlet. APL valve can be checked by opening and closing it.

In Lack's system integrity of the inner tube needs to be confirmed. It can be checked by keeping the APL valve closed and connecting the inner tubing to the patient and blowing down the tube and movement of the bag will occur if there is a leak between two tubes. The other method is to occlude both limbs and squeeze the bag with the APL valve open the breach of inner tubing will allow the air to escape via the APL valve **(Figs. 3 and 4)**.

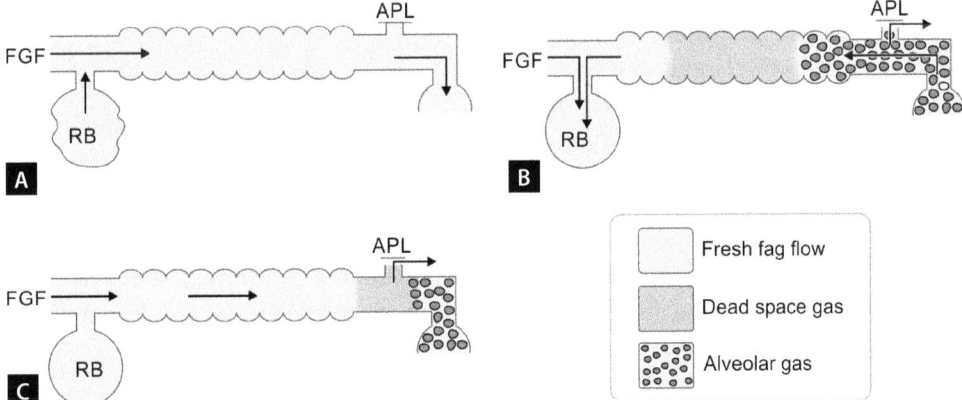

Figs. 3A to C: Functional analysis of Mapelson's A circuit—spontaneous breathing: (A) Inspiration; (B) Expiration; (C) Expiratory pause.
(APL: adjustable pressure limiting; FGF: fresh gas flow; RB: reservoir bag)

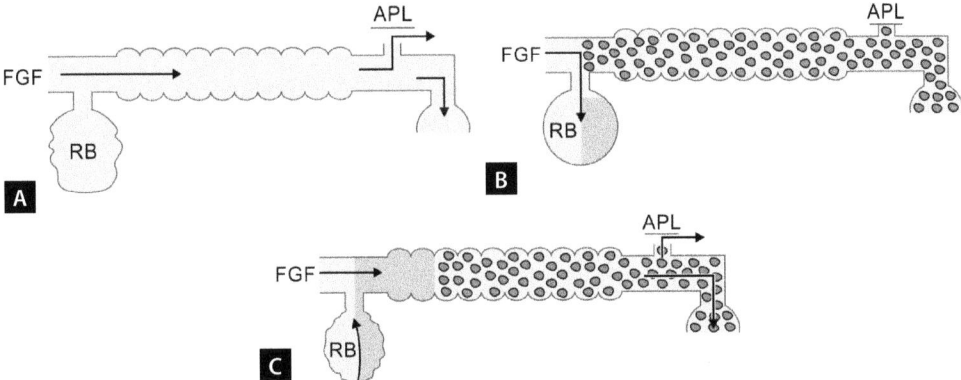

Figs. 4A to C: Controlled ventilatlation—(A) Inspiration; (B) Expiration; (C) Next inspiration.
(APL: adjustable pressure limiting; FGF: fresh gas flow; RB: reservoir bag)

Q. 10. What are the advantages and disadvantages of Mapelson's A breathing circuit?

Ans.

Advantages:
- Adequate flow causes no rebreathing and hence the best circuit for spontaneous respiration.
- Less FGF is required.

Disadvantages:
- Mechanical ventilation should not be used as the whole circuit becomes dead space.
- Theater pollution and wastage of gases by Magills system.

Q. 11. What are Mapelson's B and C circuits?

Ans. The FGF and the APL valve are on the patient end and the reservoir bag is at the machine end of the circuit. Both are the same but there is no corrugated tubing in the Mapelson's C circuit. They are not routinely used but may be used in emergency situations **(Figs. 5 and 6)**.

- *Disadvantages*:
  - High FGF is required (20–25 L/min)
  - Theater pollution is maximum
  - Wastage of gases is much

Q. 12. What is Mapelson's D system?

Ans. It has a T-piece near the patient end. FGF is supplied by a 6 mm tube near the patient end. T-piece is connected to the patient end and another limb is connected to wide-bore corrugated tubing to which reservoir bag is attached and APL valve is positioned near the bag. This circuit is most efficient during controlled ventilation **(Fig. 7)**.

Q. 13. What is Bains modification of Mapelson's D circuit and describe its working in detail?

Ans. In 1972 Bain and Sporel introduced this circuit. FGF tubing runs coaxially inside the clear transparent corrugated tubing. The Length of the circuit is 1.8 cm and can be modified according to the working requirement. The diameter of outer tubing is 22 mm and inner-tubing is 7 mm **(Fig. 8)**.

- *Technique of use:*
  - *Spontaneous respiration*: APL valve is fully opened and expired gas is exhaled out thru APL and FGF is delivered to the patient.

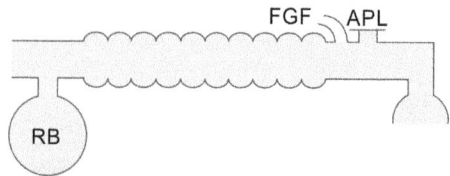

Fig. 5: Mapelson's B circuit.
(APL: adjustable pressure limiting; FGF: fresh gas flow; RB: reservoir bag)

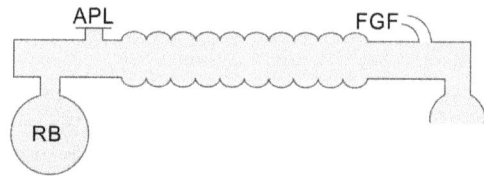

Fig. 7: Mapelson's D circuit.
(APL: adjustable pressure limiting; FGF: fresh gas flow; RB: reservoir bag)

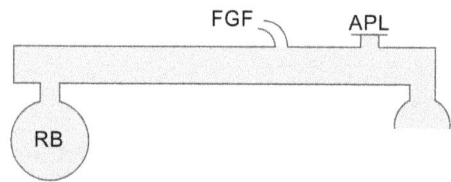

Fig. 6: Mapelson's C circuit.
(APL: adjustable pressure limiting; FGF: fresh gas flow; RB: reservoir bag)

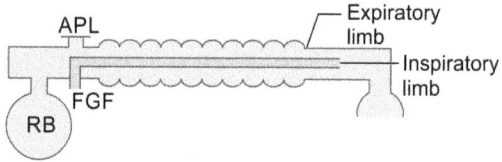

Fig. 8: Mapelson's D Bains circuit.
(APL: adjustable pressure limiting; FGF: fresh gas flow; RB: reservoir bag)

- *Controlled ventilation:* The patient is ventilated with the help of a bag while keeping the APL valve partially closed. FGF should be kept at 1.5–2 times the minute ventilation. Mechanical ventilator can be connected if required in place of reservoir bag.

Q. 14. Describe the functional analysis of Mapelson's D and its checking before use.

Ans.

- *Spontaneous respiration:* During inspiration FGF goes to the patient and during expiration, the expired gas is mixed with the FGF in the corrugated tubing and gets filled into the reservoir bag. During expiratory pause, FGF continues to fill the proximal part of the circuit. In the next breath, the patient inhales the mixed gases. If the FGF is 1.5–2 times the minute volume patient will inhale the FGF but if it is less it will inhale the mixture.
- *Controlled ventilation:* Adjustable pressure limiting valve is partly closed during expiration to facilitate the controlled ventilation. During inspiration, patient breathes FGF and during expiation, the exhaled gases are mixed with the FGF in the corrugated tubing. During expiratory pause the FGF in the tubing pushes the exhaled gases to the reservoir bag, as the bag is squeezed the exhaled gases escape via the APL valve. Depending on the FGF the patient will breathe the mixed gases or the fresh gas if the FGF is >1.5–2 times the minute ventilation or if the expiratory pause is increased in between. Recommended FGF is 70–100 mL/kg/min with a tidal volume of 10 mL/kg and a rate of 10–14 breaths/min.
- *Checking of the system:*
  - It can be checked by pressurizing the system after occluding the patient end and closing the APL valve. Easy deflation of the bag after opening the APL will check the integrity of the APL valve.
  - Checking the integrity of the outer tube wet the hands with spirit and blows through the tube and swipes the tube with wet hands. Leak in the tube will feel the air in the hand swiped.
  - Checking the integrity of inner tube setting a low flow on and occluding the inner tube and observes the flow meter indicator. If the inner tube is connected correctly and intact the indicator will fall.
  - Pathick's test—this is to check the integrity of the inner tube. Activate the oxygen flush and observe the bag. Due to the Venturi effect, the high flow from the inner tube at the patient end will create a negative pressure in the outer exhalation tubing and this will suck gas from the bag and the bag will deflate. If the inner tube is not intact, this maneuver will cause the bag to inflate slightly **(Figs. 9 and 10)**.

Q. 15. What are the advantages and disadvantages of the Bains circuit?

Ans.

Advantages:

- Lightweight as compared to other Magills circuits.
- A transparent circuit allows easy visibility of the tubes.
- Low resistance.
- It can be used in both spontaneous and controlled ventilation and can be connected to a ventilator easily.
- It is useful in patients for anesthesia in remote locations like magnetic resonance imaging (MRI) suits.
- APL valve is situated at the other end hence does not make the tube end heavy

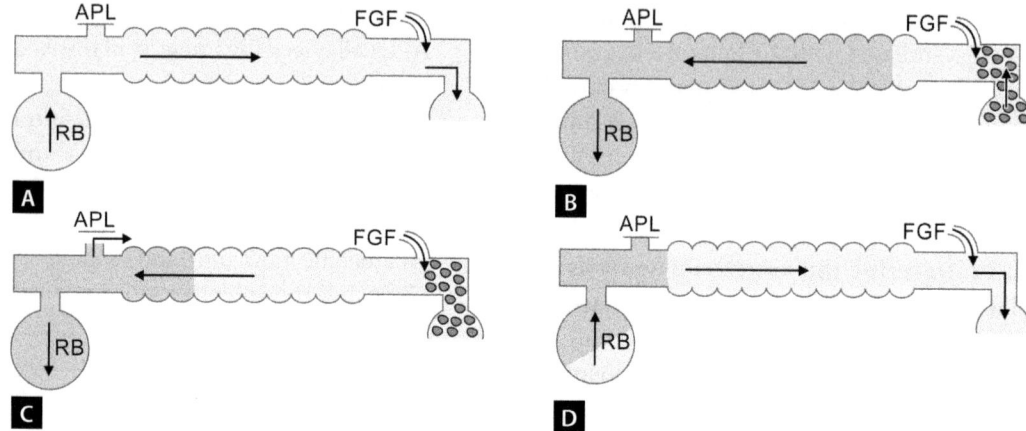

Figs. 9A to D: Functional analysis of Mapelson's D circuit—spontaneous breathing: (A) Inspiration; (B) Expiration; (C) Expiratory pause; (D) Next inspiration.

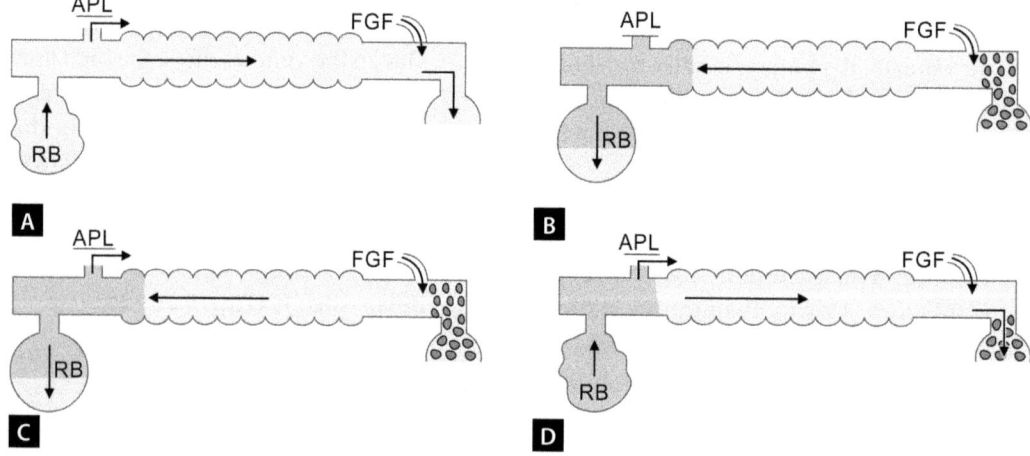

Figs. 10A to D: Functional analysis of Mapelson's D circuit—controlled ventilation with Mapelson's D circuit: (A) Inspiration; (B) Expiration; (C) Expiratory pause; (D) Next inspiration.

and exhaled gases, not near the surgical plane, hence no risk of fires.
- For easy scavenging, the scavenging valve is at the machine end.
- Some warming of the inspired gases as the inspiratory tubing is inside the expiratory tubing.

Disadvantages:
- Multiple connections make the circuit liable for wrong connections and disconnections.
- Scavenging systems are needed for preventing theater pollution.
- Higher FGF is required.
- It cannot be used in pediatric population weight <20 kg.

Q. 16. What is Mapelson's E circuit?

Ans. It is also known as Ayre's T-piece and was invented in 1937. It functions as a nonrebreathing circuit. Fresh gas flow enters via side-arm and expired gas is vented out via one side and there is no rebreathing. It does not have a bag and an APL valve. It is used mostly in spontaneously breathing patients. Rebreathing depends on the length of the expiratory limb and the fresh gas flow.

Disadvantage: Difficult for scavenging of gases and high fresh gas flow required, hence its use in anesthesia has decreased **(Fig. 11)**.

Q. 17. What is Mapelson's F circuit and where it is mostly used?

Ans. It is also known as the *Jackson Rees circuit* or Jackson Rees modification of T-piece. It has a breathing bag along with the APL valve.

It may also have a hole in the bag which can be regulated with a finger and help to release excess of gases or may be fitted with an APL valve. It has a 500 mL bag attached to the expiratory limb which helps in monitoring of respiration or assisted breathing.

It is mostly used in pediatric patients with a weight <20 kg and an age of <5 years **(Fig. 12)**.

Q. 18. What is the technique of use of Mapelson's F circuit and its functional analysis?

Ans.
- *Technique of use:* During spontaneous respiration, the valve is kept fully open. During assisted respiration, the bag is kept distended by altering the diameter of the valve with the fingers and help with assisted respiration.
- *Functional analysis:* It works like a Mapelson's D circuit. To prevent rebreathing flows required 2.5–3 times the minute ventilation during spontaneous ventilation and 1.5–2 times minute ventilation during controlled ventilation. During expiration the fresh gas and exhaled gas collect in the expiratory limb. It is replaced by fresh gas during the expiratory pause and during the next inhalation patient will inhale fresh gas both from exhaled limb and fresh gas supply. As compared to the pediatric circle system work of breathing is less. Increased in resistance when heat moisture exchanger is attached to a breathing circuit.

Q. 19. What are the advantages and disadvantages of Mapelson's E and F system?

Ans.
Advantages:
- Inexpensive
- Easy to assemble
- Low resistance (due to absence of valves).

Disadvantages:
- High fresh gas flow required
- Atmospheric pollution.

Q. 20. What are the advantages and disadvantages of Mapelson's system?

Ans.
Advantages:
- They are simple and inexpensive instruments.
- They can be easily sterilized and disinfected and easy to disassemble.
- They are light weight and easy to use and cause minimal drag on the endotracheal tube.
- Warming and humidification of gases occur in coaxial systems (Bains and Lacks).
- Length of the circuits can be modified for use in remote locations like MRI.

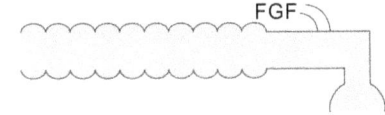

Fig. 11: Mapelson's E circuit.

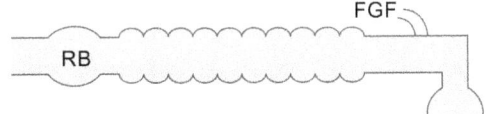

Fig. 12: Mapelson's F circuit.

- Resistance in these circuits is relatively low.
- Due to lack of CO_2 absorbent, there is no production of toxic metabolites like compound A.

Disadvantages:
- The systems require high FGF and hence higher cost.
- Scavenging of gases is difficult and hence leads to atmospheric pollution.
- It is difficult to determine optimum fresh gas flow so as to avoid wastage and rebreathing.
- There is difficulty in scavenging while using Mapelson's E and F and air dilutions can occur with it.
- Mapelson's circuits are difficult to use in patients with malignant hyperthermia as it is difficult to increase FGF enough to decrease CO_2 load.

FURTHER READING

1. Dorsch JA, Dorsch SE. Mapleson breathing system. In: Understanding Anesthesia Equipment, 5th edition. Philadelphia: Williams and Wilkins; 2008. pp. 209-21.
2. Kaul TK, Mittal G. Mapleson's breathing systems. Indian J Anaesth. 2013;57(5):507-15.

CHAPTER 51

Manual Resuscitators

Ajeet Kumar, Kunal Singh, Chandni Sinha

Q. 1. What is a manual resuscitator?
Ans.
- Manual resuscitator is a hand-held device used to provide ventilatory support and supplemental oxygenation to patients with respiratory failure or arrest.
- It is also referred to as *Ambu bag, bag valve mask apparatus,* and *self-inflating resuscitation systems.*
- It was first developed by German engineer Holger Hesse and his partner Henning Ruben in 1953 and was named as an artificial manual breathing unit (AMBU), which was manufactured and marketed since 1956 by their company. Now there are several manufacturers which produce self-inflating bag resuscitators.
- It is an integral part of resuscitation kits used in both in and out of hospital settings.

Q. 2. What are the uses of a manual resuscitator?
Ans. Ventilating by using a manual resuscitator is a basic airway management skill that allows for oxygenation and ventilation of patients until a definitive airway can be established. Various uses of manual resuscitator are:
- Ventilating patient during cardiopulmonary resuscitation
- Transport of the critically ill patients
- Administration of high flow oxygen
- Providing controlled ventilation in patients with respiratory arrest
- Augmentation of spontaneous ventilation in patients of respiratory failure.

Q. 3. What are the components of a manual resuscitator?
Ans. Manual ventilators are composed of the following parts:
- Self-refilling bag
- Nonrebreathing valve
- Bag inlet valve
- Oxygen enrichment device
- Pressure limiting device for pediatric bags.

Self-refilling bag: It is made of silicone rubber or polyvinyl chloride material and is usually oval or cylindrical in shape. The bag remains inflated in its resting state. It is compressed during inhalation and the bag reinflates to its normal position during exhalation. The rate of re-expansion of the bag determines the maximum minute volume.

Nonrebreathing valve: This valve ensures unidirectional flow of gas thus preventing the mixing of fresh gas and exhaled gases. Opening of the valve allows fresh gas flow from the self-refilling bag to enter the patient during inspiration. The patient's exhaled gases are released into the atmosphere at the end of inhalation with the closure of the valve. Various designs of this valve are available, fish mouth valve is the most commonly used valve.

Bag inlet valve: The gas inlet valve is located opposite to the nonrebreathing valve of the self-refilling bag. The gas inlet has a one-way valve, which opens during exhalation when the bag is refilling and closes when the bag is squeezed during inhalation.

Oxygen enrichment device: The purpose of reservoir is to store the oxygen during the inhalation phase and release the stored oxygen into the self-refilling bag during the exhalation. The inspired oxygen concentration of the system can be significantly increased by attaching the oxygen enrichment device.

Pressure limiting device: A pressure relief valve prevents accidental over-pressurization of the lungs and protects against barotrauma. It is typically included in pediatric versions whereas in adult resuscitators it is optional.

Q. 4. Describe the functional analysis of a manual resuscitator.
Ans. The manual resuscitator consists of a compressible self-inflating bag, an inspiratory valve, and a bag inlet valve.

When the bag is compressed by the operator it creates positive pressure. The air inside the bag then opens the inspiratory valve by pushing it downward, the expiratory port is blocked and the air within the silicone bag is delivered to the patient. At this time the inlet valve is closed due to pressure build-up inside the bag.

When the self-inflating bag is released, it re-expands creating a negative pressure inside. This pushes the inspiratory valve upward and keeps it in a close position and the exhaled air is released through the exhalation port. At the same time, the inlet valve is opened by the negative pressure created by releasing the bag and sends the oxygen into the self-inflating bag from the oxygen reservoir through the inlet valve till the bag returns to its original shape. If an oxygen reservoir is not attached to the bag, then air will be entailed into the bag from the atmosphere.

Q. 5. How do you use a manual resuscitator for ventilating patients?
Ans.
- A manual resuscitator must deliver between 400–500 mL of air to an adult patient's lungs.
- A target rate of 10 BPM should be achieved.
- High-flow supplemental oxygen, if available is connected to the reservoir bag.

Q. 6. How do you check a manual resuscitator?
Ans.
- *Visual inspection:* Manual resuscitator should be thoroughly inspected for any damage before use.
- *Leak in the bag:* It can be checked by occluding the nonrebreathing valve outlet at the patient end and then compressing the self-inflating bag. The bag should not compress easily if there is no leak.
- *Bag inlet valve:* The bag should be squeezed and the patient port should be blocked. The bag should expand immediately once the pressure is released from it.
- *Nonrebreathing valve:* The test lung is connected to the patient port, compressing the bag should open the nonrebreathing

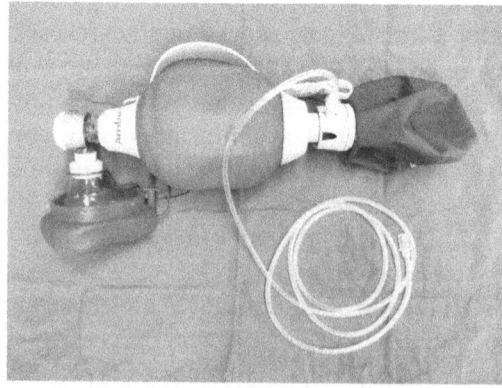

Fig. 1: Bag valve mask ventilation.

valve and the test lung should fill. When the pressure is released, the nonrebreathing valve should close and as the test lung deflates, gas should flow through the expiratory ports.
- *Oxygen reservoir:* It can be checked by multiple compression cycles without the oxygen flow to the reservoir. The reservoir should deflate and the self-inflating bag should expand.

Q. 7. What are the complications of bag valve mask ventilation (Fig. 1)?

Ans.
- Over-ventilating or hyperventilation
- Aspiration
- Barotrauma

FURTHER READING

1. Dorsch JA, Dorsch SE. Understanding Anaesthesia Equipment, 5th edition.

52. Humidification Equipment

Chandni Sinha, Abhinav Prakash, Pratik Singh

Q. 1. Explain the following terms.
Ans.
- *Humidity:* The amount of water vapor in gas.
- *Absolute humidity:* It is the mass of water vapor present in a volume of gas (milligrams of water per liter of gas).
- *Relative humidity:* It is the amount of water vapor at a particular temperature. It is expressed as a percentage of the amount that would be held if the gas were saturated.
- *Humidity at saturation:* It is the maximum amount of water vapor that a volume of gas can hold. It varies with temperature. It is 44 mg H_2O/L at a body temperature of 37°C.

Q. 2. What are the anesthetic considerations of humidification?
Ans. The upper respiratory tract in humans functions as physiological HME. During normal nasal breathing, the temperature in the upper trachea is between 30 and 33°C providing a relative humidity of approximately 98%. However, in a patient with a tracheal tube or supraglottic device, these physiological checkpoints are bypassed. Apart from this, the medical gases are also free of any water. These factors make humidification an important part of patient care during anesthesia or oxygen therapy.

Q. 3. What are the complications of inhaling dry medical gases?
Ans.
- *Respiratory tract:* Thickening of secretions which may lead to obstruction, infection, and atelectasis, impaired ciliary function, and reduced surfactant activity. It may also cause bronchoconstriction.
- *Body temperature:* Heat is lost as the airways equilibrate the temperature of the inspired gases and saturate it with water.

Q. 4. What are the types of humidification devices?
Ans.

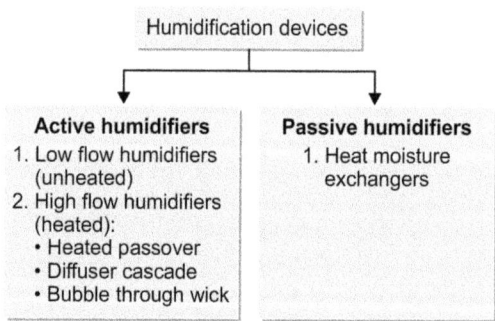

Q. 5. Describe heat moisture exchangers.
Ans. Heat and moisture exchanger (HME) is a device designed to *conserve* moisture and heat and return it to the patient via inspired gases. The exchanging medium is enclosed in a lightweight plastic housing. Some of these devices may also provide bacterial/viral filtration and those are hence called *heat*

moisture exchanging filters (HMEF). There are two types of HME. They are—(1) hygroscopic and (2) hydrophobic.

Hydrophobic HME: These have plated (to increase surface area) hydrophobic membranes with small pores. They provide excellent inspired humidity and are efficient bacterial/viral filters as well. One of the advantages is that the increase in resistance is less even when wet.

Hygroscopic HME: These are coated with moisture-retaining chemicals. Composite hygroscopic HMEs have a thin membrane that's subjected to an electric field to increase its polarity, thereby increasing its filtering efficiency. They are much more efficient than hydrophobic HME. However, their resistance increases significantly when wet.

Q. 6. What are the advantages and disadvantages of HME?

Ans.
Advantages:
- Economical, simple to use, lightweight, and noiseless
- No requirement of external energy, water, monitor, or alarm
- No risk of hyperthermia, electrical shock, or overhydration
- May provide protection from nosocomial infections.

Disadvantages:
- Limited ability to preserve temperature and humidity
- Increases dead space and can cause rebreathing especially when low tidal volumes are used
- Increased work of breathing in a spontaneously breathing patient
- Risk of occlusion due to secretions
- Can be a source of foreign particle aspiration.

Q. 7. What are unheated humidifiers?

Ans. Unheated humidifiers are also known as *passover humidifiers*, these are used to humidify oxygen that is delivered by face masks or nasal cannulas. These are bubble through devices with limited capacity to humidify. They carry a risk of being a source of nosocomial infections such as *Pseudomonas aeruginosa*.

Q. 8. What are heated humidifiers?

Ans. All heated humidifiers incorporate a device to heat the water. Broadly they contain a humidification chamber, heat source, inspiratory tube, and/or a monitor. They are of the following types:
- Heated Passover—medical gases are directed towards a reservoir of hot water.
- Diffuser cascade—similar to bubble humidifier in design, it additionally contains a heat source and increased area for gas-water interface due to the larger diffusion tower.
- Bubble through wick—it consists of a paper or cloth wick through which gases pass.

Q. 9. What are the advantages and disadvantages of heated humidifiers?

Ans.
Advantages:
- Highly efficient
- Provides adequate humidification even at high flow rates
- Some of these can be used for spontaneously breathing and tracheostomized patients.

Disadvantages:
- Bulky and complicated
- Higher maintenance costs
- Electrical and thermal hazard
- Risk of overhydration and water aspiration
- Source of nosocomial infection
- Increased work of breathing.

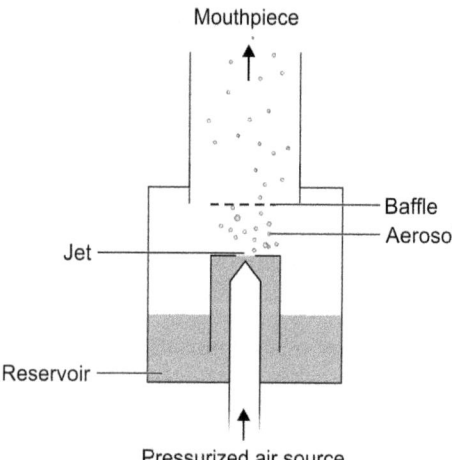

Fig. 1: Pneumatic nebulizer.

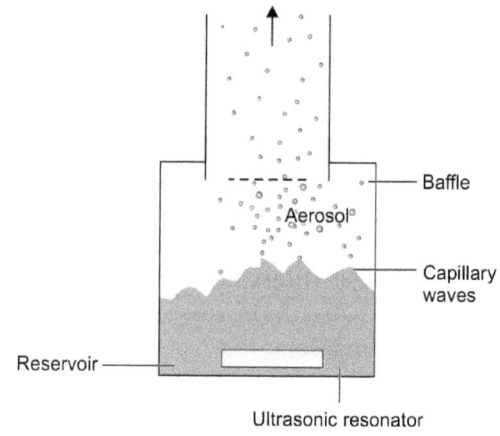

Fig. 2: Ultrasonic nebulizer.

Q. 10. What is a nebulizer? Describe the types of nebulizers.

Ans. A nebulizer is a device that emits water in the form of an aerosol mist. It can be used for humidification as well as delivery of drugs via the breathing system.

There are two types of nebulizers **(Figs. 1 and 2)**:
1. *Pneumatic nebulizer:* Pneumatic nebulizer pushes a jet of high-pressure gas into a liquid which leads to shearing forces. This breaks the water into fine particles and turns it into aerosol mist.
2. *Ultrasonic nebulizer:* The reservoir liquid is subjected to high-frequency oscillations by an electrically driven ultrasonic resonator. It does not require driving gas.

Q. 11. What are the disadvantages associated with nebulizers?

Ans.
- It can act as a source of infection via water droplets.
- There is a risk of overhydration.
- Pneumatic nebulizers require high gas flows; ultrasonic require an energy source and can be an electric hazard.
- Nebulized drugs can block the HME or tubing.

FURTHER READING

1. Davey A, Diba A. Ward's Anesthesia Equipment, 5th edition.

53

Circle System

Abhyuday Kumar, Chandni Sinha, Ajeet Kumar

Q. 1. What are the components of the circle system?

Ans.
- Carbon dioxide (CO_2) absorber canister
- Breathing bag/reservoir bag
- Pressure relief valve/adjustable pressure-limiting (APL) valve
- Inspiratory unidirectional valve
- Expiratory unidirectional valve
- Low resistant interconnecting tubing
- Y-piece
- Fresh gas flow inlet.

Q. 2. What are the advantages of the circle breathing system?

Ans.
- Allows rebreathing of gases after CO_2 absorption making it cost-effective.
- Preserves anesthetic gases and oxygen.
- Preserves heat and moisture.
- Reduces the risk of fire hazards.
- Allows low flow anesthesia.

Q. 3. What are the disadvantages of the circle breathing system?

Ans.
- There is a time lag between the change in the concentration of inhalational agents and its reflection at the patient's end while using low flows.
- There is an increased risk of hypercapnia in the presence of a desiccated absorber.
- Incompetent unidirectional valves.
- Fraction of inspired oxygen (FiO_2) monitoring is mandatory.

Q. 4. What should be the ideal position of the fresh gas inlet, reservoir bag, and APL valve for the efficient functioning of the classic circle system?

Ans.
- *Fresh gas inlet:* Upstream of the inspiratory valve and downstream of the absorber
- *Reservoir bag:* Between the expiratory valve and the absorber
- *APL valve:* Near the reservoir bag, downstream of the expiratory valve, and upstream of the absorber.

The arrangement of components of the classic circle system is shown in **Figure 1**.

Q. 5. What constitutes the dead space in the circle system?

Ans. The dead space of the circle system is from the patient to the Y-piece because of the presence of unidirectional valves. Unlike the Mapleson system, the circle system tube length does not affect the dead space.

Q. 6. What formulations are used in CO_2 absorbents?

Ans. There are various formulations used in CO_2 absorbents:
- *High alkali absorbents:* Contains a higher amount of sodium hydroxide (NaOH) and/or potassium hydroxide (KOH). When desiccated, more likely to form carbon monoxide (CO) with inhalational agents.
- *Low alkali absorbents:* Contains a reduced amount of NaOH and/or KOH.

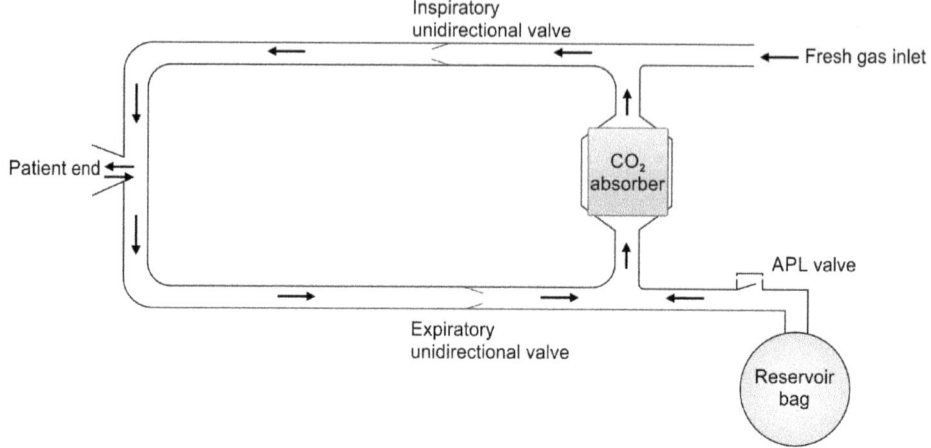

Fig. 1: Classical circle system.
(APL: adjustable pressure-limiting)

- *Alkali free absorbents:* Contains mainly calcium hydroxide $Ca(OH)_2$ with a small amount of other agents. Least likely to form CO or compound A even when desiccated.
- *Lithium hydroxide:* Does not react with anesthetic agents even when desiccated. Costly and harmful to the skin.

Q. 7. What are the components of soda lime?
Ans.
- $Ca(OH)_2$—80%
- $NaOH$—4%
- KOH—1%
- H_2O—15%
- Silica or Kieselguhr—hardening agent
- pH indicator.

Q. 8. What is the general principle on which the absorbent works?
Ans. The general principle is based on an acid neutralized by a base. CO_2, when reacts with the absorbent, it gets converted into *carbonate* and *water*. This is an *exothermic reaction*.

$$CO_2 + H_2O \rightarrow H_2CO_3$$
$$2NaOH + 2H_2CO_3 + Ca(OH)_2 \rightarrow CaCO_3 + Na_2CO_3 + 4H_2O + Heat$$

Q. 9. What indicator is used in absorbent?
Ans.

Indicator	Fresh color	Exhausted color
Phenolphthalein	White	Pink
Ethyl violet	White	Purple
Clayton yellow	Red	Yellow
Ethyl orange	Orange	Yellow
Mimosa Z	Red	White

Ethyl violet is mainly used as an indicator in newer machines (e.g., Dräger).

Q. 10. What should be the shape and size of the CO_2 absorbent?
Ans. CO_2 absorbent should provide a larger surface area and the least resistance. Therefore, they are supplied in pellets or granules. The granule size is measured by mesh number. A 4-mesh strainer has 4 openings per square inch, and 8-mesh has 8 openings per square inch. A 4-mesh granule will pass through a 4-mesh strainer but not through 8-mesh strainers. Granules used in anesthesia are usually of size between 4-mesh and 8-mesh.

Q. 11. What are the different byproducts produced when inhalation agents react with the absorbents?

Ans.

- *Phosgene:* Formed due to reaction with trichloroethylene. It is a pulmonary irritant and can cause ARDS.
- *BCDFE (bromochlorodifluoroethylene):* Formed due to reaction of soda-lime with halothane.
- *Carbon monoxide:* Formed due to reaction between desflurane and dry Baralyme. There were reports of carboxyhemoglobinemia at the start of the Monday morning operating session due to unused anesthetic machines having been left switched on over the weekend, thereby allowing drying of the Baralyme.
- *Compound A [fluoromethyl-2, 2-difluoro-1-(trifluoromethyl) vinyl ether]:* Formed due to reaction with sevoflurane on low fresh gas flows. Studies on rats showed that compound A causes acute tubular necrosis at concentrations in excess of 250 ppm. There is a practical margin of safety in humans as the concentration in low flow typically reaches only around 15 ppm. Food and Drug Administration (FDA) has set up a limit for the use of sevoflurane with a flow of 1 L/min with a 2-monitored anesthesia care (MAC) hour exposure. However, many countries have abandoned their flow restrictions.

Q. 12. How can the production of CO in the absorbers be decreased?

Ans. Emergency care research institute recommendations:

- When the machine is not in use, the gases have to be turned off.
- Change the absorbent regularly, on Monday morning, for instance.
- Change absorbent whenever the color change indicates exhaustion.
- Change all absorbent, not just 1 canister in a 2-canister system.
- If there is uncertainty regarding the state of hydration, the absorbent has to be changed.
- If compact canisters are used, consider changing them more frequently.

Q. 13. What are low flow, minimum flow, and metabolic flow?

Ans. There is no universally accepted definition of low-flow anesthesia.

Baker has classified the fresh gas flow in the following categories:

- *Medium flow:* 1–2 L/min
- *Low flow:* 500–1,000 mL/min
- *Minimal flow:* 250–500 mL/min
- *Metabolic flow:* about 250 mL/min

However, a flow of less than 2 L/min is considered as a *low-flow* by many.

Q. 14. What are the functions of the reservoir bag?

Ans.

- It allows gas to accumulate during exhalation. This permits rebreathing and allows more economical use of anesthetic gases.
- It provides means of providing assisted or controlled ventilation.
- It helps in monitoring spontaneous ventilation through visual and tactile observation.
- It protects the lungs from excessive pressure in the breathing system due to its distensible properties.

The volume of the breathing bag must be greater than the patient's inspiratory capacity. This is estimated at 30 mL/kg bodyweight.

Q. 15. Which method is used to check the integrity of the outer circuit of the circle system?

Ans. *Leak test:* The patient end of the breathing circuit is occluded, the APL valve is fully closed, and the fresh gas flow is set to zero. The breathing circuit is pressurized to 30 cm of H_2O by using the O_2 flush. Drop-in airway pressure to <30 cm of H_2O within 10 seconds indicates a leak in the system. This should be performed before every use.

FURTHER READING

1. Dorsch JA, Dorsch SE. Understanding Anesthesia Equipment, 5th Edition. Philadelphia: Lippincott/Williams and Wilkins; 2007.
2. Herbert L, Magee P. Circle systems and low-flow anaesthesia. BJA Educ. 2017;17(9): 301-5.
3. Parthasarathy S. The closed circuit and the low flow systems. Indian J Anaesth. 2013; 57(5):516-24.

CHAPTER 54

Face Masks and Airways

Prachi Agrawal, Amit Kohli

FACE MASKS

Introduction

Face masks are devices that allow the administration of gases to the patient from the breathing system without introducing any apparatus into the patient's mouth.

They are of two types:
1. Open face mask
2. Closed face mask

Open Face Mask

These are devices used to deliver supplemental Oxygen, have no tight seal and additional holes for exhalation are present. For example, Hudson mask and variable performance oxygen delivery device.

Closed/Anesthetic Face Mask

These are masks that lead to the effective administration of gases. They are made up of several materials:
- Black rubber—reusable, autoclavable, antistatic
- Silicone—reusable, autoclavable, transparent, latex-free
- PVC—disposable, clear, single-use
- Thermoplastic elastomer—copolymers of plastic and rubber; clear, single-use
- Combination of the above, e.g., silicone + polysulfone.

The dead space of a face mask depends upon the pressure applied in holding the mask and the level of inflation of the cuff.

The various parts of an anesthetic face mask are shown and described in **Figure 1** and **Box 1**, respectively.

Steps to choose the right size of face mask:
- The mask should sit over the bridge of the patient's nose with the upper border aligned with the pupils.

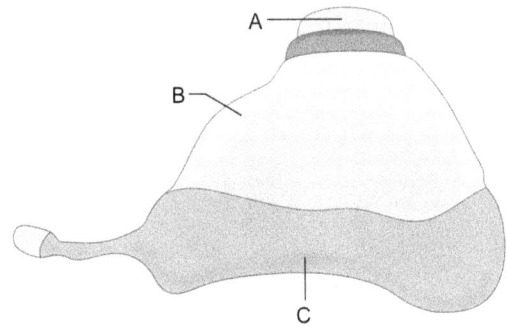

Fig. 1: Parts of an anesthetic face mask—(A) Connector, (B) Body, and (C) Seal.

BOX 1: Important parts of an anesthetic face mask (Fig. 1).

A	Orifice, connector, collar, mount (internal diameter of 22 mm)
B	Body, shell, dome [Types: (1) Transparent and (2) rubber/silicone]
C	Rim, seal, edge [Types: (1) Cushion and (2) flap]

- Sides should seal just lateral to the nasolabial folds.
- Bottom of the face mask sitting between the lower lip and chin.

Types of Face Masks

Face masks come in various sizes, shapes, and materials. There are specific face masks that facilitate additional functions.

- *Clear, disposable masks:* A transparent body allows observation for vomitus, secretions, blood, lip color, and exhaled moisture **(Fig. 2)**. A transparent mask may be better accepted by a conscious patient.
  - Anatomical rubber masks.
- *Rendell-Baker-Soucek masks* **(Fig. 3)**: Specially designed for pediatric patients, may have pacifiers/scents and have a low dead space.
- *Endoscopic masks* **(Fig. 4)**: It has a central silicone membrane removable and interchangeable with four sizes of a hole in the membrane (2, 3, 5, 10 mm), and comes in four sizes—0, 1, 2, and 3.
- Ideal for procedures such as fiber optic bronchoscopy (FOB), gastroscopy, and transesophageal endoscopy (TEE).
- *Scented masks:* The scent may be incorporated into the mask by the manufacturer or applied to the mask by the anesthesia provider.

Uses of a Face Mask (Tables 1 and 2)

- Preoxygenation
- Inhalational induction of anesthesia

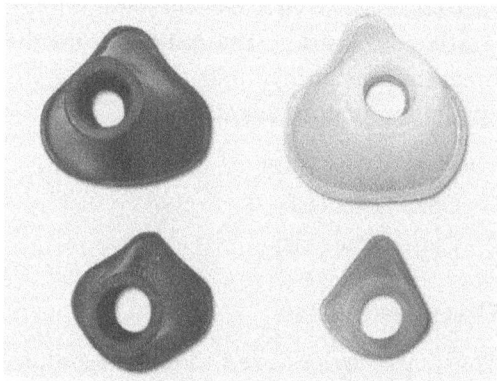

Fig. 3: Rendell–Baker–Soucek masks of various sizes—00, 0, 1, 2.

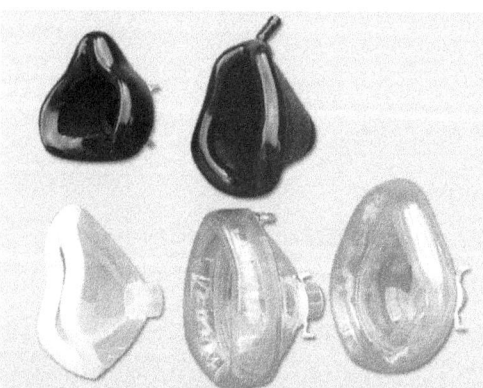

Fig. 2: A selection of face masks. *Top left:* black rubber mask with soft pliable flap; *Top right:* "anatomical" face mask in black rubber with air-filled cushion; *Bottom left:* single-use face mask with flap; *Bottom center:* single-use face mask with adjustable air-filled cushion; *Bottom right:* single-use face mask with prefilled air cushion.

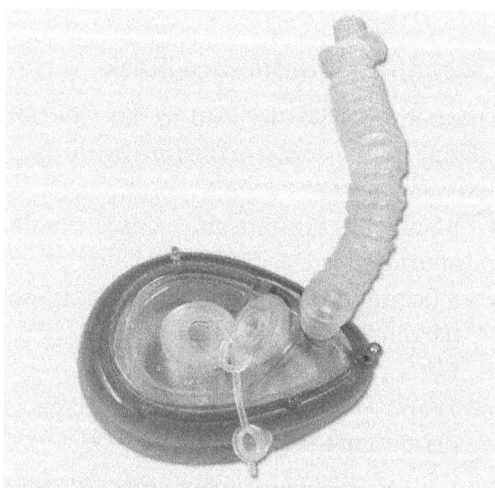

Fig. 4: Endoscopic face mask.

Chapter 54: Face Masks and Airways

TABLE 1: Indicators of a good mask fit and signs of inadequate face mask ventilation.

Indicators of good mask fit	Signs of inadequate face mask ventilation
• Tight seal • Capnography • Bag movement • Expired tidal volume	• Poor chest expansion • Patient cyanosis or low oxygen saturation • Audible gas leak or inability to generate positive pressure with the bag • Absent or poor end-tidal CO_2 trace

TABLE 2: Advantages and disadvantages of using a face mask.

Advantages	Disadvantages
• Good compliance • Low incidence of sore throat • Lesser depth of anesthesia and minimal requirement of muscle relaxant	• Higher gas flows are needed • Need airway manipulation, positioning, and are difficult to maintain for the longer durations • Higher work of breathing in spontaneously breathing patients

- Ventilation prior to intubation
- Maintenance of anesthesia
- Bag and mask ventilation (BMV) during resuscitation
- Noninvasive ventilation for respiratory failure.

Techniques of Mask Ventilation

- One-handed
- Two-handed
- Two-handed with jaw thrust
- Claw hand technique.

Demerits/Complications of Using a Face Mask

- *Skin problems:* Pressure necrosis, dermatitis
- *Nerve injury:* Pressure may lead to transient nerve dysfunction
- *Foreign body aspiration:* Loose parts of the mask, diaphragm of the endoscopic mask
- *Gastric inflation:* Because of positive pressure ventilation
- *Eye injury:* Pressure on the medial angles of the eyes and supraorbital margins may result in eyelid edema, chemosis of the conjunctiva, pressure on the supraorbital, or supratrochlear nerve, corneal injury, and temporary blindness from central retinal artery occlusion
- Latex allergy
- User fatigue
- Postoperative jaw pain.

AIRWAYS

Introduction

An airway is a device that helps to maintain the patency of the passage of air for unobstructed breathing. It can be inserted into the oropharynx or nasopharynx as adjuncts to maneuvers such as head tilt, chin lift, and jaw thrust to facilitate ventilation.

Uses of an Airway

- Prevention of upper airway obstruction.
- Serves as a bite block, and prevents tube occlusion and injury to the tongue.
- Facilitates oropharyngeal suctioning and Ryles tube insertion.
- Provides a better mask fir for ventilation.

Classification of Airways (Table 3)

- *Oropharyngeal airways:*
  - *Guedel's airway:* Size is 0–6 (**Fig. 5**)
  - *Waters' airway:* Size is 00–7
  - Connells airway
  - *Resuscitation airways:*
    - Safar's airway
    - Brook's airway
    - Gordon airway

TABLE 3: Brief description of the various oropharyngeal airways.

S. No.	Oropharyngeal airway		Description
1.	Guedel's airway, Cuffed oropharyngeal airway	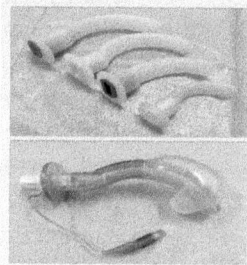	• Guedel: Most frequently used • The cuffed OPA forms a low-pressure seal and can be used for IPPV
2.	Waters' airway	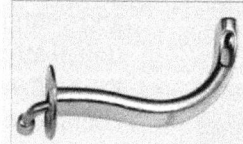	Named after Ralph Waters. Has a side hole for oxygen attachment and suctioning
3.	Connell's airway	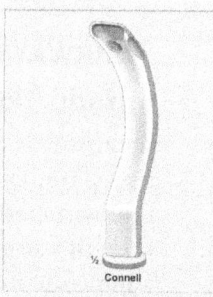	Similar to Waters, however, a port for oxygen insufflation is absent
4.	Safar's airway	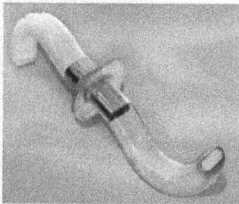	• Described in 1958 by Safar and McMahon • A modification for mouth-to-mouth respiration • Nontraumatic, and made up of soft rubber • Has two sizes of the airway, one for an adult and one for pediatrics each
5.	Brook's airway	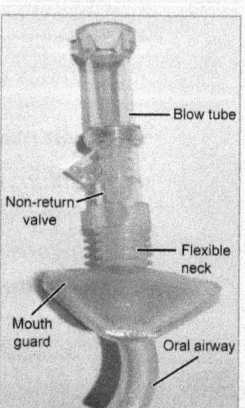	Devised by Morris Brook in 1957. It has a mouth guard, blow tube, flexible neck, and a side exit port for exhaled air to vent out

Contd...

Contd...

S. No.	Oropharyngeal airway		
6.	Gordon's airway	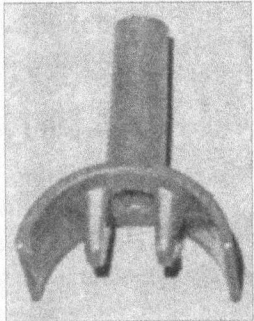	Devised by Archer Gordon. It is an interdental bite block with a flange and a mouthpiece without a valve
7.	Ovassapian airway	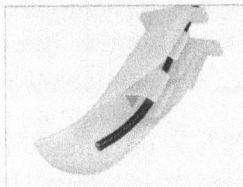	Designed for use during fiberoptic intubation. It has a guide channel and a sidewall
8.	Patil–Syracuse airway	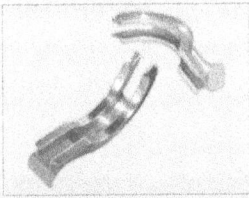	It has side ports for suction, a distal slit for fiberscope manipulation, and a lingual surface
9.	Berman's Intubating airway	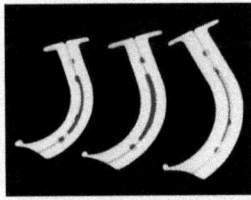	It can be split and removed from around the tube once the tube is placed
10.	Williams airway intubator	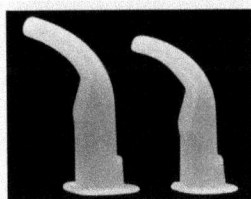	The proximal half is closed and the distal half is open on the lingual side

(IPPV: intermittent positive-pressure ventilation; OPA: oropharyngeal airway)

- Airways that aid in fiberoptic intubation:
    - Ovassapian airway
    - Patil-Syracuse airway
    - Berman's intubating airway
    - Williams airway intubator
- Nasopharyngeal airways:
    - Bardex airway

- Rusch red rubber
- Linder nasopharyngeal airway
- Binasal airway
■ *Modified airways:* Augmented supraglottic devices like laryngeal mask airway.

Oropharyngeal Airways

Parts of an Oropharyngeal Airway

The appropriate airway size is selected by measuring the length corresponding to the vertical distance between the patient's incisors and the angle of the jaw. It can be inserted by using either a tongue depressor and inserted along its concavity, or by using the rotation technique.

Nasopharyngeal Airways (Table 4)

A nasopharyngeal airway also known as a *nasal airway* or *nasal trumpet* is better tolerated than an oral airway if the patient has intact airway reflexes. It consists mainly of an airway channel and a flange that can be adjusted according to the desired length and a distal beveled end **(Fig. 6)**. The appropriate length is calculated by measuring the distance from the tragus of the ear to the tip of the nose.

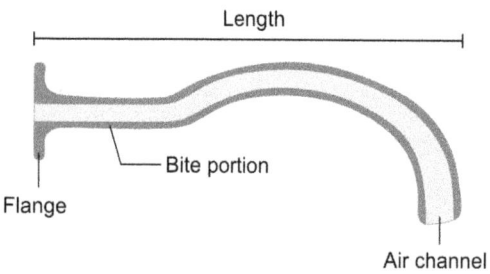

Fig. 5: Parts of the Guedel's airway.

Complications

- *Airway obstruction:* Due to wrong sized airway placement.

TABLE 4: Types of nasopharyngeal airways.

1.	Bardex airway		Made up of rubber, has a large flange (nonadjustable)
2.	Rusch red rubber		Made up of red rubber, with an adjustable flange
3.	Linder nasopharyngeal airway		Made up of plastic, has an introducer, and a leur lock system to inflate the balloon
4.	Binasal airway		Two nasal airways are connected together. It has a 15 mm adaptor for attachment to a breathing system

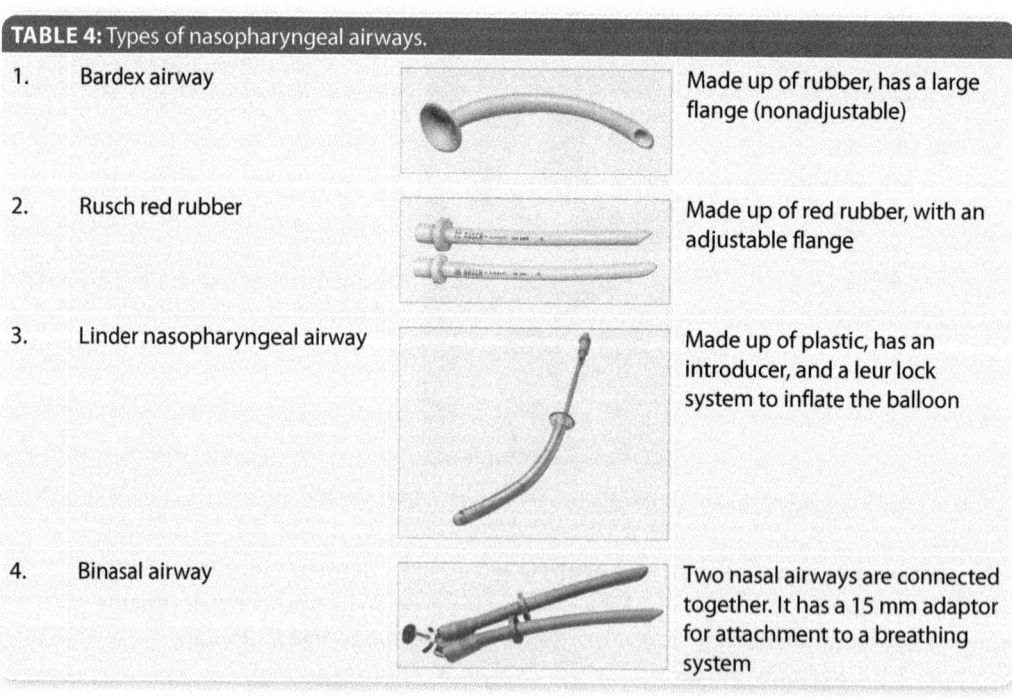

Chapter 54: Face Masks and Airways

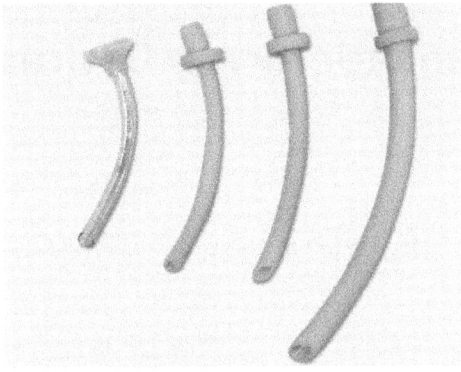

Fig. 6: Nasopharyngeal airway: Extreme left: Bardex airway made up of soft plastic, rest gradual sizes Rusch red rubber airways.

- Trauma along the passage of the airway.
- Laryngospasm and coughing if inserted in a lighter plane of anesthesia.
- Gagging and retching, due to stimulation of the posterior airways and inadvertent displacement of the airway.
- Latex allergy.

QUESTIONS

Q. 1. Nasopharyngeal airways and $EtCO_2$ maintaining uses, advantages.

TABLE 5: Indications and contraindications for the use of a nasopharyngeal airways (NPA).

Indications	Contraindications
To maintain the patency of the airway	Deranged coagulation
To apply continuous positive airway pressure (CPAP)	A basilar skull fracture
To facilitate suctioning	Pathology/deformity of the nose or nasopharynx
As a guide for a fiberscope	History of nose bleeds requiring treatment
As a guide for a nasogastric tube	
• To dilate the nasal passages in preparation for nasotracheal	
• Intubation	

Q. 2. Drawbacks of placing a nasopharyngeal airway.

FURTHER READING

1. Dorsch JA, Dorsch SE. Understanding Anesthesia Equipment, 5th Edition. Philadelphia: Lippincott/Williams and Wilkins; 2007.

CHAPTER 55

Supraglottic Airway Devices

Deepak Kumar, Abhijit Kumar, Amit Kohli

Q. 1. Describe the brief history and classification of supraglottic airway devices?

Ans. The term supraglottic airway devices (SADs) also known as extraglottic airway devices (EADs) are inserted into the pharynx to provide ventilation, oxygenation, and delivery of anesthetic gases without the need for tracheal intubation.

History: In 1981, first successful SAD was introduced by Dr Archie Brain, i.e., laryngeal mask airway (LMA)-Classic but it came into clinical practice in 1988.

Classification of Supraglottic Airway Devices

Various classification systems exist for SADs, although classification based on evolution is commonly used in clinical practice **(Tables 1 and 2)**.

Q. 2. Describe the related anatomy and clinical correlation of SADs.

Ans.

Related Anatomy and Clinical Correlation (Figs. 1A to D)

It is important for the anesthetist to be cognizant of the appropriate anatomy of the human airway as it relates to the use of the SADs. The use encompasses the placement, maintenance, removal, and overall functionality of the SADs. It also helps in understanding some of the adverse effect of these devices on the surrounding structures such as glands and their ducts, nerves, and vessels.

The ideal insertion path of an SAD is like a bolus of food proceeding along the palatopharyngeal curve; avoiding anterior structures while pressing sequentially into the hard palate, soft palate, and naso-/oro-/laryngo-/hypopharyngeal parts of the pharynx. The insertion ends with the distal cuff of the SAD occupying and impacting the hypopharynx. The ideal position of the device is achieved when its distal cuff lies in the hypopharynx, the sides lie opposite the pyriform fossae, the posterior cuff and back plate should be resting against the posterior wall of the posterior pharynx and the proximal cuff is at the base of the tongue. There may be variations in the procedure for some of the SADs, which have been described elsewhere in the later sections.

Q. 3. Describe LMA-Classic (cLMA)?

Ans.

Description (Fig. 2 and Table 3):
- It consists of an oval soft silicone inflatable mask with aperture bars (to prevent the tube from becoming obstructed by the epiglottis) that sits over the larynx.
- It has a curved airway tube connected to an elliptical mask at a 30° angle with 15 mm connector at the machine end.
- An inflating line with inflation valve and inflation pilot balloon.

Chapter 55: Supraglottic Airway Devices

TABLE 1: Donald Miller's classification (based on sealing mechanisms).

	Cuffed perilaryngeal sealers		Cuffed pharyngeal sealers		Cuffless preshaped sealers	
	Without directional sealing	With directional sealing	Without esophageal sealing cuff	With esophageal sealing cuff	Without esophageal sealing	With esophageal sealing
Devices	LMA ILMA Ambu AuraOnce Ambu Aura-I Ambu AuraGain Air-Q	PLMA LMA Supreme	CobraPLA	LT, LTS Esophageal combitube Elisha airway device	SLIPA i-gel	Baska
Sealing mechanism	Cuff surrounds the laryngeal inlet	Cuff seals at the base of the tongue	Cuff seals at the base of the tongue and esophagus		Seals outlet from pharynx at base of tongue up to the esophageal inlet	Baska mask cuff expands with each positive pressure breath

(ILMA: intubating laryngeal mask airway; LMA: laryngeal mask airway; PLMA: ProSeal laryngeal mask airway)

TABLE 2: Classification based on evolution of supraglottic airway device.

First-generation devices (simple airway tubes)	Second-generation devices (airway tubes with addition of drainage tube to reduce risk of aspiration)
• LMA Classic • LMA Flexible • Intubating LMA • Ambu AuraOnce • Ambu Aura40 • Ambu Aura-I • Ambu AuraFlex • Ambu AuraStraight • Portex SSLM • Air Q • Laryngeal tube (LT) and LT-D (disposable) • CobraPLA • SLIPA	• ProSeal LMA • LMA Supreme • i-gel • Ambu AuraGain • Laryngeal tube suction II (LTS-II) and LTSD • Gastro-LT (G-LT) • Intubating LTS (ILTS) • Air Q blocker • Combitube

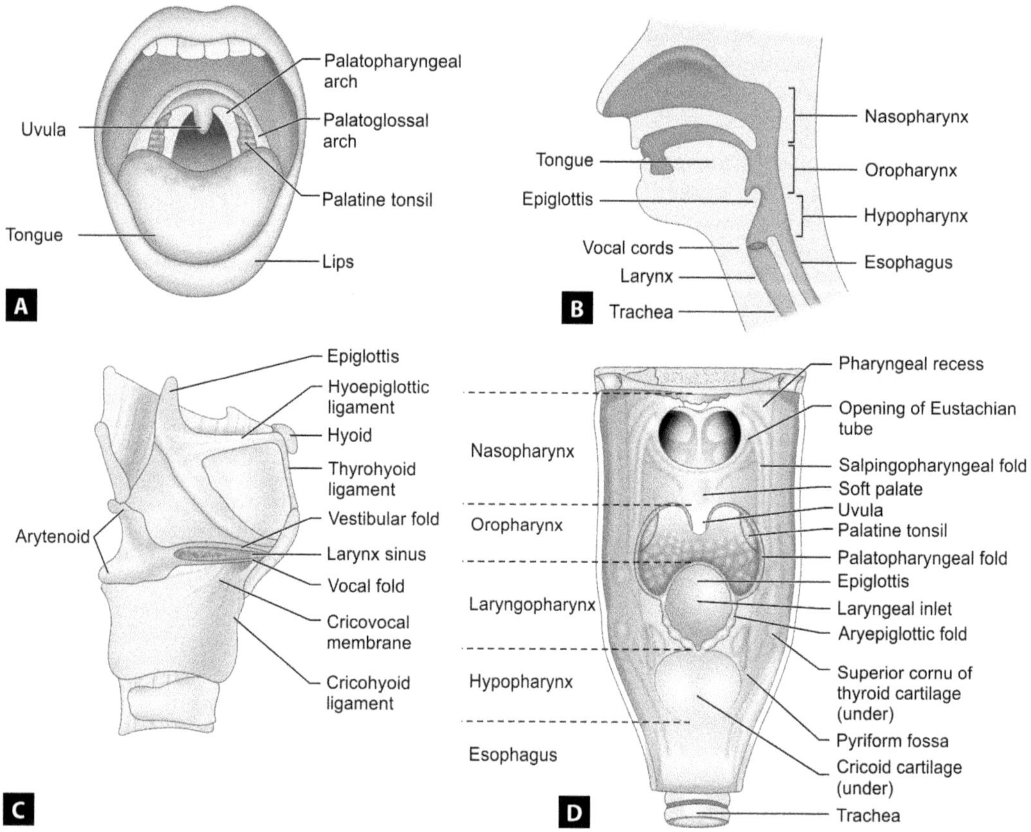

Section 3: Anesthesia Instruments

Figs. 1A to D: (A) Anterior view of oropharynx; (B) Lateral view of upper airway; (C) Right lateral view of laryngopharynx; (D) Posterior view of pharynx.

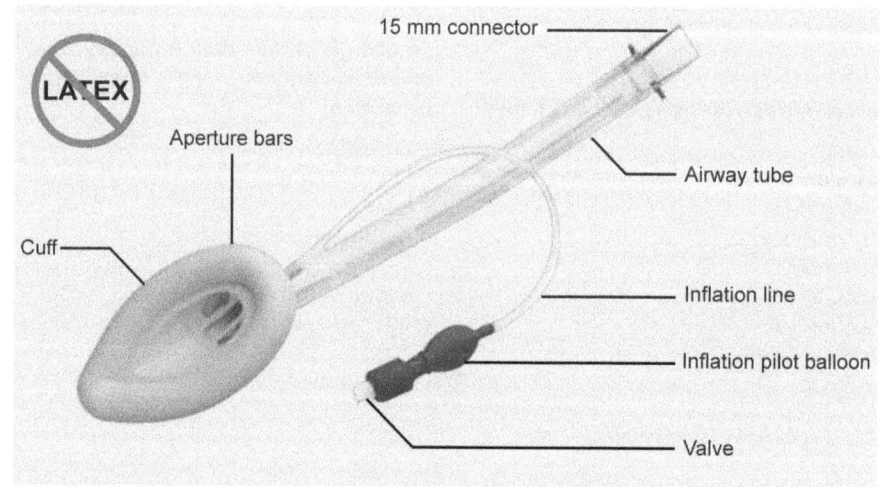

Fig. 2: Classic laryngeal mask airway (LMA).

TABLE 3: Available LMA-Classics.

LMA size	Patient size	Largest tracheal tube that can fit the LMA (ID in mm)	Largest fiberscope that fits into a tracheal tube (OD in mm)
1	Neonates/infants up to 5 kg	3.5	2.7
1.5	Infants between 5 and 10 kg	4.0	3.0
2	Infants/children between 10 and 20 kg[a]	4.5	3.4
2.5	Children between 20 and 30 kg	5.0	4.0
3	Children 30–50 kg	6.0 cuffed	5.0
4	Adults 50–70 kg	6.0 cuffed	5.0
5	Adults 70–100 kg	7.0 cuffed	5.0
6	Adults >100 kg	7.0 cuffed	5.0

[a]Size 2.5 may be more suitable for children of this size.
(LMA: laryngeal mask airway)

- It is made medical grade silicone containing no latex and can be used up to 40 times.
- There are eight sizes to fit patients from neonates to adults.
- The disadvantage of cLMA is that it does not provides any protection against pulmonary aspiration due to its low oropharyngeal seal pressure (OSP) of 10–20 cm of H_2O.

Techniques of Insertion of LMA

The techniques of insertion of laryngeal mask airway are shown in **Figures 3A to D**.

Q. 4. Describe LMA Fastrach™?

Ans. LMA Fastrach™ also known as Intubating Laryngeal Mask Airway (ILMA) **(Figs. 4 to 6)**

Description:
- LMA Fastrach™ a modification of the cLMA is in use from 1997 (Teleflex Medical, Dublin, Ireland).
- ILMA is a specially designed SAD that can be used as a conduit to facilitate intubation.
- It has been successfully used to secure airway in patients with cervical immobilization, postburn contracture neck and other difficult airway situations.
- Due to presence of metallic handle ILMA is unsuitable for use in the MRI unit.
- ILMA is available in three sizes, i.e., 3 (30–50 kg; 20 mL cuff), 4 (50–70 kg; 30 mL cuff), and 5 (70–100 kg; 40 mL cuff).

Insertion of ILMA

Clinical pearl: If the tracheal tube fails to enter the trachea, a number of maneuvers can be helpful to solve the problems.
- If resistance occur at 2 cm beyond the 15 cm mark on the endotracheal tube (ETT): Probably ETT has impacted the vestibular wall or may be having downfolded epiglottis
  Solution: Rotating the ETT may overcome the impaction or without deflating the cuff, the LMA-Fastrach should be swung outward to 6 cm and reinserted.
- If resistance is felt at 3 cm beyond the 15 cm mark on the ETT: Probably epiglottis may be out of reach of the elevating bar.
  Solution: Larger LMA should be used.

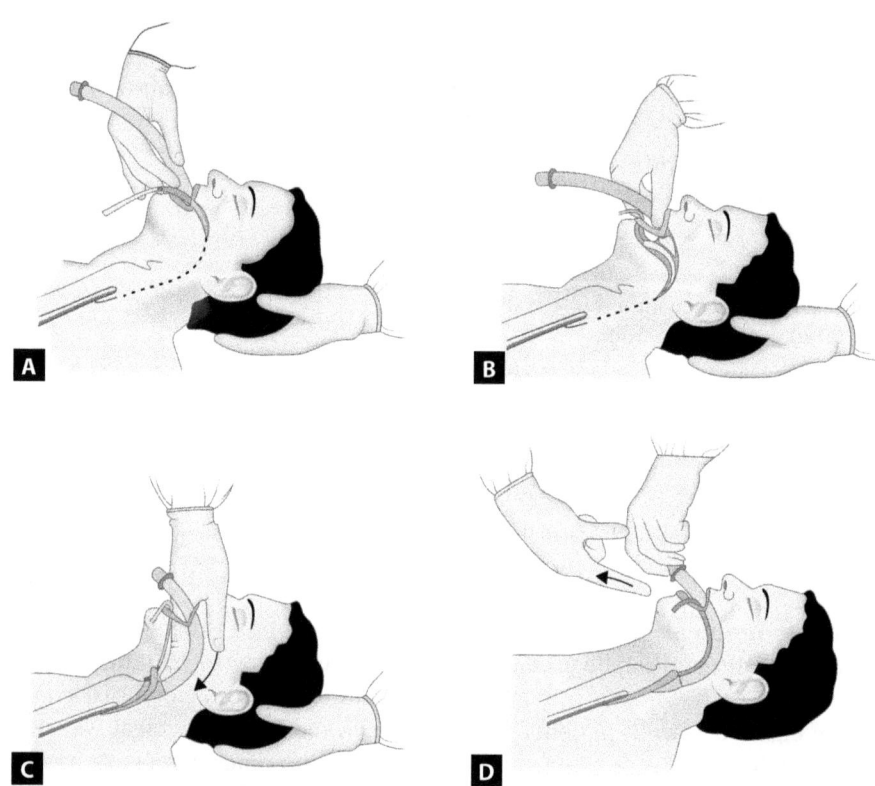

Figs. 3A to D: Insertion of a laryngeal mask airway (LMA). (A) The tip of the cuff is pressed upward against the hard palate by the index finger while the middle finger opens the mouth; (B) The LMA is pressed backward in a smooth movement. The nondominant hand is used to extend the head; (C) The LMA is advanced until definite resistance is felt; (D) Before the index finger is removed, the nondominant hand presses down on the LMA to prevent dislodgment during removal of the index finger. The cuff is subsequently inflated.

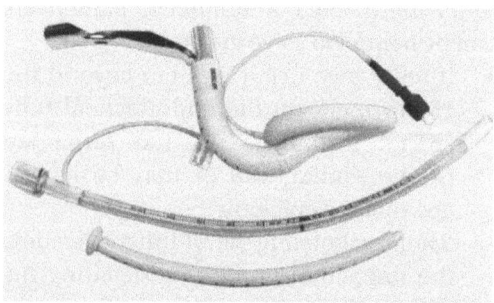

Fig. 4: *Top*: LMA-Fastrach. The tube is shorter and wider than on the LMA-Classic and has a metal handle. *Middle*: Tracheal tube designed to be used with the LMA-Fastrach. *Bottom*: Stabilizer to allow the LMA to be removed without extubating the patient.

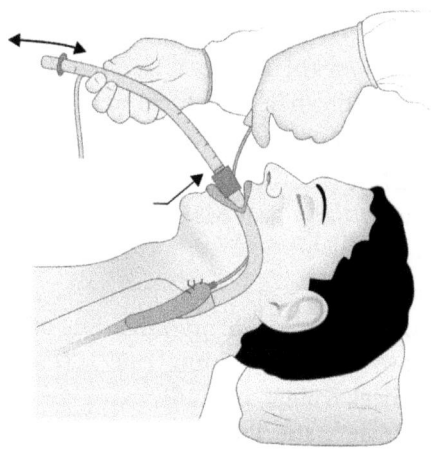

Fig. 5: Placement of an endotracheal tube (ETT) into the Intubating Laryngeal Mask Airway (ILMA).

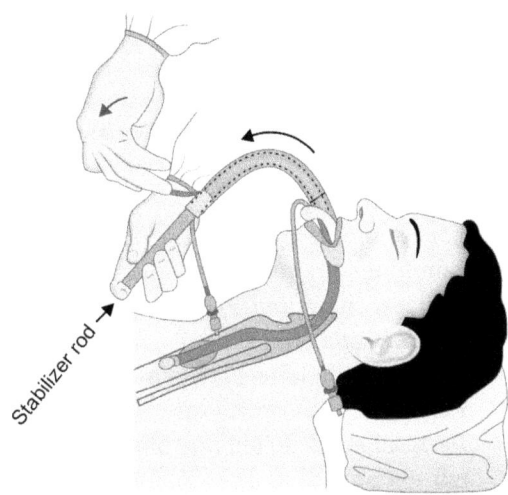

Fig. 6: Removal of the Intubating Laryngeal Mask Airway (ILMA).

- If resistance encountered at 4 cm beyond the 15 cm mark or immediately after the ETT leaves the LMA-Fastrach: Probably the LMA may be too large.
  Solution: Smaller size should be used.

Q. 5. Describe ProSeal LMA?
Ans. It is a second-generation SAD. Additional features from LMA-Classic are **(Figs. 7 and 8 and Table 4)**:

- PLMA has an additional gastric drain tube apart from an airway tube, thereby protecting the airway from aspiration from gastric regurgitation.
- Integrated bite block that protects against airway occlusion.
- PLMA has another dorsally located, cuff which helps to improve the airway seal, a particularly useful feature when positive pressure ventilation is desired. These design features were intended to achieve a greater OSP than ordinary cLMA.
- Made of medical grade silicone, this device may be reused up to 40 times.

Techniques of Insertion
- Introducer insertion technique
- Index finger insertion technique
- Gum-elastic bougie-guided insertion.

Steps for Insertion Technique
Step 1: Size selection
Step 2: Inspection
Step 3: Check deflation and inflation of cuff, then deflate
Step 4: Mounting and lubrication
Step 5: Position the airways

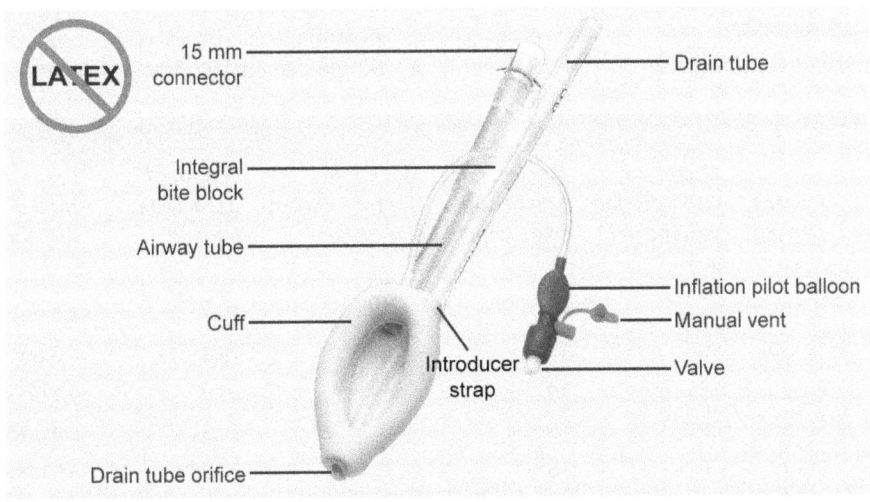

Fig. 7: ProSeal LMA.

Section 3: Anesthesia Instruments

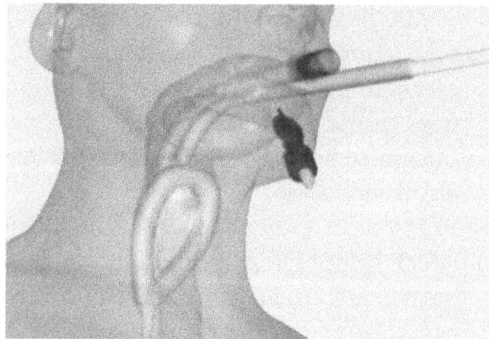

Fig. 8: Correctly positioned ProSeal laryngeal mask airway (PLMA) showing the drain tube of the PLMA in continuity with the esophagus.

Step 6: Insertion
Step 7: Cuff inflation
Step 8: Verify placement
Step 9: Securing the SAD

Confirmation of Cuff Placement

- After inflation of cuff it will pop out, smooth oval swelling in anterior part of neck, with no visible cuff in oral cavity
- Bite block-depth of insertion (should be at the level of the teeth)
- Ventilation:
  - Chest movement, compliance of bag
  - Capnography
  - Ease of ventilation
- Suprasternal notch test (Brimacombe bounce) should be present
- Able to pass orogastric tube.

Q. 6. Describe LMA Supreme (Fig. 9).
Ans.
- Introduced in 2007
- LMA Supreme is a single use device
- Combines the feature of multiple LMA devices, including ProSeal LMA, LMA Fastrach, and LMA Unique
- Seal intermediate between cLMA and PLMA
- *Parts:* Elongated cuff, bite block, fixation tab
- Anatomic curve that facilitates easy insertion
- No posterior cuff and large inflatable plastic cuff
- Fins in the mask of bowl to prevent epiglottic obstruction
- Reinforced tip—less chances of folding
- Required minimum mouth opening (approximately 1.4 cm) for insertion.

Q.7. Describe i-gel (Figs. 10 and 11 and Table 5).
Ans.
- Invented by Dr Muhammed Aslam Nasir in 2007
- Single use and truly anatomical device

TABLE 4: Available sizes of ProSeal LMA.

LMA size	Patient size (kg)	Maximum cuff inflation volume (mL)	Maximum gastric tube size (French)	Maximum fiberoptic scope size (mm)	Length of drain tube (cm)	Largest tracheal tube (ID in mm)
1	0–5	4				
1.5	5–10	7	10	–	18.2	4.0 uncuffed
2	10–20	10	10	–	19.0	4.0 uncuffed
2.5	20–30	14	14	–	23.0	4.5 uncuffed
3	30–50	20	16	–	26.5	5.0 uncuffed
4	50–70	30	16	4	27.5	5.0 uncuffed
5	70–100	40	18	5	28.5	6.0 cuffed

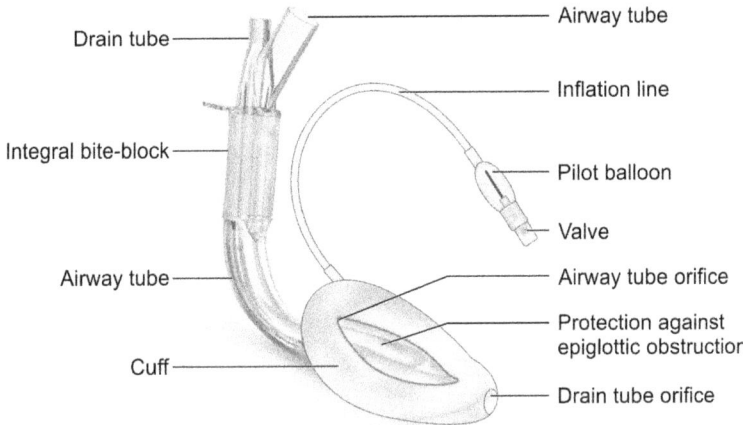

Fig. 9: LMA Supreme.

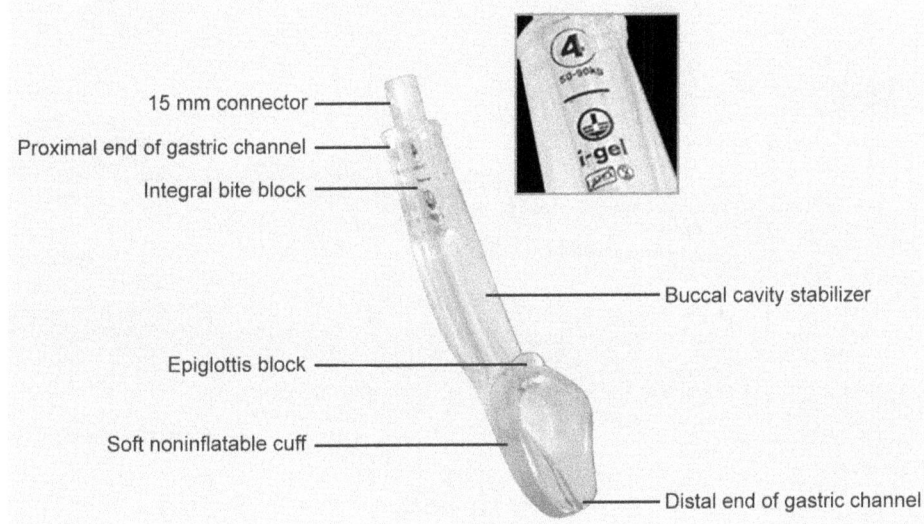

Fig. 10: I-gel.

- The i-gel has a soft, gel-like, noninflatable cuff, designed to provide an anatomical impression fit over the laryngeal inlet
- It has an integral bite block with separate channel for gastric drainage
- Contains an epiglottic rest at the anterior part of cuff which reduces the possibility of epiglottic downfolding airway obstruction
- Buccal cavity stabilizer which prevents rotation of device inside the oral cavity
- Pharyngeal seal reported is 26–30 cm H_2O.

The material of gel-like mask is made of a thermoplastic elastomer (SEBS—styrene-ethylene-butadiene-styrene) which helps to provide good laryngeal seal.

Advantages

- Noninflatable cuff has a number of potential advantages, including easier insertion, minimal risk of tissue compression, and stability after insertion (i.e., no position change with cuff inflation).

Section 3: Anesthesia Instruments

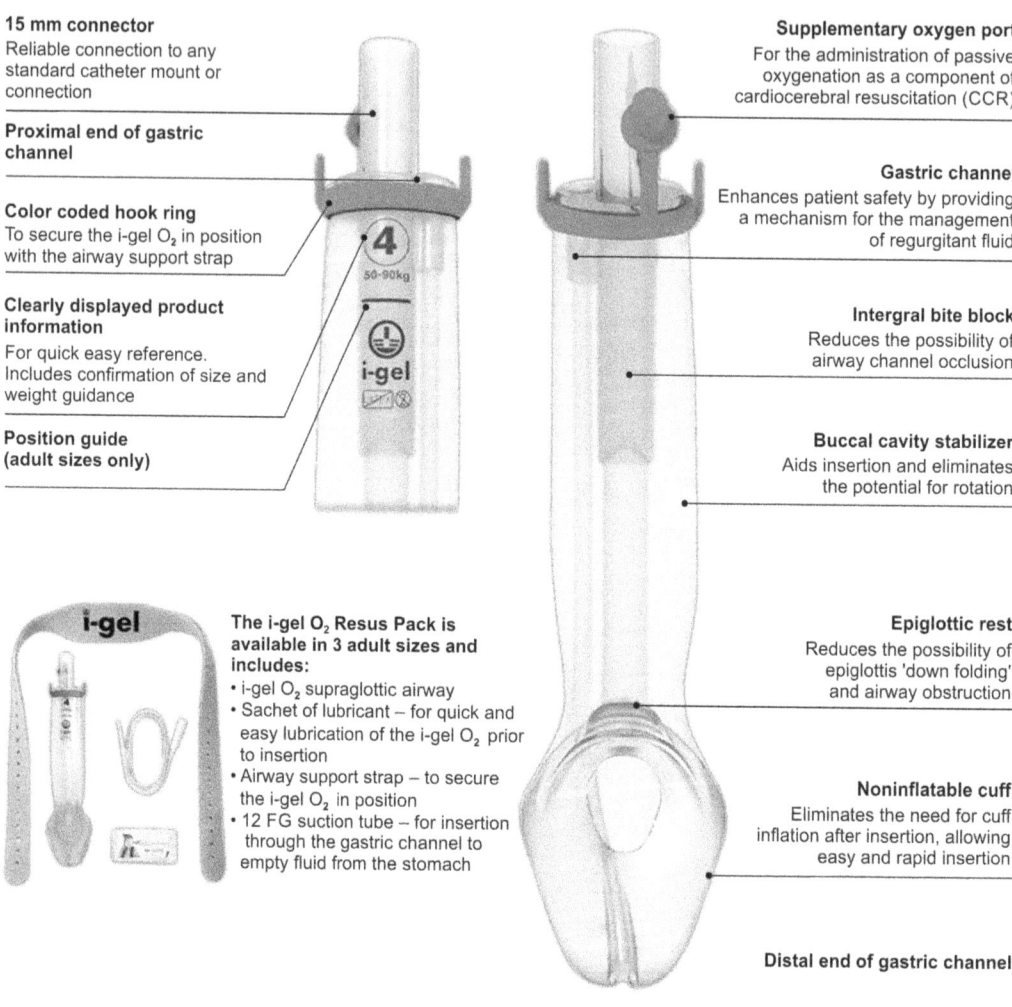

Fig. 11: I-gel O_2.

TABLE 5: Availability of different sizes.

Size	Patient size	Patient weight guidance (kg)
1	Neonate	2–5
1.5	Infant	5–12
2	Small pediatric	10–25
2.5	Large pediatric	25–30
3	Small adult	30–60
4	Medium adult	50–90
5	Large adult	90+

- Wide lumen makes it worth for both airway reserve and as a conduit for assisted intubation
- A gastric channel allows for suctioning and placement of nasogastric tube.

I-gel O_2

- Newer device which are available in three sizes (adult size)—#3, #4, #5.
- It has color coded hook ring.
- It has unique feature of supplementary O_2 port besides the airway tube and gastric

drain channel which provides passive O_2 administration by attaching standard O_2 tubing and deliver O_2 to patient.

Q. 8. Describe LMA BlockBuster (Fig. 12).
Ans.
- It is a second-generation SAD invented in 2012 (Tuoren Medical Instrument Co. Ltd., Changyuan City, China)
- High airway seal pressures (35–38 cm H_2O)
- Facilitate FOB guided or blind tracheal intubation
- Sizes #3, #4, #5

Q. 9. Describe Baska Mask (Fig. 13).
Ans.
- It is a newer SAD made of medical grade silicone introduced in 2012.
- It is available in four adult sizes (3, 4, 5, and 6) for patients ranging weight between 30 kg to >100 kg.

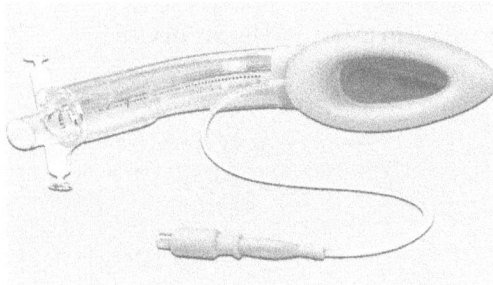

Fig. 12: BlockBuster.

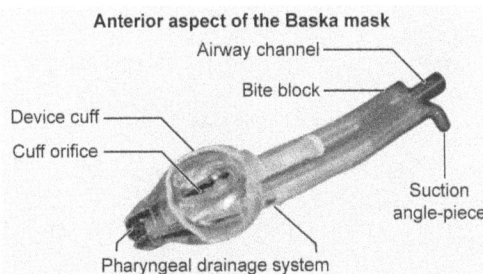

Fig. 13: Baska mask.

Components
- *Cuffless membranous bowl:* Advantage of this cuff that it inflates and deflates with each positive pressure breath during inspiration and expiration, respectively
- *Tab:* It helps to negotiate the oropharyngeal curve and helps in easy insertion of device
- Dual drainage system, i.e., an esophagus drainage inlet and side channel to drain pharyngeal contents
- Integral bite block.

Techniques of Insertion
- Lubricate the device with water soluble jelly
- Place patient head and neck in neural position
- Open the mouth of the patient
- Compress the proximal firmer parts of the mask between thumb and two fingers
- If needed, pull the tab to negotiate the palatopharyngeal curve. Once the tip of the mask crosses the curve release the tab
- The mask is advanced until resistance is encountered
- Confirm the position and fix the device.

3gLM (Fig. 14)
- Similar to Baska mask and seals the laryngeal orifice
- It consists of a noninflatable cuff which adapts to the laryngeal anatomy during pars plana vitrectomy (PPV)
- It has two gastric tube channels for drainage of gastric contents.

Q. 10. Describe LMA® Protector™ Airway (Table 6 and Fig. 15).
Ans.
- It is a single use second-generation SAD introduced in 2015. It is made of latex free silicone
- It allows separation of respiratory and digestive tracts
- Available sizes

Section 3: Anesthesia Instruments

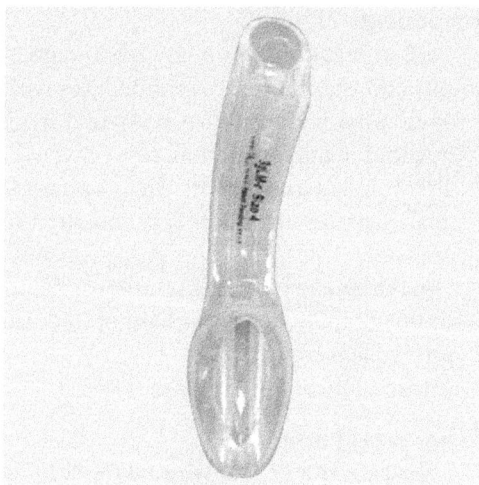

Fig. 14: 3gLM.

TABLE 6: Available sizes.

Mask size	Patient weight in kg	Maximum ETT (Id in mm)	Largest size OG tube in Fr
3	30–50	6.5	16
4	50–70	7.5	18
5	70–100	7.5	18

(ETT: endotracheal tube; OG: orogastric tube)

Components
- Dual gastric drainage channel to drain secretions around the laryngeal region and gastric content.
- Elongated cuff facilitates esophageal seal
- Airway tube is wide lumen and elliptical in cross section which allows for intubation with compatible sizes of ETT.
- Cuff pilot gives an indication of cuff pressure which is adjustable to achieve an intracuff pressure of 60 cm H_2O.
- Integral bite block.

Insertion Technique
- Place in sniffing position (extend head and flex neck)
- To facilitate the insertion of cuff of device, press the tip of the device flat against the hard palate, keep the airway tube close to the chin
- Rotate and push the device inward in a smooth circular motion till the definite resistance is felt.

Advantages
- Easy to insert and fix the device

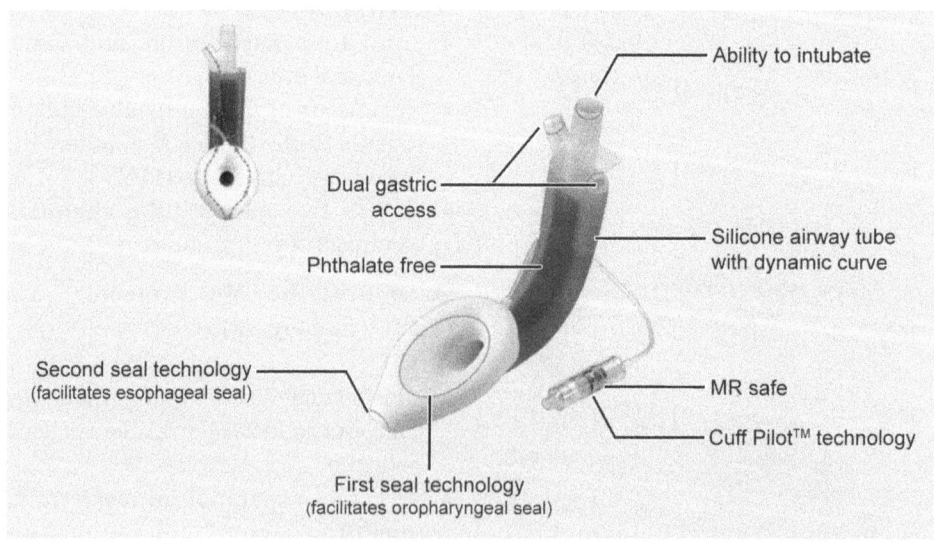

Fig. 15: LMA® Protector™ airway.

- Silicone material makes the airway tube less rigid, softer and decrease chances of trauma
- Inability to perform safe intubation provides effective option for airway replacement.

Q. 11. What are the advantages of SADs over ET Intubation?
- Ease of insertion and smooth awakening
- Decrease work of breathing
- More hemodynamic stability
- Avoid bronchial intubation
- Uses of neuromuscular blocking agents are not mandatory
- Lesser incidence of laryngospasm, coughing, and postoperative hoarse voice.

Q. 12. Elaborate different usage of SADs.
- Elective or emergency surgeries
- Supraglottic devices have been recommended as rescue airways in CVCI scenario
- Cardiopulmonary resuscitation
- Fiberoptic intubation
- Extubation and weaning in ICU
- Remote anesthesia
- Professional singers
- Supplementing regional block
- Unstable cervical spine
- Laparoscopic surgeries (preferably second-generation SADs).

Q. 13. What are the limitations of SADs usage?
- Small oral aperture (<1 cm)
- Any oropharyngeal, pharyngeal, or hypopharyngeal mass
- Esophageal pathology—caustic ingestion
- Full stomach patients
- SAD has limited value in patients of poor lung compliance.

Q. 14. Elaborate different SADs used for tracheal intubation.
- ILMA
- I-gel
- LMA BlockBuster
- Ambu Auragain
- LMA Protector.

FURTHER READING

1. Cook T, Howes B. Supraglottic airway devices: recent advances. Contin Educ Anaesth Crit Care Pain. 2011;11:56-61.
2. Dorsch JA, Dorsch SE. Practical Approach to Anesthesia Equipment, 6th edition. Philadelphia: Wolters Kluwer; 2010.
3. Endigeri A, Ganeshnavar A, Varaprasad BV, Shivanand YH, Ayyangouda B. Comparison of success rate of BlockBuster® versus Fastrach® LMA as conduit for blind endotracheal intubation: a prospective randomised trial. Indian J Anaesth. 2019;63:988-94.
4. LMA-Protector Instructions for use. Athlone, Ireland: Teleflex Medical; 2015.
5. Miller DM. Re-classification of extraglottic/supralaryngeal airway devices. In: Michalek P, Donaldson W (Eds). The i-Gel Supraglottic Airway. New York: Nova Biomedical; 2013. pp. 15-28.
6. Van Zundert T, Gatt S. The Baska Mask—a new concept in self-sealing membrane cuff extraglottic airway devices using a sump and two gastric drains. A clinical evaluation. J Obstet Anaesth Crit Care. 2012;2:23-30.

CHAPTER 56

Laryngoscopes

Anisha Singh, Abhijit Kumar

INTRODUCTION

Laryngoscope (larynx + scope) is the device that is used to visualize the larynx and related structures, mainly for insertion of endotracheal tube (ETT) into the trachea of the patient. Laryngoscopy is the technique or the procedure of visualization of larynx. This is one of the first skills the anesthesia resident intends to master upon. It is performed for diagnostic, therapeutic, and intubation purposes. Laryngoscopes are available in a wide range for their diverse use according to the indications.

HISTORY

Kirstein is often regarded as the pioneer of the first direct laryngoscopy in 1895. In 1940, Robert Macintosh and Ivan Magill designed and popularized the idea of a laryngoscope to visualize the vocal cords. Since then, newer blade designs and the latest technology have been introduced to aid and facilitate the technique of laryngoscopy.

USES

- Endotracheal intubation
- Assessment of vocal cords and larynx
- Foreign body removal
- Upper airway biopsy
- Insertion of a nasogastric tube, transesophageal echo probe, laryngeal mask airway, or throat packs.

TYPES

- Direct rigid laryngoscope
- Indirect rigid laryngoscope
- Videolaryngoscopes (VL)
- Flexible fiberoptic bronchoscopes (FFB)

DIRECT RIGID LARYNGOSCOPES

These are the conventional and universally available laryngoscopes. They are economical as well as quick to use. We need to align the visual, oral, and pharyngeal axis for their optimal use under direct vision. These contain two main parts, they are:

1. *Handle:* It is held in the nondominant hand, has a rough surface for easy grip, and contains the batteries as a power source. It is available in different sizes. For example, a short or stubby handle—for obese and pregnant patients, Patil Syracuse handles—can be locked in four different angled positions for convenient use.
2. *Blade:* It is the part that is inserted into the patient's mouth. It consists of several parts, namely—*Spatula (tongue)* which is used to compress the tongue and soft tissues, *flange* projects from side of spatula and is connected to it with help of a *web*. It helps to deflect the tissues out of line of vision and determines the cross-sectional shape of the blade. *Tip or beak* is the distal-most part, *blunt* and *thickened*

part which directly or indirectly elevates the *epiglottis*. *Base* attaches to the handle and has a slot for engaging the hinge pin of the handle. *Heel* is the end of base. *Light source* as a lamp or bulb is also situated on the blade.

Types of Blades

- *Macintosh or curved blade (Fig. 1):* This is the most common blade in use and is available in sizes numbered from 0 to 4 with increasing size of the blade according to different ages. It has a gentle curve up to the tip and is reverse "Z" in cross-section.

Various modifications of the Macintosh blade are available in the following:
- Polio blade—makes an obtuse angle to the handle
- Oxiport Macintosh blade—has an additional tube to deliver oxygen
- Tull Macintosh blade—has a suction port near the tip
- Fink blade—a wider spatula and light source is near the tip
- Bizzarri-Giuffrida blade—flangeless Macintosh to limit damage to teeth
- Flexible tip blade—a hinged tip which is controlled by a lever attached to the proximal end of blade. It is useful in difficult intubations with restricted neck movements. It is popularly known as *McCoy laryngoscope*
- *Miller (straight) blade (Fig. 2):* This is available from size 0 to 4. The spatula is straight with a slight upward curve near tip and forms "C" in cross-section.

Various modifications of Miller blade are available in the following:
- Oxiport Miller blade
- Tull Miller blade
- Mathew's blade—has a wide and flattened petaloid at the tip for difficult nasotracheal intubations
- Wisconsin blade—spatula has no curve and flange is curved to form two-third of a circle
- Flexible tip Miller blade double-angle blade—spatula has 20° and 30° angulations to improve lifting of the epiglottis.

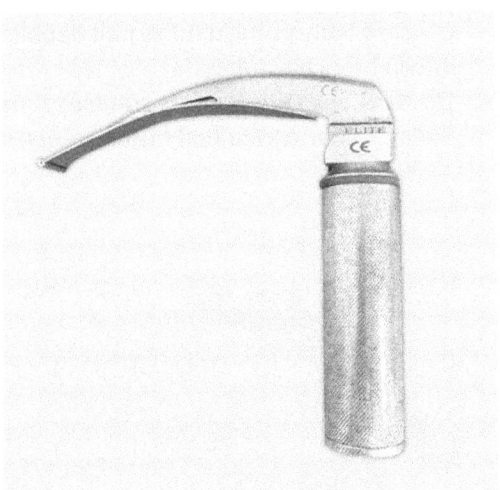

Fig. 1: Macintosh blade.

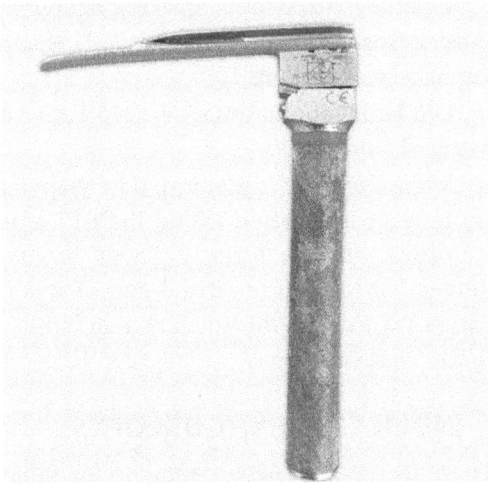

Fig. 2: Miller blade.

TECHNIQUE OF LARYNGOSCOPY

The optimal/ideal positioning for successful laryngoscopy in adults is 25–35° flexion of cervical spine and 85–90° head extension at atlanto-occipital joint, popularly known as "sniffing position" or "Boyce-Jackson" position. 8–10 cm pillow below the patient's head provides neck flexion and head extension has achieved pressure on top of the head. The handle of laryngoscope is held in nondominant left hand and mouth is opened with right hand using the scissoring action. The blade is inserted from right side of patient's mouth and advanced to shift the tongue towards the left side. Epiglottoscopy, i.e., epiglottis is visualized. When using the curved blade, its tip is inserted into the vallecula and upward force is applied along the axis of handle to lift the epiglottis in order to view the larynx. Whereas, with the straight blade epiglottis is elevated directly to view the larynx.

MANEUVRES TO AID IN LARYNGOSCOPY

Even after correct technique, certain external manipulations help to visualize the larynx and perform successful intubation.

BURP, i.e., backwards upwards rightward pressure to improve the Cormack and Lehane laryngoscopic grading.

OELM, i.e., optimum external laryngeal manipulation.

Malleable stylet is preformed in shape of "hockey stick" inserted within the ETT aids in intubation in anteriorly placed larynx. Remember to keep the distal end of stylet, within the tube to prevent accidental injury to laryngeal structures.

INDIRECT LARYNGOSCOPES

These are relatively newer laryngoscopes that do not require "line of sight" vision directly. The images from distal end of the blade are carried to the screen either through handle or optical cables. These can be either rigid or flexible fiberoptic laryngoscopes.

Indirect Rigid Laryngoscope

- *Bullard optical laryngoscope* **(Fig. 3):** This has a curved metal blade that is anatomically shaped and fiberoptic bundles are situated on the posterior aspect of the blade. The batteries are situated in the handle and working channel extends from the scope body to the distal end at the tip where light bundles terminate. It is available in three sizes—(1) pediatric, (2) pediatric long and (3) adult. Dedicated intubating or introducing stylets with a curve of 20° to left near tip is available to aid in intubation.
- *WuScope* **(Fig. 4):** This has a rigid tubular blade and flexible fiberscope that is assembled together for use. The metal blade has three detachable parts—(1) handle, (2) main blade and (3) bivalve element that assembles to form channels for tracheal tube and suction catheter. Oxygen tubing can be connected to a slot for an oxygen port. WuScope can be used to insert both tracheal tubes and double-lumen bronchial tubes.
- *UpsherScope* **(Fig. 5):** It is similar to the Bullard scope except that instead of stylet

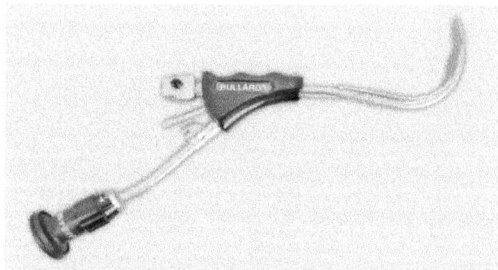

Fig. 3: Bullard optical laryngoscope.

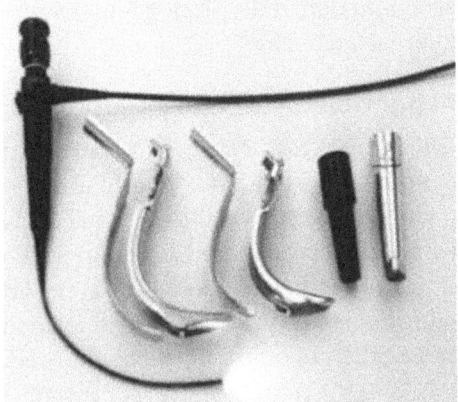
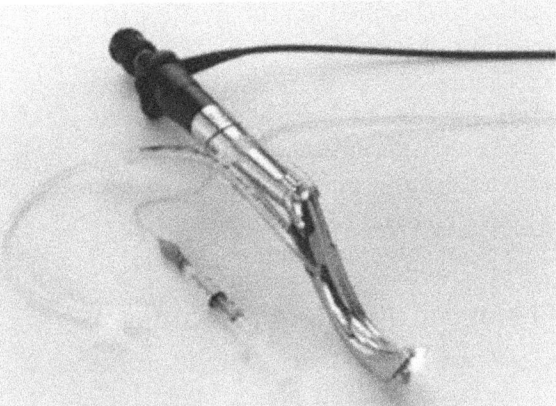

Fig. 4: WuScope

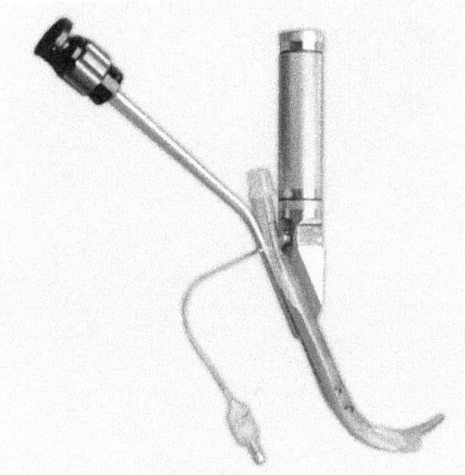

Fig. 5: UpsherScope.

it has a channel for loading tracheal tube which is situated posterior to the blade. Blade is connected to Upsher handle which has fiberoptic cable from light source. Proximal to the blade, an eyepiece with a focusing ring is present.

VIDEOLARYNGOSCOPES

These are the newer generation of laryngoscopes that utilizes the video camera technology. It does not require the line of sight vision of larynx and performs indirect laryngoscopy through slim camera chips. The images from the distal end of blade can be reflected on the attached monitor screen either through handle or fiberoptic bundles. Hence, it acts as a good teaching aid to help students master the art of successful laryngoscopy. Static images and videos can be recorded for teaching and documentation purposes. When using VL, lesser mouth opening, and neck extension is required. Also, it provides a magnified and higher resolution image of the glottis structures.

However, the hand eye-monitor coordination has a learning curve which makes intubation time-consuming even in easy cases where despite a clear view of larynx, intubation is achieved with difficulty. But this can be easily overcome by following few steps which are as follows:

Step 1: Look in mouth and insert VL till root of tongue

Step 2: Look at screen/monitor and optimize scope position

Step 3: Look in mouth and insert ETT

Step 4: Look at screen and direct ETT towards glottis and between the cords

VL can be classified according to the shape and principle used:
- Channeled VL—these have an integrated channel or slot for placement of tracheal tube to guide its insertion.
- Nonchanneled VL—these do not have channel hence requires stylet for endotracheal placement.

Channeled Videolaryngoscopes

- *Pentax airway scope* **(Fig. 6)**: It has a curved disposable plastic blade, having channels for loading both tracheal tube and suction catheter. The bulky handle has a rotating screen/monitor attached onto the top and has a flexible stem attached to it which contains the charge-coupled device camera at the tip for visualization.
- *Airtraq* **(Fig. 7)**: This device has a 90° curved insertion part in its distal third. Channels for tracheal tube and light bundles with antifog circuits are situated parallel to each other. Viewfinder or camera attached to a distant screen is used to view the image from the tip. This device has to be inserted into the oropharynx in the midline. Four sizes are available to accommodate tubes from 2.5 to 8.5 mm internal diameter.

Nonchanneled Videolaryngoscopes

- *GlideScope* **(Fig. 8)**: This has a curved plastic blade with 60° angulation at midpoint and light-emitting device along with a camera mounted at the tip which transmits image to a remote screen. It requires stylet in tube and preformed as per the curvature of the blade used.

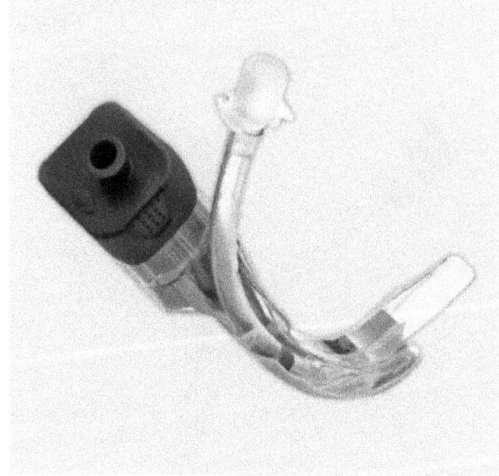

Fig. 7: Airtraq.

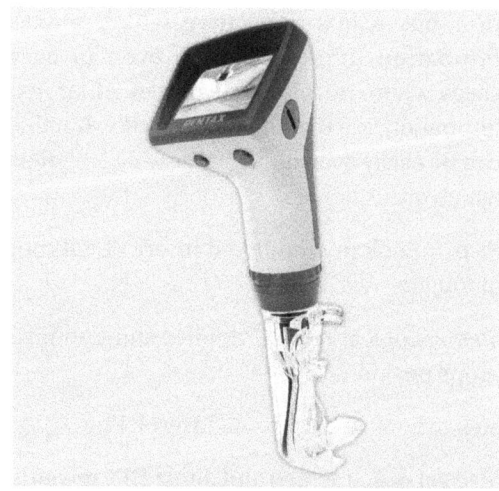

Fig. 6: Pentax videolaryngoscope.

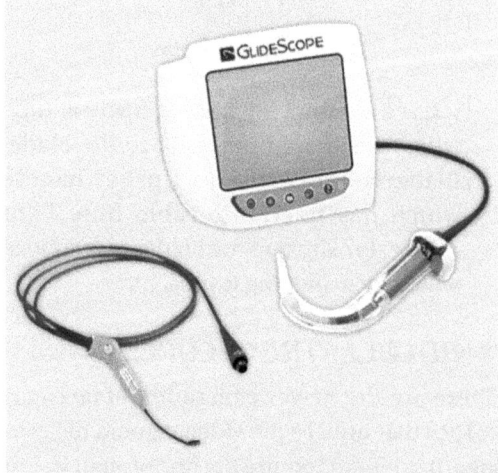

Fig. 8: GlideScope videolaryngoscope.

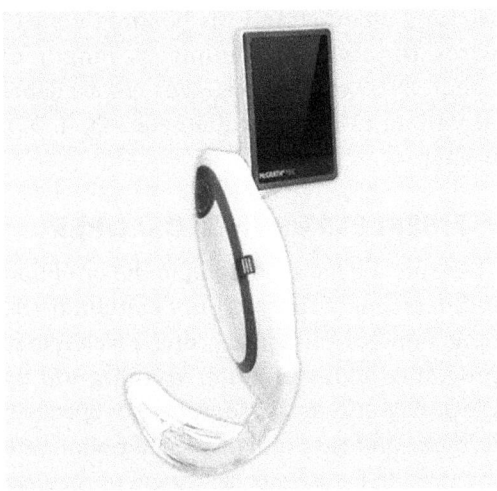

Fig. 9: McGrath videolaryngoscope.

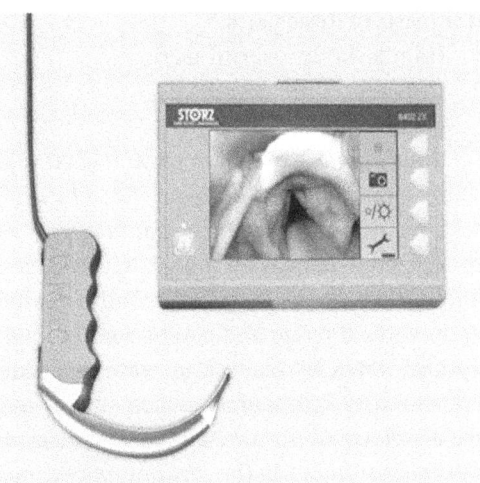

Fig. 10: C-Mac videolaryngoscope.

This device is introduced in midline of oropharynx.

Three types of GlideScope are available as follows:
1. GlideScope original—reusable, size is 2-5
2. GlideScope cobalt—reusable with a plastic sheath, size is 1-4
3. GlideScope ranger—disposable or reusable, portable, originally used in military setup.

- *McGrath series (Fig. 9):* This is a sturdy and portable laryngoscope with a disposable transparent plastic blade which covers the camera stick and its length for usage can be adjusted according to patient. The handle is robust with rechargeable batteries and a compact liquid-crystal display (LCD) screen is mounted on its top to view the laryngeal structures. This also requires a stylet in tube preshaped according to blades curvature to facilitate intubation.
- *C-Mac (Fig. 10):* This is relatively the latest VL introduced by Karl Storz with a stainless steel blade that is flattened to facilitate insertion in patients with reduced mouth opening. The laryngoscope resembles the conventional Macintosh and is connected to the display monitor via a cable. The distal lens uses a complementary metal-oxide-semiconductor (CMOS) chip which provides good vision and still images, and video recordings can be captured. It is available from size—1-4. Angulated blade, known as C-Mac. "D blade" is available in size 4 which can be used in a neutral head position because of the curvature.

FLEXIBLE FIBEROPTIC BRONCHOSCOPE

The flexible fiberoptic bronchoscope is a thin, pencil-like device that used *indirect laryngoscopy* for *endotracheal intubation*. Flexible fiberoptic bronchoscope is universally recognized as the gold standard in the awake/sedated/anesthetized "difficult to intubate" patients. Hence, it occupies a special place in the *difficult airway cart*. It is indicated in nonemergent anticipated difficult airway. It uses fiberoptic bundles to transmit images from the distal lens and these glass bundles run the length of the scope. A typical fiberoptic bundle = 10,000 glass fibers, approximately 8–10 μm in diameter.

It consists of three parts:
1. Handle/body/control section
2. Insertion cord
3. Flexible tip.

The *Handle* is the main control section of a fiberscope. It has an *eyepiece* with a *focusing ring* on its top where the camera can be connected to display an *image* on the screen. *Angulation control lever* controls the flexible tip in vertical plane and can be manipulated up and down by placing operators thumb. Ports to carry *light source, suction,* and *oxygen* are also located on the handle. *The working channel port* helps in the *instillation* of drugs.

The *insertion cord* carries the fiberoptic bundles for light and image transmission, working channel and tip bending control wires running throughout its length of about 50–65 cm. Various sizes are available according to its outer diameter—3, 4, 5.5, 6.5 mm.

FIBERLESS BRONCHOSCOPES

These are the latest addition to the invention of fiberscopes. These do not contain fiberoptic bundles and utilize camera technology providing high-resolution visualization by CMOS chip at its tip. These are battery-operated, durable, and easy to handle. They eliminate the need to focus/refocus camera or regulate the light source.

- *Flexible intubating video endoscopes (FIVE):* It is also available in disposable versions.
- *Ambu aScope* **(Fig. 12):** It is a light weight, single use flexible videoscope that has a camera at its tip and battery operated rechargeable LCD monitor. It is available in three sizes:
  1. aScope 3 slim (gray handle)
  2. aScope 3 regular (green handle)
  3. aScope 3 large (orange handle).

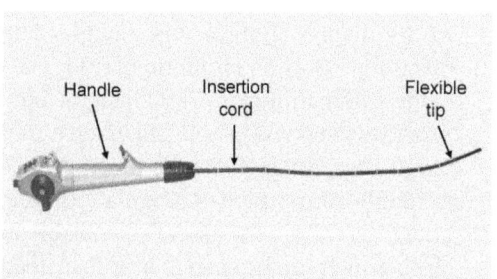

Fig. 11: Fiberscope.

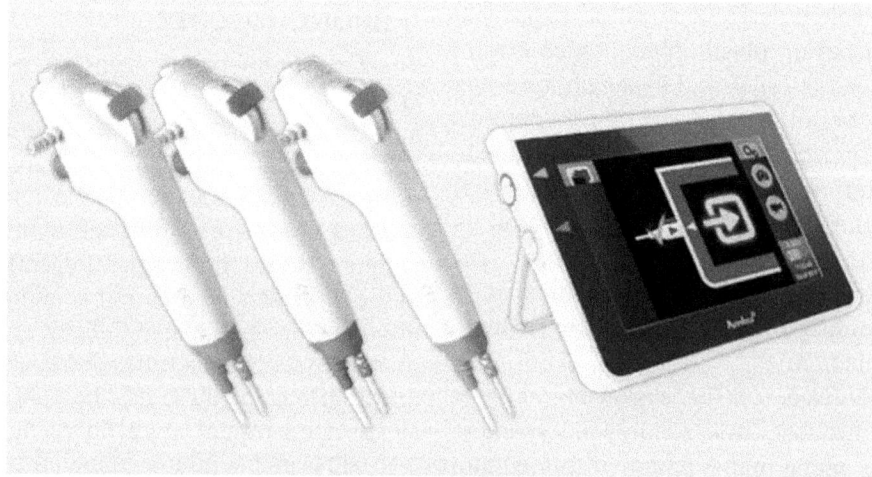

Fig. 12: Ambu aScope.

QUESTIONS

Q. 1. Compare direct laryngoscopy with video laryngoscopy.//
Q. 2. Airway USG for prediction of difficult laryngoscopy.//
Q. 3. Video laryngoscopy in a pediatric patient.//
Q. 4. Morphogenic parameters for prediction of difficult layngoscopy.//
Q. 5. Video laryngoscopy in a critically ill patient.//
Q. 6. Enumerate the components of (i) Mallampati score (ii) Extended MMP (iii) CL grading (iv) POGO scoring

FURTHER READING

1. Davey A, Diba A. Ward's Anaesthetic Equipment. Elsevier Health Sciences, 6th edition. Netherlands: Saunders; 2012.
2. Dorsch JA. Understanding anesthesia equipment. Philadelphia: Lippincott Williams and Wilkins; 2012.
3. Miller RD, Pardo M. Basics of anesthesia e-book. Gurugram, India: Elsevier Health Sciences; 2011.
4. Pieters BM, Eindhoven GB, Acott C, Van Zundert AA. Pioneers of laryngoscopy: indirect, direct and video laryngoscopy. Anaesth Intensive Care. 2015;43(Suppl):4-11.

CHAPTER 57

Endotracheal Tube

Rahil Singh, Nishant Sood

INTRODUCTION

An endotracheal tube is a device that is inserted through the oral or nasal route via the larynx into the trachea to facilitate the passage of gases and vapors to and from the lungs.

HISTORY

Since the ancient time of the Roman Civilization and present, endotracheal tubes (ETTs) have been constructed of a variety of materials including brass, reed, and steel. In 1917, Magill and Rowbotham used rubber to manufacture ETT to administer anesthesia. A protective cuff was added in 1928 by Guedel and Rowbotham to prevent aspiration. Polyvinyl chloride (PVC) was introduced in 1967 by SA Leader, and it has become the most commonly used material since then.

MATERIAL

Ideal material for ETT should have the following characteristics:
- Nonirritant and inexpensive
- Transparency to facilitate visualization of exhaled air mist, foreign bodies, and blockages
- Easy sterilization and durability with repeated sterilizations
- Nonreactive with lubricants and anesthetic agents
- Nonflammable
- Kink resistant with sufficient body to maintain its shape during insertion
- Latex-free.

It is difficult for any material to satisfy all the above-mentioned traits. Materials available for manufacturing ETT are red rubber, plastic (PVC, and more recently polyurethane), silicone, and rarely Teflon.

Red Rubber Tubes

Advantages
- Can be cleaned and sterilized for reuse
- Minimal mechanical tissue trauma.

Disadvantages
- Nontransparent.
- Repeated usage and sterilization lead to degradation and thus make them sticky and poor resistant to kinking.
- Allergenic and irritant due to coating of latex.
- Cuffs of rubber tubes are usually thick and require higher intracuff pressures which may lead to mucosal ischemia.

Polyvinyl Chloride

Advantages
- Low cost, disposable, nonirritant.
- Transparent.
- At room temperature, it provides stiffness to an ETT and thus assists with intubation

but softens at body temperature thus reducing pressure at the point of contact.
- Radiopaque lines can be embedded in PVC to facilitate visualization on a radiograph.
- The inner surface of the tube becomes smooth and nonwettable thus facilitating the passage of bronchoscope or suction catheters.

Disadvantages

Inflammable and prone to airway fires thus cannot be used in laser surgeries.

Silicone

Silicone rubber (polydimethylsiloxane) is an entirely synthetic material containing no latex derivatives, it is soft and can withstand autoclaving and therefore can be reused.

It is significantly more expensive and generally not used for disposable airway products.

Siliconized Plastic

It refers to a PVC material incorporating a very small amount of silicone oil to form a surface monolayer, intending to alter the surface characteristics of the product, for example, to decrease surface adhesion. These tubes tend to be pearlescent or opaque.

DESIGN

An endotracheal tube has two ends; a proximal end or a machine end (which gets connected to the breathing circuit) and a distal end or a patient end (which enters into the patient's trachea) **(Fig. 1)**. The tube can be shortened at the machine end if required. A typical ETT has a preformed curve, shaped like an arc of a circle with a radius of curvature of 140 ± 20 mm. This curve matches the anatomical curve of the airway and thus aids in insertion.

The distal end cut obliquely is called the *bevel* which faces to the left when held in the right hand. The bevel allows the tip of the tube to be seen passing between the vocal cords and thus facilitates insertion. A hole may be present on the wall of the tube opposite to the bevel. This is known as *Murphy's eye*. Its purpose is to provide an alternate pathway for gas flow if the bevel becomes occluded **(Figs. 2A and B)**.

Tracheal tubes which do not have Murphy's eye are called *Magill-type tubes*. The lack of Murphy's eye allows the cuff to be placed closer to the distal end of the tube thus reducing the chances of endobronchial intubation.

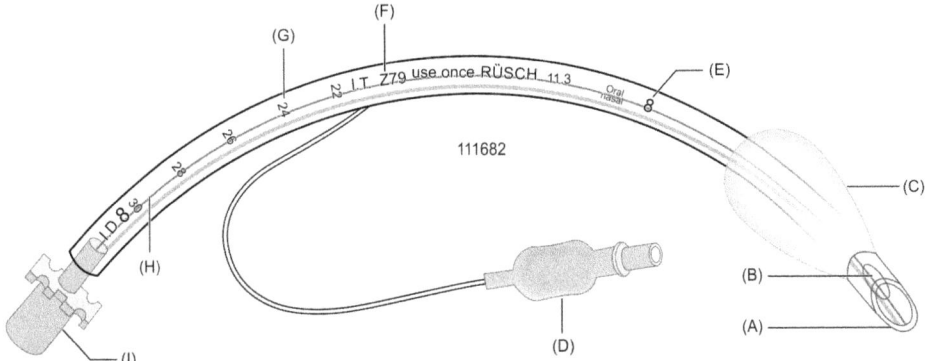

Fig. 1: (A) Bevel; (B) Murphy eye; (C) Tracheal cuff; (D) Self-sealing valve; (E) Marking to show the ID of the tube in mm; (F) Marking to show that the plastic has been tested for tissue toxicity; (G) The length of the tube in mm; (H) Longitudinal line of radiopaque material; and (I) 15 mm connector.

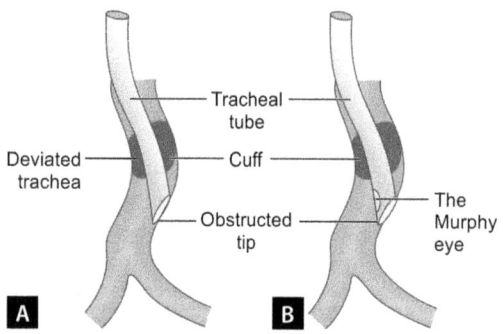

Figs. 2A and B: Bevel occlusion: Role of murphy eye.

A radiopaque line runs along the entire length of the tube so that the correct placement can be verified from the X-ray if required. A transverse black mark on some tubes marked several centimeters proximal to the cuff, designed to indicate the distance that the tube should be placed beyond the vocal cords. This black mark should remain just visible above the larynx, indicating that the tube has not been inserted too far. The distance from the tip of the bevel is also marked in centimeters on the tube wall, along with the internal diameter (ID).

CUFF SYSTEM (FIG. 3)

The cuff system serves the purpose of providing the seal between the tube and tracheal wall to prevent the passage of pharyngeal contents into the trachea and ensure no gas leaks past the cuff into the stomach during positive pressure ventilation. It includes the cuff and an inflation system which includes an inflation tube, a pilot balloon, and an inflation valve. The cuff material should be thin, soft but strong, and resistant to tearing.

The pressure on the lateral wall of the trachea when measured at the end of expiration should be approximately 20–30 cm-H_2O (15–22 mm Hg). Overinflation of the cuff leads to high pressure within the cuff which gets transmitted to the tracheal mucosa.

This problem can be avoided by the following measures:
1. The cuff should be inflated very gradually till the leak just disappears.
2. The cuff can be inflated with sterile saline or gas mixture that is identical to that and is used for anesthesia.
3. The intracuff pressure should be monitored intermittently or continuously using a cuff pressure manometer.

Types of Cuffs

High-volume Low-pressure Cuff

It has a large residual volume and diameter. It has a wider area of contact with the tracheal wall leading to equitable distribution of pressure over a large area of trachea than a specific point. The cuff adapts itself to the irregular tracheal wall. Usually used in PVC tubes.

Advantage
- Cuff-induced complications are minimal following prolonged intubation as the pressure exerted on tracheal mucosa is minimal and can be regulated.

Disadvantage
- Difficult to insert, as the cuff may obscure the view of the larynx and tip of the tube.
- The incidence of sore throat is higher than with a high-pressure cuff.
- There may be a greater likelihood of the cuff being torn during intubation especially when forceps are used.
- Less effective in preventing aspiration as the cuff may not be fully unfolded when the seal is achieved.

Low-volume High-pressure Cuff

It has a small residual volume and small diameter and requires high intracuff pressure to achieve the seal with the trachea. The area of contact of this type of cuff with the tracheal

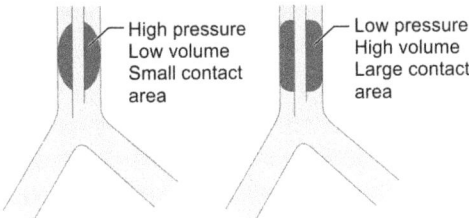

Fig. 3: Cuff system.

wall is small and it distends and deforms the trachea to a circular shape. Usually used in red rubber or reinforced tubes.

Advantages
- Better visibility of the tip of the tube and larynx during intubation.
- Better protection against aspiration.
- Lower incidence of sore throat.

Disadvantage
- Exerts high pressure on the tracheal wall thus increasing the chances of ischemic damage to tracheal wall mucosa following prolonged use.

Foam Cuff

It is a soft, low-pressure cuff with a large residual volume. It has self-inflating polyurethane foam material which replaces the air which is normally used to inflate the cuff. The cuff is actively deflated by applying suction to collapse the foam before insertion. Post intubation pilot balloon is opened to the atmosphere which allows the foam to expand and fill the cuff. The more the foam expands the lower the pressure is. The risk of aspiration is similar to that with most high-volume low-pressure cuffs.

SIZE

The widest diameter tracheal tube that would pass easily through the narrowest part of the airway is the correct size. This is to reduce the resistance to gas flow and minimize the extra work of breathing associated with the tracheal tube. In adults, the narrowest part of the airway is at the glottis; and in the pediatric population, it is the subglottis (cricoid). Again, the tube should be as short as possible to further reduce the work of breathing and to prevent the tube from entering the main bronchus (usually the right).

However, particularly in adult anesthetic practice, there is a trend towards the use of slightly smaller diameter tubes: When controlled ventilation is used, the ventilator, rather than the patient, does the work of breathing. The diameter of the tube does not determine airway pressures distal to it unless the tube is so narrow as not to allow sufficient time for passive exhalation. The larger the tube, the greater the area of contact between it and the vocal cords and the greater the likelihood of injury. Hoarseness and the incidence of sore throat are thought to increase dramatically.

Even in spontaneously breathing patients, the use of mandatory continuous capnography, by virtue of which anesthetists are able to demonstrate failing ventilation, allows greater latitude in the selection of tube size.

A size of 7 mm or 7.5 mm ID is chosen for an adult female and a size of 7.5 mm or 8 mm is chosen for an adult male patient. Pediatric ETT sizes are decided based on the age and weight of the patient **(Table 1)**. Uncuffed tubes had been in use in pediatric patients until 8–10 years of age till recently however with the development of thin polyurethane cuffs, cuffed endotracheal tubes are available in all pediatric patients.

A commonly used formula for uncuffed tube selection in patients over one year of age is:
- Age in year/4+ 4.5 mm
- The modified Cole formula: [4+ age/4] for children aged 2 and above.

Section 3: Anesthesia Instruments

TABLE 1: Tube size for children.

Recommended tube sizes for children

Age	Normal size
14 years	7.5–8
12–13 years	7–7.5
10–11 years	6.5–7
8–10 years	6–6.5
6–7 years	5.5–6
4–5 years	5–5.5
1.5–4 years	4.5–5
9–18 months	4–4.5
Full-term to 9 months	3.5–4
Premature	2.5–3

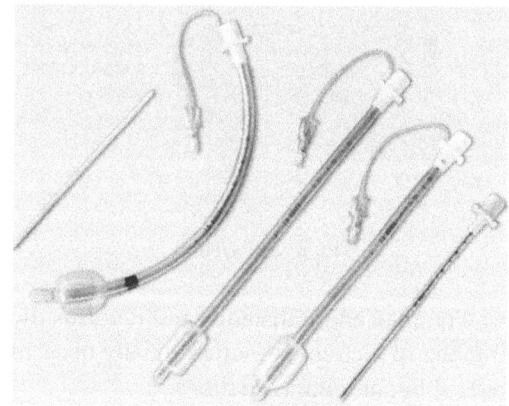

Fig. 4: Reinforced ETTs.

- Khine formula for calculating a cuffed tube size: [age/4+ 3 mm].

Micro cuff endotracheal tubes introduced for pediatric airway consist of a short, ultrathin polyurethane cuff situated away from the subglottic area (the narrowest part of the glottis in children and hence is prone to cuff induced damage). The cuff effectively seals the tracheal wall at pressures as low as 10 cmH$_2$O. The Murphy eye in these tubes is absent.

In pediatric age group: Length of the tube (cm) = [Age/2+ 12] cm.

SPECIAL TUBES

Reinforced/Armored Tubes/ Flexo-Metallic ETTs (Fig. 4)

These tubes are made up of silicon, PVC, rubber, or soft plastic. The hallmark of these tubes is a reinforcing spiral of steel or nylon wire into the wall of the tube thus making it kink resistant. The spiral however does not extend into the proximal or distal end. These tubes are very flexible with a little preformed shape and thus can be angled away from the surgical field.

Specific indication of the tube is head and neck surgery, spine surgery in the prone position, airway surgery like tracheal resection where the tube needs to be passed through the tracheostomy stoma, etc.

Disadvantages

- Due to increased flexibility either a bougie or a stylet is required to facilitate intubation. The tube may rotate on the stylet during insertion.
- It is difficult to pass the tube through the nose.
- Because of spirals, these tubes cannot be shortened in length.
- Difficult to insert through intubating laryngeal mask airway (LMA).
- Increased chances of accidental extubation due to elastic recoil force.
- The absence of Murphy's eye increases the chances of obstruction if the bevel abuts the wall of the trachea.
- Repeated sterilizations make the tube soft and sticky.

Preformed Tubes (Ring- Adair- Elwin Tubes)

This tube is named after their inventors—Ring, Adair, and Elwin (**Fig. 5**). It has a preformed

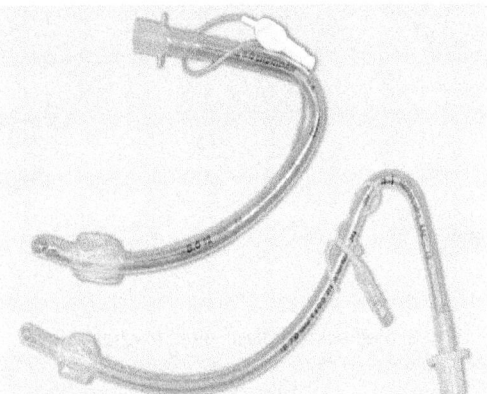

Fig 5: Preformed tubes (Ring- Adair- Elwin tubes).

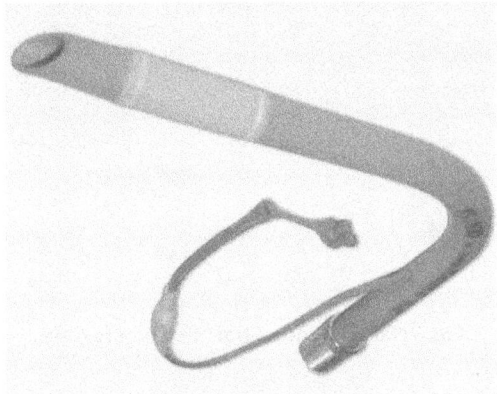

Fig. 6: Oxford tube.

bend in the tube which can be straightened during intubation. It is available in nasal and oral versions in various sizes in cuffed and uncuffed variety. When in place, the oral version rests on the patient's chin with a connector over the patient's chest and the nasal version is directed over the patient's forehead.

Advantages

- Easy to secure and the risk of unintended extubation is reduced.
- The tube can be placed away from the surgical field without using additional connectors due to the preformed curve.
- The long length allows them to be placed through a supraglottic airway device.
- The nasal version can be used for the oral intubation of patients who are to be operated on in prone positions.

Disadvantages

- Difficulty in passing a suction catheter. In an emergency, scenario suction can be done by cutting the tube at the curvature.
- Resistance is more than the similar-sized conventional tube.
- Since the length of the tube beyond the bend is fixed, a tube may be too long or too short for a given patient.

Oxford Tube (Fig. 6)

It is a right-angled (L-shaped) red rubber tube that may be cuffed or uncuffed. It is nonkinkable and thus used for airway surgeries like *palate surgery*. The internal diameter is uniform throughout but the external diameter varies so that the proximal portion in the mouth is thicker than the tracheal segment thus allowing the bigger tube to be passed through the trachea. The thicker wall at the lips prevents the compression by mouth gag.

Disadvantages

- The bevel of the tube is situated posteriorly and may abut against the tracheal wall if the head is flexed
- As with other preformed tubes distance from the bevel to the curve is fixed hence a proper sized tube must be used to avoid endobronchial intubation
- Increased resistance
- Difficult to suction
- Nontransparent.

Microlaryngeal Tracheal Surgery Tube (Fig. 7)

This tube has a small internal diameter (ID usually around 4-6 mm) but an adult-sized high-volume low-pressure cuff. The tube is

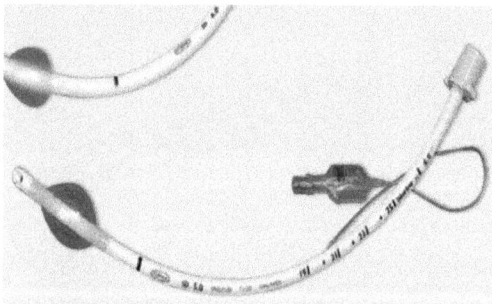

Fig. 7: Microlaryngeal tracheal surgery tube.

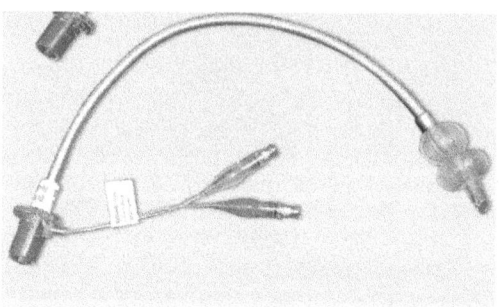

Fig. 8: Mallinckrodt "laser-flex" tracheal tubes.

designed to allow surgery around the vocal cords and is long enough for nasal intubation.

The high resistance to gas flow in these tubes virtually obligates controlled ventilation and a long expiratory phase should be used to allow complete expiration. As they are not laser resistant, they are not suitable for such surgery.

TUBES FOR LASER SURGERY

Conventional tracheal tubes of either plastic, silicone, or rubber may be damaged by the carbon dioxide, potassium titanyl phosphate (KTP), or neodymium-doped yttrium aluminum garnet (Nd: YAG) laser beam. These materials burn more fiercely in the presence of oxygen or nitrous oxide than in air and are easily ignited by a direct or indirect strike from the laser beam.

The resultant fire can produce serious upper airway burns and severe distal inhalation injury; injuries may be fatal.

Mallinckrodt "Laser-Flex" Tracheal Tubes (Fig. 8)

These single-use tubes for oral intubation are made from a gas-tight metal helix with the pilot tubes for the double cuff carried within the lumen of the airway.

The surface of the tube shaft reflects a defocused laser beam, with a lower potential for causing tissue destruction.

The tip of the tube is made of soft plastic for more atraumatic insertion. The tubes have a markedly reduced inner diameter when compared to PVC tubes. It is advised that the cuffs, which are not laser resistant, are inflated with a saline, ideally with methylene blue, to prevent ignition of the cuff and so that puncture is obvious.

The function of the proximal cuff is to protect the distal cuff and the tube must be replaced if either cuff is defective.

Foil-wrapped

An alternative approach used by some manufacturers is to spirally wrap a suitable small rubber tube with a narrow strip of silver or copper foil (this may be stippled or corrugated to disperse an incident beam).

Rusch Tubes

The characteristics of Rusch tubes are enlisted in **Box 1**.

Sheridan Tube

The characteristics of Sheridan tubes are given in **Box 2**.

Laryngectomy Tube (Fig. 9)

They are designed to be inserted into tracheostomy stoma. The J-shape allows the part of the tube external to the patient to

BOX 1: Rusch tubes.

- Sterile and single-use
- Soft white rubber tube with Murphy's eye
- Approximately 40 cm (16") long
- Hooded tip
- Two high volume cuffs (one inside the other)
- Consisting of Merocele sponge and micro-corrugated silver foil
- Laser resistant foam surrounds the lower 17 cm of tube

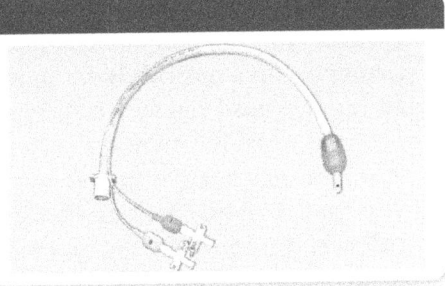

BOX 2: Sheridan tube.

- Red rubber material
- Unique embossed copper foil diffuses laser energy minimizing unintended laser damage to tissue
- Atraumatic outer covering
- Overall length is equivalent to the standard 8.0 mm tracheal tube

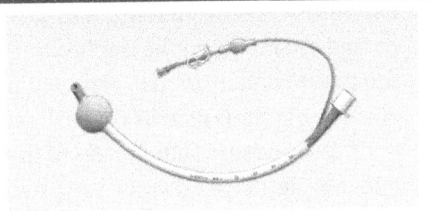

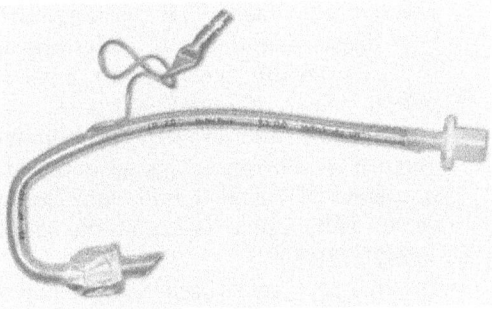

Fig. 9: Laryngectomy tube.

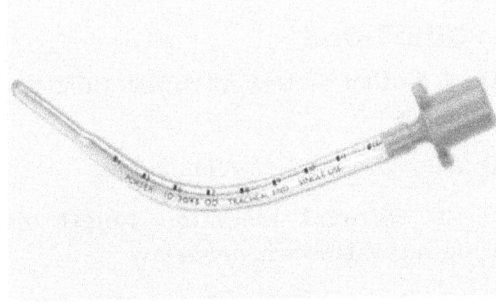

Fig. 10: Cole tube.

be directed distant from the surgical field. The curve may need to be straightened to facilitate insertion. The internal portion of the tube is short and the tip is usually cut close to the cuff to minimize the risk of bronchial intubation. The tube can be secured by either her suturing or taping it to the chest wall.

Cole Tube (Fig. 10)

It is an uncuffed tube. The patient-end has smaller ED than the rest of the parts. It has a shoulder at the junction of the tracheal end and the broad proximal end. The shoulder prevents endobronchial intubation. The size of the tube is based on the ID of the tracheal end. It is used for *neonatal resuscitation*. These tubes cannot be used for nasal intubation.

COMMON PROBLEMS WITH ENDOTRACHEAL TUBES

- Trauma to lips, teeth, tonsillar pillar, tongue, arytenoids, jaw, etc.
- Disconnection of the tube from the 15 mm International Organization for

Standardization (ISO) connector or of the connector from the catheter mount is common. This is most likely during shared airway or in head and neck surgery.

- *Leak:* In uncuffed tubes, an excessive leak indicates a larger tube is required. With cuffed tubes, a leak may arise if the cuff is at the cords. It may also indicate inadequate cuff inflation or deflation caused by cuff damage.
- Accidental extubation.
- Endobronchial placement. A tube may be passed too far down the trachea and enter the main bronchus. This can occur after correct placement when the head and neck are repositioned; flexion of the head and neck tends to advance the tube.
- Sore throat, hoarseness, and subglottic granulation tissue may occur postextubation.

QUESTIONS

Q. 1. Cuffed versus uncuffed tube for neonates.

Q. 2. Bougie vs stylet for intubation.

Q. 3. Optimal insertion length of endotracheal tubes in neonates.

Q. 4. Various formulas for length of insertion and size of ET tube.

FURTHER READING

1. Bernard WN, Cottrell, JE, Sivakumaran C, Patel K, Yost L, Turndorf H. Adjustment of intracuff pressure to prevent aspiration. Anaesthesiology. 1979;50(4):363-6.
2. Black AE, Mackersie AM. Accidental bronchial intubation with RAE tubes. Anaesthesia. 1991;46:42-3.
3. Blom H, Rytlander M, Wisborg T. Resistance of tracheal tubes 3.0 and 3.5 mm internal diameter. A comparison of four commonly used types. Anaesthesia. 1985;40:885-8.
4. Condon HA, Gilchrist E. Stanley Rowbotham: Twentieth century pioneer anaesthetist. Anaesthesia. 1986;41(1):46-52.
5. Davies RG. The importance of a Murphy eye. Anaesthesia. 2001;56(9):915.
6. Dawson P, Rosewane F, Wells D. The Montando laryngectomy tube. Can J Anaesth. 1989;36:486-7.
7. Loeser EA, Machin R, Colley J, Orr D 2nd, Bennett GM, Stanley TH. Postoperative sore throat–Importance of endotracheal tube conformity versus cuff design. Anesthesiology. 1978;49(6):430-2.
8. Loeser EA, Stanley TH, Jordan W, Machin R. Postoperative sore throat: influence of tracheal tube lubrication versus cuff design. Can Anaesth Soc J. 1980;27(2):156-8.
9. Power KJ. Foam cuffed tracheal tubes: clinical and laboratory assessment. Br J Anaesth. 1990;65(3):433-7.

58 Lung Isolation Devices

Ayushi Mahajan, Amit Kohli

INTRODUCTION

One lung ventilation (OLV) is the ability to ventilate one lung while allowing the other one to collapse either to facilitate surgical exposure or manage some diseased state. In this chapter, we will learn about the various devices which help us to achieve lung isolation.

INDICATIONS

The indications for lung isolation can be divided into *absolute* and *relative* as discussed here:

Absolute

- To prevent damage or contamination of the healthy lung
  - Lung abscess
  - Massive hemorrhage
- To control the distribution of ventilation to only one lung
  - Bronchopleural fistula
  - Major bronchial disruption
  - Unilateral lung cyst or bullae
- To facilitate single lung lavage
  - Pulmonary alveolar proteinosis.

Relative

- To improve surgical access—high priority
  - Video-assisted thoracoscopic surgery (VATS)
  - Pneumonectomy
  - Lung volume reduction surgery
  - Upper lobectomy
  - Thoracic aortic aneurysm
  - Minimally invasive cardiac surgery
- To improve surgical access—low priority
  - Esophageal surgery
  - Middle and lower lobectomy
  - Mediastinal mass reduction
  - Bilateral sympathectomies.

ANATOMICAL CONSIDERATIONS (FIG. 1)

The trachea bifurcates into the left and right *mainstem bronchus* at the level of the *carina*. The right mainstem bronchus is shorter, wider in diameter, and more vertically placed as compared to the left mainstem bronchus. The take-off of the right upper lobe bronchus is very close to the carina (1–2.5 cm), whereas the left upper lobe bronchus branches off the left main bronchus at 4–5 cm from the carina. There are considerable anatomic variations: for example, there may be an abnormal take-off of the right upper lobe bronchus directly from the trachea (0.1–2% incidence reported).

These anatomic features mean it is easier to intubate the right bronchus, especially if a blind insertion technique is used. However, it is more difficult to place a tube in the right bronchus without obstructing the upper lobe.

LUNG ISOLATION DEVICES

- Double lumen tubes (DLTs)
- Bronchial blocking (BB) devices
- Single-lumen endobronchial tubes (SLT).

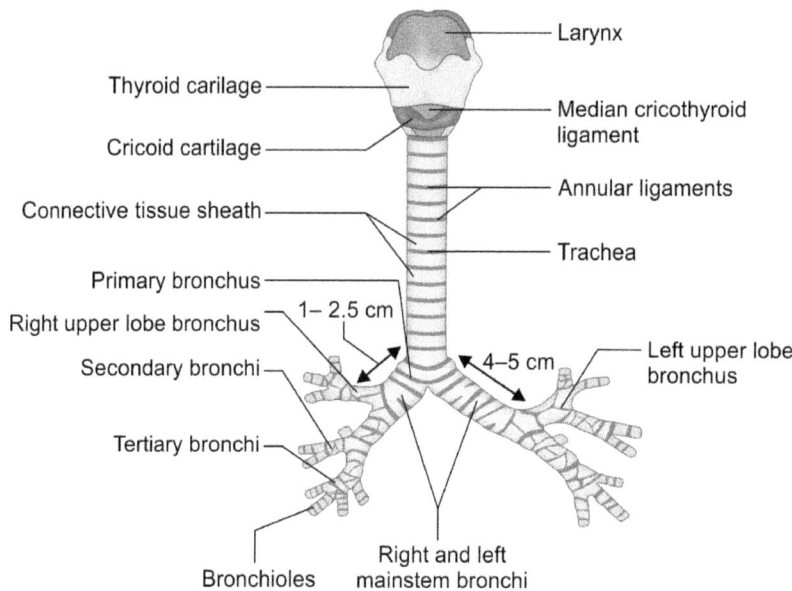

Fig. 1: Anatomy of the tracheobronchial tree. Note the distance of the right and left upper lobe bronchi from the carina.

DOUBLE LUMEN TUBES (FIGS. 2A AND B)

Double lumen tubes (DLTs) are the most common lung isolation devices used. DLTs can be either right-sided or left-sided depending upon which mainstem bronchus the tube is designed to fit. Historically, DLTs were made of reusable red rubber with high-pressure cuffs. With time disposable DLTs made of nontoxic plastic material started getting manufactured.

Components

There are several types of DLTs available, but essentially most of them share similar characteristics with minor changes. The following characteristics can be found in all DLTs:
- Two single lumen tubes bonded together, with the shorter one ending in the trachea and the longer one ending in the bronchus.
- It has two curves, a standard anterior curve, and a second curve either to the left or right to enable advancement into the respective main stem bronchus.
- High volume, low-pressure color-coded cuffs. The bronchial cuff along with its pilot balloon is mostly blue in color, whereas the tracheal cuff and its pilot balloon are clear.
- Due to the anatomical differences between the left and right mainstem bronchus as mentioned above, the right-sided Double lumen tube (DLT) has either a modified cuff with a side opening (Murphy's eye) or a slot on the endobronchial side that allows ventilation for the right upper lobe.
- Y-adapter for the proximal end which allows ventilation of both lumens through a single circuit.
- Radiographic markers near the endotracheal and endobronchial cuffs.

Specific Tubes
- *Carlens (left-sided) double-lumen tube:* It was the first clinically available DLT.

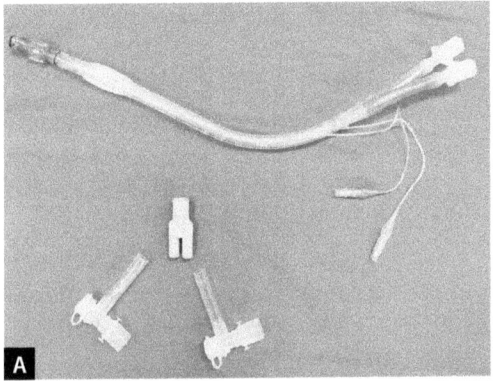

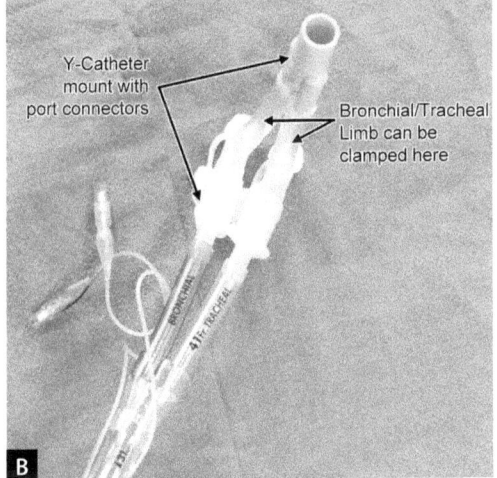

Figs. 2A and B: (A) Left sided double lumen tube (DLT); (B) Proximal end of DLT. Kindly note the connections and where the clamps can be attached.

Carlen's tubes were only left side and had a carinal hook. These tubes had a high flow resistance due to narrow lumens and were difficult to insert due to the carinal hook.
- *White (right-sided) double-lumen tube:* This was designed to fit the right mainstem bronchus and had a carinal hook.
- *Robertshaw (left and right-sided) double-lumen tube:* Initially, these were made of red rubber and came in three sizes—small, medium, and large. The carinal hook was absent which made its insertion easier. With time, red rubber has been replaced by PVC disposable material. Both left and right-sided Robertshaw tubes are available. The bronchial cuff of the right-sided Robertshaw DLT has a slotted opening in its lateral aspect.
- *Bronchocath (left and right-sided) double-lumen tube:* Both left and right-sided tubes are available. The right-sided tube has a bronchial cuff shaped like a slanted doughnut to facilitate proper placement and ventilation of the right upper lobe.
- *Sher-I-bronch (left and right-sided) double-lumen tube:* The right-sided version has two cuffs on the bronchial segment for better ventilation of the right upper lobe.
- *Silbroncho (left and right-sided) double-lumen tube:* Silbroncho DLT is made of silicone and has a wire-reinforced bronchial segment.

Choosing the Size

Adult DLTs come in sizes of 35, 37, 39, and 41 FR. Traditionally 39 FR is used in an average-sized adult male, whereas 37 FR is used in an average-sized adult female. Upper or lower sizes are used for patients larger or smaller respectively. 32 FR is available for small adults, and 26 and 28 FR for pediatric cases.

Choosing the Side

Left-sided DLTs are preferred over the right-sided ones even when the right lung needs to be isolated because of the various anatomical considerations mentioned earlier. However, there are a few indications of right-sided tubes, viz., distorted anatomy of a left main bronchus by an intrabronchial or extra-bronchial mass left pneumonectomy, or a left lung transplant.

Depth of Insertion

In adults, the depth of insertion correlates with the height of the patient. For a height of

170–180 cm, the average depth of insertion is 29 cm. For every 10 cm increase or decrease in height, DLT is advanced or withdrawn 1 cm, or it can be calculated by the formula: 12 + (patient height/10) cm.

Insertion

The tube is prepared before placement. Both the bronchial and tracheal cuffs are inflated and checked for any leaks. The tracheal cuff can be filled with up to 20 mL of air and the bronchial cuff with up to 3 mL of air. The tube is sprayed with an aerosolized silicon spray (lubricant jelly is avoided as it may cause problems in fiberscopy).

Blind Technique

Using a normal laryngoscope or a video laryngoscope, DLT is inserted with the distal curvature concave anteriorly. After the tip passes the vocal cords, the stylet is removed and the tube is rotated 90° to the side that the tube is to be put and advanced blindly till resistance is felt.

Direct Vision Technique

Double lumen tube can also be placed by inserting a fiberscope into the appropriate bronchial lumen and directing the tube over it. However, it takes more time to perform than the blind technique.

Confirming Position

Various methods have been described to confirm the right placement.

Auscultatory Method

The below example illustrates how to check a left-sided DLT.

- The tracheal cuff is inflated (5–10 mL). Bilateral air entry should be present. Unilateral air entry to either side means the depth of insertion is more than required. The tube should be withdrawn appropriately.
- The bronchial cuff is inflated (1–3 mL)
- The tracheal lumen is clamped. Air entry should be present only on the left side. Bilateral air entry at this stage means the bronchial opening is still in the trachea. Advance the tube further. If only right-sided air entry is present, it means the tube is in the wrong bronchus. Withdraw the tube and reinsert.
- The tracheal lumen is unclamped and the bronchial lumen is clamped. Air entry should be present only on the right side.

Flexible Endoscopy Technique

Flexible endoscopy is the most accurate method to determine the correct placement of the DLT. Most DLTs easily accommodate 3.6–4.2 mm outer diameter fiberscope.

For left-sided DLTs
- Insert the fiberoptic bronchoscope (FOB) through the tracheal lumen and visualize the carina.
- Identify the blue-colored endobronchial cuff as a thin crest within the left main bronchus but not herniating over the carina after inflation.

For right-sided DLTs
- In addition to the above steps, insert the FOB through the endobronchial lumen and ensure Murphy's eye is aligned with the right upper lobe bronchus.

The advantages and disadvantages of DLT are mentioned in **Table 1**.

BRONCHIAL BLOCKING DEVICES

In some instances, the use of DLT is not possible. An alternate method to achieve lung isolation in such cases is by using bronchial blockers (BBs). There are many different types of BBs available that can be used either

TABLE 1: Advantages and disadvantages of bronchial blocker and DLTs.

Devices	Advantages	Disadvantages
Double lumen tube (DLT)	• Quickest to place • Large lumen facilitates suctioning • Best device for absolute lung separation	• Size selection is more difficult • Difficult to place in difficult airway patients • It cannot be used where nasal intubation is required • Not optimal for postoperative mechanical ventilation • Potential laryngeal or bronchial trauma • Smaller sizes are not available, cannot be used in <12 years old patient
Bronchial blocker (BB)	• Size selection easy • Can be used in an already intubated patient • Easier to place in difficult airway patients • Less traumatic • More optimal for continued postoperative ventilation • Selective lobar lung isolation is possible • Nasal intubation possible • Can be used in a patient with a tracheostomy • Can be used in an already intubated patient	• Small channel for suctioning • Slow lung deflation • High maintenance device (dislodgement or loss of seal during surgery is seen more) • More time is needed for positioning • Less satisfactory lung separation

in conjugation with a standard SLT or with a modified SLT with integrated blockers.

Devices

- Univent bronchial blocking tube
- Arndt endobronchial blocker (WEB)
- Cohen tip deflecting bronchial blocker
- Embolectomy (Fogarty) catheter.

Univent Bronchial Blocking Tubes

It is a silastic SLT with an attached chamber for a bronchial blocker along with the concave side of the tube. The blocker has a high-pressure, low-volume cuff. The blocker has a small lumen along its entire length which helps to deflate the lung and can be used for suctioning. At the proximal end of the blocker, there is a lumen cap that needs to be blocked during normal two lung ventilation. Univent tubes are available in many sizes **(Fig. 3)**.

Before the placement of the Univent tube, tracheal and bronchial cuffs are checked for any leaks. The tube is lubricated, and the tip of the BB is withdrawn inside the chamber. After direct laryngoscopy, the tube is placed and the tracheal cuff is inflated, FOB is passed through the tube, and under direct vision, the BB is advanced into the desired bronchus.

The Univent blocker (Uniblocker) is available independent of the entire tube and can be used with the standard endotracheal tubes coaxially or para-axially.

Arndt Bronchial Blocker

Arndt bronchial blocker that is shown in **Figure 4** is also known as a *wire-guided bronchial blocker (WEB)*. It has two parts:
1. A blocking catheter with a low-pressure, high-volume cuff and a nylon guidewire that extends from the proximal to the distal end of the blocker and exits as a loop snare. The snare loops around the tip of FOB and guides the blocker into the desired bronchus.

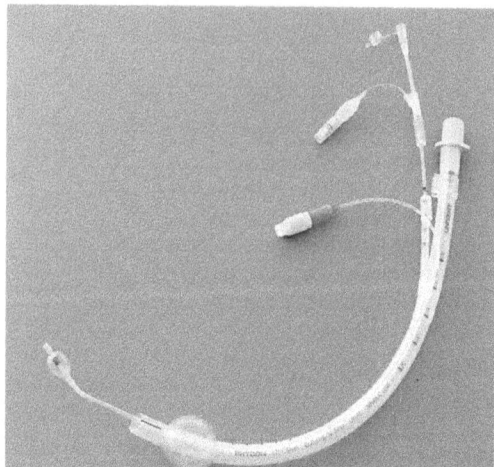

Fig. 3: Univent tube.

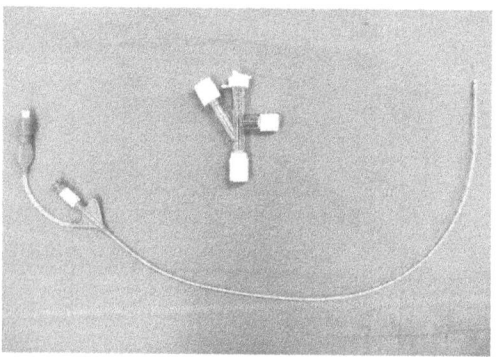

Fig. 4: Arndt bronchial blocker.

2. A multiport adapter that has a 15 mm ET tube connector, a ventilation port, a bronchoscopy port, and a blocker port.

Cohen Tip-deflecting Bronchial Blocker

It has a high-volume, low-pressure blue balloon at the tip. There are side holes between the tip and the balloon which help to evacuate gas from the lung during deflation or insufflate the gas in the lungs during inflation. The blocker has a rotating wheel that deflects the soft tip by >90° and hence directs it into the desired bronchus.

Embolectomy (Fogarty) Catheter

Embolectomy (Fogarty Catheter can be used as a Bronchial Blocker. Ready availability in most operating suites is an advantage. However, the main disadvantage is that the occlusion balloon is high-pressure, low-volume, and it is impossible to do suction or insufflation through it.

Advantages and disadvantages of BB are mentioned in **Table 1**.

SINGLE LUMEN BRONCHIAL TUBES

Another option for lung isolation is to use a single lumen tube to intubate the desired main stem bronchus. It can be done with the conventional single lumen tube or especially available endobronchial tubes with an angulated distal tip. This method is however hardly ever used except in rare cases of emergency surgery, very difficult airway, or in pediatric patients whose airways are too small for DLTs or bronchial blockers.

FURTHER READING

1. Aoun NY, Velez E, Kenney LA, Trayner E. Tracheal bronchus. Respir Care. 2004;49(9): 1056-8.
2. Bahk JH, Oh YS: Prediction of double-lumen tracheal tube depth. J Cardiothorac Vasc Anesth. 1999;13(3):370-1.
3. Benumof JL. The position of a double-lumen tube should be routinely determined by fiberoptic bronchoscopy. J Cardiothorac Vasc Anesth. 1993;7(5):513-4.
4. Boucek CD, Landreneau R, Freeman J, Strollo D, Bircher NG. A comparison of techniques for placement of double-lumen endobronchial tubes. J Clin Anesth. 1998;10(7):557-60.
5. Chow MY, Go MH, Ti LK. Predicting the depth of insertion of left-sided double-lumen endobronchial tubes. J Cardiothorac Vasc Anesth. 2002;16(4):456-8.

CHAPTER 59

Devices for Difficult Airway Management

Ridhima Sharma, Ripon Choudhary

INTRODUCTION

Difficult airway management (DAM) requires anesthesiologists and critical care clinicians to respond promptly with an apt evaluation of specific scenarios. Therefore, it is prudent to have organized information regarding the DAM devices and device-oriented guidance for DAM. This will aid the practitioners to select the safest and most efficacious strategy. Based on literature search and DAM device information, various devices can be chosen according to the device-oriented strategy and anatomical difficulty faced. Apart from the conventional devices, the neo-options include; supraglottic airway device (SAD), video laryngoscope (VLS), and flexible fiberoptic scope (FOS). Therefore, knowledge of these devices is an essential key to the successful management of difficult airways and saving a life.

INCIDENCE

Overall, the advancement in the DAM devices has lowered the incidence of airway-associated complications. However, the intricacy to complete ventilatory failure is devastating and challenging. The incidence of the *cannot intubate and cannot oxygenate (CICO)* is approximately 0.02–0.02% cases, contributing to 25% of all anesthesia-related deaths. In another study, 5%, 18%, 0.004–0.008% of patients were difficult to oxygenate, intubate, and cannot be oxygenated/intubated respectively. Hence, strong recommendations exist for early management before desaturation. The incorporation of advanced monitoring including capnography also had a great role.

Q. 1. What is the definition of a difficult airway?

Ans. The American Society of Anesthesiologists (ASA) defined a difficult airway as the clinical situation in which a conventionally trained anesthesiologist experiences difficulty with mask ventilation, difficulty with tracheal intubation, or both.

Q. 2. How would you define difficult mask ventilation?

Ans. According to the ASA, it is defined as a clinical situation in which it is not feasible for the unassisted anesthesiologists to maintain oxygen saturation >90% using 100% oxygen and positive pressure mask ventilation in a patient whose oxygen saturation was >90% before the anesthesiologist intervention or inability to prevent or reverse the signs of inadequate ventilation during positive pressure ventilation.

Q. 3. How would you define difficult laryngoscopy?

Ans. It is defined as; the inability to view the glottis opening using a conventional curve blade laryngoscope, corresponding to a Cormack and Lehane grade III or IV view.

Q. 4. What is the definition of difficult endotracheal intubation?

Ans. Intubation is called difficult when the trained anesthesiologist needs more than three attempts or >10 minutes for successful endotracheal intubation.

Q. 5. What is Lemon law?

Ans. The *LEMON* law represents five rapid, reproducible components for the assessment of the airway.

1. *L* = Look externally (facial trauma, large incisors, beard or mustache, and large tongue)
2. *E* = Evaluate the 3-3-2 rule (incisor distance <3 fingerbreadths, hyoid/mental distance <3 fingerbreadths, thyroid to-mouth distance <2 fingerbreadths) **(Fig. 1)**
3. *M* = Mallampati (Mallampati score ≥3)
4. *O* = Obstruction (presence of any condition that could cause an obstructed airway)
5. *N* = Neck mobility (limited neck mobility).

Predictors of the difficult airway: There are various clinical tests and models for the prediction of difficult laryngoscopy and intubation. Among all these, Cormack-Lehane grading is the most predicted model recounted to describe difficult laryngoscopy. Based on the laryngoscopy view obtained four grades are classified. They are as follows:

- *Grade I:* Entire glottis is completely visible
- *Grade II:* Only the posterior commissure is visible
- *Grade III:* Only the tip of the epiglottis is visible
- *Grade IV:* No glottic, structures are visible.

Higher Cormack–Lehane grade conglomerate with difficult intubation; (grades III and IV).

Another most commonly qualitative assessment method in the airway examination is termed as modified Mallampati classification. To perform this test, the patient is asked to be seated in a position with his head in a neutral position with his mouth wide open and his tongue protruding to its maximum. This 4-category classification is described as:

- *Class 1:* Visualization of the soft palate and uvula.

- Mouth opening ≥ 3 fingers
- Tip of the chin to the hyoid bone ≥ 3 fingers
- Hyoid bone to the tip of the thyroid cartilage ≥ 2 fingers

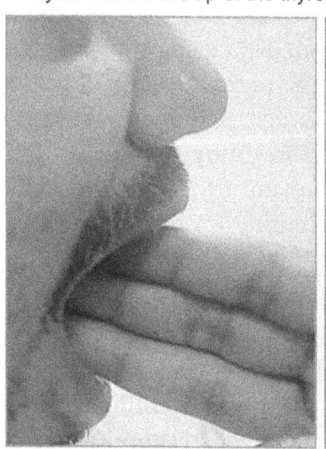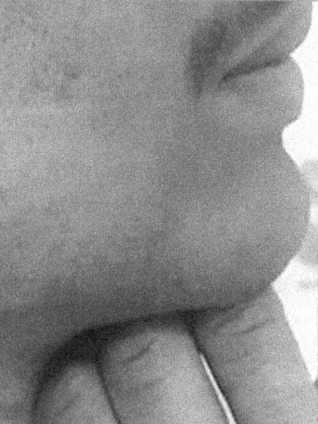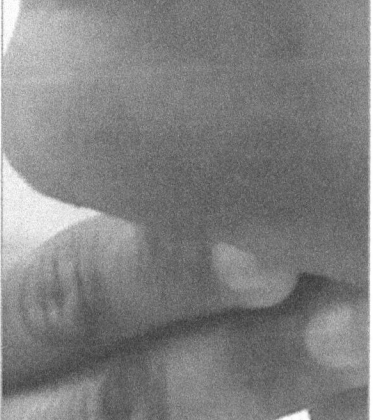

Fig. 1: Lemon law; 3-3-2 rule.

TABLE 1: Findings suggestive of difficult airway management.

Parameters	Accepted Value	Significance
Interincisor distance	>3 cm	Easy insertion of laryngoscope (gap >3 cm)
Sternomental distance	<12.5 cm	Difficult laryngoscopic intubation
Thyromental distance	>5 cm or >3 fingerbreadth	Suggestive easy alignment of axes and optimal position of the larynx
Hyomental distance	Grade 1: >6 cm Grade 2: 4.0–6.0 cm Grade 3: <4.0 cm	Grade 3, suggestive of impossible laryngoscopy and intubation

- *Class 2:* Visualization of the soft palate and tonsillar pillars.
- *Class 3:* Visualization of the soft palate only.
- *Class 4:* Visualization of the hard palate only.

In addition to this, findings suggestive of difficult airway management include; short thyromental distance (6 cm), protruding or prominent maxillary incisors, and limited neck extension **(Table 1)**.

Q. 6. What are the criteria for difficult bag-mask ventilation?
Ans. There are two easy indices to predict difficult bag-mask ventilation and can be easily remembered by the following mnemonics:
1. BONES
    - Bearded individual
    - Obesity [body mass index (BMI) >26 kg/m^2]
    - No teeth
    - Elderly (age >55 years)
    - Snorer

   Patients having two or more of these criteria will have difficult mask ventilation.
2. MOANS
    - Mask seal can be difficult or impossible
    - Obesity (BMI>26kg/m^2) or upper airway obstruction
    - Advanced age
    - No teeth
    - Snorer.

Q. 7. Which scoring system can be used for the evaluation of any new directly visualizing intubating device?
Ans. *Percentage of glottic opening (POGO) scoring:* This scoring is used, while directly visualizing with a laryngoscope or any other similar modifications. The scoring is as follows:
- Entire glottis was seen—100% score
- No glottis seen (not even the arytenoids)—0% score
- The only lower third of the vocal cords and the arytenoids visible—33% score.

Q. 8. Enumerate commonly used options/alternative devices to conventional rigid laryngoscopes and tracheal intubation.
Ans. Commonly used optional devices for rigid laryngoscope and tracheal intubation are as follows:
- Fiberoptic (flexible) aided intubation
- Intubating laryngeal mask airway, LMA C Trach™, LMA (classic) guided endotracheal intubation (ETI)
- Gum elastic bougie aided ETI
- Rigid (indirect) fiberoptic laryngoscopes (Bullard's, Wu-Scope, Upsher's) guided ETI
- Retromolar scope aided intubation
- Pharyngeal airway Xpress guided ETI
- Retromolar ETI
- C-Arm guided ETI.

Q. 9. List the devices which should be available in the difficult airway cart.
Ans.

Devices for difficult airway cart

- Face mask all sizes
  - *Different sizes airways:* Nasopharyngeal; #6, 7, 8 (adult), #3, 4, 5 (pediatric)
  - *Guedels oropharyngeal airway:* #7, 8, 9, 10, 11 (adult), #3, 4, 5, 6 (pediatric)
  - *Endotracheal stylets:* #14 F Mallinckrodt (adult), # 6, 8 F (pediatric)
  - *Bougie:* Eschmann gum elastic #10 and 15 F, 65 cm (adult)
- Manual resuscitation bag with reservoir, oxygen tubing, and connectors to connect to cylinder or wall outlet oxygen sources
  - *Laryngoscope:* Two sets (minimum) including a video laryngoscope
  - *Laryngoscope blades:* Curved Macintosh, straight Miller, McCoys flexible blade; 3 and 4, 3 and 4, and 3 respectively (adult), #1 and 2 straight millers (pediatric)
  - *Magill's forceps:* Two different sizes
  - *Suction catheter:* All sizes
  - *Endotracheal tubes:* #5.0, 6.0, 6.5, 7.0, 7.5, 8.0ID (Adult), #2.5, 3.0, 3.5, 4.0, 4.5 ID (pediatric)
  - *Laryngeal mask airway (LMA):* Different sizes (#3, 4, 5) adult and (#1, 1.5, 2, 2.5) pediatric including intubating LMA (ILMA)

Contd...

- Flexible fiberoptic laryngoscope
  - Transcricothyroid membrane jet ventilation: #12, 14 Gauge IV catheter (2 inches), jet ventilation hose with Luer-lock connector, and J-wire or epidural catheter for the retrograde catheter.
- Percutaneous tracheostomy set
  - Surgical cricothyroidotomy equipment: Scalpel (#3 scalpel handle), blade (#11), ET tube (6.0), cuffed tracheostomy tube (#4, 6, 8, and 10), tracheal retractor hook
- End-tidal CO_2 measurement devices, tube exchanger
  - Miscellaneous items: Bite block, spare batteries, equipment for spraying local anesthetics Bullard indirect scope, Retromolar scope.

Q. 10. What does the ideal difficult airway trolley (DAT) look like?

- Top workspace with 4–5 drawers **(Fig. 2)**
- Trolley to be mobile
- Robust
- It should be stocked in a logical sequence
- Labeled clearly
- Easy to clean
- Documents attached to the trolley; Difficult Airway Society (DAS)/local modified institutional guidelines

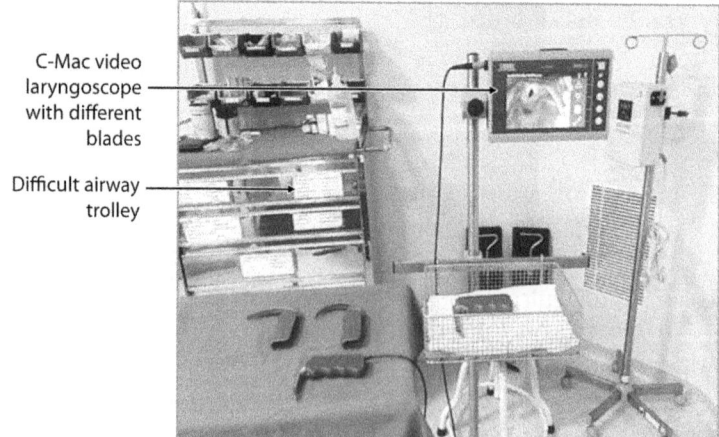

Fig. 2: Difficult airway trolley and C-Mac video laryngoscope.

- Checklist for the restocking purpose
- Daily checking logbook
- Reproducible

Q. 11. What devices can be used for cannot ventilate, cannot intubate situation (CVCI) from the DAT?

Ans. Refer Drawer 4 and 5 in the Table on next page.

Q. 12. What are the devices used stepwise for unanticipated difficult intubation according to DAS guidelines?

Ans. According to the DAS guidelines, the plan and devices used for unanticipated difficult intubation are as follows (Flowchart 1):

Step 1: Laryngoscopy and tracheal intubation
- Two or more attempts [oxygen saturation (SpO_2) ≥95%] may be made after the initial intubation failure
- Immediately call for help
- Ensure oxygenation all the time in between attempts by proper mask ventilation
- Ensure adequate depth of anesthesia throughout the procedure
- Subsequent attempts to be made by the experienced personnel
- Consider different techniques or technology.

Step 2: LMA (second generation)
- Attempt a second-generation supraglottic device (SGD) to maintain ventilation and oxygenation
- Not more than two attempts with SGD insertion with mask ventilation, using 100% oxygen.
- In case of device failure, consider an alternative type of SGD
- With a successful insertion of SGD, the type of surgery decides the further course, if not emergency; wake up the patient, in case surgery is necessary and can be performed with the device; continue the surgery, in case surgery, is not safe with SGD; attempt using fiberoptic intubation to secure definitive airway or surgical airway.

Step 3: Reverse and wake the patient
- Final attempt at mask ventilation using optional techniques/adjuncts, if there is a difficulty in mask ventilation.
- Ensure complete neuromuscular blockade before proceeding to cricothyroidotomy.
- Maintain oxygenation using an anesthesia circuit or pressure-regulated jet ventilation.

Step 4: Emergency surgical or needle cricothyroidotomy
- Cricothyroidotomy to be performed, depending upon the user's practice and immediate availability of instruments.
- Cricothyroidotomy is the procedure of choice, not tracheostomy.

Q. 13. Enumerate steps of needle and surgical cricothyroidotomy.

Ans.

Needle Cricothyroidotomy

- Needle cricothyroidotomy involves the insertion of the needle through the cricothyroid membrane into the trachea in an emergency, when a definitive airway cannot be achieved (Fig. 4).
- Percutaneous transtracheal oxygenation (PTO) is performed by placing large-caliber cannula (#12–14G) for adults and (#16–18G) in children; through the cricothyroid membrane into the trachea.
- After confirmation by aspirating the air in a syringe, the steel shaft of the Intra-Cath is removed and the cannula is fully inserted into the trachea in a caudal direction and firmly held.
- The cannula is connected to the oxygen source at 12–15 L/min (40–50 psi) with a Y-connector or side hole cut in the oxygen tubing attached between the plastic cannula and oxygen source.

Devices according to plan	Contents	Side of the trolley	Adjuvants	Miscellaneous
Top of trolley	• Flexible intubating fiberscope • Portable score with battery light source • Single used fiberscope: Ambu aScope	• Bougies (adult/pediatric) • Airway exchange catheter **(Fig. 3)** • Aintree intubation catheter		• DAS intubation guidelines (laminated) • Local-algorithms Checklist for restocking • Logbook for daily checking procedures
Drawer 1: Plan A • Optimize head position • Bougie • Alternative laryngoscope **(Fig. 3)**	• Short handle laryngoscope • McCoy blade and/or straight blade video laryngoscope	Bougie (ideally)on side of the trolley		
Drawer 2: Plan B • LMA • Followed by fiberoptic tracheal intubation through LMA	• LMA #3,4,5 and /or second-generation device #3, 4, 5 • ILMA: #3, 4, 5	Intubating catheter (ideally on side of the trolley	*Fibreoptic adjuvants* • Berman/Ovassapien airways • Mucosal atomization devices • Fiberscope-compatible angle connector • Nasal sponge • 4% lignocaine • 10% lignocaine	
Drawer 3: Plan C • Bag-mask ventilation +/− airway adjuncts • Supraglottic airway device	• Facemasks; of various sizes • Oropharyngeal/nasopharyngeal airways of various sizes • LMA/Proseal LMA —#3, 4, 5			
Drawer 4: Plan D • Surgical cricothyroidotomy	• The large bore cannula device • Scalpel (number 20 blade) • Tracheal dilator or tracheal hook Bougie • Cuffed tracheal tubes #6 and 7			
Drawer 5—Plan D • Cannula cricothyroidotomy	• Kink-resistant jet ventilation cannula, e.g., Ravussin (VBM) • High and/or low-pressure ventilation system, e.g., Manujet III (VBM) Ventrain (Ventinova)			

Chapter 59: Devices for Difficult Airway Management

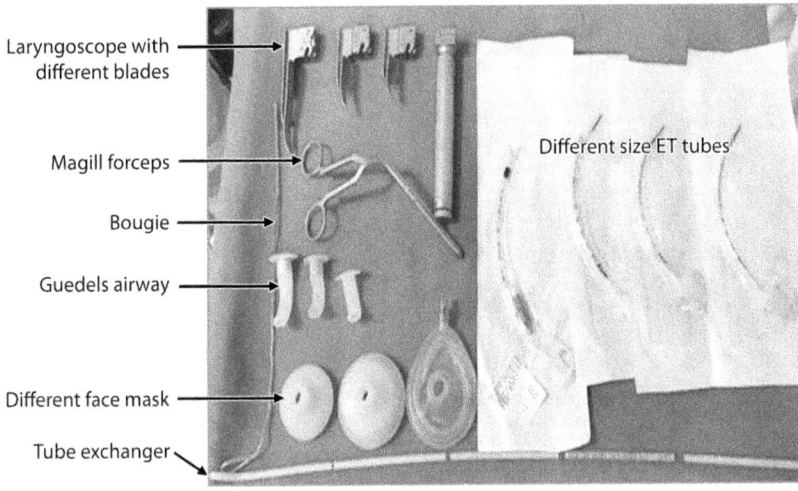

Fig. 3: Difficult airway trolley.

Flowchart 1: Difficult Airway Society 2016 algorithm for unanticipated difficult airway management.

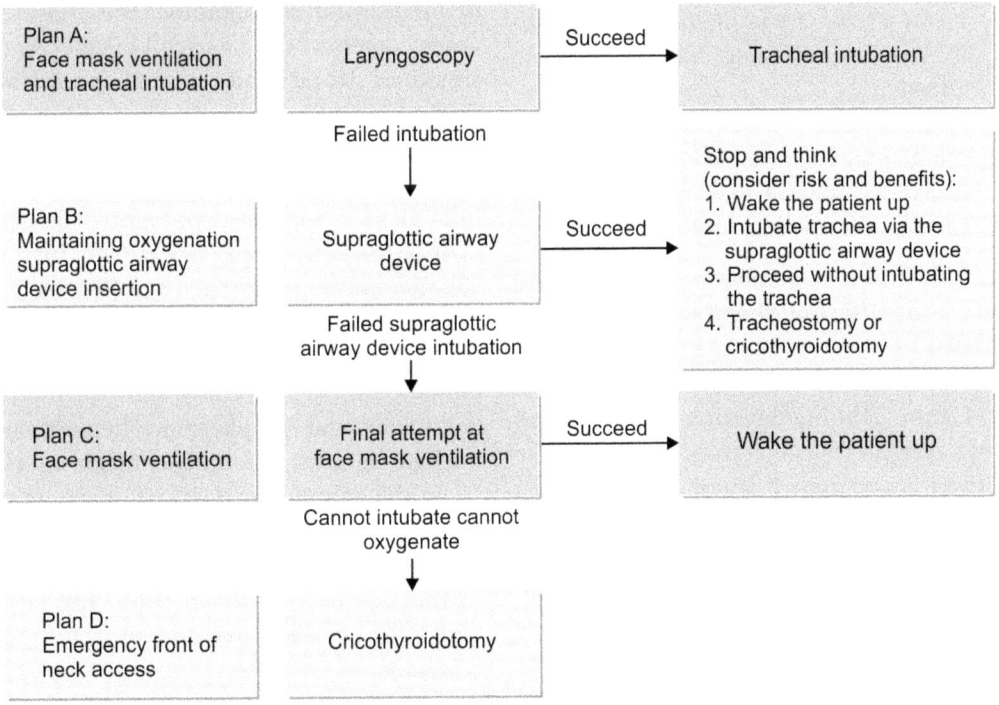

- Intermittent insufflation is done—1 second on and 4 seconds off. It can be achieved by keeping a thumb on the hole of the tubing or over the end of the Y-connector.

- This technique can be used for 30–45 minutes. During 4 seconds oxygen is not delivered under pressure, so exhalation occurs. Due to inadequate exhalation,

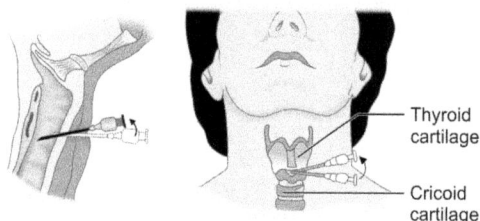

Fig 4: Needle cricothyroidotomy.

CO_2 accumulates slowly and limits this technique used for longer periods.

SURGICAL CRICOTHYROIDOTOMY

- Identify the cricothyroid membrane
- Make a skin incision over the cricothyroid membrane transversely
- Insert a scalpel handle or hemostat into the incision and rotate it 90° to open the airway
- Properly sized, cuffed endotracheal tube/tracheostomy tube to be inserted properly into the membrane incision, directing the tube into the trachea (distally).

Q. 14. Describe transnasal humidified rapid insufflation ventilatory exchange (THRIVE).

Ans. Preoxygenation is done using oxygen at 70 L/min, continued during induction and after muscle relaxant, until the definitive airway is secured. It increases the apnea time and can be considered whenever the option is available. In research, the author concluded that the use of this technique can decrease the incidence of severe hypoxia from 21 to 0%. However, it may cause airway trauma, gastric distension, and hypercarbia acidosis.

Q. 15. Describe the role of ultrasound sonography (USG) in difficult airway management.

Ans. Ultrasound (US) has emerged as an important reliable tool for the assessment

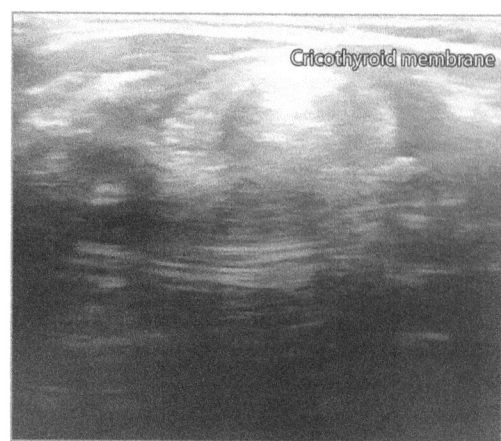

Fig. 5: USG showing airway anatomy.

of airway structure. Thorough knowledge of ultrasound sonography (USG)-guided airway anatomy can be useful in emergency situations. Ultrasound can aid in predicting difficult laryngoscopy by measuring the anterior neck soft tissues, even in obese patients also. The distance can be measured from the skin to the anterior aspect of the skin at three levels including—vocal cords, thyroid isthmus, and suprasternal notch **(Fig. 5)**.

The identification of anterior neck structure in USG may facilitate percutaneous dilatational tracheostomy and can inhibit potentially fatal complications; hemorrhage, tracheal stenosis, and injury to major vessels.

In the coming era, USG can become an important tool in the armamentarium of difficult airway management and expertise in this device can aid in achieving rapid and effective definitive airway in difficult scenarios.

Things to Remember

- Clearly labeled trolley can:
  - Serve as a visual guide
  - Prompt one to move along the strategy if not making progress.

- *What is most important is providing?*
  - The right equipment
  - In the right amount
  - In the right place
  - At the right time
- *PLAN:* Know what you need
- *COMMUNICATE:* Know who you need
- *PREPARE:* Have what you need
- *TRAIN:* Do what you need

FURTHER READING

1. Benumof JL, Dagg R, Benumof R. Critical hemoglobin desaturation will occur before return to an unparalyzed state following 1 mg/kg intravenous succinylcholine. Anesthesiology. 1997;87(4):979-82.
2. Gil KS, Diemunsch PA. Fiberoptic and Flexible Endoscopic-Aided Techniques. Benumof and Hagberg's Airway Management, 3rd edition. Amsterdam: Elsevier Inc; 2012.
3. Gupta A, Sharma R, Gupta N. Evolution of videolaryngoscopy in pediatric population. J Anaesthesiol Clin Pharmacol. 2021;37(1):14-27.
4. Hartle A, Anderson E, Bythell V, Gemmell L, Jones H, McIvo D, et al. Checking Anaesthetic Equipment 2012: association of anaesthetists of Great Britain and Ireland. Anaesthesia. 2012;67(6):660-68.
5. Henderson JJ, Popat MT, Latto IP, Pearce AC, Difficult Airway Society. Difficult Airway Society guidelines for management of the unanticipated difficult intubation. Anaesthesia; 2004:59(7):675-94.
6. Jaber S, Monnin M, Girard M, Conseil M, Cisse M, Carr J, et al. Apnoeic oxygenation via high-flow nasal cannula oxygen combined with non-invasive ventilation preoxygenation for intubation in hypoxaemic patients in the intensive care unit: the single-centre, blinded, randomised controlled OPTINIV trial. Intensive C are Med. 2016;42(12):1877-87.
7. Law JA, Broemling N, Cooper RM, Drolet P, Duggan LV, Griesdale DE, et al. The difficult airway with recommendations for management–part 2–the anticipated difficult airway. Can J AnestSh. 2013;60(11):1119-38.
8. Patel A, Nouraei SR. Transnasal Humidified Rapid-Insufflation Ventilatory Exchange (THRIVE): a physiological method of increasing apnoea time in patients with difficult airways. Anaesthesia. 2015;70(3):323-9.
9. Roth D, Pace N, Lee A, Hovhannisyan K, Warenits A, Arrich J, et al. Bedside tests for predicting difficult airways: an abridged Cochrane diagnostic test accuracy systematic review. Anaesthesia. 2019;74(4):915-28.
10. Stickles S, Carpenter CR, Gekle R, Kraus CK, Scoville C, Theodoro D, et al. The diagnostic accuracy of a point-of-care ultrasound protocol for shock etiology: a systematic review and meta-analysis. CJEM. 2019;21(3):406-17.

60. Gas Monitoring Equipment

Abhishek Singh

TYPES OF MONITORING

There are two types of monitoring being used for clinical purposes, they are:
1. Diverting (sidestream)
2. Nondiverting (mainstream).

Nondiverting Monitoring

It measures the gas concentration by utilizing the sensor which is located directly in the gas stream. Nondiverting monitors can measure only oxygen and carbon dioxide. Mainstream oxygen sensor utilizes electrochemical technology while carbon dioxide sensors use infrared technology.

Advantage of Mainstream Sensors

- The mainstream carbon dioxide (CO_2) sensors have a fast response and the waveform have better fidelity.
- Since no gas is removed for analysis, there is no need to increase fresh gas flow or scavenge these gases.
- Accumulation of water and secretion from the patient does not pose any significant problem. Although, sometimes it may interfere with CO_2 monitoring.
- Standard gas is not needed for calibration purposes.
- Such sensors use a lesser number of disposable items than diverting ones.

Disadvantages of Mainstream Sensors

- CO_2 mainstream sensors are required to be placed close to the patient for getting the correct value. The weight of the sensor causes traction on the breathing system and may cause disconnection.
- It may prone the circuit to leaks and obstruction.
- Optical sensors for CO_2 are costly and susceptible to damage.
- It is limited to measuring O_2 and CO_2 only.
- Some instances of thermal damage and pressure injury have been reported with mainstream CO_2 sensors.

Sidestream Monitoring

Such monitoring system uses a pump to aspirate gas from the circuit at the sampling site and transport it to the sensor in the main unit through a sampling tube. Such sensors are zeroed at room air and are calibrated by using a gas of known composition. In order to reduce contamination by water and particulate matter, various devices such as traps, filters, and hydrophobic membranes have been used in such monitors. The accuracy of sidestream monitors decreases with long sampling lines and increased respiratory rates. The sampling flow rate should not be <150 mL/min. The low flow rate may cause elevated baseline and low peak readings while the high flow rate may result in incorrect end-tidal readings.

Advantages of Sidestream Sensors

- The zeroing and calibration of such sensors are usually automatic.

- Added dead space is usually less than mainstream sensors.
- Several gases can be analyzed simultaneously.
- There is less chance of cross-contamination between the patients.
- They are better suited for use in a location where the patient is away from the monitor. For example, the magnetic resonance imaging (MRI) suite.

Disadvantages of Sidestream Sensors

- The leaks, sampling tube obstruction, and failure of aspirator pump can hamper functioning of the sensor.
- Blood, secretion, water, and particulate matter can obstruct tubing.
- Problem with scavenging of aspirated gas.
- Need for a constant supply of calibration gas.
- Higher numbers of disposable items are used in these monitors.
- Dilution of aspirated gas by air or fresh gas from a machine may lead to an erroneous reading.
- Some delay in analysis is expected in side stream analyzers.

TECHNOLOGY USED FOR GAS MONITORING

Infrared Analysis

It is based on the principle that a gas molecule consisting of two or more different atoms, for example, CO_2 containing carbon and oxygen atoms has a specific and unique infrared absorption spectrum. Since the amount of infrared radiation absorbed is directly proportional to the concentration of the absorbing molecule; therefore, the concentration of the gas can be determined by comparing the infrared absorbance of the gas with that of a known standard.

Two types of infrared technology are being used nowadays, they are:
1. *Blackbody radiation:* It is one of the most commonly used infrared technology. It uses a heated element as a source of infrared light. A filter is used to remove the undesired infrared radiation from the emitter. The analyzer selects the appropriate infrared wavelength and the sensor detects the transmitted infrared light and converts it into electrical and displays the concentration of the agent.
2. *Microstream technology:* It uses laser-based technology for generating infrared light which matches the absorption spectrum of CO_2. The infrared emitting sours is electronically controlled in such a way that measurements are repeated every 25 ms which results in a very rapid response time. The amplitude of the signal which is received by the detector depends upon the amount of radiation absorbed by the gas molecule which is displayed as the concentration.

Advantages of Infrared Analysis

- It has the ability to analyze multiple gases simultaneously.
- There is no need for gas scavenger as the gases can be returned to the breathing system if needed.
- They are lightweight, small, and have a compact design.
- They have a quick response time and short warm uptime.
- Nowadays, these units only require periodic calibration of up to 0.25 seconds with a standard gas mixture.
- There is a lack of interference due to presence of other gas during the measurement.

Disadvantages of Infrared Analysis

- It cannot measure oxygen and nitrous oxide.

- Presence of ethanol, methanol, ether, acetone, etc., can cause spuriously high-volatile anesthetic reading.
- Presence of water vapor may cause raised CO_2 and volatile agent reading.
- In presence of a rapid respiratory rate, it has a slow response time.

Oxygen Analyzer

Oxygen analyzer is a crucial part of the anesthesia workstation. They monitor oxygen concentration either at a common gas outlet or in the inspiratory limb of the circle system. The three most commonly used techniques of measuring oxygen concentration consist of galvanic, polarographic, and paramagnetic techniques.

Paramagnetic Oxygen Analyzer

Oxygen is a paramagnetic molecule due to the presence of an unpaired electron in its outer orbit that gets attracted to the magnetic field. This forms the basic mechanism on which the paramagnetic oxygen analyzer works. The analyzer consists of two chambers (sampling and reference chamber) with a sensitive pressure transducer in between two chambers. Sampling chamber receives gas from the patient end via sampling line while the reference chamber receives room air. The electromagnet creates a rapidly changing magnetic field which causes oxygen molecules to get attracted and agitated. This leads to the development of pressure on either side of the transducer and pressure difference is proportional to oxygen partial difference between a sample and reference gas. The partial pressure is calibrated for oxygen concentration in percentage. These analyzers are highly sensitive and rapid, allowing measuring of oxygen concentration on breath-to-breath basis.

Galvanic Oxygen Analyzer

This type of analyzer works on the principle of a chemical phenomenon by oxygen molecules. Oxygen diffuses through the electrolyte and membrane to a cathode that is connected to the lead anode through an electrolyte solution. It creates an electrical current that is directly proportional to partial pressure of oxygen in the sampled gas. These analyzers are connected to the inspiratory limb of the breathing circuit and require 100% oxygen and room air for calibration. These analyzers have a limited life span because of the depletion of the battery due to continuous exposure to oxygen.

Polarographic Oxygen Analyzer

They work on a similar principle like that galvanic cell but oxygen molecules move across Teflon membrane and resultant current flow between the platinum anode and silver cathode. The current is directly proportional to partial pressure of oxygen in the sampled gas. It is usually attached to the inspiratory limb of the breathing circuit and has a life span of approximately 3 years.

Use of oxygen analysis:
- Detection and prevention of hypoxic mixture being given to the patient.
- It can be used for detecting disconnection and leaks in the circuit.
- End-tidal oxygen concentration is used to monitor the adequacy of preoxygenation.

Piezoelectric Absorption

This technique uses piezoelectric compounds such as quartz and its resonance property is used for analyzing anesthetic agent concentration. It consists of two quartz crystals, one coated with silicone-based oil while the other remains uncoated, are placed between two electrodes. The oil-coated quartz crystal absorbs the halogenated anesthetic agents. This changes the resonant frequency of the crystals which is directly proportional to the concentration of the vapor. They have a fast response time but are limited by their inability to differentiate individual anesthetic gases.

Refractometry

In this technique, monochromatic light is emitted from the source and is focused on the screen. It results in the creation of a typical band pattern that depends on the light beam arriving in or out of phase of each other which further depends upon the gas concentration and its refractive index. Rayleigh refractometers consist of a series of prism which spilt the light beam through control and sampling tubes. These devices are calibrated for a particular gas. These analyzers do not give breath-to-breath analysis but they are useful tools to calibrate vaporizer output and detect environmental anesthetic gas exposure.

FURTHER READING

1. Dorsch, JA, Dorsch SE. Understanding Anesthesia Equipment, 5th edition. Philadelphia: Lippincot Williams & Wilkins;2012.

61. Spinal and Epidural Needles

Richa Saroa, Sanjeev Palta, Umang Sharma, Amitesh Chugh

INTRODUCTION

Spinal and epidural needles are specially designed medical-use needles employed for regional anesthetic techniques, to provide intraoperative anesthesia and analgesia, postoperative analgesia in patients undergoing surgery, intrathecal injection of cytotoxic drugs/antibiotics, or obtaining cerebrospinal fluid (CSF) tap for lab analysis. Spinal-epidural techniques of anesthesia have become increasingly popular and various types of needles have become commercially available based on the length, gauge, and tip designs.

SPINAL NEEDLES

History

Initially, hypodermic needles with short and sharp bevels were utilized till an Irish surgeon Francis Rynd introduced hollow needles with a trocar and cannula.

Corning, an American neurologist, injected cocaine between the lumbar spinous processes in the epidural space of a dog in 1885. In 1898, August Bier, a German surgeon first performed spinal anesthesia successfully in a human subject.

In 1891, Quincke demonstrated a lumbar tap using a beveled cutting needle. In 1926, Greene used an atraumatic needle that passed between dural fibers without cutting them. Finally, pencil tip conical needles were introduced by Whitacre in 1951. In 1987, Sprotte made some modifications to the Whitacre needle.

Parts of the Spinal Needle

A spinal needle consists of a shaft, plastic hub, tip/orifice, and stylet. It usually has a length of 10 cm from the tip to the hub. The pediatric needles are usually smaller with a length of 5 cm (**Fig. 1**).

Features of a Spinal Needle

Needle gauge: The accepted standards for the needle gauge are derived from Standard Wire Gauge (SWG) which is used to measure the electrical wires. For instruments, the standard gauge was described by Holzapfel and Stubs in 1847; who described it in inches. Gauges are usually taken as multiples of 4/1,000 of an inch and therefore increasing the gauge usually represents a decrease in the diameter (**Fig. 2**). The spinal needle is available from 19–30 G but the most commonly used is 22–27 G. Needle size is identified by a number, a Gauge symbol, and a fraction that

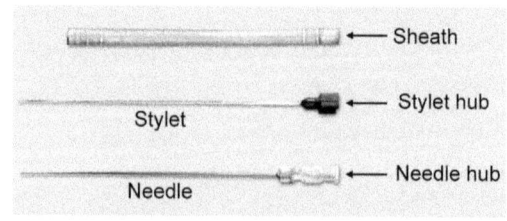

Fig. 1: Parts of a spinal needle.

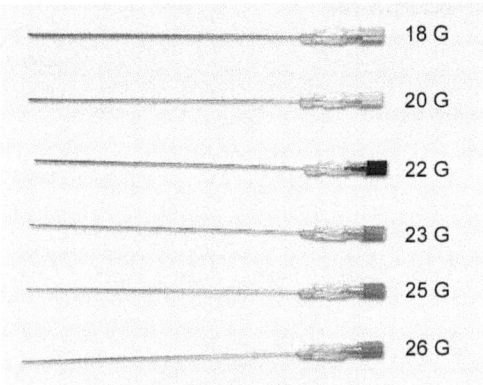

Fig. 2: Needle gauge.

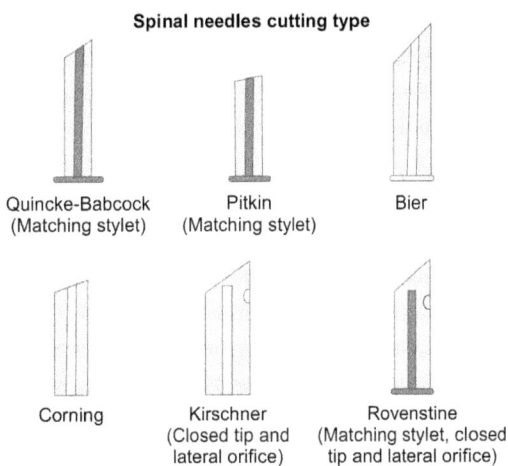

Fig. 3: Needle tip.

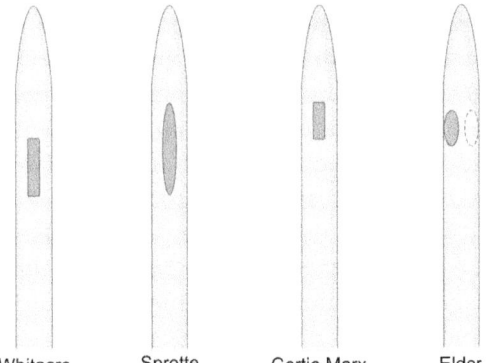

Fig. 4: Dura noncutting/atraumatic/pencil-point needle.

represents the length of the needle. The needle Guage (27-29 G) usually needs an introducer for insertion and performance of the block.

Needle tip: Spinal needles can be categorized into two types based on the design of the bevel **(Figs. 3 and 4)**.
- *Cutting type*
  It includes:
  - Quincke-Babcock needle—it is considered the standard spinal needle. It has a sharp tip and a cutting bevel
  - Pitkin needle—it has a sharp point and a short bevel
  - Bier's needle
  - Corning needle
  - Kirschner needle
  - Rovenstine needle
- *Dura noncutting/atraumatic/pencil-point needle:* These needles separate the dural fibers; give a better tactile sensation of penetrating tissue layers, and decrease the chances of postdural-puncture headache (PDPH).
  - Whitacre needle—it has a sharp pencil point type of bevel with no cutting edge
  - Sprotte needle
  - Gertie Marx needle
  - Eldor needle

Orifice location: While earlier needles had an orifice at the tip of the needle, the introduction of closed-end needles (dura separating) led to the development of a lateral orifice near the tip. The first tapering, noncutting needle with lateral orifice was introduced by Haraldson in 1951. It was designed primarily for a better dural click for appreciation during the performance of the block. It was shown to improve CSF flow, cause less trauma, lead to a better spread of local anesthetic, decreased needle deformation, and reduced the chances of postdural puncture headache. However, the distance between the tip and the orifice (1 mm) has been reported to cause paresthesias secondary to spinal cord contact which has always been a matter of research with no discrete conclusions.

Material: Initially the spinal needles were made of platinum, gold, iridized gold, steel, and nickel/silver alloy that were sterilized and reused. Presently the needles are usually disposable needles made of stainless steel alloys with a combination of iron, carbon, and chromium with the needle hubs made from plastic that is primarily joined to the needle shaft with the help of adhesives.

Spinal needles used for spinal catheter insertion: In an attempt to prolong the spinal anesthesia, continuous spinal anesthetic techniques were employed using 20 G microcatheters in subarachnoid space introduced through a 17 G epidural needle. However, usage of the same was associated with an increased incidence of PDPH. Therefore, the use of smaller microcatheters (28-32 G) placed through 25-26 G spinal needles was introduced into the clinical practice. The disadvantage of the use of microcatheters is increased resistance to the placement of drugs, kinking, shearing, and breakage of catheters.

EPIDURAL NEEDLES

History

While epidural anesthesia was administered for the first time by a Spanish surgeon, Fidel Pagés in 1921 using a sharp edge needle, it was Edward B Tuohy, who replaced the sharp edge of the needle with a directional tip designed by Ralph H Huber and popularized the use of Tuohy's needle for epidural anesthesia. Since the time of introduction and performance of the first epidural, various types of needles were introduced for single-shot epidural anesthesia. The first use of a catheter in epidural space was

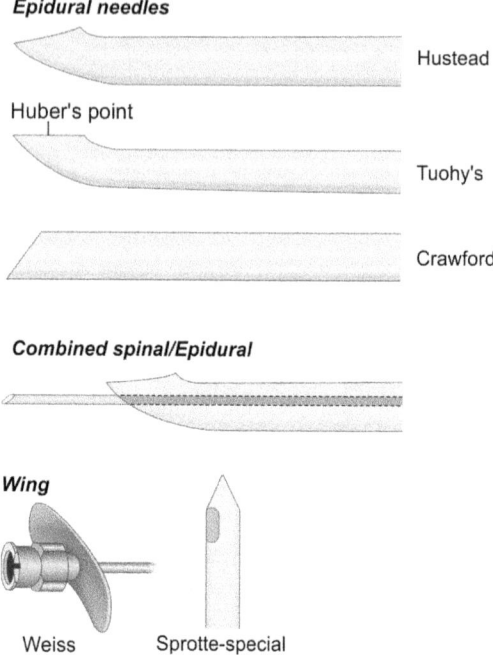

Fig. 5: Types of epidural needles.

done by a Cuban anesthetist, Manuel Curbelo in 1949, and the technique of continuous epidural anesthesia was demonstrated by Philip Bromage, in 1961.

Types of Epidural Needles (Fig. 5)

- The Tuohy's needle (most commonly employed)
- The Hustead needle
- Crawford Needle
- Weiss needle
- Sprotte Spezial needle
- Others—Wagner's needle, Cheng needle, Crawley needle, Folds needle, Bell's needle (historical purpose).

PARTS OF TUOHY'S NEEDLE (FIG. 6)

The needle is 10 cm in length with an actual needle length of 8 cm and the hub constitutes

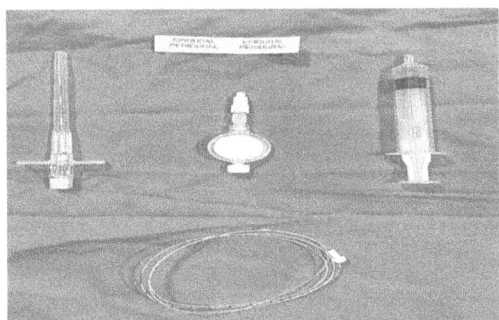

Fig. 6: Epidural set (Tuohy's needle).

2 cm. The needle is marked and graded at every 1 cm interval which is used to calculate the distance between skin and epidural space. Epidural needles are available in the sizes of 16 G to 19 G for adults with a 20 G catheter and pediatric epidural needle is available as 19 G needles with the epidural catheter of 22 G. The needle is generally made up of iron (69%), chromium (18%), nickel (9%), manganese (1.5%) silicone (0.5%), and molybdenum (0.2–2.5%).

Design: The tip of the needle which is commonly called the *Huber's point*, is beveled and curved by 15–30°, which allows the needle to abut against the dura while inserting through the ligamentum flavum and thus preventing dural puncture and also allowing identification of the dural space by creation of negative pressure. It also facilitates catheter direction during insertion which can be cephalad or caudal. The Hub of the needle can be with or without wings. The wings to the epidural needle were added by Jess Weiss. Wings help in the controlled insertion of the needle and provide a better grip.

Catheter and filter: The catheter in a 16 G epidural needle set is a transparent tubing of 1 mm external diameter and 0.55 mm internal diameter with a length of 100 cm. The epidural catheter has three lateral eyes that are present 1 cm proximal from the tip of the catheter. Though single port catheters are available too but multiport catheters are the most frequently employed these days. The lateral eyes are present in different directions to allow uniform distribution of the drug in the epidural space. However, the multiport catheters may be associated with the multicompartment block. It is usually made of nylon, Teflon, polyurethane, and silicone and is designed in such a way to pass easily through the needle. Wire reinforced catheters with fewer coils at the tip provide more flexibility and offer an advantage of lesser paresthesia and perforation of dura as well the epidural vessels.

The catheters are manufactured in a way that they have good tensile strength/stiffness and are kink-resistant for appropriate placement in the epidural space. The use of polyvinyl chloride (PVC) catheters was described by Fowlers in 1949. The catheter is marked till the distance of 20 cm with well-defined markings at regular intervals of 1 cm each from 5 to 15 cm that enables the placement of the epidural catheter in the epidural space at desired length precisely. While marking of 10 cm is represented by a double bar mark, 15 and 20 cm are represented by three and four marks at the catheter respectively. The proximal end is connected to a Luer lock that has distinct connectors to differentiate it from other catheters, especially the intravascular catheters, and thus safeguard it from accidental drug administration.

Filter: It is the hydrophilic component with a 0.2-micron mesh that helps filter microbes and foreign bodies during epidural drug administration.

Caution should be taken regarding accidental dural puncture as epidural needles having a larger bore leads to a higher incidence of postdural puncture headache and therefore use of loss of resistance syringes with low resistance plunger with air or saline is recommended to identify the epidural space.

COMBINED SPINAL EPIDURAL TECHNIQUE

It has gained more popularity in recent times in view of performing the anesthetic techniques through different routes that combine the advantages of both techniques while reducing the complications at the same time. The first needle through needle technique was described by Coates in 1982. While spinal anesthesia provides rapid onset of block, the epidural can be utilized to augment the block or the duration of the anesthesia and also provide excellent postoperative analgesia.

The commercially available needle through needle sets comprises of an epidural needle that has an eye known as "Backeye" along the curvature of the epidural needle to allow the passage of the spinal needle for subarachnoid block. The presence of Backeye also ensures dural puncture away from the epidural catheter and allows the spinal needle to follow a straight course **(Fig 7)**. The epidural needle acts as an introducer for the spinal needle till the epidural space is identified and then the subarachnoid block is performed with the spinal needle provided with a combined spinal epidural set (CSE).

Certain commercially available sets have Luer locks that allow fixation of the spinal needle to the epidural needle and help in the stabilization of the spinal needle. This also requires an extension of the spinal needle beyond the epidural needle that may be variable and can result in either block failure or nerve damage as a consequence of too short or too long extension respectively. However, the use of a spinal needle without a fixation lock may be more difficult to use and perform the block. Most commonly 16 G Tuohy's needle is inserted and fixed in the

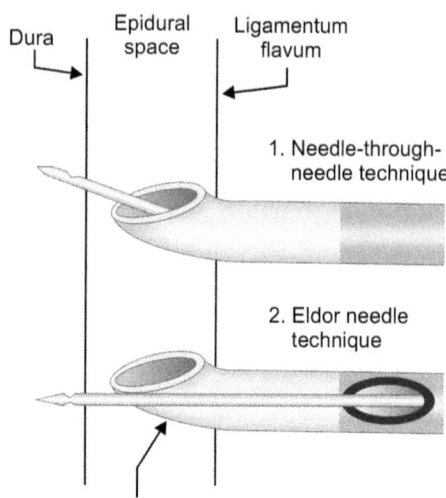

Fig. 7: Combined spinal epidural needle set.

epidural space and a 26 G spinal needle is introduced through it into the subarachnoid space. The spinal needle available with CSE sets is usually a noncutting needle (mostly Whitacre) and is longer (about 13 cm) in length in comparison to the standard spinal needles (10 cm). Certain Double-barreled needles have also been manufactured where the sleeve for both epidural and spinal needles lies side by side and both are performed through different barrels **(Fig. 7)**.

The risk of damaging the epidural catheter with the spinal needle, failure of the spinal needle to advance through the Backeye leading to failed block, longer spinal needle puncturing the anterior aspect of the dura leading to more CSF leak with resultant postdural puncture headache and higher incidence of paresthesias are certain disadvantages reported with the use of the combined spinal epidural needle.

The availability of a wide range of spinal and epidural needles has made the central neuraxial techniques to be performed more effortlessly. The choice of needle for performing the block depends upon the expertise and comfort of the anesthesiologist who should select the needle tailored to the needs of the patient.

QUESTIONS

Q. 1. Post dural puncture headache (PDPH). Incidence, methods of prevention, management.

Q. 2. Rapid sequence spinal. Indications, advantages.

Q. 3. Spinal catheters. Continous spinal analgesia.

Q. 4. USG-guided epidural and spinal anesthesia.

Q. 5. Management of spinal anesthesia induced hypotension.

Q. 6. Approach to failed spinal anesthesia in cesarean section.

Q. 7. Low dose spinal, unilateral spinal, segmental spinal.

Q. 8. Pediatric spinal and epidural needles, techniques, drug used, dosages, advantages, contraindications.

Q. 9. Metabollic changes that occur during spinal.

Q. 10. Epidural and spinal in a scoliotic patient.

Q. 11. Continous epidural anesthesia and analgesia.

Q. 12. Influence of epidural anesthesia on thromboembolism and prevention of deep vein thrombosis.

Q. 13. Epidural electric stimulation.

Q. 14. Maternal fever, epidural fever (Epidural labor).

Q. 15. Caudal epidural.

FURTHER READING

1. Barash PG, Cullen BF, Stoelting RK, Cahalan MK, Stock MR, Ortega R. Clinical Anesthesia, 7th edition. Philadelphia: Wolters Kluwer Health, 2013.
2. Calthorpe N. The history of spinal needles: getting to the point. Anesthesia. 2004;59(12): 1231-41.
3. Dorsch, Jerry A, and Susan E. Dorsch. 1999. Understanding anesthesia equipment. Baltimore: Williams and Wilkins.
4. Gropper MA, Miller RD. Miller's Anesthesia, 9th edition. Philadelphia: Elsevier; 2020.
5. Martini JA, Bacon DR, Vasdev GM. Edward Tuohy: The man, his needle, and its place in obstetric analgesia. Reg Anesth Pain Med. 2002;27(5):520-3.
6. Xu H, Liu Y, Song W, Kan S, Liu F, Zhang D, et al. Comparison of cutting and pencil-point spinal needle in spinal anesthesia regarding postdural puncture headache: a meta-analysis. Medicine (Baltimore). 2017;96(14): e6527.

Patient-controlled Analgesia Pumps

CHAPTER 62

Richa Saroa, Sanjeev Palta, Puja Saxena, Parul Sood

INTRODUCTION

Patient-controlled analgesia (PCA) has been utilized to optimize pain relief since 1971, with the first commercially available PCA pump launched in 1976. The primary goal of PCA is effective and adequate analgesia that is primarily controlled by the patient and delivered through programmable infusion pumps that can be modified by the prescriber. The PCA can be accomplished through various techniques where the drugs can be administered in a preset manner with the schedule in the form of a predetermined bolus dose of medication that is offered on-demand at the press of a button that is usually integrated into the infusion pump. The bolus so offered can be administered alone or coupled with a background infusion of the medication. The technique was developed initially for the relief of pain in labor, but the use of PCA has extended for use in the treatment of acute or chronic pain, acute postoperative pain, labor pain, intraoperative analgesia, and sedation and analgesia in critical care set up and also in patients undergoing procedures at remote locations. (1) PCA can be administered through various routes viz., intravenous, epidural, peripheral nerve catheter, and transdermally as tailored to the needs of the patients. The most commonly employed drugs for use with PCA include either opioids or local anesthetics as a single agent or in combination. However, other drugs like analgesics from the phencyclidine group (ketamine), α-2 agonists (dexmedetomidine), lignocaine, magnesium, droperidol, and ketorolac have also been employed for PCA with varied results. Since the development of the first available commercial pump in 1976, PCA devices have undergone enormous technological advancement in terms of sophistication, programmability, flexibility, transportation, and ease to utilize these devices.

PHARMACOKINETICS OF PATIENT-CONTROLLED ANALGESIA

The variability in response to opioid administration in the postoperative period especially with increased mobilization and physiotherapy is one of the major limitations of the analgesic techniques that heralded the era of PCA. The ability to titrate the drug concentration to an individual need and achieve a constant plasma concentration of the analgesic drug without any abrupt changes in the mean effective drug concentration has revolutionized the practice of patient-controlled analgesia. The underlying principle of PCA where the patient primarily controls the dose of analgesia has led to optimal analgesia and a better recovery profile. Patient-controlled analgesia (PCA) also offers and advantage of maintaining minimum effective analgesic concentrations

(MEAC) without reaching the maximal toxic concentration (MTC). The pharmacokinetic principle has primarily been studied with opioids as a prototype considering the steep sigmoid curve followed by the dose of the opioid analgesics **(Fig. 1)**.

PHYSIOLOGY

The PCA can be administered and practiced through various routes, the primary modalities being through intravenous (IV) catheters, central venous catheters, peripheral venous catheters, central neuraxial catheters (both epidural and spinal) with epidural catheters being more commonly employed for the continuous infusions and transdermal patches through iontophoresis. Administration through the peripheral veins makes it an easy option to provide adequate analgesia even after moderate surgeries and in patients where placement of blocks, either peripheral or central neuraxial blocks, is either not possible or contraindicated secondary to one or the other reason. Epidural catheters placement along the thoracic to the lumbar region provides wide dermatomal coverage and thus offers an advantage of planning the postoperative analgesia according to the site of surgery that makes the PCA site-specific and allows analgesia pertaining to particular dermatomal distribution. Similarly, the placement of catheters adjacent to the peripheral nerves allows continuous analgesia, however, the fixation of catheters through subcutaneous tunneling or appropriate fixation through adhesive tapes is mandatory to avoid the displacement of the same with movement. And therefore, visual inspection and checks in all the routes of administration before administration of bolus or in case of breakthrough pain are necessary to avoid the failure of PCA.

INDICATIONS

Patient-controlled analgesia is a lucrative option of analgesia for acute and chronic postoperative pain, labor analgesia, and in critical care setups. Patient-controlled

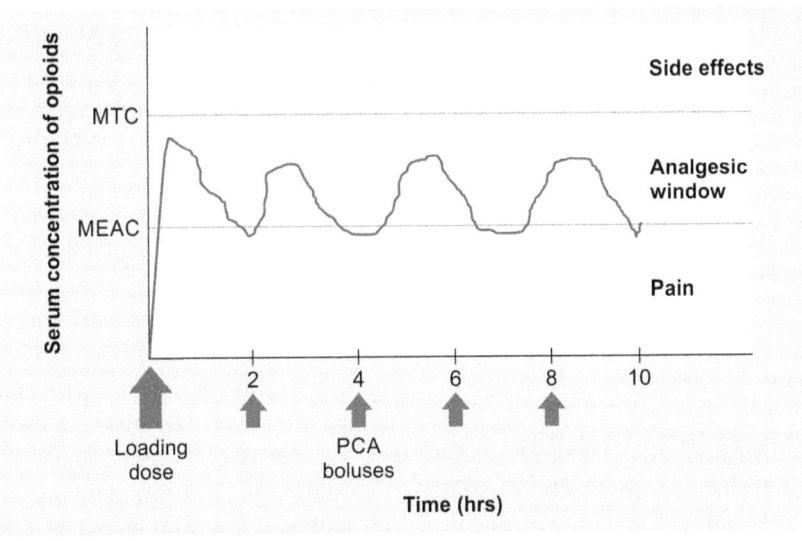

Fig. 1: Pharmacokinetic principle of patient-controlled analgesia (PCA) pumps.

analgesia (PCA) carries an inherent advantage by delivering predetermined boluses at fixed time intervals or at the behest of the patient and thus contributes to reducing the workload of the working staff. The maintenance of constant and effective concentration of the analgesic has shown to have better outcomes and better quality of life indices in the perioperative period. Effective labor analgesia that allows the mother to self-administer a bolus of analgesic regimen (local anesthetic with opioid primarily through epidural route) during uterine contractions, contributes to better maternal-child relations, and the mother is not exhausted resulting in adequate analgesia and is able to cater to the needs of the child especially breastfeeding.

CONTRAINDICATIONS

Patient-controlled analgesia is absolute contraindicated through the following:
- Inability of the patient to understand the concept behind PCA
- Infections at the site of PCA placement
- Allergic reactions to the medication
- Burns or trauma in the area of PCA placement
- Pre-existing neural deficits in the area of distribution of nerve catheter placement.
- Raised intracranial pressure especially if a neuraxial blockade is planned
- The PCA may be undertaken with caution and after thorough assessment in patients with chronic kidney disease or underlying congenital bleeding disorders, patients receiving anticoagulants, and those with a history of sleep apnea.

EQUIPMENT (PCA PUMPS)

The patient-controlled analgesia is usually practiced through a PCA pump that is a programmable computerized machine that delivers the analgesic in a predetermined dosage as or continuous infusion with intermittent boluses as specified by the treating pain physician **(Figs. 2A to C)**. In simpler terms, the PCA pumps dispense the medications into the patient's body in a controlled manner. The majority of available delivery systems are electronic pumps which are a simplified version of the Cardiff Palliator introduced in 1976. The PCA pumps can be both electronic and disposable and also may be large or small-volume pumps. Irrespective of the type and volume, all pumps have integral components, i.e., medication chamber/reservoir, locking device, programmable function either through buttons or touch, display screen, and a push-button that is patient enabled (patient control module).

The *medication chamber/reservoir* may be reusable or disposable and the capacity may vary as per the manufacturer **(Fig. 3)**. While the reusable pumps usually make use of the disposable syringes and the type of syringe can be selected from the menu, usually 50 mL is commonly employed for the same. The disposable chambers usually have a capacity of 100–200 mL and a small capacity enables them as to be used for ambulatory anesthesia. The disposable devices usually do not deliver for >0.5 mL every six minutes even if the demand button is pressed continuously. The reservoir usually fills up again in six minutes and acts as a locking interval in disposable pumps. In these pumps since a fixed amount of drug is delivered with fixed volume, the concentration of the drug needs to be altered if higher dosages are required to be administered. The electronic pumps are more flexible in terms of dosing and timing of the drug administered. The syringes or the cassettes with pumps usually are provided with antireflux/antisiphoning valves to prevent the reflux of the drug back into the pump or excessive drainage secondary to the gravity.

Chapter 62: Patient-controlled Analgesia Pumps

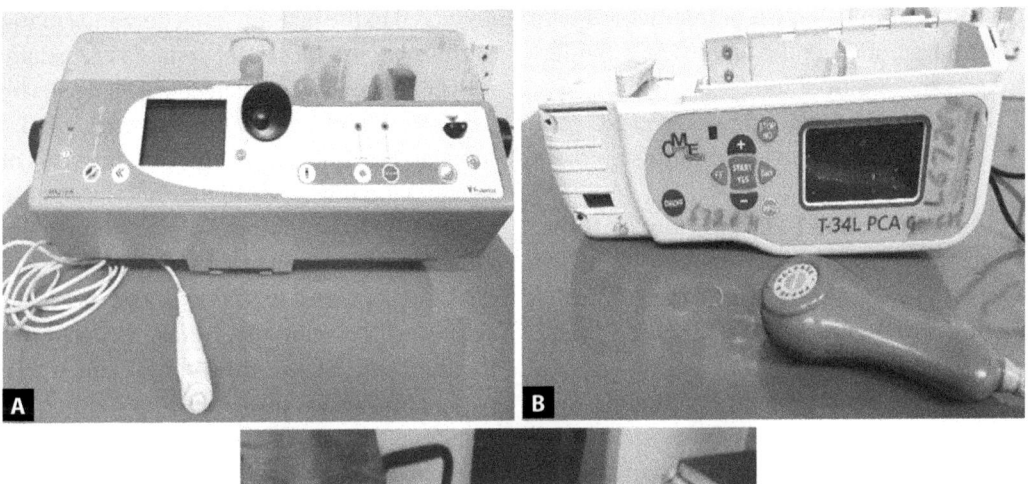

Figs. 2A to C: Electronic patient-controlled analgesia (PCA) pumps.

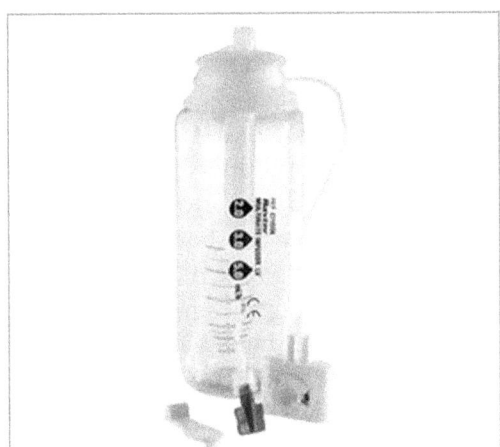

Fig. 3: Disposable elastomeric patient-controlled analgesia (PCA) pump.

The *locking device* is either a key or lock mechanism as inbuilt with most of the electronic models of PCA pumps that make it "tamper-proof" in terms of the inability to access the medication without a key. The newer versions have a lock-enabled screen function or have passwords for unlocking the pump mechanisms and making changes to the set programs. The features of the locking device serve as a safety feature that does not allow anyone to tamper with the specified programs and also alter the dosing schedule once it is preset as customized to a particular patient.

Programmable functions/Modes: Nearly all the PCA pumps offer a programed function of either a demand mode or continuous infusion with demand mode most commonly. While a fixed dose is self-administered intermittently in the prior mode, a constant

background infusion is complemented with demand duration in the latter. The other less frequently employed modes include:
- Infusion demand mode where a successful number of demands are administered as a bolus.
- Preprogrammed variable rate infusion with demand dosing—the infusion is preprogrammed to continue till a stipulated time after which only demand mode is active.
- Variable-rate feedback infusion with demand dosing where the inbuilt microprocessor unit cumulatively assesses the patient demands and modifies the infusion rate.

For all the modes the basic variables that have to be adjusted are initial loading dose, demand dose, lockout interval, background infusion rates, and dose to be administered over one hour and maximal permissible dose over four hours.

The *initial loading dose* is usually decided by the programmer who may be a physician or nurse anesthetist or anesthetist and depends upon multiple factors such as patient's age, comorbidities, psychological attributes of a patient, opioid dependency, proficiency to use of the PCA pumps.

The *demand dose* also known as the incremental or PCA dose is the additional analgesic dose delivered with the press of the push button. Ideally, the demand dose should be such that one dose should be able to provide effective analgesia. However, the demand dose so offered may be too high to cause side effects or toxicity, and therefore demand dosages are allowed to be delivered at certain intervals with a lock-out interval that allows spaced delivery of the analgesic drug. All the PCA pumps usually display the number of demanded doses requested by the patients and the number of demands successfully delivered to the patient. If the demands made outnumber the successful demands, it usually is a pointer to enhanced needs of analgesia by the patient and may require the change in the infusion rates or the dose/lockout intervals of the demand dosages and thus acts as a guide to alter the bolus dosages of analgesic being prescribed.

The *lock-out interval* is the interval during which no demand dose is delivered irrespective of the number of times the patient pushes the push button for additional analgesia. This mode serves as a safety feature to avoid excessive dose by continual demand and also in patients who inadvertently push the button thinking it to be a nurse call button and also accidental push-button usage by the family and visitors. The lock-out interval should ideally be based on the maximal dose-effect before permitting another dose to prevent overdosing and therefore the onset of analgesia with a particular drug is taken into account while prescribing a lock-out interval. Hence, a drug with early onset of action like fentanyl may have a lesser lock-out interval as compared to morphine which requires a longer lock-out time interval. In usual practice, the lock-out interval usually varies from 5–10 minutes for commonly employed opioid analgesics. Another useful concept that defines lockout interval is the rate of distribution of a drug between the plasma and brain wherein the bolus of the drug should coincide with the peak effect of the drug after it is leaving the brain, i.e., *negative flux* which requires more inflow of the drug to maintain the brain concentration. The relationship between the demand dose and lock-out interval also carries significance as in with a higher demand dose longer lock-out interval is required and a lower lock-out with low demand dosages is needed though the efficacy of one over the other is still debatable.

The *background infusion* is the continuous infusion of analgesic that is administered round the clock to the patient at a constant rate regardless of whether the patient demands an additional dose or not. Though the concept of background infusion has been associated with oversedation and side effects of opioids and should be sparingly used routinely. It may be more suitable in patients with high opioid requirements or opioid dependence or patients with episodes of awakening during the night. In children, background infusions have been shown to provide good pain relief even through the night but it demands vigilance and monitoring to prevent hypoxemia secondary to opioid overdosage. Also with newer microprocessor controlled machines that deliver variable rate infusion, as a result, the complications have been reduced even with background infusions.

The *one and four-hour cumulative analgesic doses* are intended to administer a limited analgesic dose over a period of one hour and the total permissible dose in four hours which is usually calculated by the maximal dose of the analgesic drug that can be administered over these time intervals taking into account their total duration of action and half-life. This concept was introduced again as a safety measure to avoid overdosage of the analgesic drug. However, it may not be effective in certain patients in whom higher or additional dosages are required for adequate analgesia. This has been circumvented by the microprocessor-driven PCA devices which allow programming and variation of the dose as required for the patient.

The *display screen* is usually well lit to display the mode, program, continuous infusion rate, demand dose, and lock-out interval clearly displayed. Usually, the total amount of drug administered, and the dose are also displayed on the screen. The number of successful as well as unsuccessful demand dosages can be accessed in the machine. However, any variation to the above said can only be made after unlocking the machine.

The *push button* is a handheld compressible knob that is attached to the PCA pump and delivers the demand dose once it is compressed down and released for the next dose. It is mandatory to explain the usage of the push button to the patient before prescribing and initiating the PCA regimen as there have been reports where the push button has been mistaken for the nurse call buttons or emergency activation buttons triggering repeated boluses and side effects of the analgesic drugs. There have also been reports of inadequate analgesia even after using push buttons which have been noted due to coiling or tethering of the cord in the railings or the clamping of the cord in the pump while closing it and in magnetic resonance imaging (MRI) suites/hyperbaric chambers.

With a number of commercially available PCA pumps certain operational features that should be considered during the evaluation of the same are given in **Box 1**.

PRESCRIBING THE PATIENT-CONTROLLED ANALGESIA REGIMENS

Choice of opioids: Though all opioids have been used successfully with PCA, morphine, and fentanyl have been utilized most frequently for the same, especially for intravascular PCA (IV PCA). Amongst the entire range of opioids, μ-opioid receptor agonists (morphine, fentanyl, hydromorphone, meperidine, sufentanil, alfentanil, and remifentanil), agonist-antagonists (butorphanol, nalbuphine, pentazocine), and partial μ-opioid receptor agonists (buprenorphine) have been employed for the PCA regimen with equianalgesic and equipotent dose compared to a standard dose of morphine. It is imperative to know the relative equipotent dosages of opioids like morphine

> **BOX 1:** Patient-controlled analgesia (PCA) pumps.
>
> *As concerned to the programmer usage:*
> - The programmability of the machine
> - Terminology utilized for various functions/programs
> - Flexibility
> - Easy distinguishability from other infusion devices
> - Good visual display
> - Select rate and dosing limits (as customized to the patient)
> - Downloading capability
> - Lightweight, portable
> - Protection against tampering
> - Locking facility(manual/electronic)
> - Battery back up
>
> *As concerned with the operability of the device:*
> - Pump mechanism
> - Modes available
> - Regulatory approval for use in patients
> - Fail-safe device
> - Alarm and indicator system (power failure, safety limits, disconnection, occlusion, incorrect syringe)
> - Impedance protection
> - Type of mounting
> - Data storage and retrieval
> - Availability of disposables (cassettes/tubings)

and also take into consideration the intensity and duration of action of the opioid so chosen before initiating PCA for effective analgesia.

The initial loading dose should ideally be administered in the postanesthesia care unit till the pain scores are <4 as bolus doses. A continuous infusion of opioids is usually not initiated at the start. Multimodal analgesia should always be considered to enhance analgesia while reducing the side effects especially respiratory depression with the use of opioids at the same time. If the pain scores are >4, either a bolus dose by a physician or a demand dose can be self-administered. The pain scores of >4 also act as a pointer to increasing the demand dose as titrated to effective analgesia. In patients where repeated administration fails to keep pain scores <4, the opioid infusion rate may be considered starting from the lowest possible rate. The continuous infusion rate should be able to cater to 50% of the analgesic/total opioid requirement. The total percentage may be increased in opioid-dependent patients or chronic patients but the rates have to be individualized to a particular patient as per the standard institutional protocol. Other routine opioid medications for the patient should be avoided when the patient is receiving an opioid PCA.

For neuraxial PCA, either continuous basal infusions with a low concentration of local anesthetic with an opioid as an adjuvant may be initiated and bolus dosages may be set to achieve pain scores <4. In case of inadequate analgesia, either the basal rate may be increased which carries an inherent risk of motor blockade or bolus doses may be increased. The concentration of local anesthetics needs to be kept in check and the PCA pumps mandate frequent checks to ascertain the optimal position of the catheter which may get displaced causing inadequate analgesia or misplaced in subarachnoid space causing catastrophic complications.

It is mandatory to document the initial settings, bolus/demand dosing, and the basal rates if nay on the top of the charts of the patients. It is also important to document the drugs being used in PCA pumps for any inadvertent errors. It is also a good practice to label as "on PCA PUMP" by the bedside for safety and monitoring purposes.

Other medications that have been used with IV PCA pumps with varying results include naloxone, clonidine, magnesium, ketorolac, lidocaine, and droperidol.

Complications

The complications are primarily related to the inherent mechanisms of either the equipment or the pharmacological agents used for analgesia not to forget that errors committed by medical personnel can also lead to undesirable effects. The incidence of respiratory depression with the use of PCA pumps in hospitals with acute pain services (APS) has been reported to be 0.1–0.8% in comparison to the risk of 0.2–0.9% for respiratory depression following intermittent intramuscular analgesia and 1.7% with continuous IV opioid infusions.

Complications about PCA usually include the problems of "run-away pumps", failure of antireflux valves, incorrect syringe placement, PCA by proxy, and machine tampering.

Runaway pumps are a mechanical error resulting from incorrect delivery of drugs through the pump at incorrect time intervals. The dose so administered may also vary with each delivery leading to lethal overdosing thereby signifying appropriate and continuous monitoring in patients on PCA.

Antireflux valves prevent the opioid medication from flowing up into the intravenous fluid infusion line leading to delivery of medication to the patient at once in case the intravenous line is flushed, resulting in overdose. Uncontrolled siphoning of syringe contents has been reported secondary to failure of the damaged drive mechanism to retain the syringe plumber, cracked glass PCA syringes, and improperly secured PCA cassettes. Hence the use of an antireflux valve and antisiphon valves is strongly recommended in PCA pumps.

If the syringe containing the drug is damaged or incorrectly placed, it can potentially empty on account of gravity and deliver the entire drug to the patient at once. To prevent this, lines should be cross clamped when changing the syringe and pumps should be equipped with antisiphon valves to be kept level up to or below the intravenous catheter in the patient.

PCA by proxy is when the attendant or some other person presses the button rather than the patient, believing that the patient is in pain leading to severe respiratory depression. So the attendants must be counseled beforehand before commencing the PCA pump.

Other causes of equipment-related problems include patient tampering and the use of pumps close to the MRI machine or in a hyperbaric chamber as explained earlier too.

Errors committed by medical personnel including nursing staff have also been reported. These errors in many instances have led to over sedation resulting from the programming of incorrect bolus dose size, incorrect drug concentrations, incorrect background infusions, and background infusions when none were ordered. To prevent tampering with PCA pumps, access to the pump, key/code and the drug should be accessible only to dedicated health care personnel. The devices should be regularly screened.

Complications of epidural and indwelling nerve catheter PCA include incorrect placement of catheter, infection, catheter dislodgement, allergic reaction, and short/long term neural damage.

Side effects of PCA administration may also be due to medications especially opioids that can occur irrespective of the route of administration or mode of delivery and usually includes nausea, vomiting constipation, pruritus, urinary retention, sedation, confusion, or delirium that can be managed using agents commonly employed for treatment of individual side effects otherwise. The most dreaded complication that is of major concern is respiratory depression which needs utmost vigilance on the part of the team of residents and nursing staff dedicated to the use of PCA pump and needs to be managed immediately by supporting airway and breathing or oxygen administration if the need arises.

Monitoring of PCA: The use of PCA pumps in an establishment demands optimal safety and efficacy that is implemented

> **BOX 2:** Monitoring of patient-controlled analgesia (PCA).
>
> - Continuous education program for medical and the nursing staff caring for patients using PCA.
> - Ensuring protocolized approach to using a uniform regimen in PCA pumps at all the places
> - Clear instructions and assignment of services related to PCA including
>   - Ensuring availability of medical personnel capable of dealing with emergencies if any.
>   - Ensuring minimum standards of monitoring with the use of PCA—(pulse rate, non-invasive blood pressure, respiratory rate, motor blockade with neuraxial PCA)
>   - Protocolized approach to handling the side effects in a stepwise manner (Pharmacological agents)

by education, local guidelines, and monitoring which is supervised by the acute pain team or the team undertaking the PCA prescription. Therefore, uniform guidelines and continuous monitoring by the APS team have been laid down to prevent complications that can jeopardize the safety of the patient (Box 2).

The patients should be monitored frequently by the nurses and resident doctors to assess pain and sedation levels every two hours for the first 24–48 hours considering the highest risk of hypoventilation and hypoxemia during this time interval. Patients should also be assessed for pain by using standard numeric or behavior scales as well as by evaluating the number of demands for medication. A dedicated team of nurses and resident doctors should set up the PCA pumps and should ensure smooth functioning of the pump and are responsible for refilling/altering the medications to avoid complications and reduce the side effects.

CONCLUSION

PCA has been established as a safe and effective method of excellent and adequate analgesia that is useful even in busy, understaffed wards. It has gained popularity primarily due to the availability of sophisticated PCA pumps that are either manual or microprocessor-controlled and cater to the analgesic requirement of the patient, providing a pain-free environment and enhancing the speedy recovery as well. However, the use of these devices demands utmost vigilance and monitoring standards to avoid potential side effects and complications. The prehand knowledge of working of the model of an individual pump along with commonly employed terminology and modes should be understood beforehand and should be uniformly adapted to avoid potential errors.

QUESTIONS

Q. 1. Intravenous Vs epidural routes of PCA.

Q. 2. PCA and PCEA in ERAS.

Q. 3. PCA in pediatric patients.

Q. 4. Oral PCA. What is PCoA®?

FURTHER READING

1. Aguirre J, Del Moral A, Cobo I, Borgeat A, Blumenthal S. The role of continuous peripheral nerve blocks. Anesthesiol Res Pract. 2012;2012:560879.
2. Chumbley G, Mountford L. Patient-controlled analgesia infusion pumps for adults. Nurs Stand. 2010; 25(8):35-40.
3. End of Life/Palliative Education Resource Center. Fast Fact and Concept #085: Epidural Analgesia. Wisconsin: Medical College of Wisconsin; 2019.
4. Grass JA. Patient-controlled analgesia. Anesth Analg. 2005;101(5 Suppl): S44-61.
5. Macintyre PE. Safety and efficacy of patient-controlled analgesia. Br J Anesth. 2001;87(1): 36-46.
6. Mann C, Ouro-Bang'na F, Eledjam JJ. Patient-controlled analgesia. Curr Drug Targets. 2005;6(7):815-9.
7. Pastino A, Lakra A. Patient Controlled Analgesia. In: StatPearls [Internet]. Treasure Island (FL): StatPearls Publishing; 2021.

CHAPTER 63

Cleaning and Sterilization

Chandni Sinha, Abhinav Prakash, Ajeet Kumar

Q. 1. Define the following terminologies.
Ans.
- *Antimicrobial:* A chemical or material capable of destroying or inhibiting the growth of microorganisms.
- *Antiseptic:* A chemical germicide that has antimicrobial activity and that can be safely applied to living tissue.
- *Asepsis:* A process that prevents contact with microorganisms.
- *Bactericide:* A chemical agent that kills bacteria.
- *Bacteriostat:* An agent that will prevent bacterial growth but does not necessarily kill the bacteria. Bacteriostatic action is reversible.
- *Biological indicator:* A sterilization-process monitoring device consisting of a standardized, viable population of microorganisms (usually bacterial spores) that are known to be resistant to the mode of sterilization being monitored. It indicates whether or not conditions were adequate for sterility.
- *Disinfection:* Process capable of destroying most microorganisms but, as ordinarily used, not bacterial spores.
- *Sanitization:* Process of reducing the number of microbial contaminants to a relatively safe level.
- *Sanitizer:* A low-level disinfectant.
- *Sterilization:* Process capable of removing or destroying all viable forms of microbial life, including bacterial spores, to an acceptable sterility assurance level.

Universal precautions: Recommendations made by the Centers for Disease Control and Prevention (CDC) that healthcare workers consider blood and certain body fluids to be potentially infectious for bloodborne pathogens and use protective barriers and workplace practices to reduce the risk of exposure. In 1996, universal precautions were incorporated into standard precautions, which expanded the coverage to anybody fluid that may contain contagious microorganisms.

Q. 2. Explain various types of disinfection.
Ans.
- *High-level disinfection:* A procedure that kills all organisms with the exception of small number of bacterial spores and certain prions. Most high-level disinfectants can produce sterilization with sufficient contact time.
- *Intermediate-level disinfection:* A procedure that kills vegetative bacteria, including *Mycobacterium tuberculosis*, most fungi, and viruses but not bacterial spores.
- *Low-level disinfection:* A procedure that kills most vegetative bacteria (but not *M. tuberculosis*), some fungi, and viruses but no spores.

Q. 3. What is the important step before disinfection/sterilization?
Ans. Cleaning is the first step. It involves the removal of gross debris, rinsing, and then drying from the product to be sterilized. This is an important step because dirt over instruments may hinder the action of

sterilants/disinfectants. Some instruments require disassembly during cleaning. Commercial automated cleaners with ultrasonic waves are also available.

Q. 4. What are the various methods of disinfection/sterilization?
Ans.
- Pasteurization
- Steam sterilization (autoclaving)
- Dry heat sterilization
- Chemical disinfection and sterilization
- Gas sterilization
- Radiation sterilization
- Gas plasma sterilization.

Q. 5. Compare the advantages and disadvantages of the above methods?
Ans. The advantages and disadvantages of disinfection/sterilization are given in **Table 1**.

Q. 6. Explain various methods by which heat is used for disinfection and sterilization.
Ans.

Pasteurization
Named after French microbiologist Louis Pasteur, it involves the immersion of equipment in water at a high temperature (usually <100°C) for a specified period of time. For example, 70°C for 30 minutes. Centers for Disease Control and Prevention (CDC) guidelines refer it to as a *high-level disinfection process*. The contact time required is inversely proportional to temperature.

Steam Sterilization/Autoclaving
It involves using saturated steam under pressure. Pressure on its own has a negligible sterilizing effect but works to increase the boiling point of water within the chamber.

The time needed to achieve sterilization is inversely proportional to temperature. Some of the combinations include 121°C for 15 minutes, 126°C for 10 minutes, 134°C for 3.5 minutes, and a few seconds at 150°C. Items are dried in the postexposure phase, which involves exhausting the chamber to the atmosphere and circulating filtered air or drawing a deep vacuum.

Monitoring of Autoclave
- *Mechanical indicators:* These include time, temperature, and pressure monitors.
- *Chemical indicators:* These are divided into various classes from Class I to Class V. Increasing class indicates more sensitivity. Chemical indicators give quick results and are inexpensive. One of the most common examples is autoclave tape, which is a class I indicator.
- *Biological indicators:* These are standard preparations of spores that are placed alongside the load to be autoclaved. A positive indicator is suggestive of possible sterilization failure. One of its major disadvantages is the time needed for incubation.

Dry Heat Sterilization
Although a slow process, its main use lies in its noncorrosive nature. Convection hot air sterilizers use forced air for heat transfer.

Q. 7. What do you understand by chemical sterilization?
Ans. This method involves immersing the item in a solution containing the chemical disinfectant. Automated systems such as STERIS are available which provide the full cycle of disinfection, rinsing, and drying. Chemical sterilization is especially useful for items that are heat sensitive.

Q. 8. List various types of chemical agents, their spectrum, and advantages/disadvantages.
Ans. Various types of chemical agents and their advantages and disadvantages are listed in **Table 2**.

Chapter 63: Cleaning and Sterilization

TABLE 1: Advantages and disadvantages of the methods of disinfection/sterilization.

Method	Advantages	Disadvantages
Pasteurization	• Simple, inexpensive • Lower temperature is less damaging • No residues or fumes	• Heat may damage sensitive materials • Chance of contamination during drying and packaging
Autoclaving	• Simple, inexpensive • No residues or fumes • Kills all viruses, bacteria, spores	Steam can damage sensitive equipment
Dry heat	• Useful for items sensitive to moist heat • No corrosion of metallic instruments	Slow method
Chemical	Simple, inexpensive, quick	• Residues can be tissue irritants • Risk of contamination during packaging • Environmental pollution • Occupational health hazard
Gas sterilization	• Suitable for items that are heat/moisture sensitive • Reliable as it penetrates all parts • Risk of recontamination is eliminated as items are prepacked • Multiple items can be sterilized at once	• Long processing time • Fire and explosion hazard • Risk of exposure to employees • Expensive • Cannot sterilize devices with petroleum-based lubricants
Radiation sterilization	• Item can be prepackaged; no risk of contamination till the package is opened • Kills all microorganisms, including spores • Suitable for thermolabile items • No risk of retained radioactivity	• Impractical for everyday use • Expensive
Gas plasma sterilization	• Short processing time • No toxic residues; safe for workers and environment	• Small size of the sterilizing chamber • Certain items such as cellulose materials, paper, linens, powders, liquids, and implants cannot be sterilized • Inferior penetration as compared to EO

(EO: ethylene oxide)

Q. 9. How is ethylene oxide (EO) used for sterilization?

Ans. Ethylene oxide (EO) is a colorless gas with a sweet odor. It kills bacteria, fungi, virus, and spores. It can penetrate narrow crevices of instruments and through permeable bags. Since blood and other proteinaceous materials act as hindrance to EO, items must be thoroughly cleaned, rinsed and dried before packaging. Items are placed in wire baskets/metal cans and then loaded in the sterilizer. Automatic sterilizers may require 1.5–6 hours. It is recommended to maintain a relative humidity between 35–70% and temperature between 18–32°C throughout processing and storage facility. After sterilization, process of aeration is used to reduce the level of EO to a safe level.

Q. 10. What do you understand by critical, semicritical and noncritical items?

Ans. *Critical items*: These include equipment that enters sterile tissue, for example, vascular catheters, and regional block needles. These items must be sterile.

TABLE 2: Various types of chemical agents, their spectrum, and advantages/disadvantages.

Class	Spectrum	Advantages	Disadvantages
Glutaraldehyde	Bacteria, tubercle bacillus, virus, fungi, spores (±)	• Noncorrosive with most equipment • Active in presence of organic material • Extensive shelf life can be used for long after activation • High-level disinfection	• Evaporates at room temperature → exposure to healthcare personnel • Requires activation (made alkaline)
Orthophthaldehyde	Bacteria, tubercle bacillus, virus, fungi, spores (±)	• Faster disinfection • Minimal odor • No activation required • High-level disinfection	• Eye and mucous membrane irritant • Dermatitis on repeated contact
Quaternary ammonium compounds	Bacteria, virus, fungi	• Quick acting • Relative nontoxic, noncaustic	• Ineffective against mycobacteria, hydrophilic virus, spores • Inactivated by organic matter
Phenolics	Bacteria, tubercle bacillus, virus, fungi	• Active in presence of organic matter • Very stable, retain activity after drying or mild heating	• Corrosive to metals, can damage plastics, rubber • May damage skin, mucous membrane
Alcohols	Bacteria, tubercle bacillus, virus(±), fungi (±)	Short contact time required Inexpensive	• Inactive against spores, hydrophilic virus • Flammable
Iodophores	Bacteria, tubercle bacillus, virus, fungi	• Effective against most microorganisms • Low toxicity	Inactive against spores, mycobacteria and certain fungi
Peroxide-based compounds	Bacteria, fungi, virus, spores	• Wide spectrum of activity • Not inactivated by organic matter • No restriction on disposal	• Requires careful storage as it is inactivated by heat and light • Can damage rubber, plastic, metals • Skin and eye irritant
Formaldehyde	Bacteria, tubercle bacillus, virus, fungi	• Noncorrosive • Not inactivated by organic matter • High level disinfectant	• Flammable and highly toxic fumes • Eye, skin and respiratory tract irritant • Probable carcinogen

Semicritical items: These equipment do not pierce mucous membrane, for example, laryngoscope blades, face masks, oral and nasal airways, etc. They should undergo sterilization/high-level disinfection.

Noncritical items: These come into contact with intact skin, for example, stethoscopes, blood pressure cuffs, etc. These items need only cleaning followed by intermediate or low-level disinfection.

TABLE 3: Decontamination of anesthesia equipments.

Items	Comments
Anesthesia carts and anesthesia machine	Items that require different levels of disinfection should be kept in separate drawers. Clean covering should be placed at the top of the cart, and cleaned in between the cases and at the end of day with *germicide*. Empty the drawers and clean the surface with germicide at least once a month
Gas cylinders	Wash the cylinder with soap and water or spray with germicide before taking inside the theater
Anesthesia ventilator	Treat the external surface same as anesthesia machine. Bellows and tubing can be sterilized using EO
Unidirectional valves, APL, and water trap	Clean and disinfect periodically. Some APL valves can be autoclaved/pasteurized
Absorbers	Canisters should be disassembled, cleaned and then autoclaved or EO sterilized
Reservoir bags	If reusable, then high-level disinfection/sterilization using chemical disinfection/EO sterilization
Breathing system and Y-piece	Prefer disposable tubing. If reusable, clean, and sterilize/high-level disinfection. Y-piece should be thoroughly cleaned, sterilized using EO or plasma sterilization
Scavenging equipment	Clean periodically and chemical disinfection
Face mask and airways	Prefer disposable. If reusable, clean, rinse, and then sterilize/high-level disinfection using EO, autoclaving, chemical, or pasteurization
Tracheal and double lumen tubes	Always prefer disposable tubes. In case if required, EO sterilization may be used
LMAs	Manufacturer's instructions to be followed for different types. Autoclave if reusable and heat tolerant
Bougies	Single use or high-level disinfection
Laryngoscope blades	Handle should be cleaned and disinfected. If reusable, blades should be sterilized with EO, plasma, or chemical sterilization
Flexible endoscopes	Should be sterilized/high-level disinfection using EO/chemical disinfection
Stylets	Disposable. If reusable, autoclave, EO, plasma, or chemical sterilization
Oxygen masks	Disposable
BP cuffs	Periodic chemical disinfection or EO. Clean if visibly contaminated in between the cases or at the end of the day
Stethoscopes	Clean with alcohol swabs

(APL: adjustable pressure-limiting; BP cuffs: blood pressure cuff; EO: ethylene oxide; LMAs: laryngeal mask airway)

Q. 11. How will you decontaminate anesthesia-related equipment?

Ans. The process of decontamination of various anesthesia-related equipment is given in **Table 3**.

FURTHER READING

1. Davey A, Diba A. Ward's Anesthetic Equipment, 6th edition.
2. Dorsch JA, Dorsch SE. Understanding Anaesthesia Equipment, 2012.

SECTION 4

ICU Instruments

- **Percutaneous Tracheostomy**
  Akhilesh Gupta, Devang Bharti
- **Oxygen Delivery Devices**
  Anshu Gupta, Akhilesh Gupta
- **Ventilators, Modes of Ventilator, and Ventilator Graphics**
  Nitin, Akhilesh Gupta
- **Deep Vein Thrombosis: Mechanical Pump**
  Devang Bharti, Akhilesh Gupta
- **Jet Ventilation**
  Akhilesh Gupta, Shubhi Singhal
- **Ultrasound Machine**
  Himanshu Bhasin, Akhilesh Gupta
- **Rapid Infusion Pumps**
  Akhilesh Gupta, Jyoti Singh
- **Automated Chest Compressor Machine**
  Jyoti Singh, Akhilesh Gupta
- **Extracorporeal Membrane Oxygenation**
  Devang Bharti, Akhilesh Gupta
- **Renal Replacement Therapy**
  Gourav Mittal
- **Defibrillators**
  Shubhi Singhal, Akhilesh Gupta
- **Intra-abdominal Pressure Monitoring**
  Anshu Gupta, Akhilesh Gupta
- **Esophageal Pressure Manometry**
  Akhilesh Gupta, Himanshu Bhasin

CHAPTER 64

Percutaneous Tracheostomy

Akhilesh Gupta, Devang Bharti

Q. 1. What is a percutaneous tracheostomy?
Ans. Percutaneous tracheostomy (PCT) is a type of tracheostomy which involves the insertion of a tracheal cannula through the anterior tracheal wall, followed by the insertion of a guidewire, and dilation of the created stoma till it is large enough for the placement of a tracheostomy tube.

Q. 2. What are the advantages of tracheostomy over endotracheal intubation in intensive care unit patients?
Ans. The following are the advantages of tracheostomy over endotracheal intubation in intensive care unit (ICU) patients:
- Improved patient comfort
- Decreased need for sedation
- Shorter length of stay in ICU
- Decreased airway resistance
- Decreased work of breathing
- Better airway clearance
- Decreased chances of kinking
- Better oral care
- Comfortable to feed the patients.

Q. 3. What are the advantages of PCT over surgical tracheostomy?
Ans. Advantages of PCT over surgical tracheostomy are:
- Better procedural safety
- Can be performed at the bedside
- Shorter procedural time
- Decreased cost of the procedure
- Decreased incidence of surgical site infection
- Reduced blood loss
- Decreased incidence of tube blockage
- Lower rate of tube displacement.

Q. 4. What are the disadvantages of PCT over surgical tracheostomy?
Ans. Disadvantages of PCT over surgical tracheostomy include:
- Increased incidence of hypoxemia
- Prolonged learning curve
- Cannot be performed in patients with difficult front of neck anatomy such as thyroid mass, cysts and obese patients with short necks leading to difficulty in appreciation of landmarks.

Q. 5. What are the indications of PCT?
Ans. Indications of PCT are:
- Long-term airway protection (e.g., after traumatic brain injury)
- Need for prolonged intubation
- Prolonged respiratory failure
- Facilitation of weaning in a difficult to wean patient
- Upper airway obstruction
- Pulmonary toilette.

Q. 6. What are the contraindications for PCT?
Ans. Contraindications for PCT are:
- Refusal of consent
- PCT site infection
- Distorted neck anatomy
- Severe coagulopathies
- Mobile and compressible airway, as in children

- Airway emergencies
- Previous neck surgery or trauma
- Unstable cervical spine
- Known difficult airway
- Tracheomalacia
- Need of FiO_2 >0.6 or positive end-expiratory pressure (PEEP) >10 cm H_2O.

Q. 7. What are the complications of PCT?
Ans. The following complications have been attributed to PCT:
- Incorrect tracheostomy tube placement
- Subcutaneous emphysema
- Pneumothorax
- Pneumomediastinum
- Trauma to the trachea and surrounding structures
- Hemorrhage
- Foreign body in trachea (e.g., tracheal dilator, fractured guidewire, etc.)
- Tracheal stenosis
- Tracheomalacia
- Tracheoesophageal fistula.

Q. 8. How will you prepare a patient for PCT?
Ans. Preparation of a patient for PCT includes:
- *Preprocedural assessment:*
  - *History:* A detailed medical history should be taken from the patient with an emphasis on the underlying pathology, estimated length of stay in ICU, need for intubation, indication for PCT and any contraindication of PCT. Details regarding previous endotracheal intubation and/or history of PCT/surgical tracheostomy should be elicited. The size of an endotracheal tube in situ, ventilatory settings, and need for suctioning should also be noted. A detailed medication history should also be elicited.
  - *Examination:* General physical examination of the patient should be undertaken and vital parameters duly noted. A local examination of the neck should be performed after placing a roll beneath the patient's shoulders for optimal neck extension. This position not only facilitates the identification of various landmarks but also allows for the proper assessment of suprasternal length of the trachea. The neck should be inspected for the presence of any lesions, rash, pustules, or any other signs of local infection. Any restriction in neck extension or presence of excessive subcutaneous fat in the neck should be recorded. The hyoid cartilage, thyroid cartilage, cricothyroid membrane, cricoid cartilage, and tracheal rings distal to the cricoid cartilage are all assessed by palpation.
- *Investigations:*
  - Hemoglobin
  - Coagulation profile [prothrombin time (PT), activated partial thromboplastin time (aPTT), international normalized ratio (INR)]
  - Ultrasonography/computed tomography neck
  - Renal function tests
- *Preprocedural optimization:*
  - Therapeutic anticoagulation should be withheld
  - Reversal of coagulation abnormalities
  - Optimization of hemoglobin level
  - Informed consent
  - Peripheral IV access should be secured.

Q. 9. List the equipment required for performing PCT?
Ans. The following equipment should be kept ready before performing PCT:
- Fiberoptic bronchoscope
- Percutaneous dilatational kit, including.
  - 22G needle and syringe
  - 1.32 mm guidewire

- 8F guiding catheter
- 11F punch dilator
- 18F, 21F, 24F, 28F, 32F, 36F and 38F dilators
  (Or Ciaglia's Blue Rhino/Blue Dolphin Kit)
- Tracheostomy tubes of different sizes
- Shoulder rolls
- Difficult airway cart
- Sterile equipment—gowns, drapes, gloves, forceps, sponges, etc.

Q. 10. What are the various techniques of PCT?

Ans. The Seldinger technique, i.e., the initial puncture of the anterior tracheal wall and passing of the guidewire, forms the basis of PCT. Subsequent dilation of the trachea may be undertaken using different techniques:
- Ciaglia's serial dilation technique
- Blue Rhino single dilation technique
- Griggs forceps technique
- Translaryngeal tracheostomy
- Blue Dolphin balloon dilation technique.

Q. 11. Describe the Seldinger technique of PCT.

Ans. Before starting the procedure, monitors; including electrocardiography (ECG), pulse oximetry (SpO_2), capnography ($EtCO_2$), and noninvasive blood pressure (NIBP) are attached and patient is sedated. Muscle relaxation is often employed in the form of nondepolarizing muscle relaxants. Ventilator settings are modified to increase FiO_2 to 1.0 and to ensure optimal minute ventilation.

The patient is positioned supine and neck extension is achieved by placing a roll under the shoulders. The neck is palpated to identify the landmarks—thyroid notch, cricoid cartilage, and tracheal rings. The area over the second and third tracheal rings is cleaned and draped, and the site of incision is infiltrated with *2% lignocaine* and *1:200,000 adrenalines*.

A flexible fiberoptic bronchoscope is inserted inside the endotracheal tube with its tip positioned just distal to the distal end of the tube so as to transilluminate the anterior trachea. The cuff of the endotracheal tube is deflated and the tube along with the bronchoscope is withdrawn till the transillumination is at the selected site of incision. The cuff of the tube is reinflated and optimal ventilation is ensured. The tip of the bronchoscope is then withdrawn inside the tube and a 1.5-2 cm horizontal midline incision is made over the selected site. Curved artery forceps are used for blunt dissection to expose the pretracheal fascia. Further dissection may be achieved by gently rotating the finger in the incision to identify the intercartilaginous area.

An introducer needle with an overlying catheter sheath is connected to a saline-filled syringe. The needle is then guided into the tracheal lumen under continuous suction. The intratracheal placement of needle is indicated by aspiration of air bubbles and may be confirmed by direct visualization by a bronchoscope. The catheter sheath is passed into the trachea and the needle is withdrawn. A guidewire is then placed inside the trachea and its placement is confirmed by bronchoscopic visualization.

Q. 12. Describe Ciaglia serial dilation technique for tracheal dilation.

Ans. A short rigid dilator is placed over the intratracheal guidewire so as to facilitate the subsequent placement of an 8F guiding catheter over the guidewire. Further, dilators of increasing size (11F, 18F, 21F, 24F, 28F, 32F, 36F, and 38F) are used sequentially to increase the size of tracheal stoma. Each dilator is introduced with a twisting motion, after liberal application of lubricating jelly, and is usually passed three times in and out of the stoma. Finally, when the stoma is large enough, a tracheostomy tube with a trocar is passed through it inside the trachea. The trocar is then removed and the tube is left in situ.

Q. 13. Describe the Ciaglia blue rhino single dilation technique.

Ans. Ciaglia blue rhino single dilation technique employs the use of a single conical dilator instead of multiple serial dilators. The large conical dilator is passed over the guidewire using a curved hand motion, till the black skin line is visible just inside the trachea. The dilator is then removed and a tracheostomy tube with a trocar is introduced through the tracheal lumen. The final position of the tube is confirmed using the bronchoscope.

Q. 14. How will you care for a post-tracheostomy patient?

Ans. Immediately after tracheostomy, optimal ventilation should be reconfirmed by checking for adequate expiratory volume. The neck should be palpated to identify any air leak or subcutaneous emphysema.

Obtaining a post-tracheostomy chest radiograph is a prevalent practice, although various studies suggest that it should be reserved only for patients who underwent difficult and complicated PCT or for PCTs without fiberoptic guidance.

The tracheal stoma should be kept clean and dry, and optimal tracheal suction should be performed to avoid ulceration at the tracheostomy site. Very tightly bound sutures may result in pressure ulceration.

All supplies to replace a tracheostomy tube should be available at bedside of the patient. These include tracheostomy tube of same size and one size smaller, suction catheter, scissors, gloves, replacement ties, water-based lubricant, etc. Emergency airway equipment including direct laryngoscope, endotracheal tube, manual resuscitator and masks should also be readily accessible.

Q. 15. When can tube exchange be perfomed after PCT?

Ans. There are different practices around the world for this. Too early removal can cause loss of airway due to collapse and creation of false tract. So any exchanges need to be perfomed only after 48 to 72 hours, even better with the help of a bougie or airway exchange catheter. If a situation arises that need change of tracheostomy tube before 2 days, it is better to intubate the patient and carry on the procedure.

■ FURTHER READING

1. Dixon LM, Mascioli S, Mixell JH, Gillin T, Upchurch CN, Bradley KM. Reducing tracheostomy-related pressure injuries. AACN Adv Crit Care. Winter 2018;29(4):426-31.
2. Ghattas C, Alsunaid S, Pickering EM, Holden VK. State-of-the-art: percutaneous tracheostomy in the intensive care unit. J Thorac Dis. 2021;13(8):5261-76.
3. Khan RM. Airway management, 7th edition. Hyderabad: Paras Medical Publishers; 2020.
4. Mehta C, Mehta Y. Percutaneous tracheostomy. Ann Card Anaesth. 2017;20(Suppl):S19-25.
5. Mitchell RB, Hussey HM, Setzen G, Jacobs IN, Nussenbaum B, Dawson C, et al. Clinical consensus statement: tracheostomy care. Otolaryngol Head Neck Surg. 2013;148(1):6-20.
6. O'Toole TR, Jacobs N, Hondorp B, Crawford L, Boudreau LR, Jeffe J, et al. Prevention of tracheostomy-related hospital-acquired pressure ulcers. Otolaryngol Head Neck Surg. 2017;156(4):642-51.
7. Yeo WX, Phua CQ, Lo S. Is routine chest X-ray after surgical and percutaneous tracheostomy necessary in adults: a systemic review of the current literature. Clin Otolaryngol. 2014;39(2):79-88.

CHAPTER 65

Oxygen Delivery Devices

Anshu Gupta, Akhilesh Gupta

Q. 1. What are the indications of oxygen therapy?

Ans. Treatment or prevention of hypoxemia is the most common indication for oxygen therapy.

Q. 2. What are the causes of hypoxia?

Ans. *Hypoxia may result from a:*
- Decrease in any of the determinants of oxygen delivery (DO_2)
- Arterial hypoxemia

  Oxygen delivery (DO_2) = cardiac output (L/min) × arterial oxygen content = cardiac output (L/min) × (arterial partial pressure of oxygen (PaO_2) × hemoglobin concentration of arterial blood × saturation of hemoglobin with oxygen)

  For a healthy 70 kg, patient's cardiac output (L/min) value is approximately 5 L/min, arterial oxygen content per 100 mL of blood (mL/dL) is approximately 20 mL/dL with hemoglobin of 15 g/dL.

  Therefore, DO_2 is approximately 1,000 mL/min in a healthy 70 kg adult.

The causes of hypoxia are:
- *Decrease in oxygen delivery (DO_2):*
  - Oxygen delivery is out of proportion to demand, e.g., anemia, low cardiac output, hypoxemia, or abnormal hemoglobin affinity (e.g., carbon monoxide toxicity).
- Failure of oxygen use at the tissue level (e.g., shock) or at the cellular level (e.g., cyanide poisoning).
- *Arterial hypoxemia:*
  - Defective ventilation
    - Respiratory center depression drugs such as narcotics, anesthetics, and sedatives, cerebral infarction, cerebral trauma.
    - Neuromuscular disorders such as myasthenia gravis, Guillain–Barré syndrome, brain or spinal injuries polio, porphyria, and botulism.
    - Airway obstruction chronic obstructive pulmonary disease—acute severe asthma.
    - Restrictive defects: Interstitial lung disease, kyphoscoliosis, ankylosing spondylitis bilateral, and diaphragmatic palsy—severe obesity.
  - Impaired diffusion and gas exchange
    - Pulmonary edema
    - Acute respiratory distress syndrome
    - Pulmonary thromboembolism
    - Pulmonary fibrosis
  - Ventilation-perfusion (V/Q and Q) abnormalities
    - Chronic obstructive pulmonary disease
    - Pulmonary fibrosis
    - Acute respiratory distress syndrome
    - Thromboembolism.

Q. 3. What is the final goal of oxygen therapy?

Ans. Treatment or prevention of hypoxemia is the most common indication for oxygen therapy, and the final goal of effective treatment is avoidance or resolution of tissue hypoxia.

Q. 4. How are the oxygen therapy devices classified?

Ans. Oxygen delivery systems are generally classified as:
- Low-flow or variable-performance devices
- High-flow or fixed-performance devices.

Q. 5. Why low-flow systems are known as variable-performance devices and high-flow as fixed-performance devices?

Ans. Low-flow systems provide lower oxygen flows than the actual inspiratory flow. It is because when the patient inspires, the oxygen is diluted with room air, and the degree of dilution depends on the inspiratory flow. With low-flow devices final concentration of oxygen delivered depends on the ventilatory demands of the patient, the size of the oxygen reservoir, and the rate at which the reservoir is filled. They are therefore called *variable performance devices* as they deliver variable inspiratory oxygen fraction (FiO_2).

High-flow systems provide the entire inspiratory demand. High-flow systems use reservoirs or very high-flow rates to meet the large peak inspiratory flow demands and the exaggerated minute volumes of the patient. They do not depend on the patient's respiratory effort. Constant high-flow rates and reservoir are essential to meet the patient's peak inspiratory flow. Flows 3-4 times the measured minute volume (30-40 L/min) is often necessary. Regardless of the patient's respiratory pattern, high-flow systems are expected to deliver predictable, consistent, and measurable high and low FiO_2 values. Some high-flow systems also can control the humidity and temperature of the delivered gases.

Q. 6. Give examples of low-flow devices. How will you calculate FiO_2 a variable performance device delivers?

Ans.
- Six low-flow devices include the nasal cannula, simple face mask, partial rebreathing mask, nonrebreathing mask, and tracheostomy mask.
- Low-flow systems produce FiO_2 values from 21 to 80%.
- The FiO_2 depends on the size of the oxygen reservoir, oxygen flow, and the patient's ventilatory pattern [e.g., tidal volume (VT), peak inspiratory flow, respiratory rate, minute ventilation]. With a normal ventilation pattern, these devices deliver a relatively predictable and consistent FiO_2 level.
- The following examples are theoretical estimates of a FiO_2 produced by a low-flow system (e.g., nasal cannula) in two clinical conditions at two different flow rates.
- The example for estimation of FiO_2 from a low-flow system is based on the standard normal patient and ventilatory pattern.
- For the FiO_2 calculation, we estimate the anatomic reservoir for a nasal cannula which consists of the nose, nasopharynx, and oropharynx, and it is about one-third of the entire normal anatomic dead space (including trachea), i.e., 150 mL ÷ 3 = 50 mL
- We calculate the FiO_2 of the nasal cannula at oxygen flow rate of 6 L/min assuming VT of 500 mL, respiratory rate of 20 BPM, inspiratory (I) time of 1 second, and expiratory (E) time of 2 seconds.

$$\text{Flow rate 6 L/min} = 6{,}000 \text{ mL}/60 \text{ s}$$
$$= 100 \text{ mL/s}$$

I:E ratio assumed to be 1:2 in a normal respiratory pattern, rate = 20 breaths/min, 100% oxygen provided/s is 100 mL: Inspiratory time = 1 second volume inspired oxygen

If the terminal 0.5 second of the 2 second expiratory time has negligible gas flow, the anatomic reservoir (50 mL) completely fills with 100% oxygen, assuming an oxygen flow rate of 100 mL/s.

In nasal cannula, there is no mechanical reservoir, Oxygen from anatomic reservoir 50 mL flow/sec (0.5 second end-expiratory pause × 100 mL/s)

Therefore inspired room air = 0.20 × [500 − (100 + 50)]
Inspired room air (0.20 × 350 mL) = 70 mL
Inspired oxygen = 50 + 100 + 73
= 223 mL of 100% oxygen
Inspired FiO_2 = 223 mL of oxygen/500 mL
= 0.44% at 6 L/min

- At flow rate of 2 L/min with same respiratory parameters:

Flow rate 2 L/min = 2000 mL/60 s
= 33 mL/s

Oxygen from anatomic reservoir = 17 mL Flow/sec (0.5 second end-expiratory pause × 33 mL/s)
Oxygen from room air = 450 mL (500 − 17 + 33) of 21% oxygen (room air) = 95 mL of 100% oxygen
100% oxygen inspired = 17 + 33 + 95 mL
= 145 mL
FiO_2 = 145 mL of oxygen/500 mL = 0.29%

Q. 7. Name the low-flow devices you know about.
Ans.
- Nasal cannula (prongs)
- Nasal catheters
- Transtracheal catheter
- Face mask
- Partial rebreathing mask
- Nonrebreathing mask
- Tracheostomy mask.

Q. 8. Describe nasal cannula.
Ans. Nasal cannula is low-flow and variable performance oxygen delivery device **(Fig. 1)**. It consists of two soft prongs attached to O_2 supply tubing. It delivers a FiO_2 of 0.28–0.44 at a flow rate of 2–6 L/min. Nasopharynx acts as a reservoir.

The approximate FiO_2 delivered at various flow rates are mentioned in **Table 1**:

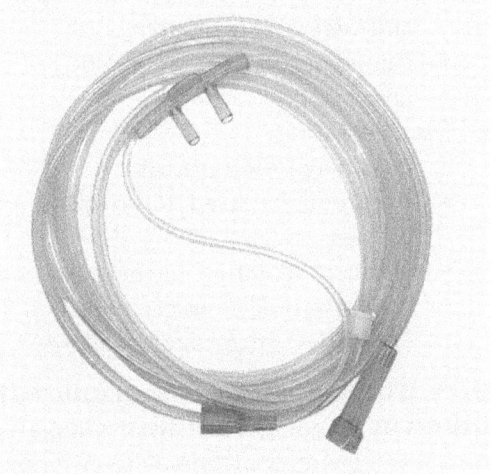

Fig. 1: Nasal cannula.

TABLE 1: The approximate FiO_2 delivered at various flow rates.

Flow rates (L/min)	FiO_2
1	0.24
2	0.28
3	0.32
4	0.36
5	0.40
6	0.44

Q. 9. Can we increase FiO$_2$ of nasal cannula by increasing flow >6 L/min?
Ans. No, we cannot increase FiO$_2$ if the flow is >6 L/min.

Q. 10. Discuss merits and demerits of nasal prongs over other devices.
Ans.
- *Advantages:*
  - Ideal for patients on long-term oxygen therapy
  - Lightweight and comfortable
  - The patient is able to speak, eat, and drink
  - Ideal for patients requiring a small amount of oxygen for a long time
  - It does not increase the dead space and there is no rebreathing.
  - Humidification is not required
  - Low cost.
- *Disadvantages:*
  - It cannot provide FiO$_2$ >0.4.
  - It cannot be used for respiratory distress
  - It causes irritation in the nose and cannot be used in nasal obstruction
  - FiO$_2$ varies with respiratory efforts.

Q. 11. What is a nasopharyngeal catheter? Discuss its advantages and disadvantages.
Ans. It is a low-flow oxygen delivery device with variable performance **(Fig. 2)**. They are soft tubes with several distal holes. Prior to insertion, the size is measured which is equal to the distance from the ala nasi to the tragus. After lubrication, it is inserted into the anterior naris just above the uvula. Deep insertion can cause air swallowing and gastric distension. It should not be used when a nasal mucosal tear is suspected because of the risk of surgical emphysema. Oxygen flows of 2-3 L/min can be used to provide FiO$_2$ 35-40%. It must be repositioned every 8 hours.

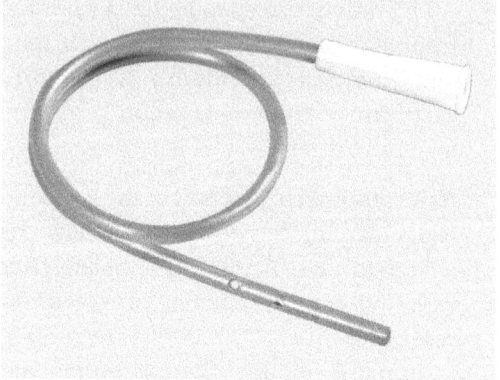

Fig. 2: Nasopharyngeal catheter.

Advantage:
- Same as nasal cannula. No advantages over the nasal cannula.

Disadvantages:
- It is invasive in nature so maybe discomforting for the patient.
- It may be obstructed by mucous and has to be checked and changed regularly.
- Insertion has to be accurately in the oropharynx.

Q. 12. Describe the oxygen face mask.
Ans. It is a low-flow variable performance device. It is a transparent mask provided with side holes and has a reservoir capacity of 100-250 mL. Face mask fits over the mouth and nose of the patient and consists of exhalation ports (holes on the side of the mask) through which the patient exhales CO$_2$ (carbon dioxide). These holes should always remain open. The mask is held in place by elastic around the back of the head, and it has a metal piece to shape over the nose to allow for a better mask fit for the patient. Humidified air may be attached if concentrations are drying for the patient. It is used when a moderate amount of O$_2$ is needed **(Fig. 3)**.

It is used when a moderate amount of O$_2$ is to be delivered. It can carry up to 5-10 L of O$_2$/min with FiO$_2$ 0.35-0.55. It slightly

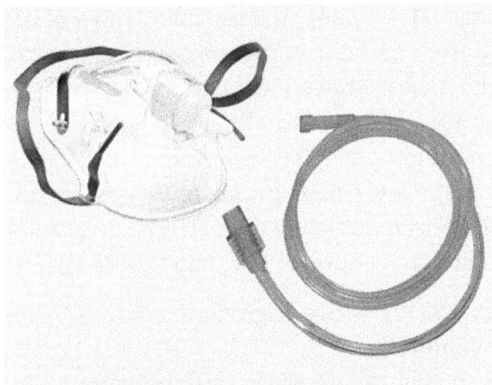

Fig. 3: The oxygen face mask.

TABLE 2: Change of FiO$_2$ and flow rate with O$_2$ flow/min.

O$_2$ flow rate (L/min)	FiO$_2$
5–6	0.4
6–7	0.5
7–8	0.6

increases dead space and there is little rebreathing. Rebreathing of CO$_2$ can occur with O$_2$ flow rates of <2 L O$_2$ L/min or if minute ventilation is very high. Flow rates >8 L/min do not increase FiO$_2$ **(Table 2)**.

Advantages:
- It is a less expensive device for delivering oxygen up to 0.6 FiO$_2$.
- Can be used in mouth breathers.

Disadvantages:
- It is uncomfortable for the patient
- It requires a tight seal
- It does not deliver high FiO$_2$
- FiO$_2$ varies with breathing efforts
- It interferes with eating, drinking, communication
- It is difficult to keep in position for long
- Chances of rebreathing are high.

Q. 13. What is a partial rebreathing mask? Explain.

Ans. It is a low-flow; variable performance device which consists of a face mask with a

TABLE 3: Flow rate of FiO$_2$ with partial rebreather mask.

Flow rate (L/min)	FiO$_2$
6	0.6
7	0.7
8	0.8
9	0.8+
10	0.8+

reservoir bag of 600 mL to 1 L capacity to deliver FiO$_2$ >60%. It can deliver FiO$_2$ of 0.60–0.80 in a patient with a normal respiratory pattern with the mask fitting properly.

The oxygen flows directly into the reservoir bag. The side port entrain the room air and exits the gases exhaled. The 33% of exhaled air fills the reservoir bag. This exhaled air contains very little CO$_2$ as this volume of exhaled air is mainly the anatomic dead space. During inspiration, the bag should not deflate completely because then room air will be entrained and there will be a decrease in FiO$_2$. In each breath during inspiration, during inspiration first, the gas from the reservoir bag (expired gas) and fresh gas are inhaled. Thus it is called a *partial rebreathing mask*. For high FiO$_2$ and adequate CO$_2$ evacuation, the reservoir bag should remain inflated and fresh gas flow should be high at least >8 L/min during the entire respiratory cycle **(Table 3)**.

Advantages:
- It is possible to deliver higher FiO$_2$ with a face mask.
- It can be used during transportation where the oxygen supply is low.

Disadvantages:
- Oxygen cannot be given for a longer time as humidification cannot be done.
- Difficult to apply in claustrophobic patients and orally taking patients.

Q. 14. What is a nonrebreathing mask?
Ans. A nonrebreathing mask is a low-flow effort-dependent device. It is a face mask with a reservoir bag and three unidirectional valves. Two are present on each side port of the face mask to prevent room air entrainment and one between the reservoir bags and face mask to prevent exhaled gases from entering the reservoir bag **(Fig. 4)**. The bag must be inflated throughout the respiratory cycle so that the highest CO_2 can be evacuated and the highest FiO_2 is delivered. To keep the bag inflated and achieve minimum room air entrainment fresh gas flows are kept between 10 and 15 L/min so that FiO_2 between 0.80 and 0.90 can be attained. At a fresh gas flow of 15 L/min, FiO_2 of 1 can be achieved.

There is also a safety valve present which entrains room air if fresh gas flow and reservoir volume cannot meet the ventilatory demands, this valve opens. If this safety valve is not present and one of the unidirectional valves must be removed if ventilatory demands cannot be met so that room air can be entrained. If it meets the respiratory demands and the reservoir bag remains inflated and the mask is fitted tightly then FiO_2 up to 1 can be delivered at flows of 15 L/min **(Table 4)**.

Q. 15. What are high-flow devices? Give examples.
Ans. High-flow devices are fixed performance devices that do not depend on a patient's effort for meeting patient peak inspiratory flow demands. High-flow systems deliver predictable, consistent, and measurable high and low FiO_2 values regardless of the patient's respiratory pattern. These devices use a high-flow rate to meet the patient's peak inspiratory flow. Flows of 30–40 L/min (or 3–4 times the measured minute volume) are often used. High-flow system can deliver warm and humidified gases. Examples include Venturi masks, high-flow nasal cannula, and manual resuscitator bags.

Q. 16. Describe Venturi mask?
Ans. These are high-flow and fixed performance oxygen delivery devices. It uses gas entrainment to provide the FiO_2 but does not depend on patient's efforts to meet the oxygen demands. Venturi mask uses the Bernoulli principle to deliver a predetermined and fixed concentration of oxygen to the patient. This principle is based on the phenomenon by which when a high velocity of gas moves through a narrow orifice there are shearing forces that creates a negative pressure relative to the surrounding gases around the orifice. This allows the ambient air to be entrained and mixed with the oxygen flow until the pressures are equalized.

The FiO_2 is dependent on the air-entrained. The lesser entrainment of air causes higher

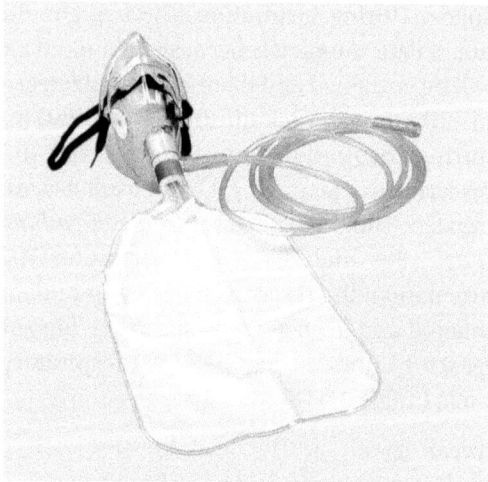

Fig. 4: Nonrebreathing mask.

TABLE 4: Flow rate and FiO_2 with nonrebreathing mask.

O_2 flow rates (L/min)	FiO_2
10	0.80–0.85
12	0.85–0.90
15	0.90–1.00

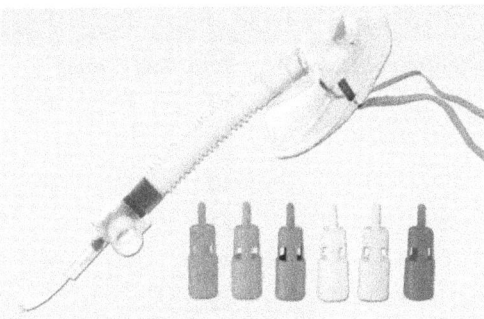

Fig. 5: Venturi mask.

FiO$_2$ delivery. This can be used to provide variable FiO$_2$ by altering the size of the gas orifice or entrainment port size **(Fig. 5)**. These masks are of two types:
1. Venturi mask with fixed FiO$_2$ delivery—it is color-coded and it has jets that deliver known FiO$_2$ with a known flow of oxygen.
2. Venturi mask with variable FiO$_2$ delivery—in these Venturi mask adjustment of the entrainment port can be done to allow variation in FiO$_2$ at different known flows of oxygen.

A fixed FiO$_2$ model, which requires specific inspiratory attachments that are color-coded and have labeled jets that produce a known FiO$_2$ with a given flow; and a variable FiO$_2$ model **(Fig. 5)**, which has a graded adjustment of the air entrainment port that can be set to allow variation in delivered FiO$_2$.

To use any air entrainment device properly to control the FiO$_2$, the standard air-oxygen entrainment ratios and minimum recommended flows for a given FiO$_2$ level must be used **(Table 5)**.

The minimum total flow requirement should result from entrained room air added to the fresh oxygen flow and equal 3–4 times the minute ventilation. This minimal flow is required to meet the patient's peak inspiratory flow demands. As the desired FiO$_2$ increases, the air-oxygen entrainment ratio decreases with a net reduction in total gas flow. The higher the desired FiO$_2$, the greater the probability of the patient's needs exceeding the total flow capabilities of the device.

Q. 17. How do you decide how much air will be entrained by the venture mask?

Ans. The amount of air entrained by a particular Venturi mask (color-coded) or at a particular FiO$_2$ setting depends on the settings made by the manufacturer. The total gas flow will be the sum of the oxygen flow and the amount of air entrained **(Table 5)**.

Entrained air flow is given by the equation:

$$\text{Entrained air flow} = [O_2 \text{ flow from wall} \times (1 - FiO_2)] \div (FiO_2 - 2)$$

Any back pressure or suction will change the entrainment ratio and more air will be entrained. Therefore when the air entrainment will be high the FiO$_2$ will decrease **(Table 6)**:

TABLE 5: Flow rate and FiO$_2$ with Venturi mask.

FiO$_2$ provided by the Venturi valve	Oxygen flow to the valve (L/min)	Amount of air-entrained (L/min)	Total flow to patient (L/min)
0.24	2	51	53
0.28	4	41	45
0.31	6	41	47
0.35	8	37	45
0.40	10	32	42
0.60	15	15	30

TABLE 6: Total gas flows with variable FiO_2.

FiO_2 (L/min)	Oxygen flow (driving) (L/min)	Air flow (entrained) (L/min)	Total flow (L/min)
1.0	10	0	10
0.6	10	10	20
0.6	20	20	40
0.5	10	17	27
0.5	15	25	40
0.4	10	30	40
0.24	2	38	40

Q. 18. Describe the manual resuscitator bag.

Ans. Manual resuscitation bags are used primarily for resuscitation and manual ventilation of ventilator-dependent patients. Manual resuscitators consist of a compressible self-expanding bag, a bag refill valve, and a patient intake valve (nonrebreathing valve). It may also have a pressure-limiting device, positive end-expiratory pressure (PEEP) valve, and mechanism for scavenging expired gases.

- *Self-inflating bag:* It is made up of silicone. The bag expands during expiration. If the volume of oxygen from the delivery source is inadequate to fill the bag, then room air is entrained. The rate at which the bag reinflates will determine the maximum respiratory rate. This bag can be attached to an O_2 source to deliver the FiO_2 of 1.
- *The respirable gas inlet:* It has several components:
  - Bag refill (intake) valve: It is a one-way flap valve that is fitted to the inlet of the self-inflating bag. When the bag is squeezed, the gas pressure inside the bag causes the flap valve to close. This prevents the escape of gas back through the inlet. When the bag is released, its self-inflating characteristics cause entrainment of fresh gas from the respirable gas inlet. This may normally be either air, oxygen, or a mixture of both.
  - *A small-bore nipple:* This is mounted on the inlet, to allow oxygen supply to be attached.
  - *A reservoir system:* The inlet may be fitted with a reservoir system that stores the oxygen supply. Use of a reservoir significantly increases the oxygen concentration in the inspiratory air. With each bag compression, up to 100% of oxygen can be delivered to the patient if the oxygen flow rates are greater than the volume given to the patient. The reservoir assembly for the resuscitators consists of a valve unit and either an inflatable bag or an elongated wide bore hose (popular in pediatric resuscitators).

The size of the reservoir may limit the oxygen delivered. If the volume of the reservoir is less than that of the bag, the inflowing oxygen may not be sufficient to make up the difference and room air will be drawn in. A large reservoir makes the resuscitator more cumbersome. The reservoir assembly is attached to the wide-bore connector in the rear of the intake valve.

The valve unit consists of an overflow valve to prevent overfilling from too high a flow of oxygen and an entrainment valve to entrain air if the bag collapses due to underfilling. When the bag is not filling, i.e., during squeezing and in the fully expanded state, the oxygen inflow will initially partly fill the ventilation bag and partly flow out through the open end of the intake valve and fill the reservoir bag.

During bag re-expansion there is negative pressure in the ventilation bag which causes the inlet valve to open and oxygen from the reservoir enters the bag. If the ventilation bag is not squeezed, and the mask is not held tightly over a patients face, oxygen will flow continuously through the lip membrane of the patient valve.

However, if the mask is held tightly in place, or when patient valve is connected to a tracheal tube, excess oxygen will escape through the outlet membrane of the reservoir valve until the ventilation bag is squeezed. During ventilation if the reservoir bag remains flat it indicates that there is no oxygen supplementation.

- *Demand valve:* A demand valve connecting a compressed gas source to the self-expanding bag will consistently provide a high inspired oxygen concentration. A negative pressure in the bag triggers a flow of oxygen, which stops at the preset pressure. If the demand valve gets stuck or the oxygen supply depleted, the bag will not refill.
- *Patient valve (nonrebreathing valve):* It is also known as *direction control valve*. The valve should have a transparent housing which will enable the user to check the valve function during use. The valve ensures that during the inspiratory phase the gas flows from the bag into the patient port only and during expiratory phase the exhaled gases escape from the expiratory port without mixing with the fresh gas stored in the bag.

The inspiratory port is the opening through which gas enters the valve from the bag. Expiratory port is the opening through which exhaled gases pass to the atmosphere. The expiratory port may have a tapered 30 mm connector for attachment of the transfer tube of a scavenging system.

The patient valve has a standard 15 (ID)/22(OD) mm patient end which connects to all standard masks or tube adaptors. The adult masks and the pediatric circular mask size 2, fit outside the patient valve connector.

All other (pediatric) sizes fit inside, to reduce the dead space. During inspiration, as the self-inflating bag is pressed, the valve directs the gas from the bag to the patient. At the same time, expiration port is blocked. When the squeezing of the bag is stopped and the bag is released, the expiration port opens and allows exhalation of the gases to the atmosphere. The valve may have means to prevent air intake so that a spontaneously breathing patient will inhale only from the bag.

A patient who breathes spontaneously can inhale oxygen through the resuscitator with minimal resistance. The capacity of the valve is 5–7 mL.

These bags can deliver a FiO_2 of >0.90 and VT values up to 800 mL when oxygen flows to the bag are 10–15 L/min. Factors that promote the highest FiO_2 level include the use of an oxygen reservoir, connection to an oxygen source, and slow rates of ventilation that allow the bag to refill completely. Positive end-expiratory pressure (PEEP) valves can also be used along.

Q. 19. What are the disadvantages of a manual resuscitator (Fig. 6)?

Ans.

- *High airway pressure:* If excessive force is used to compress the bag in intubated patients.

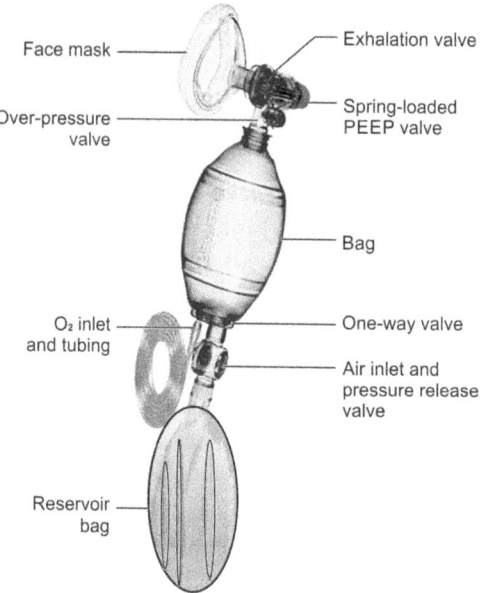

Fig. 6: Typical bag-valve-mask ventilation. (PEEP: positive end-expiratory pressure)

- Barotrauma can occur due to the use of high tidal volume.
- Rebreathing can occur if the nonrebreathing valve is stuck in the inspiratory position or is improperly assembled.
- Low delivered oxygen concentration may occur due to oxygen flow, detached, or defective oxygen tubing or problems with the oxygen enrichment device.

Q. 20. What is high-frequency nasal cannula (Fig. 7)?

Ans. It is a high-flow oxygen delivery device that gives a fixed performance. It can provide humidified gas flows up to 50 L/min while achieving 72–100% FiO_2. These high-frequency nasal cannula (HFNCs) generate mild to moderate levels of continuous positive airway pressure (CPAP) in nasal-breathing and mouth-breathing patients and reduce anatomic dead space by washing out room air from the upper airway. It does not require a face mask, unlike most other high-flow systems, and therefore patients can verbally communicate and eat in a normal manner.

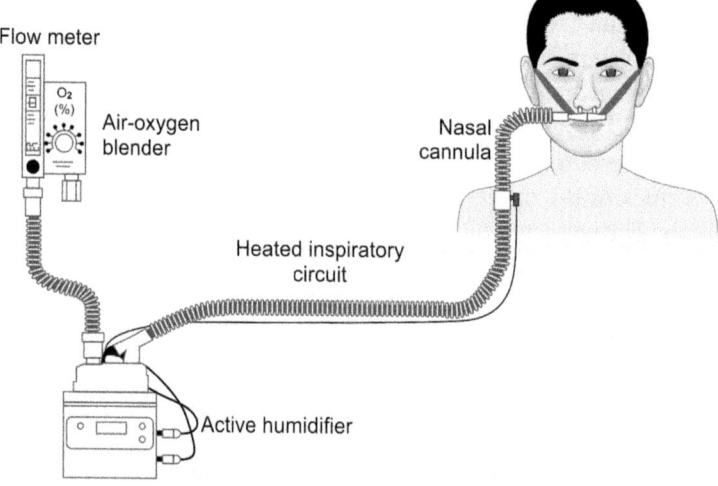

Fig. 7: High-frequency nasal cannula.

The high-flow adult cannula and precision flow appear similar to a regular nasal cannula at the patient interface. The nasal high-flow employs small-diameter corrugated tubing throughout the length of the supply tubing to achieve flow rates up to 50 L/min.

QUESTION

Q. 1. How can HFNC be used through a tracheostomy tube?

FURTHER READING

1. Dorsch JA, Dorsch SE. Understanding Anaesthesia Equipment, 2012.
2. Davey A, Diba A. Ward's Anesthesia Equipment, 6th edition.
3. Kacmarek R, Stoller J, Heuer A. Egan's Fundamentals of Respiratory Care, 12th edition.

CHAPTER 66

Ventilators, Modes of Ventilator, and Ventilator Graphics

Nitin, Akhilesh Gupta

Q. 1. What are the indications for using mechanical ventilation?

Ans. Indications for mechanical ventilation include but are not limited to:
- Apnea or bradypnea with impending respiratory arrest
- Acute lung injury or acute respiratory distress syndrome
- Respiratory muscle fatigue
- Impaired level of consciousness [preferably Glasgow Coma Scale (GCS) ≤8]
- Hemodynamic instability requiring high-dose inotropic support
- Neuromuscular disorders.

Ventilatory support can be either invasive or noninvasive depending on the severity and type of condition.

Q. 2. How to decide between invasive and noninvasive ventilation (NIV) as initial ventilation?

Ans. Noninvasive ventilation is considered as the initial ventilation modality provided to the patient who had patent airway refluxes, hemodynamically stable, proper seal formation (no fascial anomaly), and not at high risk of aspiration (e.g., hemoptysis, hematemesis, vomiting, and intestinal obstruction). It is indicated in conditions of acute hypercapnic respiratory failure [(e.g., acute exacerbation of asthma or chronic obstructive pulmonary disease (COPD)], acute hypoxemic respiratory failure [e.g., acute respiratory distress syndrome (ARDS) and pneumonia] and special conditions like postextubation, weaning, chest trauma, etc., proper monitoring is essential to evaluate the improvement with NIV and prompt decision should be made at the earliest in case NIV fails to achieve the required goals.

Invasive ventilation is advocated in patients with hemodynamic instability on presentation or during NIV ventilation, failed NIV trials, has risk of aspiration and poor neurological status.

Q. 3. Enumerate the difference between bilevel positive airway pressure (BiPAP) and continuous positive airway pressure (CPAP)? What are the advantages and indications of using noninvasive modes of ventilation?

Ans. During CPAP, continuous positive pressure is applied throughout inspiration and expiration in a spontaneously breathing patient. For application of CPAP, patient should have healthy lungs to sustain eucapnic ventilation.

During BiPAP, one can independently regulate the positive pressure during the inspiratory (IPAP) and expiratory (EPAP) phase of respiration. While IPAP improves ventilation, EPAP helps in alveolar recruitment.

Advantages of NIV:
- Cost-effective
- Easy to wean from NIV
- Does not require personnel trained in airway management

- Aids in alveolar recruitment and prevent them from collapsing
- Allows tight control of inspired oxygen concentration and airway pressures
- Better tolerated.

Indications:
- Acute hypoxemic respiratory failure
- Acute hypercapnic respiratory failure
- Special conditions such as obstructive sleep apnea, preoxygenation, postextubation, and chest trauma.

Q. 4. What is the difference between pressure and volume control mode of ventilation?
Ans. Both pressure and volume control modes are defined by the primary mechanism employed for gas delivery during inspiratory phase of respiration.

During pressure control ventilation, the inspiratory pressure assist is set on the ventilator and tidal volume is delivered to achieve the set inspiratory pressure. Factors affecting the impedance and compliance of either lung or chest wall or both will have direct impact on the generated tidal volume. The airway pressure and inspiratory time are prefixed. It is time-triggered, time-cycled, and pressure limited.

Whereas in volume-controlled ventilation, tidal volume is preset, while the inspiratory airway pressure varies with each cycle. It is time-triggered and volume-cycled.

Q. 5. What is volume-targeted assist control (AC) mode of mechanical ventilation. How does this work? How does it differ from synchronized intermittent mandatory ventilation (SIMV) or pressure control (PC)?
Ans. In assist control ventilation, the tidal volume and respiratory rate are decided by the treating physician on the basis of patient profile. The ventilator delivers the set tidal volume at the given respiratory rate per minute. Patient-triggered breaths over and above the set respiratory rate are supported by the ventilator to reach the set tidal volume which is then delivered to the lungs.

In SIMV mode of ventilation, one has to set a target respiratory rate and tidal volume to be delivered at the patient end. The patient-triggered breaths are also delivered over the set respiratory rate but the tidal volume of these patient-triggered breaths depends on the inspiratory effort and the set pressure support in the ventilator. Unlike AC ventilation, the machine does not ensure the same tidal volume as is set for the time-triggered breaths from the ventilator. Synchronized intermittent mandatory ventilation mode is again of two types namely (1) volume targeted and (2) pressure targeted.

In pressure control mode, the peak inspiratory pressure and desired respiratory rate are set on the ventilator. Factors affecting the compliance of the respiratory system will unduly increase the airway pressure there by impairing generation of required tidal volume. The tidal volume received by the patient varies based on the compliance of the respiratory system and the airway resistance.

Q. 6. How does the clinician decide the tidal volume which needs to be set on the ventilator in volume AC mode of ventilation?
Ans. The tidal volume is decided based on the patient's weight. This however is contrary to the fact that size and volume of lung are largely decided by the height. Therefore, the volume and size of the lungs is largely a function of the height of the person. Therefore, the patient's ideal body weight is considered for calculating the tidal volume.

To calculate the ideal body weight in kilograms, one can use the following formulas:

Men: [(Height in inches − 60) × 2.2] + 50
Women: [(Height in inches − 60) × 2.2] + 45

Normal tidal volume is of 8–10 mL/kg of ideal body weight. Choose lower tidal volume of 6–8 mL/kg in COPD or asthma patients to reduce the chances of air trapping and barotrauma. As per ARDS net protocol, tidal volume of 4–6 mL/kg should be used for ventilation.

Q. 7. How is lung-protective mechanical ventilation (LPMV) achieved?

Ans. Lung-protective mechanical ventilation (LPMV) is implemented to decrease the incidence of lung injury following barotrauma or volutrauma. It was initially started for patients who presented with ARDS, but current consensus advocates its us in all patients who are on mechanical ventilation. It should be implemented right from the time of intubation till the time the patient is weaned off from the ventilator.

The key components of LPMV strategy are as follows: (1) a tidal volume of 4–8 mL/kg predicted body weight (PBW), (2) a plateau pressure (P_{Plat}) of <30 cm H_2O, (3) a driving pressure of <15 cm H_2O, (4) an appropriate PEEP level that sustains the lung open at end exhalation, and (5) an FiO_2 that maintains the PaO_2 between 55 and 80 mm Hg or a SpO_2 between 88 and 95%.

Q. 8. What does "static" pressures represent on the ventilator?

Ans. The static or "plateau" pressure is indicative of the total compliance of the respiratory system that includes the lung, chest wall as well as the abdomen). It depicts the pressure required to inflate the lung with each successive inspiration. Any pathology which is likely to affect the compliance of the respiratory system will also have its repercussions on the static pressures.

To observe the static pressures on ventilator, one needs to activate the inspiratory pause and only then can the ventilator run its algorithm and display the static pressure.

Q. 9. What does "peak" pressures represent on the ventilator?

Ans. The peak pressure is indicative of increased resistance anywhere from the ventilator tubings till the segmental bronchi. Factors like mucous plugs, blood clots, bronchospasm, kinking of endotracheal tube, etc. increase the resistance in the pathways with resultant increase in the airway pressures. Peak pressure is displayed with each breath delivered by the ventilator. Certain factors may simultaneously impair the peak and static airway pressures. Also the reason for increased peak airway pressure may be an external factor which has no correlation with the lung compliance.

Q. 10. When do you plan to start weaning in an intubated patient?

Ans. Following prerequisites should be considered before planning weaning in a patient on mechanical ventilation.

To begin with the patient should have fully recovered from the underlying primary etiology or at least a significant improvement should have occurred, responsible for the need for mechanical ventilation. Thereafter, the patient should be able to maintain adequate oxygenation aiding minimal support (e.g., PaO_2 >80 mm Hg on an FiO_2 of 0.5 and PEEP <8.0 cm H_2O).

Lastly, there should not be any acid-balance imbalance requiring high ventilatory support. Patients on high ventilatory support have higher than normal minute ventilation because of which there are very high chances of patient going into muscle fatigue. If higher levels of minute ventilation are required, the ventilatory demands on the patient may be high and they are at risk of tiring if the support is withdrawn. Rapid shallow breathing index (RSBI) is a simple and effective tool which is calculated by dividing the respiratory rate by tidal volume in liters. Rapid shallow breathing index <105 should be considered for weaning.

Q. 11. How do you determine if the patient is ready to be removed from the ventilator support?

Ans. Several different variables under the umbrella of "weaning parameters" should be considered before terminating the ventilatory support of any patient.

Vital capacity was >10 mL/kg is indicative of good respiratory efforts at patient end and the increased likelihood of success weaning off the ventilator. As no single parameter is definitive indicator of success of discontinuation of mechanical ventilation, they are usually supplemented by spontaneous breathing trial (SBT).

During SBT, patient is placed on CPAP, T-piece or a low level of pressure support and is monitored for 30–120 minutes wherein they breathe spontaneously. An arterial blood gas analysis is performed at the end of SBT. During successful SBT, the patient appears comfortable, maintains a good respiratory rate (<25 breaths/minute), sufficient tidal volume is achieved (>5 mL/kg), and maintains stable vital signs including heart rate, blood pressure, and SaO_2. The arterial blood gas should also be within normal and relatively stable oxygenation. Successful SBT lasting for minimum of 30–60 minutes increases the likelihood of successful discontinuation of mechanical ventilation.

FURTHER READING

1. Goligher EC, Ferguson ND, Brochard LJ. Clinical challenges in mechanical ventilation. Lancet. 2016;387:1856-66.
2. Ferrer M, Esquinas A, Arancibia F, Bauer TT, Gonzalez G, Carrillo A, et al. Noninvasive ventilation during persistent weaning failure: a randomized controlled trial. Am J Respir Crit Care Med. 2003;168:70-6.
3. Ferguson ND, Cook DJ, Guyatt GH, Mehta S, Hand L, Austin P, et al. High-frequency oscillation in early acute respiratory distress syndrome. N Engl J Med. 2013;368:795-805.
4. Young D, Lamb SE, Shah S, MacKenzie I, Tunnicliffe W, Lall R, et al. High-frequency oscillation for acute respiratory distress syndrome. N Engl J Med. 2013;368:806-13.
5. Murias G, Lucangelo U, Blanch L. Patient-ventilator asynchrony. Curr Opin Crit Care. 2016;22:53-9.
6. Amato MB, Meade MO, Slutsky AS, Brochard L, Costa EL, Schoenfeld DA, et al. Driving pressure and survival in the acute respiratory distress syndrome. N Engl J Med. 2015;372:747-55.
7. Guérin C, Reignier J, Richard JC, Beuret P, Gacouin A, Boulain T, et al. Prone positioning in severe acute respiratory distress syndrome. N Engl J Med. 2013;368:2159-68.
8. Santiago VR, Rzezinski AF, Nardelli LM, Silva JD, Garcia CS, Maron-Gutierrez T, et al. Recruitment maneuver in experimental acute lung injury: the role of alveolar collapse and edema. Crit Care Med. 2010;38:2207-14.
9. Kallet RH. A comprehensive review of prone position in ARDS. Respir Care. 2015;60:1660-87.
10. Protti A, Cressoni M, Santini A, Langer T, Mietto C, Febres D, et al. Lung stress and strain during mechanical ventilation: any safe threshold? Am J Respir Crit Care Med. 2011;183:1354-62.
11. Graves C, Glass L, Laporta D, Meloche R, Grassino A. Respiratory phase locking during mechanical ventilation in anesthetized human subjects. Am J Physiol. 1986;250: R902-9.

Deep Vein Thrombosis: Mechanical Pump

Devang Bharti, Akhilesh Gupta

Q. 1. What is deep vein thrombosis?
Ans. Deep vein thrombosis (DVT) is defined as a clot formation (thrombosis) within the deep veins of the body, especially of the lower limb or pelvis. It is a fairly common phenomenon with a reported incidence of 100 per 100,000 individuals. At times this thrombus dislodges from these deep veins and embolizes to cause obstruction of the pulmonary artery or its branches, leading to pulmonary embolism (PE), which is a life-threatening condition. Around one-third of all the patients with DVT develop PE.

Q. 2. What is Virchow's triad?
Ans. Rudolf Virchow first described the phenomenon of DVT in 1846. He implicated three factors in the development of DVT— (1) venous stasis, (2) vascular injury, and (3) hypercoagulability, known as *Virchow's triad*. Venous stasis is the most important factor for the development of DVT, but stasis alone seems to be insufficient to cause thrombosis. However, the presence of vascular injury or hypercoagulability greatly increases the likelihood of clot formation.

Q. 3. Describe the pathogenesis of DVT.
Ans. The blood flow is significantly slowed in pockets adjacent to valves in the deep veins of the leg. With this stasis of blood, oxygen concentration declines with a consequent rise in the hematocrit. This leads to downregulation of antithrombotic proteins (such as thrombomodulin, endothelial protein C receptor, etc.) and upregulation of procoagulants (such as P-selectin, etc.) ensuring a hypercoagulable microenvironment. When this hypercoagulable environment gets coupled with vascular injury or hypercoagulability, DVT ensues.

Q. 4. What are the risk factors for the development of DVT?
Ans. The following are the risk factors for DVT:
- Advanced age
- Smoking
- Obesity
- Surgery, especially orthopedic surgery
- Trauma
- Prolonged immobilization
- Past history of a thromboembolic event
- Malignancy
- Pregnancy
- Antiphospholipid antibody syndrome
- Hormonal therapy/oral contraceptive pills
- Varicose vein
- Chronic medical conditions:
  - Cardiac:
    - Hypertension
    - Heart failure
    - Atherosclerosis
    - Dyslipidemia

- Renal:
  - Renal failure
  - Renal transplantation
  - Nephrotic syndrome
  - Microalbuminemia
- Endocrine:
  - Polycystic ovary syndrome
  - Diabetes mellitus
- Respiratory:
  - Asthma
  - Chronic obstructive pulmonary disease (COPD)
- Hematological:
  - Polycythemia vera
  - Paroxysmal nocturnal hemoglobinuria
  - Hyperhomocysteinemia
- Rheumatological:
  - Rheumatoid arthritis
  - Systemic lupus erythematosus (SLE)
  - Behcet's disease
  - Antineutrophil cytoplasmic antibodies (ANCA)-associated with vasculitis
- Inflammatory bowel disease
- Sepsis
- COVID-19
- Tuberculosis.

Q. 5. What are the clinical manifestations of DVT?

Ans. A patient with DVT may present with the following signs and symptoms:
- Pain in the affected limb
- Limb edema
- Tenderness
- Calf pain on dorsiflexion of the foot—Homans sign
- Reddish purple discoloration of the limb
- Cramps
- Paresthesia
- Pruritus
- Venous ulcers.

Q. 6. How will you diagnose DVT?

Ans. If left untreated, DVT may lead to catastrophic complications like PE. Thus, there is a need for prompt diagnosis and treatment. The first step in diagnosing is to assess the risk of development of DVT in a patient. Clinical features related to the disorder should be actively looked for, especially in patients having risk factors for the development of DVT.

- *Wells scoring system (Table 1):* Various scoring systems have been developed for diagnosing DVT. Wells scoring system is one of the most commonly used systems.
  - Wells score >2: High-probability group, likelihoods for developing DVT—53%
  - Wells score = 1–2: Moderate-probability group, likelihoods for developing DVT—17%

TABLE 1: Criteria description of the Wells scoring system.

Wells score criteria description	Points
Active Cancer (treatment within last six months or palliative)	+1 point
Calf swelling ≥3 cm compared to asymptomatic calf (measured 10 cm below tibial tuberosity)	+1 point
Swollen unilateral superficial veins (nonvaricose, in symptomatic leg)	+1 point
Unilateral pitting edema (in symptomatic leg)	+1 point
Previous documented DVT	+1 point
Swelling of entire leg	+1 point
Localized tenderness along the deep venous system	+1 point
Paralysis, paresis, or recent cast immobilization of lower extremities	+1 point
Recently bedridden ≥3 days, or major surgery requiring regional or general anesthetic in the past 12 weeks	+1 point
Alternative diagnosis at least as likely	–2 points

(DVT: deep vein thrombosis)

- Wells score <1: Low-probability group, likelihoods for developing DVT—5%
- *D-dimer assay:* D-dimer is a fibrin degradation product. It has a high sensitivity and low specificity for diagnosing DVT. It is a helpful tool to rule out DVT in the low-risk patients.
- *Coagulation profile:* It is useful to rule out hypercoagulability.
- *Ultrasonography:* Three main modalities are often used—(1) compression ultrasonography, (2) duplex Doppler ultrasonography, and (3) color Doppler ultrasonography.
- *Contrast venography:* Gold standard.
- *Computed tomography (CT) venography.*
- *Magnetic resonance (MR) venography.*

Q. 7. How can DVT be prevented?

Ans. Deep vein thrombosis (DVT) prophylaxis can be prevented in the form of mechanical methods and pharmacological agents:
- Mechanical methods
  - Vena cava filters
  - Graded compression stockings
  - Pneumatic compression devices
  - Venous foot pumps
  - Neuromuscular electrical stimulation
- Pharmacological agents (NOACs)
  - Unfractionated heparin (UFH)
  - Low molecular weight heparin (LMWH)
  - Vitamin K antagonists (warfarin)
  - Factor Xa inhibitors (fondaparinux).

Q. 8. What are pneumatic compression devices? How do they work?

Ans. Pneumatic compression devices are mechanical devices used to improve the venous return from lower extremities and thus, prevent DVT. They employ the use of sleeves or cuffs which are to be worn around the lower limbs. These sleeves are intermittently filled with air at a preselected pressure leading to milking of blood out of the foot and leg. Intermittent release of pressure allows the blood to enter back into these veins. Thus, the overall circulation of blood is improved in these areas relieving the venous stasis and preventing the development of DVT.

A typical pneumatic compression device consists of the following parts **(Fig. 1)**:
- *Pneumatic pump:* It is an electrical pump that inflates the sleeves with compressed air.
- *Air valve:* It ensures the unidirectional flow from the pump to the sleeves.
- *Microcontroller unit (MCU):* It controls the pump. It has a power switch for turning the pump on or off. Additionally, it may also have an interface to control the inflating pressure and duration of the compression cycle.
- *Pipes or tubing:* These pipes connect the pump to the sleeves, allowing the passage of compressed air, and hence, inflation of these sleeves.
- *Sleeve:* It is the garment that is worn over the limb and maybe of a calf or thigh length. It consists of two parts:
  1. *Inflatable bladder:* The air enters this bladder causing it to inflate and exert pressure on the limb.

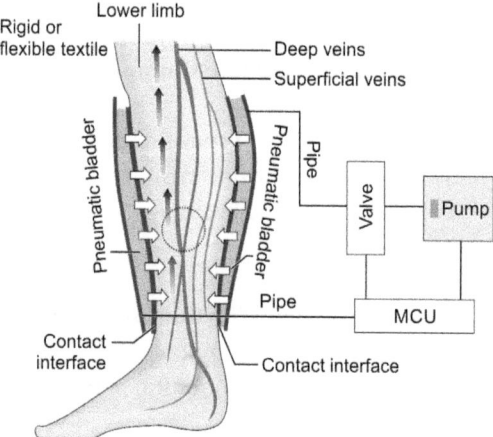

Fig. 1: Parts of a typical pneumatic compression device.
(MCU: microcontroller unit)

2. *Shells:* These are laminated over the inflatable bladder and come in direct contact with the limb. They may be rigid or flexible. These shells transmit the pressure developed in the bladder onto the lower limb.

Intermittent pneumatic compression devices apply a compression pressure of 35–55 mm Hg, and the compression cycles last from 10–35 seconds. The deflation period varies from 20 seconds to one minute, to allow adequate leg refilling. Recently, a device that detects the postcompression refill of the leg veins has been introduced. Its usage increases the total expelled blood volume by 75%.

Q. 9. What are the contraindications to the use of pneumatic compression devices?
Ans. Following are the contraindications of pneumatic compression devices:
- Thrombosis of leg vein
- Fracture of lower limb bones
- IV access (only) on leg
- Severe dermatitis, burns, or any other skin condition of the leg
- Unable to achieve proper fit due to patient size
- Limb ischemia due to PVD.

QUESTION
Q. 1. What is CUS?

FURTHER READING
1. Badireddy M, Mudipalli VR. Deep Venous Thrombosis Prophylaxis. In: StatPearls [Internet]. Treasure Island (FL): StatPearls Publishing; 2022.
2. Caprini JA. Mechanical Methods for thrombosis prophylaxis. Clin Appl Thromb Hemost. 2010;16(6):668-73.
3. Meier KA, Clark E, Tarango C, Chima RS, Shaughnessy E. Venous thromboembolism in hospitalized adolescents: an approach to risk assessment and prophylaxis. Hosp Pediatr. 2015;5(1):44-51.
4. Stone J, Hangge P, Albadawi H, Wallace A, Shamoun F, Knuttien MG, et al. Deep vein thrombosis: pathogenesis, diagnosis, and medical management. Cardiovasc Diagn Ther. 2017;7(Suppl 3): S276-84.
5. Toker S, Hak DJ, Morgan SJ. Deep vein thrombosis prophylaxis in trauma patients. Thrombosis. 2011;505373.
6. Weinberger J, Cipolle M. Mechanical prophylaxis for posttraumatic VTE: stockings and pumps. Curr Trauma Rep. 2016;2: 35-41.
7. Zhao S, Liu R, Fei C, Guan D. Dynamic Interface Pressure Monitoring System for the Morphological Pressure Mapping of Intermittent Pneumatic Compression Therapy. Sensors (Basel). 2019;19(13): 2881.

CHAPTER 68

Jet Ventilation

Akhilesh Gupta, Shubhi Singhal

Q. 1. What is jet ventilation?
Ans. Jet ventilation is characterized by a rapid flow of compressed gases delivered to the patient by a high-pressure jet ventilator through a nozzle. It is a versatile, safe, and effective technique being used for various elective and emergency indications.

Q. 2. What are the various types of jet ventilation?
Ans. There are three types of jet ventilation are as follows:
1. *Low-frequency jet ventilation:* It is also known as normo-frequent jet ventilation. Ventilation is provided using a small tidal volume (1–3 mL/kg) at a frequency of 0.1–0.5 Hz followed by passive expiration. It is usually applied via hand-triggered devices.
2. *High-frequency jet ventilation:* It involves ventilation through a high-pressure jet at a supraphysiological frequency of 1–10 Hz followed by a passive expiration. It is usually administered using specialized equipment.
3. *Superimposed high-frequency jet ventilation:* It is a combination of the above two types in which a continuous high-frequency stream is superimposed over low-frequency jet ventilation.

Q. 3. What is "bulk flow" ventilation?
Ans. *Bulk flow* or *convective ventilation* is responsible for gas exchange during normal or low-frequency jet ventilation. During bulk flow, the tidal volume exceeds the dead space which leads to bulk or mass flow of gases into and out of the lung. The alveolar ventilation, V_A, can be calculated by the following formula:

$$V_A = f \times (V_T - V_D)$$

Where f is the ventilatory rate, V_T is the tidal volume, and V_D is the dead space.

Q. 4. What is the physiology of ventilation during high-frequency jet ventilation?
Ans. High-frequency jet ventilation utilizes tidal volumes which are less than the total dead space (equipment dead space + anatomical dead space). Consequently, bulk flow plays a very limited role in ventilating the alveoli. The following mechanisms ensure adequate ventilation during high-frequency jet ventilation:
- *Pendelluft ventilation/collateral ventilation:* Following inspiration, there is redistribution of inspired gas from full, fast-filling units to slower-filling units, augmenting gas exchange. This redistribution of inspired air occurs because of regional variations in airway resistance and compliance causing some areas of the lung to fill or empty more rapidly than others. Such variation in time constants (resistance-compliance) leads to a phase lag between neighboring lung units and causes gas to flow from one alveolus

to another. This redistribution leads to the augmentation of gas exchange.
- *Taylor dispersion/convective streaming/enhanced molecular diffusion:* It occurs as a result of the asymmetrical velocity profile of the inspired gas front as it moves through the bronchial tree. In laminar flow, molecules in the central zone, having higher velocities, diffuse to lateral zones, with lower velocities. During turbulent flow, as in larger airways, eddy currents produce a similar radial mixing effect.
- *Cardiogenic mixing:* It is the enhancement of gas exchange and diffusion by the mechanical agitation of the lung units lying in close proximity of the beating heart.
- *Bulk flow:* It may partially contribute to gas exchange as the leading stream of high-pressure gas may actually reach alveoli lying in close vicinity.

Q. 5. What are the indications for jet ventilation?

Ans. Indications of jet ventilation:
- Emergency, life-saving measures in "cannot intubate", "cannot ventilate" scenario. Jet ventilation may be applied using a transtracheal cannula in such scenarios
- Partial airway obstruction
- Preemptive use during direct laryngoscopy in anticipated difficult airway cases
- Diagnostic laryngoscopy
- Vocal cord surgeries
- Airway surgeries (carinal resections, resection of tracheal stenosis, tracheal reconstruction, etc.)
- Thoracic surgeries
- To the nondependent lung during one-lung ventilation
- For administering lung-protective ventilation [e.g., in acute respiratory distress syndrome (ARDS)]
- Radiofrequency ablation
- Lithotripsy.

Q. 6. What are the contraindications of Jet ventilation?

Ans. Contraindications to the use of jet ventilation are:
- Significant damage to the cricoid cartilage
- Complete upper airway obstruction
- Airway obstruction below the level of vocal cords which renders exhalation is difficult
- The foreign body which may be distally lodged
- Obesity or poor pulmonary compliance
- Severe tracheal stenosis
- Risk of excessive bleeding during the procedure
- Risk for aspiration.

Q. 7. What are the advantages of jet ventilation (Table 1)?

Ans. Advantages of jet ventilation:
- Reduced peak airway pressure
- Less mucosal trauma (as compared to endotracheal tube insertion)
- Less hemodynamic compromise [compared to intermittent positive-pressure ventilation (IPPV)]
- Cardiac output may be augmented using electrocardiographic (ECG) synchronization
- Reduced antidiuretic hormone (ADH) production and fluid retention
- Minimal surgical field movement
- Improved visibility and surgical access
- Decreased incidence of airway fire during light amplification by the stimulated emission of radiation (LASER) surgery
- It may be used for emergency transtracheal jet ventilation
- Good for low resistance large volume airway leak
- Good for airway surgery.

TABLE 1: Three approaches for jet ventilation along with their advantages and disadvantages.		
Technique	Advantages	Disadvantages
Supraglottic	Tubeless field	• Rapid increase in airway pressure • Reliance on surgeon for adequate ventilation • No PAWP/ETCO$_2$ monitoring • Vocal cord movement • No control of FiO$_2$
Transtracheal	• Tubeless field • Control FiO$_2$	• Incomplete control of ventilation • Contraindicated in tight stenoses • No PAWP/ETCO$_2$ monitoring
Subglottic	• Minimal increase in airway pressure • Control FiO$_2$ • PAWP/ETCO$_2$ monitoring	Catheter in surgical field

(ETCO$_2$: end-tidal carbon dioxide; PAWP: pulmonary arterial wedge pressure)

Q. 8. What are the disadvantages of jet ventilation (Table 1)?

Ans. Disadvantages of Jet ventilation:
- Risk of barotrauma
- No airway protection
- Cooling and drying of inspiratory gases
- Efficacy of gas exchange is less predictable, especial concern in obesity, chronic obstructive pulmonary disease (COPD)
- Delivered FiO$_2$ is multifactorial
- Increase in effective dead space
- Contamination of expired gas flow by surgical debris
- Inhalational anesthesia is often impractical
- Contamination of operating room air
- Continuous end-tidal carbon dioxide (CO$_2$) monitoring is not feasible
- Pressure measurements are unreliable
- High gas flow is required
- There is a need for active humidification
- Requires specialized training and communication.

Q. 9. What complications are associated with the use of Jet ventilation?

Ans. Complications associated with jet ventilation are:
- Barotrauma
  - Pneumothorax
  - Pneumomediastinum
  - Pneumopericardium
  - Pneumoperitoneum
  - Subcutaneous emphysema
- Malposition of catheters
  - Gastric distension
  - Gastric rupture
- Aspiration
- Inadequate ventilation
- Dysrhythmias
- Necrotizing tracheobronchitis
- Increased incidence of necrotizing enterocolitis in neonates
- Inadequate gas exchange (hypoxemia, hypercapnia) in patients with severe lung pathology (predominantly restrictive).

Q. 10. What are the various approaches for Jet ventilation? Enlist their advantages and disadvantages.

Ans. Jet ventilation can be applied using three approaches **(Table 1)**:
1. Supraglottic approach
2. Transtracheal approach
3. Subglottic approach

Q. 11. Describe the equipment used for jet ventilation.

Ans. High-frequency jet ventilators consist of the following components:
- *Ventilator (Fig. 1):* They deliver warm, humidified gases at a frequency of 1–10 Hz.

Chapter 68: Jet Ventilation

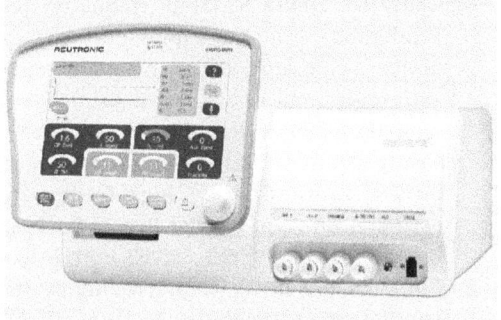

Fig. 1: Ventilator.

The continuous flow of gases is broken into square wave pressures by a high-frequency flow interrupter. This flow interrupter is usually an electrical solenoid valve, but can also be a fluidic or rotating cylinder valve. Pressure, frequency, inspiratory time, and the composition of gases are all adjustable. The ventilator is equipped with alarms and automatic shutdown devices to discontinue as flow in the presence of inadvertent high airway pressures.

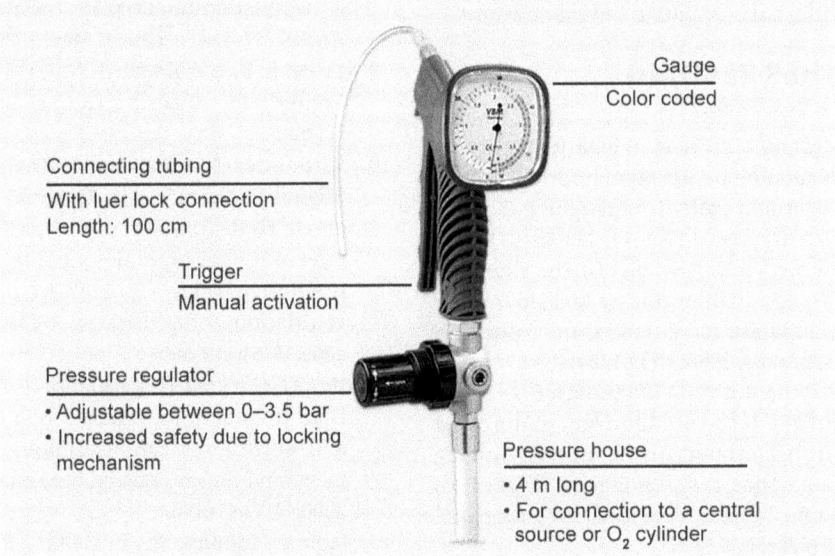

Gauge
Color coded

Connecting tubing
With luer lock connection
Length: 100 cm

Trigger
Manual activation

Pressure regulator
- Adjustable between 0–3.5 bar
- Increased safety due to locking mechanism

Pressure house
- 4 m long
- For connection to a central source or O_2 cylinder

Fig. 2: Hand/manual trigger device.

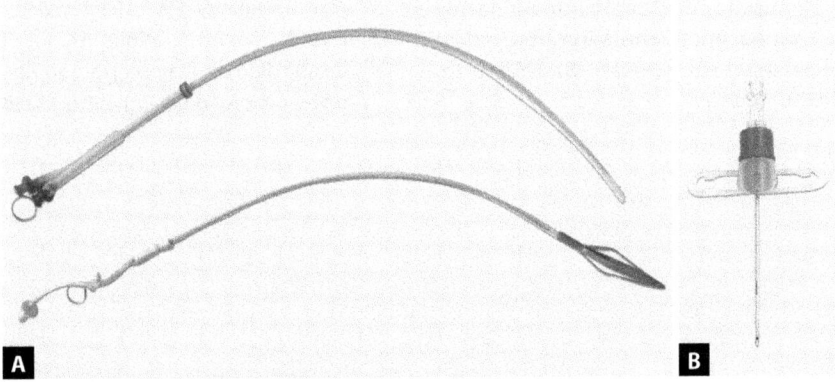

Figs. 3A and B: Catheters.

Various hand-triggered devices are also available for administering low-frequency jet ventilation **(Fig. 2)**.
- *Catheters **(Figs. 3A and B)**:* These can be used alone or through an endotracheal tube and can be placed supra or subglottic. Jet cannulas are also available to be used for transtracheal approach. These catheters may be made up of metal or plastic. They usually have two ports, one for ventilation and other for intratracheal pressure monitoring and/or intermittent end-tidal carbon dioxide measurement.

FURTHER READING

1. Abe K, Oka J, Takahashi H, Funatsu T, Fukuda H, Miyamoto Y. Effect of high-frequency jet ventilation on oxygenation during one-lung ventilation in patients undergoing thoracic aneurysm surgery. J Anesth. 2006;20(1):1-5.
2. Biro P, Eyrich G, Rohling RG. The efficiency of CO_2 elimination during high-frequency jet ventilation for laryngeal microsurgery. Anesth Analg. 1998;87(1):180-4.
3. Biro P, Spahn DR, Pfammatter T. High-frequency jet ventilation for minimizing breathing-related liver motion during percutaneous radiofrequency ablation of multiple hepatic tumours. Br J Anaesth. 2009;102(5):650-3.
4. Brice JW, Davis WB. High-frequency ventilation in the adult. Clin Pulm Med. 2004;11(2):101-6.
5. Buczkowski PW, Fombon FN, Lin ES, Russell WC, Thompson JP. Air entrainment during high-frequency jet ventilation in a model of upper tracheal stenosis. Br J Anaesth. 2007;99(6):891-7.
6. Canty DJ, Dhara SS. High frequency jet ventilation through a supraglottic airway device: a case series of patients undergoing extra-corporeal shock wave lithotripsy. Anaesthesia. 2009;64(12):1295-8.
7. Chang HK. Mechanisms of gas transport during ventilation by high-frequency oscillation. J Appl Physiol Respir Environ Exerc Physiol. 1984;56(3):553-63.
8. Conlon CE. (2012). High Frequency Jet Ventilation—Anaesthesia Tutorial of the Week 271. [online]. Available from: https://resources.wfsahq.org/atotw/high-frequency-jet-ventilation-anaesthesia-tutorial-of-the-week-271/ [Last accessed May, 2022].
9. Evans E, Biro P, Bedforth N. Jet ventilation. Contin Educ Anaesth Crit Care Pain. 2007;7(1):2-5.
10. Fernandez-Bustamante A, Ibañez V, de Miguel E, Germán MJ, Mayo A, Alfaro JJ, et al. High-frequency jet ventilation in interventional bronchoscopy: factors with predictive value on high-frequency jet ventilation complications. J Clin Anesth. 2006;18(5):349-56.
11. Ihra G, Gockner G, Kashanipour A, Aloy A. High-frequency jet ventilation in European and North American institutions: developments and clinical practice. Eur J Anaesthesiol. 2000;17(7):418-30.
12. Jaquet Y, Monnier P, Van Melle G, Ravussin P, Spahn DR, Chollet-Rivier M. Complications of different ventilation strategies in endoscopic laryngeal surgery: a 10-year review. Anesthesiology. 2006;104(1):52-9.
13. Putz L, Mayné A, Dincq AS. Jet ventilation during rigid bronchoscopy in adults: a focused review. Biomed Res Int. 2016;4234861.

CHAPTER 69

Ultrasound Machine

Himanshu Bhasin, Akhilesh Gupta

Q. 1. What is the principle of the generation of ultrasound waves?

Ans. Ultrasound waves are generated when a strong electrical field is applied to an array of *piezoelectric crystals* located on the transducer surface. Piezoelectric crystals start vibrating when an electrical stimulus is applied.

This results in the production of sound waves and is called the *converse piezoelectric effect*.

Each crystal generates an ultrasound wave and the summation of all these waves produces an ultrasound beam.

The waves are generated in an intermittent train called pulses.

Q. 2. What do you understand by the term attenuation coefficient?

Ans.
- As the ultrasound beam travels through different tissue layers, the amplitude of the wave signal reduces, and the depth of penetration increases due to:
  - Absorption (conversion of acoustic energy to heat)
  - Reflection and scattering at interfaces.
- The attenuation caused by each tissue is represented by its attenuation coefficient.
- Tissues like bone have a high attenuation coefficient and severely limit beam transmission.
- Attenuation also varies with the frequency of the ultrasound wave.
- High frequency waves are attenuated to a greater extent and thus have lesser tissue penetration and vice versa.

Q. 3. How do ultrasound waves create images of tissues?

Ans. Ultrasound waves are inaudible sound waves of very high frequency. For ultrasound machines used in clinical practice, emit frequencies in the range of 2–15 MHz. When ultrasound waves contact different tissues, these waves are reflected back to the probe as "echoes" of varying intensities. The intensity of the echo corresponds to the brightness of the image. Bright areas of the image are called *hyperechoic* and dark areas are called *hypoechoic*. Increasing the gain of an image will increase its brightness.

Q. 4. How do liquid, air, and bone appear on ultrasound?

Ans. Liquids do not reflect ultrasound waves so they appear black or anechoic and allow waves to pass to tissues beneath them (so-called "good acoustic windows"). Whereas gas-filled structures block the transmission of ultrasound waves, that is why lung ultrasound is actually based on the interpretation of artifacts. Bones and other calcified structures strongly reflect ultrasound waves, so appear very bright, and cast a dark "acoustic shadow" behind them. Muscles, other soft tissues, and solid organs have moderate brightness.

Q. 5. What are the components of an ultrasound scanner?
Ans.
- *Pulser:* Applies high amplitude voltage to energize crystals
- *Transducer:* Converts mechanical to electrical energy and vice versa
- *Receiver:* Receives and amplifies weak signals
- *Memory:* Stores video display
- *Display:* Displays ultrasound signals in a variety of modes.

Q. 6. What are the different probes available for critical care ultrasonography, and when would you use each probe?
Ans. Ultrasound probes contain piezoelectric crystals that convert electrical energy to sound waves of a particular range of frequencies. In general, higher frequency ultrasound waves produce a greater resolution of tissues but penetrate poorly, while lower frequency waves penetrate deeper structures but give less resolution.
- Phased array probes (also called sector array or "cardiac" probes)—are low-frequency probes (2-4 MHz) that image over a small area and are therefore well suited for imaging between rib spaces in cardiac and thoracic ultrasound.
- Curved array probes (also called a convex array)—are also low-frequency (2-6 MHz) but image over a wider area and are ideal for abdominal or pelvic imaging.
- Linear array probes—these have the highest frequency (7-15 MHz) and offer the highest resolution and are best for vascular imaging and superficial structures.

Q. 7. Describe the imaging modes most commonly available in ultrasound machines.
Ans.
- *A (amplitude) mode:* The transducer sends a single pulse of ultrasound into the medium and waits for the returned signal. The distance between the echoed spikes can be calculated by dividing the speed of the ultrasound in the tissue (1,540 m/s) by half the elapsed time.
- *B (brightness) mode:* Supplies a two-dimensional image. When the wave meets the first wall, a part of the wave is reflected back into the probe. However, this time, instead of a bump, the strength of the returning wave is recorded by a bright dot. The brightness of the dot represents the strength of the returning wave.
- The stronger the strength the brighter the dot. The B scan is the commonest mode of ultrasound used in Anesthesia.
- *Doppler mode:* At a stationary position, the sound frequency is constant. If the sound source moves toward the sound receiver, a higher-pitched sound occurs. If the sound source moves away from the receiver, the received sound has a lower pitch.
- This is known as the Doppler principle and is applied in the use of ultrasound.
- *M (motion) mode:* It is a time-motion display of the ultrasound wave along an ultrasound line.

Q. 8. What do you mean by echogenicity and resolution?
Ans.
- Echogenicity:
  - When an echo returns to the transducer, its amplitude is represented by the degree of brightness of a dot on display (echogenicity)
  - Strong specular reflection produces bright dots (hyperechoic)
  - Weaker diffuse reflections produce gray dots
  - Hypoechoic shadows, e.g., solid organs
  - No reflection produces dark dots (anechoic shadows)

- Nerves exhibit the phenomenon of anisotropy—a phenomenon where the echogenicity of the nerve varies with the angle of insonation.
- *Resolution:* Resolution refers to the ability of an ultrasound machine to distinguish two structures that are close together as separate:
  - *Spatial resolution* determines the degree of image clarity: Spatial resolution is influenced by axial and lateral resolution.
  - *Axial resolution* refers to the ability to distinguish two structures that lie along the axis of the ultrasound beam as separate.
  - *Lateral resolution* refers to the resolution of objects lying side by side, i.e. perpendicular to the beam axis.

Q. 9. What are the uses of ultrasound in anesthesia and intensive care unit (ICU)?

Ans.
- Ultrasound-guided nerve blocks:
  - Regional anesthesia
  - Chronic pain
- Ultrasound guidance for vascular access
- Diagnostic modality:
  - Pleural/pericardial effusion
  - Intra-abdominal hemorrhage
  - Perforated hollow viscus
  - Trauma patients
- Monitoring:
  - Transesophageal echocardiography
  - Cardiac output monitoring
  - Transthoracic echocardiography.

FURTHER READING

1. Khanna P. Ultrasound in Critical Care, 1st edition. 2019.

CHAPTER 70

Rapid Infusion Pumps

Akhilesh Gupta, Jyoti Singh

Q. 1. How will you define shock? What is the cornerstone of the management of shock?

Ans. Shock is defined as the condition of inadequate tissue perfusion caused by impaired cardiac function, vasodilation, and hypovolemia. The body may initially compensate for shock by various mechanisms maintaining normal blood pressure but the development of hypotension demonstrates a decompensated state which is associated with increased morbidity and mortality. Rapid intravenous infusion of blood products and fluid is needed in such circumstances to improve cardiac function, correct hypotension, restore circulating intravascular volume, correct organ perfusion, and to reverse shock. Early fluid therapy and hemodynamics optimization have been shown to improve the outcome in shock patients. The Frank-Starling curve helps us to explain the basis of fluid resuscitation during the early phases of shock since many of the patients are in the preload-dependent area of the curve. Various techniques and devices have been recommended for the rapid administration of fluid.

Q. 2. Mention various methods of rapid fluid infusion.

Ans. Various methods are as follows:
- *Infusion pumps*—they are generally used in an acute care setting. They can provide a maximum flow rate of 1,000 mL/h, which is considered insignificant for rapid correction of acute hypotension during the initial stages of resuscitation.
- *Gravity*—gravity infusion is commonly used for fluid resuscitation, but in this method, it must be recognized that fluid flow is highly dependent upon luminal diameter, tubing length, and the position of the patient's extremity. According to Poiseuille's law, the fluid flow rate will be greater in large-bore catheters with a shorter length. Gravity-dependent flow through the standard intravenous catheter will be very slow for conditions requiring fast intravenous fluid resuscitation.
- *Pressure infusion*—hanging a pressure cuff around the bottle of intravenous fluid or blood products helps in increasing the infusion speed. But this method does not attain a high infusion speed and requires the cuff to be continuously reinflated for maintaining the flow.
- *Manual syringe infusion*—they work on the principle of "push-pull" for rapid fluid infusion. They are generally used in pediatric patients and in urgent situations when large-bore intravenous access and rapid infusers are not available. There are certain demerits of this method such as two-handed operation, user fatigue, distraction, accidentally withdrawing blood from the patients, and risk of infection.

- Rapid infusers—they are considered as the fastest method of intravenous fluid delivery and they can achieve a rate up to 1 L/min.

Q. 3. Describe various types of rapid fluid infusers.

Ans.
- *Rapid infusion system (RIS):* It was developed in the 1980s for use in liver transplantation surgery. It was able to deliver intravenous fluid at rates up to 1,200 mL/min, with the help of a roller pump that has an inbuilt safety mechanism for detecting air and rise in infusion pressure. But the subsequent data showed that patients treated with RIS received excessive intravenous fluid which resulted in electrolyte and pH imbalance, coagulopathy, and third space fluid accumulation. Therefore, new rapid infusion devices with better safety features have been developed and are now commercially available.
- *Level 1 H-1,200:* It pressurizes the chamber around the fluid reservoir to push it rapidly. It warms the intravenous fluid by a countercurrent mechanism in which warm water circulates around the infusion tubing. It limits infusion pressure to approximately 300 mm Hg. It reduces the flow or even stops it when the resistance in the tubing causes pressure to rise above the set level.
- *Belmont rapid infuser (RI-2)*—this rapid infuser uses a roller pump mechanism similar to RIS to achieve faster flow. It warms the fluid or blood by passing it through heating elements. It also limits infusion pressure to approximately 300 mm Hg and same as level 1 H-1200 slowing or stopping the flow if the resistance causes pressure to rise above this level.
- *Thermacor 1,200*—also uses the roller pump mechanism to achieve faster flow. It uses a highly efficient conduction temperature-controlled heating mechanism for warming intravenous fluid flowing through it. The limit of infusion pressure is the same as the two above-mentioned infuser pumps. It comes with a ShurGard Vortex air trapping system which captures air in the circuit even when the pump is working at a maximum rate. It can also be used in the pediatric population as it is designed to have options for slower flow rates, lower fluid pressure, and small bolus volume.
- *LifeFlow rapid infuser*—it is a single-use and hand-operated device which allows healthcare professionals to administer recommended fluid bolus quickly and efficiently. It has a 10 mL syringe that automatically recoils and fills. It is compatible with cannulas of varying sizes. It can infuse fluid and blood products at a rate up to 250 mL/min.

Q. 4. What are the complications related to rapid infusion and devices of rapid infusion?

Ans.
- *Complications related to rapid infusion with rapid infusers:*
  - Air embolism
  - Hypervolemia or over transfusion
  - Overheating of fluids
  - Hypothermia
  - Hemolysis
  - Complications due to rapid blood transfusions such as hyperkalemia, hypocalcemia, transfusion-related reactions, and transfusion-related acute lung injury (TRALI)
  - Electrical shock.

- *Complications related to the device:*
  - High cost
  - Complexity—size, weight, and need for electricity which make these devices difficult to use during pre-hospital and in-hospital transport.
  - Frequent staff training—in operation theaters and emergency places frequent staff training is required.

FURTHER READING

1. ScienceDirect. (2019). Rapid Infusion System. [online] Available from: https://www.sciencedirect.com/topics/nursing-and-health-professions/rapid-infusion-system [Last accessed May, 2022].
2. Piehl MD, Park CW. When minutes matter: rapid infusion in emergency care. Curr Emerg Hosp Med Rep. 2021;9(4):116-25. (2021).

CHAPTER 71

Automated Chest Compressor Machine

Jyoti Singh, Akhilesh Gupta

Q. 1. What do you understand about cardiopulmonary resuscitation (CPR) and what is the mechanism by which it helps in saving a life?

Ans. Cardiopulmonary resuscitation (CPR) is an emergency lifesaving procedure. The procedure consists of chest compressions often combined with artificial ventilation in an effort to manually preserve circulation of blood to keep brain and heart function intact until further means are taken to restore spontaneous blood circulation and breathing.

Kouwenhoven et al., suggested that during CPR, the heart is compressed between the sternum and spine, resulting in increased intraventricular pressure, closing of the atrioventricular valves, and ejection of blood into the lungs and aorta. During the relaxation phase, negative intrathoracic pressure caused by expansion of the thoracic cage facilitates blood return, and aortic pressure results in aortic valve closure and coronary perfusion. This has come to be known as the cardiac pump theory of blood flow during CPR. Echocardiography supports this theory that shows a reduction in ventricular size and mitral valve closure with chest compression during the early stage of CPR.

The objective of CPR is to delay tissue death and extend the brief window of opportunity for successful resuscitation without permanent brain damage.

Q. 2. Give a brief history of CPR and the automatic CPR machine.

Ans. In 1891 first case of closed cardiac massage by Dr Friedrich Maass was reported in Germany. In 1901 first open cardiac massage was performed until 1957 it was continued till Dr James Jude and electrical engineers William Kouwenhoven introduced closed cardiac massage.

In the 1960s first mechanical CPR device was introduced which used a piston-based mechanism, also known as a *thumper*. The compressions were powered by electricity or compressed gas, while compression rate and depth were controlled electronically.

Q. 3. What is an automatic CPR machine? Mention the method of use and parts of the automated CPR machine.

Ans. For successful cardiopulmonary resuscitation, we need perfect uninterrupted chest compressions, interruption degrades the chance of a successful outcome of the patient. An automated CPR machine is designed for resuscitation, which provides quality CPR chest compression automatically without interruption

Automatic CPR machines perform effective, customized, hands-free CPR. They allow medical professionals to concentrate on other life-saving procedures and provide improved access to the patient.

The AutoPulse is an automated, portable, battery-powered cardiopulmonary resuscitation device. It is a chest compression device composed of a constricting band (**Fig. 1**) or a motorized piston (**Fig. 2**) and a half backboard that is intended to be used as an adjunct to CPR during advanced cardiac life support by professionals health care providers. Some automated CPR machines also have in-built ventilators. The compression band compresses the heart as well as the rest of the thorax, while the motorized piston puts the load directly on the heart, sparing the rest of the thorax.

The patient's head, shoulder, and upper back should lie flat upon the base unit, with the controls for the AutoPulse beside the patient's left ear. The base unit can be augmented for cervical spine support. The unit contains the control computer, the rechargeable battery, and the motors that operate the LifeBand. The LifeBand is an adjustable strap that covers the entire rib cage. When the patient is strapped in and the start button is pressed, the LifeBand pulls tight around the chest, and proceeds to rhythmically constrict the entire rib cage, pumping the heart. The LifeBand can be placed over defibrillator pads. The LifeBand is disposable and designed for single use only for sanitary reasons.

The AutoPulse measures chest size and resistance before it delivers the unique combination of thoracic and cardiac chest compressions. The compression depth and force vary per patient. It runs in a 30:2, 15:2 or continuous compression mode which is user selectable.

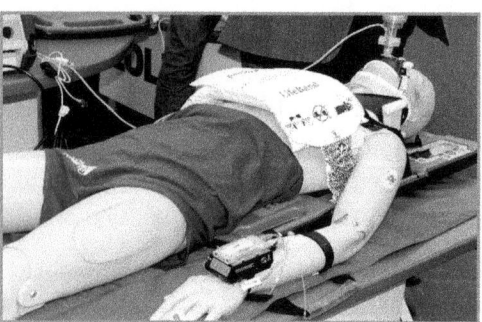

Fig. 1: AutoPulse.

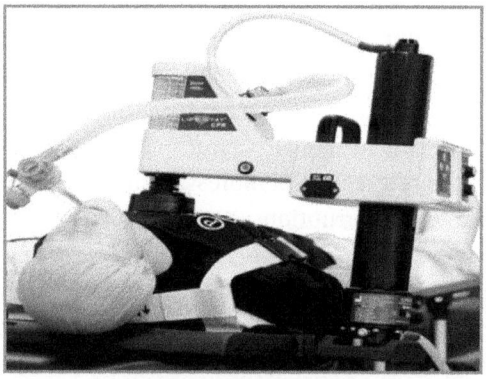

Fig. 2: Motorized piston.

Q. 4. What are the benefits of an automated CPR machine over manual CPR?
Ans.
- *Uninterrupted CPR that does not quit:* Automated CPR machine never quits, and provides perfect uninterrupted CPR for as long as needed. Interruption of CPR degrades the chances of successful defibrillation.
- *Increased patient access:* No need to work around people providing chest compression (and breaths). If necessary, mechanical CPR can be paused and resumed with the push of a button, maintaining nearly complete access to the patient throughout the resuscitation effort.
- *Reduces the risk to the patient and the caregivers:* Rescuers must pause compression so that they themselves do not get defibrillated. Rescuer fatigue degrades the quality of CPR over time. Automated CPR machines outsource the task of CPR to the machine which suffers neither fatigue nor electrical shock.

- *Make CPR during transport possible:* High quality cardiac compression in transport is extremely difficult, but automated CPR device can be securely applied to the patient throughout transportation, avoiding any interruption in life-saving CPR.
- *Saves manpower:* Frees up the staff for other vital tasks, such as administration of medicines.
- Lightweight and easy to use.

Q. 5. Mention disadvantages of automated CPR machine over manual CPR.
Ans.
- The device takes time to set up.
- An incorrectly aligned device might actually perform poorer compression than a rescuer because a rescuer corrects their own position.
- There may be higher chances of rib fractures with a machine, apart from other injuries, such as liver, lung, spleen, stomach lacerations, and mediastinal or aortic trauma.

Q. 6. What are some recommendations for use of an automated CPR machine?
Ans.
- Where CPR will be prolonged, and consistent quality will be required.
  - Cardiac arrest due to hypothermia
  - Cardiac arrest following thrombolysis for pulmonary embolism (PE) or myocardial infarction (MI)
- Use where rescuers are few or untrained
  - Prehospital setting
  - Rural and regional setting

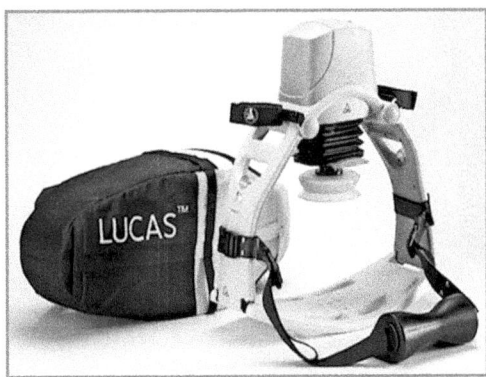

Fig. 3: Lund University Cardiopulmonary Assist System (LUCAS) CPR device.

- Where space is limited
  - Aeromedical retrieval
  - Ambulance transport
  - Interventional radiology suite.

Q. 7. Mention different medical brands of automated CPR machine.
Ans.
- Wellife automated CPR machine
- Defibtech emergency medical services (EMS) chest compressor machine, Lifeline ARM Automated Chest Compression (ACC)
- Electromedics LUCAS chest compression system
- Electromedics LUCAS CPR device **(Fig. 3)**
- Zoll AutoPulse CPR Device
- Schiller mechanical chest compression CPR device.

FURTHER READING

1. LUCAS CPR device.
2. Zoll catalogue (auto CPR).

CHAPTER 72

Extracorporeal Membrane Oxygenation

Devang Bharti, Akhilesh Gupta

Q. 1. What is extracorporeal membrane oxygenation?

Ans. Extracorporeal membrane oxygenation (ECMO) or extracorporeal life support is a technique based on cardiopulmonary bypass which provides prolonged cardiac and respiratory support to the patients with cardiorespiratory failure refractory to the conventional treatment. It allows gas exchange and pumping of the blood to be done outside of the human body. It is a supportive therapy used to buy time for the treatment of underlying pathology.

Q. 2. What are the indications for the use of ECMO?

Ans. Indications of ECMO:
- Indications for cardiac support:
  - Cardiogenic shock:
    - Acute coronary syndrome (ACS)
    - Severe intractable cardiac arrhythmias with hemodynamic instability, refractory to other treatment modalities
    - Drug toxicity causing myocardial depression
    - Anaphylaxis
    - Cardiac trauma
    - Sepsis with severe myocardial depression
    - Pulmonary embolism
    - Acute myocarditis
  - Failure of weaning after cardiopulmonary bypass
  - Chronic cardiomyopathy
  - Severe pulmonary hypertension (after pulmonary endarterectomy)
  - Graft failure after cardiac or cardiopulmonary transplantation
  - As a bridge to cardiac or cardiopulmonary transplantation
  - Postcardiac arrest—as a part of advanced life support
  - Local anesthetic toxicity
- Indications for respiratory support:
  - Acute respiratory distress syndrome (ARDS):
    - Infective pneumonia
    - Aspiration pneumonitis
    - Alveolar proteinosis
  - Status asthmaticus
  - Massive pulmonary hemorrhage
  - Airway obstruction
  - Pulmonary contusion
  - Severe inhalational injury
  - Graft failure after pulmonary transplantation
  - Bridge to pulmonary transplantation
  - Congenital diaphragmatic hernia (CDH)
  - Meconium aspiration syndrome.

Q. 3. What are the contraindications to ECMO?

Ans. The following are contraindications to ECMO:
- Disseminated malignancy
- Brain death

- Unrecoverable heart in a patient who is not a candidate for cardiac transplantation
- Unwitnessed cardiac arrest
- Prolonged cardiopulmonary resuscitation (CPR) with poor tissue perfusion
- Unrepaired aortic dissection
- Severe aortic regurgitation
- Emphysema
- Cirrhosis
- Chronic renal failure (CRF)
- Advanced age
- Peripheral vascular disease
- Contraindication for anticoagulation (relative contraindication).

Q. 4. What complications are associated with the use of ECMO?

Ans. Complications associated with ECMO are:
- Hemorrhage
  - At the cannulation site
  - At surgical site
  - Intracerebral
  - Pulmonary
- Decannulation
- Dissection
- Thromboembolism
- Heparin-induced thrombocytopenia
- Infection/sepsis
- Hypovolemia
- Capillary leak syndrome
- Air embolism
- Hypertension
- Arrhythmia
- Oliguria
- Electrolyte disturbances
- Hemolysis
- Coronary/cerebral hypoxia
- Pump failure
- Failure of gas exchange
- Coagulopathy.

Q. 5. What are the different techniques of ECMO?

Ans. Extracorporeal membrane oxygenation (ECMO) may be set up using three different techniques:
1. *Venoarterial ECMO (VA-ECMO):* Blood is pumped from the venous to arterial circuit while allowing gas exchange and hemodynamic support.
2. *Venovenous ECMO (VV-ECMO):* Blood is taken from and returned to the venous circuit after facilitating gas exchange. Hemodynamic support is not provided.
3. *Arteriovenous ECMO (AV-ECMO):* Facilitates gas exchange by using patient's own arterial pressure to pump the blood from the arterial to venous circuit.

Q. 6. Describe venoarterial ECMO.

Ans. In venoarterial ECMO (VA-ECMO) blood is drained from the venous circulation and returned back to the arterial circulation. It facilitates both, gas exchange, as well as hemodynamic support and is used in patients with compromised cardiac and respiratory functions. Blood is commonly drained from inferior vena cava (IVC) or right atrium (RA). This is achieved centrally by sternotomy or peripherally via an internal jugular vein (IJV) or femoral vein. Blood is returned either centrally to ascending aorta or peripherally to femoral artery. VA-ECMO decreases the cardiac workload and consequently, the myocardial oxygen demand. It ensures adequate systemic tissue perfusion with oxygenated blood.

Q. 7. What is venovenous ECMO?

Ans. Venovenous (VV) ECMO is employed for improving gas exchange in patients with preserved cardiac function. Blood is taken from and returned back to large veins like femoral vein or jugular vein (or both). A dual-chamber cannula may also be used which allows drainage from inferior and superior vena cava and return to the right atrium.

Q. 8. What is an atrioventricular pump-less assist device?

Ans. Atrioventricular (AV) pump-less assist device is another name for AV-ECMO. It involves a membrane oxygenator device integrated into a pump-less arteriovenous circuit, usually established by cannulating the femoral artery and vein. This device is mainly utilized for removing CO_2 from the blood in patients with good cardiac pump function.

Q. 9. What are the various components of an ECMO circuit?

Ans. A typical ECMO circuit consists of the following components **(Fig. 1)**:

- *Pump:* It drives the blood through a membrane oxygenator. Different types of pumps in use are roller, centrifugal, etc.
- *Membrane oxygenator:* It is also known as membrane lung/artificial lung. They allow a gaseous exchange to take place. Their surface area may vary from 0.4 to 4.5 m^2. Various types of membrane oxygenators are available for use:
  - *Microporous hollow-fiber oxygenators:* They are highly efficient at the gas exchange, offer low resistance to blood flow, and are easy to prime. But their use is associated with multiple complications such as plasma wetting, decreased gas exchange, unpredictable performance, etc.
  - *Microporous hollow-fiber membranes coated with thin siloxane layers:* Decreased incidence of plasma wetting and increased bioavailability.
  - *Spiral wound silicone-membrane oxygenator:* They are commonly used nowadays.
- *Heat exchanger:* It can either be separate or integrated with the membrane oxygenator. It consists of a warm water

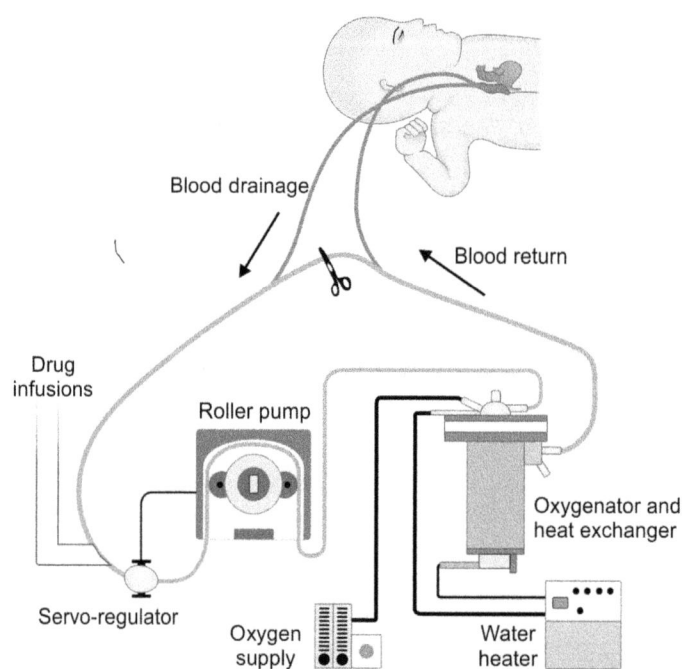

Fig. 1: Extracorporeal membrane oxygenation (ECMO) circuit with components.

bath (42°C) which warms the blood by counter-current mechanism before it renters the body. It also acts as the last port to catch any bubbles which may have inadvertently formed in the blood.
- *Bladder:* A silastic bladder with a capacity of around 35 mL is placed at the lowest point on the venous side. This bladder is kept in a bladder box with a feedback switch that turns off the pump in case the bladder collapses from impaired return or hypovolemia.
- *Bridge:* It is a direct connection between afferent drainage and an efferent oxygenated circuit. It acts as a bypass in case a patient requires isolation from the circuit.
- Polyvinyl chloride (PVC) connector tubing.

FURTHER READING

1. Chauhan S, Subin S. Extracorporeal membrane oxygenation–an anaesthesiologist's perspective–Part II: clinical and technical consideration. Ann Card Anaesth. 2012;15(1):69-82.
2. Martinez G, Vuylsteke A. Extracorporeal membrane oxygenation in adults. Contin Educ Anaesth Crit Care Pain. 2012;12(2):57-61.
3. Shekar K, Mullany DV, Thomson B, Ziegenfuss M, Platts DG, Fraser JF. Extracorporeal life support devices and strategies for management of acute cardiorespiratory failure in adult patients: a comprehensive review. Crit Care. 2014;18(3):219.
4. Shimamoto A, Kanemitsu S, Fujinaga K, Takao M, Onoda K, Shimono T, et al. Biocompatibility of silicone-coated oxygenator in cardiopulmonary bypass. Ann Thorac Surg. 2000;69:115-20.
5. Watanabe H, Hayashi J, Ohzeki H, Moro H, Sugawara M, Eguchi S. Biocompatibility of a silicone-coated polypropylene hollow fiber oxygenator in an in vitro model. Ann Thorac Surg. 2000;69(1):115-20.

CHAPTER 73

Renal Replacement Therapy

Gourav Mittal

INTRODUCTION

Renal replacement therapy is one of the most frequently utilized modalities among critically ill patients, as acute kidney injury (AKI) remains the most common complication among these patients. The scope of this modality is now growing beyond replacement as a supportive therapy. However, one can administer this modality in different ways but hemodialysis either intermittent or continuous is the most common type.

For AKI, hemodialysis prescription and way of administration are different than that of chronic kidney disease (CKD) patients. Following are a few concerns that explain why this is different:

- AKI in intensive care unit (ICU), diagnosed with formulas that are being used for CKD, stable clearance is the prerequisite for using these formulas. In an acute care setting, clearance often fluctuates and is further complicated by different drugs used for patient care management.
- Hemodynamics, often sick patients requiring vasopressor support put a check on using intermittent hemodialysis.
- Vascular access is easy to find in CKD patient, whereas AKI vascular access and flow rate often limit the efficiency of hemodialysis.

Various indications of dialysis are depicted in **Flowchart 1**.

Various types of renal replacement therapies are given in **Figure 1**.

Various sub-techniques of hemodialysis are given in **Table 1**.

Before we proceed to more technicality, we first understand two basic process which any of above technique uses:
1. Convection—hemofiltration/ultrafiltration (UF)
2. Diffusion

Convection: Process that occurs due to pressure gradient irrespective of solute gradient (water and solvent drag). Ultrafiltrate comes out having same composition as of plasma, therefore concentration of solute will not change much. If we replace ultrafiltrate fluid with fluid, then it will dilute the plasma concentration of solutes known as hemofiltration **(Fig. 2)**.

Diffusion: Solute moves from area of high concentration to lower one through the semipermeable membrane.

Molecular weight of solute determines which process will clear them out effectively **(Table 2)**.

OTHER IMPORTANT COMPONENTS OF DIALYSIS SETUP

- *Anticoagulation:* Often required to prevent clotting inside the circuit and helps in prolonging the life of the filter.
  - Heparin

Chapter 73: Renal Replacement Therapy

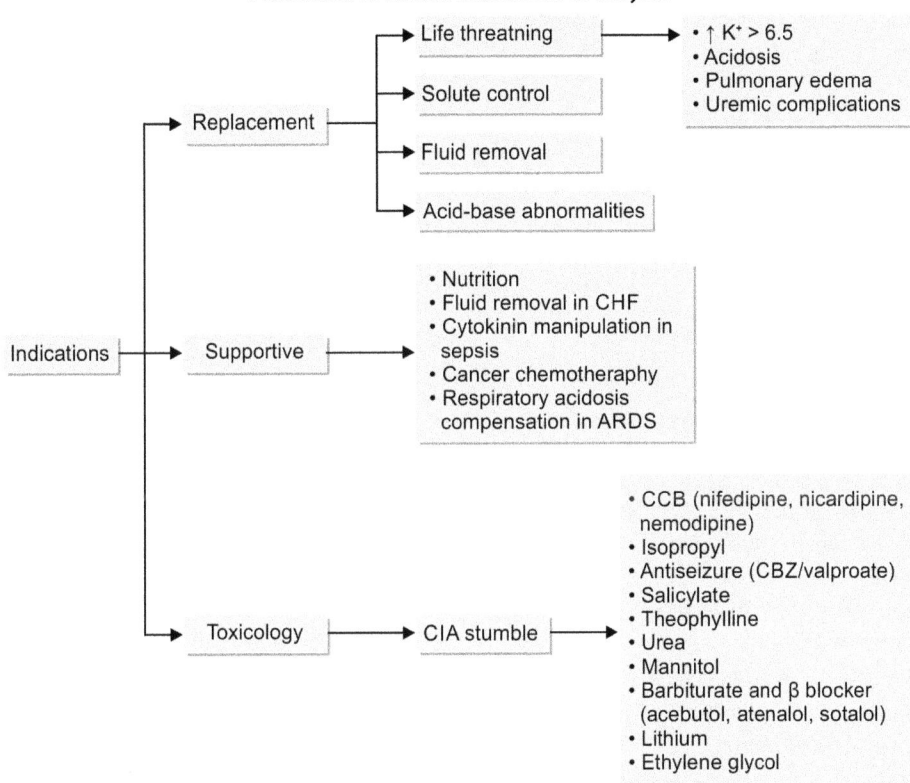

Flowchart 1: Various indications of dialysis.

(ARDS: acute respiratory distress syndrome; CBZ: carbamazepine; CCB: calcium channel blocker: CHF: congestive heart failure)

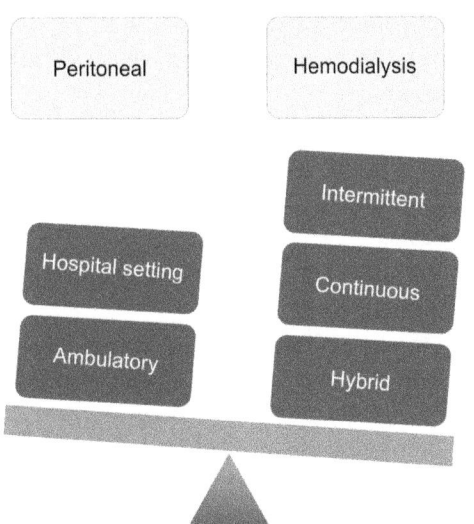

Fig. 1: Different types of hemodialysis modalities.

TABLE 1: Various sub-techniques of hemodialysis.

Intermittent	Continous	Hybrid
IHD	• CVVH • CVVHD • CVVHDF • SCUF • CAVHD	• Sustained low efficiency dialysis (SLED) aka PIRRT • SLEDD-F (diafilteration) • SCD • AVVH (accelerated venovenous hemofilteration)

(CAVHD: continuous arteriovenous hemodialysis; CVVH: continuous venovenous hemofiltration; CVVHD: continuous venovenous hemodialysis; CVVHDF: continuous venovenous hemodiafiltration; IHD: intermittent hemodialysis; PIRRT: prolonged intermittent renal replacement therapy; SCD: slow continuous dialysis; SCUF: slow continuous ultrafiltration)

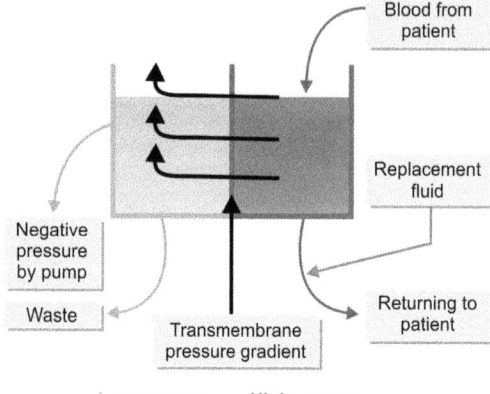

Fig. 2: Process of convection and hemofiltration.

TABLE 2: Molecular size and weight.	
Small <500 Dalton: Urea, amino acid, and creatinine	C = D
Medium 500–5,000 D B12 inulin, and vancomycin	C > D
Large molecule 5,000–50,000 D macroglobulin and cytokines	C/adsorption
Large protein >500,000 D albumin	Minimal

- Low molecular weight heparin (LMWH)
- Citrate
- Hirudin.

Anticoagulant, which can be given regionally, i.e., give prefilter and neutralize postfilter is often selected to prevent systemic side effects of anticoagulation and preserving filter life.

Citrate is the most commonly employed regional anticoagulation. Please note that citrate gets metabolized in the liver so in patients with the altered liver function, it should be used cautiously.
- Membrane of filter
  - Cellulose
  - Substituted cellulose
  - Cellulosynthetic
  - Synthetic—often biocompatible.

- Dialysis fluid:
  - *Bicarbonate:* Though more physiological but it requires fresh preparation making it a little difficult to use practically.
  - *Acetate:* Often leads to respiratory and vascular compromise, vasodilation, and increased oxygen demand.
  - *Citrate:* Add-on benefit of anticoagulation, but citrate toxicity is the main concern.
  - *Lactate:* Confounding in case of sepsis, not for liver failure or patients with lactic acidosis.

Hemodynamics often possess a greater challenge to intensivists as an indication of dialysis governs how fast one needs to get rid of the primary concern while hemodynamics directs the feasibility of the technique.

Table 3 provides some information for the same.

After knowing basic about various modalities, now a little bit about physics involved.

Filtration fraction = Ultrafiltrate rate/plasma flow rate = Unfractionated heparin (UFH)/Blood flow (1-hct).

Why do we need to know about filtration fraction?

The most important component of dialysis is the filter, to preserve its efficacy and prolong its life filtration, fraction should be <20%.

Various ways by which one can reduce filtration fraction:

Decrease ultrafiltrate rate	Often reduces efficacy if one does
Increasing blood flow rate	Does not want to compromise
Prefilter replacement fluid	Add diffusion

How to prescribe intermittent hemodialysis (IHD)/continuous renal replacement therapy (CRRT)?

Before writing a prescription, some principles and terminologies intensivists should know which govern solute removal.

Solute removal largely depends upon dialyzer perspective, patient perspective, and access recirculation.

TABLE 3: Preferable modality according to indication along with hemodynamic status

Goal	Hemodynamic	Preferred
Fluid removal	Stable Unstable	Intermittent SCUF
Urea clearance	Stable Unstable	IHD CRRT
Severe hyperkalemia	Stable Unstable	IHD IHD
Severe metabolic acidosis	Stable Unstable	IHD CRRT
Severe hyperphos-phatemia	Stable Unstable	CRRT CRRT
Brain edema	Stable/unstable	CRRT

(CRRT: continuous renal replacement therapy; IHD: intermittent hemodialysis; SCUF: slow continuous ultrafiltration)

- Dialyzer perspective:
  - Extraction ratio
  - Clearance

Extraction ratio:
= Inlet − Outlet/Inlet

Depending on the blood flow rate (Qb), the higher it is, the lower will be extraction ratio. Usually targets to achieve 60%.

Clearance:
= Extraction ratio × Blood flow rate

Largely depends upon blood flow rate and mass transfer area coefficient (K_0A).

Blood flow:
Although a low blood flow rate increases the extraction ratio, but it paradoxically slows down the clearance. Urea production is continuous while dialysis removes it from the body, therefore, slowing the rate more urea will be added to blood than its clearance. We need to have an adequate blood flow rate that gives us optimal clearance rather than the highest extraction ratio.

K_0A:

Composed of two components: Coefficient of dialyzer membrane for the given solute (K_0), the total effective surface area of membrane (A).

TABLE 4: Efficacy of various modalities for control of fluid/solute.

Techniques	Use in unstable	Solute	Fluid removal	Anticoagulant need
PD	Yes	++	++	No
IHD	Possible	++++	+++	Y/N
IHF	Possible	+++	+++	Y/N
Hybrid	Possible	++++	++++	Y/N
CVVH	Yes	+++/++++	++++	Y/N
CVVHD	Yes	+++/++++	++++	Y/N
CVVHDF	Yes	++++	++++	Y/N

(CVVH: continuous venovenous hemofiltration; CVVHD: continuous venovenous hemodialysis; CVVHDF: continuous venovenous hemodiafiltration; IHD: intermittent hemodialysis; IHF: intermittent hemofiltration; PD: peritoneal dialysis)

If we fix the extraction ratio, theoretically increasing the blood flow rate should increase the clearance in the same proportion according to the above formula. But it reaches a plateau, as it also depends upon the specific capacity of the membrane.

Nomogram predicts the clearance according to blood flow rate and K_0A of the membrane **(Fig. 3)**.

Most commonly we use membranes with K0A 800–1,200. We can see above 400–450 mL/min clearance become plateau and also at lower blood flow rates <200 mL/min, clearance remains the same irrespective of membrane used.

Now we calculate the solute clearance rate:

Clearance × concentration (inlet concentration)

This solute clearance rate will be affected by:
- Red blood cell (RBC) effect
- Body water effect
- Dialysate flow rate
- Molecular weight of solute in concern.

Red blood cell effect: The more is the RBC mass, the less will be the hematocrit. As far as urea is concerned, it is equally distributed among plasma and hematocrit but as creatinine/PO_4 is not readily distributed there, use plasma flow rate for these molecules.

Body water effect: About 93% of plasma and 72% of RBC are water. For urea, it is ok to use blood flow rate but for creatinine, use plasma flow rate to calculate clearance. The more is the hematocrit, the less will be the clearance at a given blood flow rate.

Dialysate flow rate: For IHD, as we need adequate clearance in a shorter period and also want to be efficient enough to sustain its effect for 48 hours. We afford wastage of dialysate (less extraction ratio) therefore for IHD dialysate, flow rate must be 2–3 × the blood flow rate.

For CRRT, as it is a continuous process, we want maximum efficiency with minimum wastage of resources. In CRRT, we keep the dialysate flow rate 1/5th of the blood flow rate.

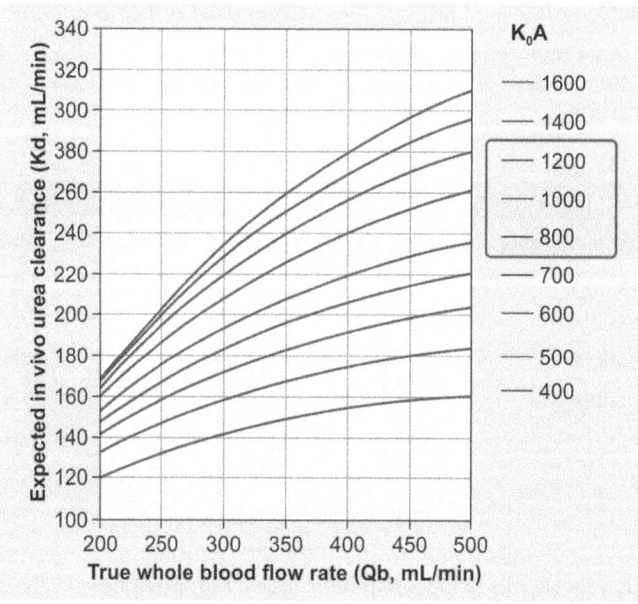

Fig. 3: Expected clearance based on filter property (K_0A) and blood flow rate.

Molecular weight: Large molecule clearance depends on membrane pore size rather than the flow rate of plasma or dialysate. Flux is used to define clearance for large molecules [K (UF)]. It is a property of membrane, a membrane with low K_0A can have high flux.

Patient perspective:
- Weekly serum nitrogen profiling
- Urea removal indices
- Urea inbound/rebound

Urea is continuously produced, so alone urea concentration will not reflect the true efficacy of dialysis. Two indices are defined to calculate efficacy.

Urea reduction rate (URR)
= Predialysis urea concentration – Postdialysis/Predialysis concentration

Kt/V
Where K is the clearance of solute, t is the session duration, and V is the volume of distribution of urea.

For efficient dialysis, we should try to achieve urea reduction ratio (URR) > 70% and Kt/V >1.

But we cannot replace the entire volume at once (obviously we cannot pour out the whole blood volume) similar to the analogy that we want to clean the water of a tank having fish, but we cannot take out the whole water at once, fishes will die and the whole purpose of purification gets defeated.

Now as urea production is a continuous process, the more you prolong your dialysis session, the less efficiently it will clear of urea. URR does not take this parameter into consideration moreover dialysis accompanies some amount of UF. UF reduces the volume of distribution by affecting the concentration (ultrafiltrate has the same composition as plasma) so its effect will not reflect in URR, while it will change Kt/V **(Fig. 4)**. Therefore, Kt/V reflects a more accurate prediction of dialysis efficacy.

Urea inbound/Rebound: Usually urea gets sequestrated in muscle, as blood flow to muscle is sluggish more in critically ill, it comes very slowly from muscle to blood.

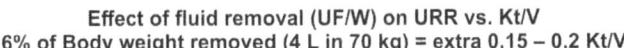

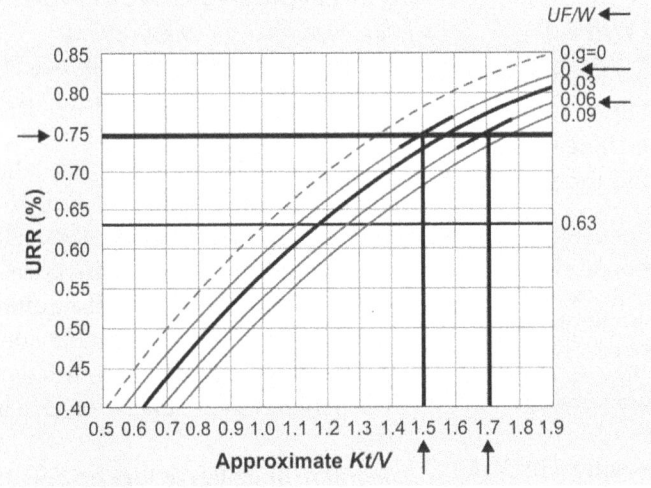

Fig. 4: Relationship between URR and Kt/V taking ultrafiltrate into consideration.

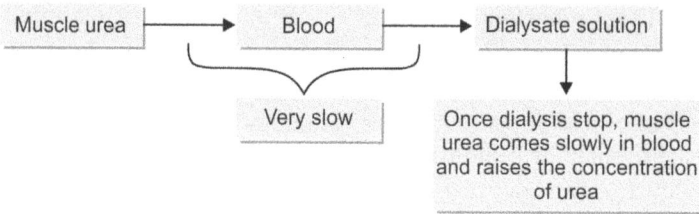

Because of this concept of equilibrated Kt/V comes into existence.

eKt/V values were deducted from a sample taken 30 minutes postdialysis. Its value will be less than standard Kt/V.

Access recirculation: It is important to know this while taking a sample at the end of the session, when the blood flow rate is less purified blood enters the dialysis inlet and factiously decreases the concentration of urea and increases URR.

To counter this either of the following can be practiced:
- Slow down blood flow to 100 mL/min (not zero—increase clotting) for 10-20 seconds, then take a sample.
- Keep blood flow the same but completely shut dialysate flow to zero for 3 minutes and then draw the sample.

Hemodialysis Prescription Writing

For intermittent hemodialysis: Eight factors need to define for effective dialysis. Details of some aspects will be discussed here however detailed explanation is beyond the scope of this book.

- Session length
- Blood flow rate

  } Determines efficacy, length will depend on urea concentration and clearance required while blood flow rate often limited by access capacity

- Dialyzer membrane → usually with K_0A 800–1,200
- Dialysate solution composition → bicarbonate, sodium, potassium, calcium, magnesium, dextrose, phosphate—their concentration depends on patient's plasma concentration—rule of thumb avoid sudden change in concentration of plasma
- Dialysate flow rate → as discussed should be around 2-3 × blood flow rate
- Dialysate temperature → 35-37°C
- Anticoagulation - often omitted is blood flow rate >250 mL/min otherwise heparin
- Fluid removal → depend upon patient volume status
  - Pulmonary edema + → 4 L
  - Normovolumic → 2-3 L
  - Collapsing SVC → nil UF

Rule: Try to keep ultrafiltration rate (UFR) @10 mL/kg/hr.

Now we have two scenarios, which show how we can customize our prescription.

1. Patient having blood urea nitrogen (BUN) >100 and also having fluid overload condition.

   If you run full session dialysis, adequate fluid will be removed but if urea concentration decreases more, chances of disequilibrium syndrome arise. If we opt for 2-hour dialysis, disequilibrium syndrome can be prevented but adequate fluid removal increase ultra-filtration rate. The patient will not tolerate such a higher rate.

   Solution: Run dialysis for first 2 hours only UF and then 2 hours UF + dialysis.

2. Patient have hyperkalemia but normovolemic/hypovolemic

   Run dialysis in the first 2 hours with nil UF (hyperkalemia is life-threatening), then run UF.

Sample for IHD prescription: 26-year-old 70 kg male presented with septic shock. While recovering from shock, develops AKI BUN 60 mg/dL, creatinine 3.4, and nil urine output. Cumulative fluid balance is +14 L. Difficulty in weaning was noticed as he often develop pulmonary edema during weaning. On two-dimensional (2D) echo grade 2 left ventricular diastolic dysfunction (LVDD) observed. Dialysis can improve a patient's condition. Prescribe IHD instruction.

Check for contraindication for anticoagulation, if nil heparins are preferred.

Volume status - volume overload—UF around 4L

Now delivering $Kt/V = 1.5$

V calculated from Watson formula let it be a 40 L

$Kt/V = 1.5$, $Kt = 1.5 \times 40 = 60$ L

We have internal jugular vein (IJV) as access for dialysis which supports a blood flow rate of 300 mL/min and we are using a membrane with $K_0A = 1,000$

Using the above nomogram, we can have K at 300 mL/min with the membrane of 1,000 = 210 mL/min

Time required = $60 \times 1,000/210 = 285$ min = 4.7 hours

Continuous renal replacement therapy prescription: **Table 5** and **Figure 5** depict various modalities as well basic line diagram for continuous venovenous hemodiafiltration (CVVHDF).

Prescription: 70 kg man

Dose recommended 30 mL/kg/hour and blood flow rate Qb= 150 mL/min
= 2,100 mL/hr.

TABLE 5: Important characteristics of various hemodialysis modalities.

	IHD	SLED	SCUF	C-HF	C-HD	C-HDF
Membrane permeability	Variable	Variable	High	High	High	High
Anticoagulation	Short	Long	Continuous	Continuous	Continuous	Continuous
Blood flow rate (mL/min)	250–400	100–200	100–200	200–300	100–300	200–300
Dialysate flow rate (mL/min)	500–800	100	0	0	16–35	16–35
Filtrate (L per day)	0–4	0–4	0–5	24–96	0–4	24–48
Replacement fluid (L per day)	0	0	0	22–90	0	23–44
Effluent saturation (%)	15–40	60–70	100	100	85–100	85–100
Solute clearance mechanism	Diffusion	Diffusion	Convection (minimal)	Convection	Diffusion	Diffusion+ convection
Urea clearance (mL/min)	180–240	75–90	1.7	17–67	22	30–60
Duration (hr)	3–5	8–12	Variable	>24	>24	24

(C-HD: slow continuous hemodialysis; C-HF: slow continuous hemofiltration; C-HFD: slow continuous hemodiafiltration; IHD: intermittent hemodialysis; SCUF: slow continuous ultrafiltration; SLED: sustained low-effifiency dialysis)
Source: Modified from Metha RL. Continuous renal replacement therapy in the critically ill patient. Kidney Int. 2005;67:781-95.

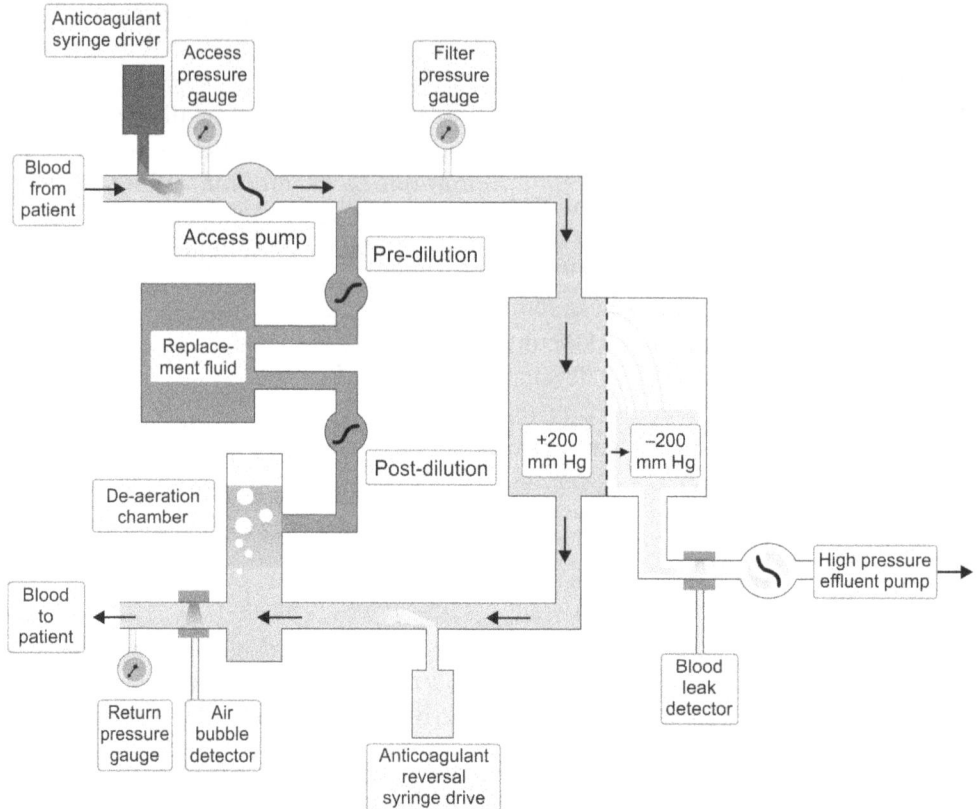

Fig. 5: Continuous venovenous hemodiafiltration (CVVHDF) line diagram.

Now suppose we only use filtration, i.e., CVVHF.

Filtration fraction = UFR/Plasma flow rate
2,100/60 × 150 × 0.7 = 35/105 = 33.3%

This is too high, have to keep it <20%, options are to increase blood flow rate usually not feasible so add diffusion along with convection, i.e., CVVHDF.

2,100 mL/hour

1,000 mL via convection, therefore FF = 1,100/60 × 150 × 0.7 = 17.4%

Use replacement fluid as 30:70 (300 mL prefilter, 700 mL postfilter)

100 mL/hour UF = 2.4 L/24 hours

1,000 mL via dialysis

Regional citrate anticoagulation is preferred with frequent monitoring of ionized calcium/total calcium ratio.

COMPLICATIONS WITH RENAL REPLACEMENT THERAPY

Two most important complications are as follows:
1. Disequilibrium syndrome
2. Intradialytic hypotension

Disequilibrium syndrome: Long-standing increased urea acts as an effective osmole, suddenly lowering of its concentration leads to reverse osmotic shift and fall in intracellular pH of cerebral cell.

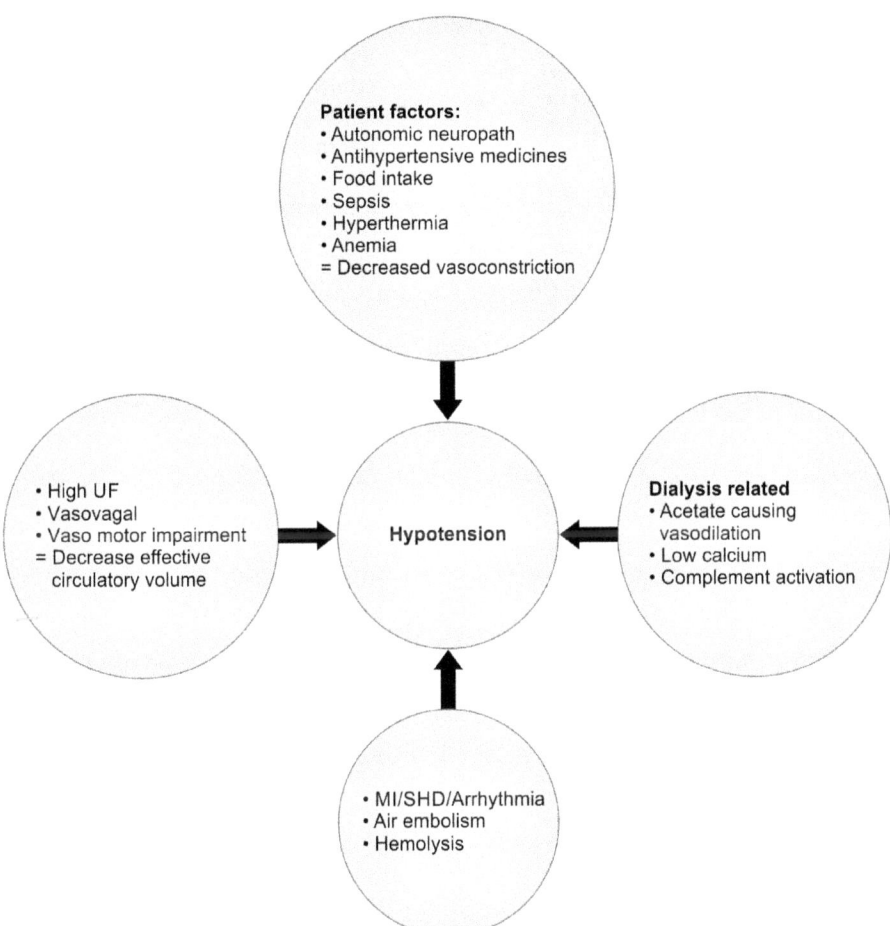

Fig. 6: Possible etiology behind intradialytic hypotension.
(MI: myocardial infarction; SHD: structural heart disease; UF: ultrafiltration)

Risk factors: The first dialysis, marked increase in urea (>175 mg/dL), CKD, severe metabolic acidosis, pre-existing neurological issues, hyponatremia, and sepsis.

Signs/symptoms: Headache, nausea, vomiting, disorientation, and seizure. If it occurs immediately, start intracranial pressure (ICP)-lowering measures.

Prevention: Slow first dialysis with shorter duration or sodium profiling.

Hypotension: Frequently encountered complication often troubles intensivist as either one has to slow down dialysis or cut down the session duration; both of these lead to reduced efficacy and will not be able to deliver Kt/V, etiology behind this is explained in **Figure 6**.

Prevention:
- Avoid food immediate before or after dialysis
- Withhold antihypertensive medications
- Maintain normal calcium
- Frequent cardiac evaluation and temperature monitoring
- Midodrine can be used.

FURTHER READING

1. Bagshaw SM, Wald R. Acute kidney injury: timing of renal replacement therapy in AKI Nat Rev Nephrol. 2016 Aug;12(8):445-6.
2. Mehta RL. Indications for dialysis in the ICU: renal replacement vs. renal support, Blood Purif. 2001;19 (2):227-32.
3. Mehta Y, Sharma J, Mehta C. Text book of Critical Care: Including Trauma and Emergency Care. p. 4211.
4. Prowle, JR, Bellomo, R. Continuous renal replacement therapy: recent advances and future research. Nat. Rev. Nephrol. 2010;6(9): 521-9.
5. Rabindranath K, Adams J, Macleod AM, Muirhead N. Intermittent versus continuous renal replacement therapy for acute renal failure in adults. Cochrane Database of Syst Rev. 2007;18(3): CD003773.

74 Defibrillators

Shubhi Singhal, Akhilesh Gupta

Q. 1. What is a defibrillation?
Ans. Defibrillation refers to the passing of an electrical current across the myocardium to depolarize the muscle, so as to convert a dysrhythmia back into a normal sinus rhythm. The device used for passing this current is known as a defibrillator.

Q. 2. What is cardioversion? How is it different from defibrillation?
Ans. Like defibrillation, cardioversion also involves the passing of an electrical current across the myocardium to convert dysrhythmia into a sinus rhythm. The key difference between the two is that whereas defibrillation involves asynchronous delivery of energy, in cardioversion delivery of shock is synchronized with the QRS complex.

Q. 3. What are the indications of defibrillation and cardioversion?
Ans.
- Indications of defibrillation:
  - Ventricular fibrillation
  - Pulseless ventricular tachycardia
- Indications of Cardioversion:
  - Hemodynamically unstable patient with:
    - Supraventricular tachycardia
    - Atrial fibrillation
    - Atrial flutter
    - Ventricular tachycardia with a pulse.

Q. 4. What are the contraindications of defibrillation and cardioversion?
Ans.
- Contraindications of defibrillation:
  - Presence of pulse
  - Asystole
  - Pulseless electrical activity
  - Obvious signs of death
  - Do not resuscitate order
- Contraindications of cardioversion:
  - Arrhythmia due to digitalis toxicity
  - Sinus tachycardia

Q. 5. What complications are associated with defibrillation and cardioversion?
Ans. Complications of defibrillation and cardioversion:
- Chest wall burns
- Myocardial tissue injury
- Inadvertent shock delivery to the healthcare provider.

Q. 6. What are various types of defibrillators?
Ans. Defibrillators could be manual or automated. As the name suggests, while using manual defibrillators, the operator analyses the cardiac rhythm and based on his judgment regarding the need of shock, delivers the shock manually. The energy delivered is also selected manually by the operator. Automated defibrillators analyze the rhythm and need of delivering the shock automatically. These could be of different types, viz., automated external defibrillators (AEDs), wearable cardioverter

defibrillator (WCD), implantable cardioverter defibrillator (ICD), etc.

Defibrillators are also classified as external or internal based on the location of a device and the electrodes. External defibrillators are external devices that need to be transferred to the patient at the time of need. The electrodes/pads need to be applied on the bare chest of the patient for cardiac rhythm assessment and delivery of a shock. Internal or implantable devices are implanted inside the body of the patient with electrodes attached directly to the myocardium.

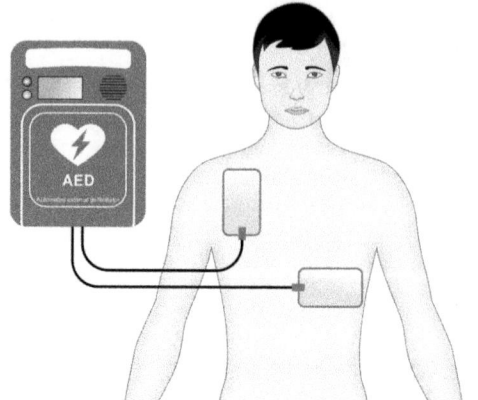

Fig.1: Automated external defibrillators (AEDs) and AED pads placement.

Q. 7. How do you select energy for defibrillation?

Ans. Defibrillators may be monophasic or biphasic. When using a monophasic defibrillator, energy is set at 360 J for the first shock. Biphasic rectilinear waveform producing defibrillators should be set at an energy level of 120 J for the first shock. While an energy level of 150–200 J is suggested for biphasic truncated exponential waveform producing defibrillators. If the type of waveform of the biphasic defibrillator is unknown an energy level of 200 J should be used.

Q. 8. What is an AED?

Ans. Automated external defibrillator (AED) are external devices that independently analyze the cardiac rhythm, once the electrodes/pads are correctly placed on the bare chest of the patient by the operator. Most of these devices provide audio (and/or visual) prompts to assist the operator. This feature ensures that even a minimally trained bystander may use the device in case of an emergency.

An AED typically consists of an AED machine, two leads, and two defibrillating pads as shown in **Figure 1**. The AED machine usually contains an on/off button and a shock delivery button. As soon as an AED is turned on, it prompts the operator to attach the pads. One of the pads is placed on the right side of the chest, just below the clavicle, while the other one is placed on the lower left side of the chest, laterally, below the left nipple. After correct placement of the pads, the AED analyses the rhythm and determines the need of the shock, if a shock needs to be delivered, the AED charges its internal battery and prompts the operator to ensure that no one is touching the patient and then instructs the operator to initiate the delivery of the shock. The shock may be delivered by pressing the shock delivery button. After delivery of the shock, it again instructs the operator to resume chest compressions.

Contemporary AEDs use biphasic waveforms that give two sequential lower-energy shocks totaling 120–200 J.

Q. 9. What is an ICD?

Ans. Implantable cardioverter defibrillator (ICD) is a small, automated device capable of detecting the patient's cardiac rhythm and accordingly cardiovert, defibrillate or pace the heart **(Fig. 2)**. The device consists of a generator, which contains a computer chip or circuitry with random-access memory

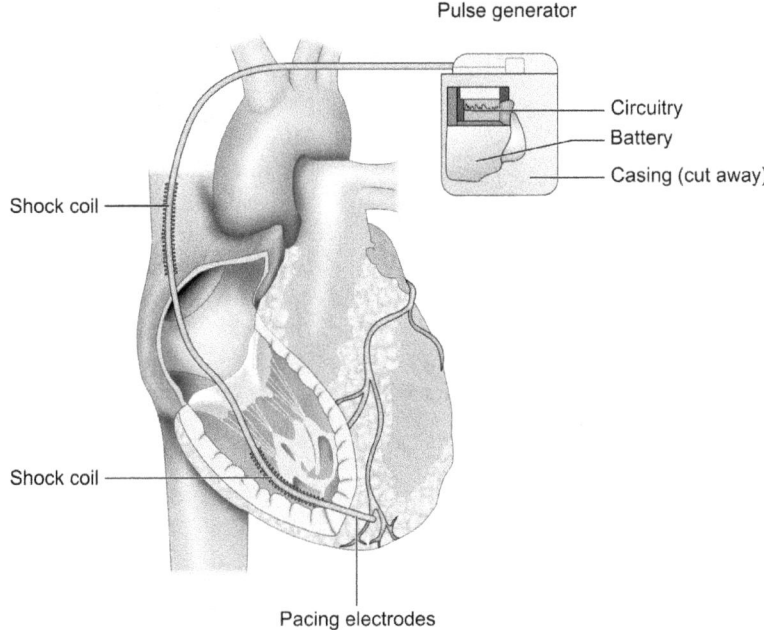

Fig. 2: Implantable cardioverter defibrillator (ICD).

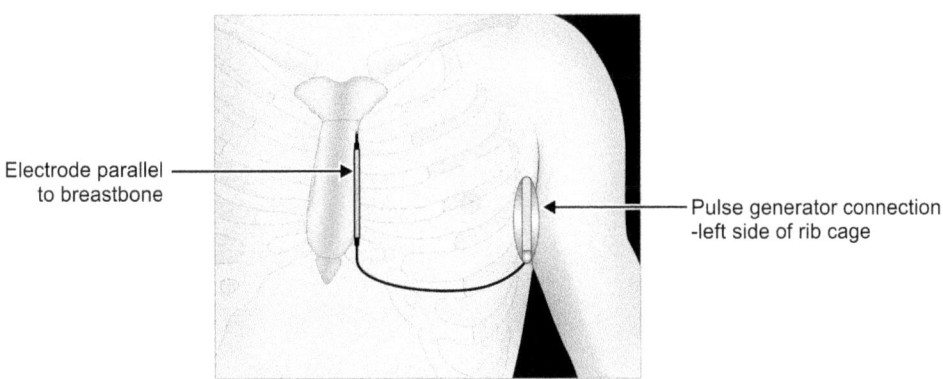

Fig. 3: Subcutaneous implantable cardioverter-defibrillator (S-ICD).

[RAM (memory)], programmable software, a capacitor, and a battery. It senses and analyses the rhythm and generates energy for cardioverting, defibrillating, or pacing the heart. This generator/analyzer is connected to the heart via electrodes/wires that pass through a vein to the right chambers of the heart. This lead usually lodges in the apex or septum of the right ventricle.

The newly developed Subcutaneous implantable cardioverter-defibrillator (S-ICD) (subcutaneous implantable cardioverter) provides protection from sudden cardiac arrest with the ability to pace the left ventricle from multiple sites near-simultaneously with Multipoint Pacing, without touching the heart or vasculature **(Fig. 3)**. Unlike transvenous ICDs, the S-ICD uses a subcutaneous electrode and analyzes the heart rhythm, rather than individual beats—to effectively sense, discriminate, and convert VT/VF.

FURTHER READING

1. Braga A, Cooper R. Physical principles of defibrillators. Anaesth Intens Care Med. 2018; 19(6):329-31.
2. Cakulev I, Efimov IR, Waldo AL. Cardioversion: past, present, and future. Circulation. 2009;120(16):1623-32.
3. Delhomme C, Njeim M, Varlet E, Pechmajou L, Benameur N, Cassan P, et al. Automated external defibrillator use in out-of-hospital cardiac arrest: current limitations and solutions. Arch Cardiovasc Dis. 2019;112(3): 217-22.
4. Minczak BM. Defibrillation and Cardioversion. In: Roberts JR (Ed). Roberts and Hedges' Clinical Procedures in Emergency Medicine and Acute Care, 7th edition. Gurugram, India: Elsevier; 2018. pp. 238-57.
5. Nichol G, Sayre MR, Guerra F, Poole J. Defibrillation for ventricular fibrillation: a shocking update. J Am Coll Cardiol. 2017; 70(12):1496-509.

75. Intra-abdominal Pressure Monitoring

Anshu Gupta, Akhilesh Gupta

Q. 1. What is intra-abdominal pressure (IAP)?
Ans. Intra-abdominal pressure is the measurement of pressure inside the abdominal cavity.

Q. 2. What is the normal IAP?
Ans. In a general population, normal IAP varies between 5 and 7 mm Hg. In obese patients, it is considered between 7 and 14 mm Hg due to effect of abdominal adipose tissue. It is suggested to look for trends of increase in IAP, rather than absolute value.

Intra-abdominal hypertension (IAH): IAP >12 mm Hg

Q. 3. What is abdominal compartment syndrome (ACS)?
Ans. Abdominal compartment syndrome:
- Sustained IAP >20 mm Hg
- With or without abdominal perfusion pressure (APP) >60 mm Hg
- Associated with injury in abdominopelvic compartment requiring urgent intervention.

Q. 4. What is the correlation between IAP and APP and mean arterial pressure (MAP)?
Ans. APP = MAP − IAP

Abdominal pressure should be >60 mm Hg.

Q. 5. What are the types of ACS?
Ans. Abdominal compartment syndrome can be of three types:
1. *Primary ACS:* It is associated with injury or disease in the abdominal pelvic region and it requires early surgical intervention or interventional radiological procedure.
2. *Secondary ACS:* It is associated with conditions that do not originate in the abdominopelvic region.
3. *Recurrent ACS:* It is associated with redevelopment of ACS following previous medical or surgical intervention of primary or secondary ACS.

Q. 6. What are the factors which affect IAP?
Ans. The factors which affect IAP are:
- *Gravity:* Patients in ICU are usually nursed in the semirecumbent position which affects the measurement of IAP.
- *Uniform compression:* It includes abdominal and diaphragmatic contractions, mechanical ventilation, and abdominal binding which changes IAP.
- *Shear deformation:* It depends on the shape stability of tissues and degree of deformation.

In view of above factors, abdomen behaves as a hydraulic liquid-filled container.

Q. 7. What are the physiological factors which affect the IAP?
Ans. The physiological factors which affect IAP are:
- Obesity
- Pregnancy
- Liver cirrhosis with ascites.

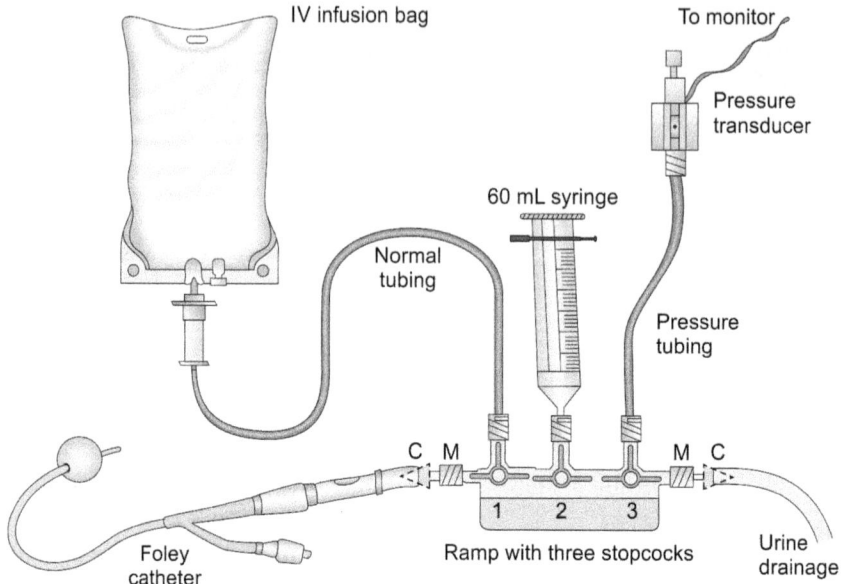

Fig. 1: Technique of measuring intra-abdominal pressure (IAP).

Q. 8. How is IAP measured?
Ans. Technique of measuring IAP **(Fig. 1)**:
- In a patient who is at risk of development of ACS, 4 hourly IAP measurement should be done.
- 25 mL of sterile saline is instilled into bladder.
- It is measured in the supine position via bladder at end expiration.
- Zero reference point is taken in midaxillary line at the level of superior iliac crest.
- Ensure that abdominal muscle contractions are absent.

Q. 9. What are the effects of raised IAP?
Ans. Raised IAP leads to constrictions of abdominal capillaries which decrease blood flow to the abdominal organs.

IAP >13 mm Hg restrict gut organs perfusion.

Q. 10. What are the contraindications in measurement of IAP?
Ans.
- Pediatric patients
- Bladder dysfunction.

Q. 11. What is the triangle perspective in managing IAP?
Ans. There is a triangle based on the management of IAP **(Fig. 2)**.
- *Intra-abdominal pressure:*
  - Look for physiological causes for increase IAP
    - Pregnancy
    - Liver cirrhosis with ascites
  - Minimal effect of increase IAP with positive end-expiratory pressure (PEEP)
  - Increase in IAP will lead to organ dysfunction.
- *Organ dysfunction:*
  - Duration of IAP.
  - Severity and impact of organ dysfunction.
  - One of the first sign of organ dysfunction is inability to ventilate.
  - Acute kidney injury is a common sequelae even at IAP as low as 12 mm Hg.
  - Other organ dysfunctions post increase IAP are metabolic failure, hemodynamic instability, and gastrointestinal failure.

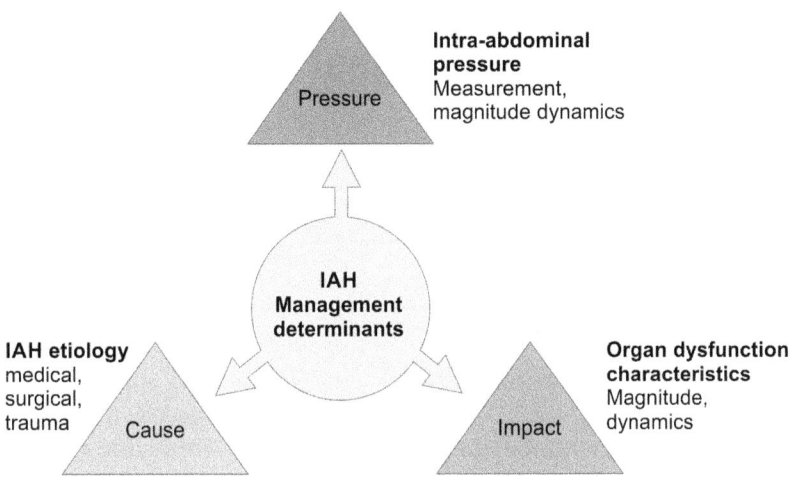

Fig. 2: Triangle based on the management of intra-abdominal pressure (IAP).
(IAH: intra-abdominal hypertension)
Source: De Laet IE, Malbrain MLNG, De Waele JJ. A clinician's guide to management of intra-abdominal hypertension and abdominal compartment syndrome in critically Ill patients. Crit Care. 2020;24(1):97.

- *Etiology:*
  - *Increase intraluminal volume:* This is seen in scenarios such as gas insufflation post gastroscopy and severe constipation.
  - *Increase extraluminal volume:* This is seen in abdominal disease such as pancreatitis and fluid overload post resuscitation.
  - *Decreased abdominal wall compliance:*
    - Body habitus
    - Abdominal wall concerns such as tight sutures, prone positioning, burns, and hematoma
    - Comorbidities which cause capillary leak.

FURTHER READING

1. De Laet IE, Malbrain MLNG, De Waele JJ. A clinician's guide to management of intra-abdominal hypertension and abdominal compartment syndrome in critically Ill patients. Crit Care. 2020;24(1):97.
2. Khot Z, Murphy PB, Sela N, Parry NG, Vogt K, Ball IM. Incidence of Intra-abdominal hypertension and abdominal compartment syndrome: a systematic review. J Intensive Care Med. 2021;36(2):197-202.
3. Kimball EJ. Intra-abdominal hypertension and abdominal compartment syndrome: a current review. Curr Opin Crit Care. 2021;27(2):164-8.
4. Kirkpatrick AW, Roberts DJ, De Waele J, Jaeschke R, Malbrain ML, De Keulenaer B, et al. Intra-abdominal hypertension and the abdominal compartment syndrome: updated consensus definitions and clinical practice guidelines from the World Society of the Abdominal Compartment Syndrome. Intensive Care Med. 2013;39(7):1190-206.
5. Montalvo-Jave EE, Espejel-Deloiza M, Chernitzky-Camaño J, Peña-Pérez CA, Rivero-Sigarroa E, Ortega-León LH. Abdominal compartment syndrome: current concepts and management. Rev Gastroenterol Mex (Engl Ed). 2020;85(4):443-51.
6. Rogers WK, Garcia L. Intra-abdominal hypertension abdominal compartment syndrome and the open abdomen. Chest. 2018;153(1):238-50.

76 Esophageal Pressure Manometry

Akhilesh Gupta, Himanshu Bhasin

Q. 1. What is esophageal pressure measurement?
Ans. Esophageal pressure measurement is a tool for monitoring to assess transpulmonary pressure and the risk of ventilator-induced lung injuries (VILI) as well as optimize ventilator settings in a mechanically ventilated patients.

Q. 2. How esophageal pressure is monitored?
Ans. Steps of monitoring esophageal pressure:
- *Checking and insertion of catheter:*
  - Check the balloon of the catheter with initial inflation and deflation which prevents adhesion of balloon with the catheter
  - Apply local anesthetic gel in nose and oropharynx and lubricate the tip of esophageal manometer
  - Place the patient in semirecumbent position with head tilted forward
  - Measure the distance of catheter from nostril to ear to the xiphoid
  - The catheter is pushed down from nostril or mouth to the depth of 50–60 cm so that the tip lies in the stomach.
- *Placing the esophageal catheter at correct position:*
  - The esophageal balloon is inflated and is connected to the pressure transducer linked to the dedicated monitoring device or the pressure port of the ventilator.
  - At that level, position in the stomach is confirmed by the positive pressure deflection during repeated manual pushes in the epigastric region.
  - The balloon is then slowly withdrawn till the cardiac artifacts start appearing on the pressure tracings indicating the position of balloon in the lower third of the esophagus.
- *Inflation of esophageal balloon:*
  - The esophageal balloon is then inflated with nonstressed volume to accurately measure esophageal pressure. The balloon should fit the esophageal wall and do not stretch it
  - Nonstressed volume is the adequate filling volume, neither causing underestimation of P_{es} due to low filling volume nor overestimation of P_{es} due to the elastance of esophagus.
  - Overinflation results in inaccurately high measured pressures secondary to the compliance of the balloon, while underinflation causes dampening of waveform variation.

Q. 3. What are the ways by which correct positioning of esophageal catheter is confirmed?
Ans. Correct positioning of esophageal catheter is confirmed by following ways:
- Chest X-rays with the guidewire
- Presence of cardiac artifacts on the esophageal waveform

- There should be equivalent changes in esophageal and airway pressures when dynamic end-expiratory occlusion test is performed.

Q. 4. Is there some variations in the type of esophageal catheters?

Ans. Some esophageal catheters have a second balloon that rests in the stomach and measure gastric pressure. This helps in assessment of transdiaphragmatic pressure which is the difference between gastric pressure and P_{es}.

Q. 5. How esophageal catheter can be utilized in various scenarios?

Ans.

Scenario 1: The patient is comatose, deeply sedated, paralyzed, and the ventilator is providing positive-controlled ventilation. Machine insufflation leads to positive deflection due to an increase in P_{es} **(Fig. 1)**.

Scenario 2: Patient is actively breathing. The respiratory effort leads to a negative swing due to a decrease in P_{es} **(Fig. 2)**.

Scenario 3: Patient triggers the breath but does not sustain effort (as in assisted ventilation), there is an initial negative swing followed by a positive deflection **(Fig. 3)**.

Q. 6. What are the clinical applications of esophageal manometry in ICU and OT?

Ans. Esophageal manometry is used in the following conditions:
- *Uses in passive conditions:* The esophageal pressures are used in the sedated and paralyzed patients.
  - Interpretation of pressure displayed: P_{es} is a surrogate master of P_{pl}. It helps in setting of positive end-expiratory pressure (PEEP) to prevent atelectasis in mid to dependent lung regions.
  - The esophageal manometry can be uses in operating room. P_{es} can be used as a guide to mechanical ventilation in patients in increased abdominal pressure, scoliosis, and pleural effusion.
  - P_{es} can be used to measure extramural pressures, which in turn helps

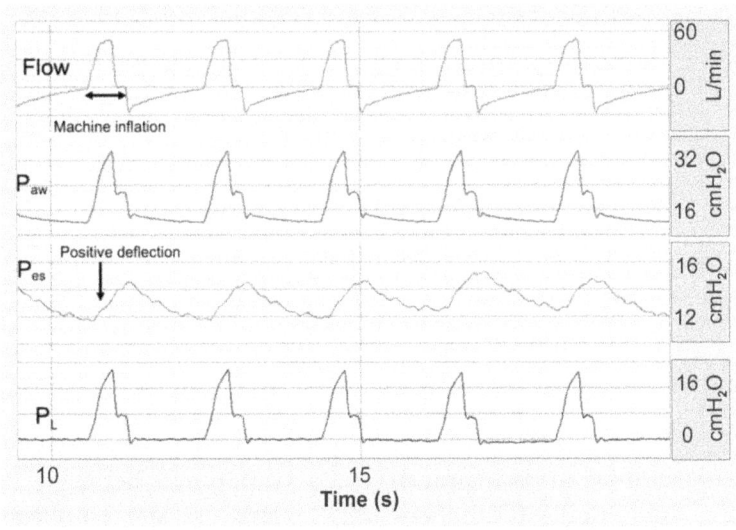

Fig. 1: Scenario 1.
Source: Pham T, Telias I, Beitler JR. Esophageal manometry. Respir Care. 2020;65:772-92.

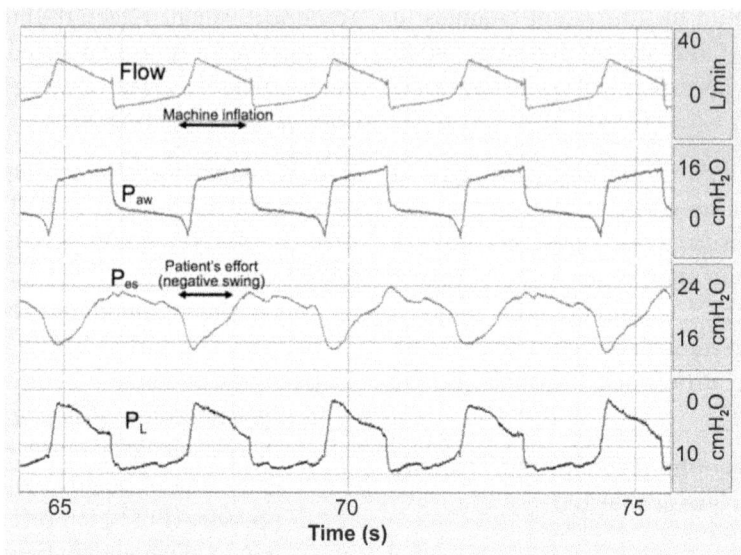

Fig. 2: Scenario 2.
Source: Pham T, Telias I, Beitler JR. Esophageal manometry. Respir Care. 2020;65:772-92.

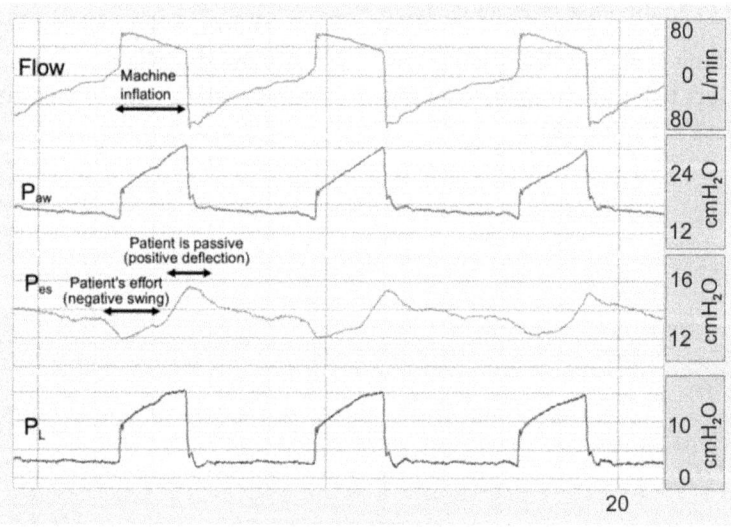

Fig. 3: Scenario 3.
Source: Pham T, Telias I, Beitler JR. Esophageal manometry. Respir Care. 2020;65:772-92.

in measurement of transmural pressure. The Frank-Starling law takes into account transmural filling pressures. Transmural pressure is difference between intravascular pressure and esophageal pressure. Hence, esophageal pressure helps in prevention of pulmonary edema.

- P_{es} is used in patient triggered or assisted mechanical ventilation:
  - In a patient who is breathing spontaneously, P_{es} helps in assessment of respiratory muscle effort.
  - It helps in prevention of patient-ventilator asynchrony
  - Weaning from mechanical ventilation
  - Measurement of auto-PEEP
  - During spontaneous breathing P_{es} can be used to assess respiratory muscle effort and work of breathing (WOB) generated by the patient.
  - Obese patients or patients with increased abdominal pressure, scoliosis, spondylitis, fibrothorax, or pleural effusion also have altered chest wall mechanics.

Q. 7. What are the limitations of esophageal monitoring?

Ans. The limitations of esophageal pressure monitoring are:
- *Esophageal spasm, transmission of heart beat:* Changing the angle of the bed to more seated position or withdrawing the catheter by few centimeter can decrease artifacts
- P_{es} in the supine subject is higher than Pes in other conditions. In the supine position, the mediastinal content compressed the esophagus and generated an artifact overestimating P_{es}
- Respiratory mechanics
- Mechanical properties of the balloon
- Large pleural effusion
- Increased abdominal pressure.

FURTHER READING

1. Baydur A, Behrakis PK, Zin WA, Jaeger M, Milic-Emili J. A simple method for assessing the validity of the esophageal balloon technique. Am Rev Respir Dis. 1982;126:788-91.
2. Bellani G, Laffey JG, Pham T, Fan E, Brochard L, Esteban A, et al. Epidemiology, patterns of care, and mortality for patients with acute respiratory distress syndrome in intensive care units in 50 countries. JAMA. 2016;315:788-800.
3. Chiumello D, Cressoni M, Colombo A, Babini G, Brioni M, Crimella F, et al. The assessment of transpulmonary pressure in mechanically ventilated ARDS patients. Intensive Care Med. 2014;40:1670-8.
4. Gulati G, Novero A, Loring SH, Talmor D. Pleural pressure and optimal positive end-expiratory pressure based on esophageal pressure versus chest wall elastance: incompatible results. Crit Care Med. 2013;41:1951-7.
5. Mauri T, Yoshida T, Bellani G, Goligher EC, Carteaux G, Rittayamai N, et al. Esophageal and transpulmonary pressure in the clinical setting: meaning, usefulness and perspectives. Intensive Care Med. 2016;42:1360-73.
6. Mojoli F, Chiumello D, Pozzi M, Algieri I, Bianzina S, Luoni S, et al. Esophageal pressure measurements under different conditions of intrathoracic pressure. An in vitro study of second generation balloon catheters. Minerva Anestesiol. 2015;81:855-64.
7. Mojoli F, Lotti GA, Torriglia F, Pozzi M, Volta CA, Bianzina S, et al. In vivo calibration of esophageal pressure in the mechanically ventilated patient makes measurements reliable. Crit Care. 2016;20:98.
8. Niknam J, Chandra A, Adams AB, Nahum A, Ravenscraft SA, Marini JJ. Effect of a nasogastric tube on esophageal pressure measurement in normal adults. Chest. 1994;106:137-41.
9. Pelosi P, D'Andrea L, Vitale G, Pesenti A, Gattinoni L. Vertical gradient of regional lung inflation in adult respiratory distress syndrome. Am J Respir Crit Care Med. 1994;149:8-13.
10. Pelosi P, Goldner M, McKibben A, Adams A, Eccher G, Caironi P, et al. Recruitment and derecruitment during acute respiratory failure: an experimental study. Am J Respir Crit Care Med. 2001;164:122-30.

11. Staffieri F, Stripoli T, De Monte V, Crovace A, Sacchi M, De Michele M, et al. Physiological effects of an open lung ventilatory strategy titrated on elastance-derived end-inspiratory transpulmonary pressure: study in a pig model. Crit Care Med. 2012;40:2124-31.
12. Talmor D, Sarge T, Malhotra A, O'Donnell CR, Ritz R, Lisbon A, et al. Mechanical ventilation guided by esophageal pressure in acute lung injury. N Engl J Med. 2008;359:2095-104.
13. Washko GR, O'Donnell CR, Loring SH. Volume-related and volume-independent effects of posture on esophageal and transpulmonary pressures in healthy subjects. J Appl Physiol. 2006;100: 753-8.
14. Yoshida T, Brochard L. Ten tips to facilitate understanding and clinical use of esophageal pressure manometry. Intensive Care Med. 2018;44:220-2.

SECTION 5: Resuscitation

- **Cardiopulmonary Resuscitation**
  Ajay Singh, Michelle Shirin Lazar

CHAPTER 77

Cardiopulmonary Resuscitation

Ajay Singh, Michelle Shirin Lazar

"The goal of cardiopulmonary resuscitation (CPR) is to achieve the best possible outcomes for individuals who are experiencing a life-threatening event."

INTRODUCTION

Recommendations for adult basic life support (BLS) and advanced cardiovascular life support have been combined in the 2020 *American Heart Association (AHA) Guidelines* for cardiopulmonary resuscitation (CPR) and Emergency Cardiovascular Care. The 2020 guidelines are a revision of the guidelines for adult, pediatric, and neonatal resuscitation science and systems of care.

Following significant improvements in the survival of both adults and pediatric individuals suffering an out-of-hospital cardiac arrest (OHCA), the outcomes plateaued since 2012, while that of in-hospital cardiac arrest (IHCA) continued to improve. The outcomes of IHCA were found to be significantly better than that of OHCA. The variation in the survival rates was attributed to the strength of the chain of survival which depicts the sequence of critical actions that must occur to maximize the possibility of survival following a cardiac arrest. An extra link was added to the previous version in order to provide extra emphasis on the importance of recovery for the improvement of the outcomes. **Figure 1** comprises the American Heart Association (AHA) chains of survival with the new sixth link added to each chain.

BASIC AND ADVANCED LIFE SUPPORT

General Concepts

According to the Center for Disease Control (CDC), heart disease continues to be the leading cause of death in the United States

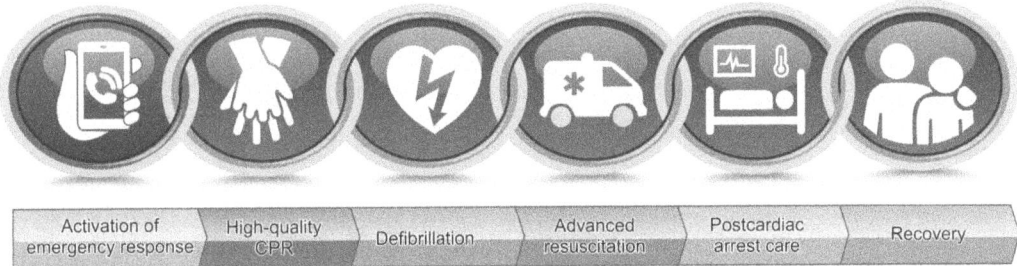

Fig. 1: Adult out-of-hospital chain of survival.
(CPR: cardiopulmonary resuscitation)

responsible for over six Lakhs deaths per year. Research has been done over the years to improve the techniques of response to such life-threatening situations in order to improve the outcomes. These systematic responses designed constitute the chain of survival which begins with BLS continuing to Advanced Life Support (ALS), postcardiac arrest care, and recovery. The chain of survival provides the victim with the best probability to return to a healthy life.

The heart is the primary pumping organ that pumps blood to the vital organs—the heart, brain, and the rest of the body as well. The blood delivers oxygen to the body and returns carbon dioxide which is then released out by the lungs. Cessation of the hearts' functions leads to a pause of blood supply to the entire body. The heart and brain become quickly damaged due to lack of oxygen and the person becomes unconscious. Basic life support (BLS) constitutes actions that slow this damage to vital organs until the cause of the arrest can be determined and corrected. It improves the victim's chance of survival until advanced care becomes available.

Key points of BLS:
- Steps of chain of survival should be quickly started.
- High-quality chest compressions should be delivered.
- Automated external defibrillators (AED) to be used appropriately whenever available.
- Rescue breathes are to be provided.
- Teamwork and effort.
- Quick actions to find the cause of arrest and its treatment.

Chain of Survival

The chains of survival in the **Figures 1 to 4** states the step to be taken while resuscitating an adult who has suffered an arrest. Each link

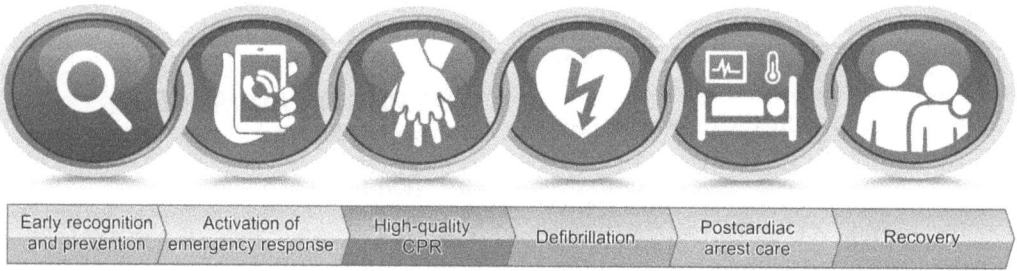

Fig. 2: Adult in-hospital chain of survival.

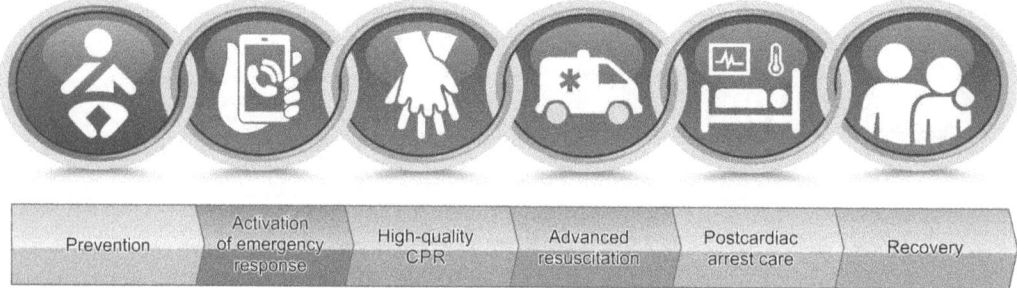

Fig. 3: Pediatric out-of-hospital chain of survival.

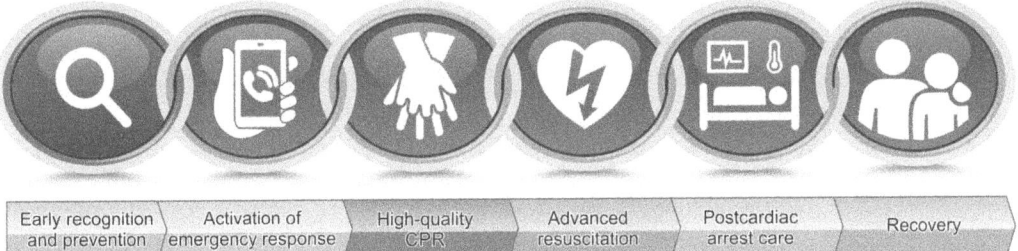

Fig. 4: Pediatric in-hospital chain of survival.

describes an action during resuscitation that is critical to successful outcomes. If any link is broken, the possibility of a good outcome is decreased. The pediatric chain of survival differs from the adult due to the fact that most emergencies that trigger the arrest in children and infants are usually respiratory in origin.

- *Immediate recognition of cardiac arrest and activation of the emergency response system:* The victim in cardiac arrest should be recognized based on unresponsiveness and absence of a palpable pulse and normal breathing. Once recognized, the emergency response team should be activated, or at least someone else should be asked to do it.
- *Early CPR with an emphasis on chest compressions:* High-quality CPR should be started immediately after cardiac arrest, as it improves the chances of survival of the victim. Chest compressions can be provided by bystanders also who have no training and they may also be guided by the emergency response team over the telephone.
- *Rapid defibrillation with an AED:* Rapid defibrillation in combination with high-quality CPR can double or triple the chances of survival. Defibrillation with an AED or manual defibrillator should be done as soon as the device is available.

The AED is a lightweight, portable device that is easy to operate and can identify lethal heart rhythms and deliver the required shock to terminate the lethal rhythm and allow the normal rhythm of the heart to resume.

- *Advanced resuscitation:* Advanced life support (ALS) bridges the transition from BLS to the more advanced care. ALS can occur both "in and out" of the hospital. Interventions such as:
  - 12 lead electrocardiogram (ECG)
  - Cardioversion
  - Obtaining a vascular access
  - Administration of appropriate drugs
  - Placing an advanced airway constitutes effective ALS
- *Multidisciplinary postcardiac arrest care:* After there is a return of spontaneous circulation (ROSC), the next link is to provide a multidisciplinary postcardiac arrest care to the patient. This particularly focuses on preventing another episode of cardiac arrest and also specific therapies tailored to the patient to improve long-term survival and outcomes. It may be provided in an intensive care unit (ICU) or a cardiac suite.
- *Recovery:* This link was added in the newer AHA guidelines and specifies the need to address the treatment, surveillance, and rehabilitation that needs to be provided to cardiac arrest survivors and their caregivers at hospital discharge. It also includes the need to address the sequelae

of cardiac arrest and optimize transitions of care to independent physical, social, emotional, and role function.

The chain of survival for an in-hospital cardiac arrest differs from out-of-hospital cardiac arrest by the first link which states that the cardiac arrest in the hospital usually occurs as a result of serious respiratory or circulatory conditions that may get worse. These arrests can be predicted, and prevented by close monitoring, prevention, and early detection and treatment of these pre-arrest conditions.

BASIC LIFE SUPPORT FOR ADULTS

Basic life support (BLS) focuses on performing multiple tasks simultaneously. The simultaneous and choreographed steps include chest compressions, managing the airway, delivering rescue breaths, using the AED, and working as a team. The coordinated efforts of the team of rescuers can save valuable time and help prevent damage to the heart and brain.

One Rescuer Basic Life Support for Adults (Flowchart 1)

- Ensure scene safety—move the victim out of water/traffic or any such possible surroundings.
- Ensure rescuer safety [wear adequate personal protective equipment (PPE)]

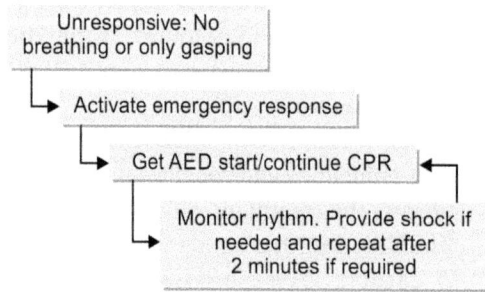

Flowchart 1: One rescuer—basic life support.

(AED: automated external defibrillators; CPR: cardiopulmonary resuscitation)

- Assess the victim—pulse and breathing
- Check to see if the person is breathing. Gasping or agonal breathing doesn't count as breathing.
- Check the carotid pulse on the side of the neck. Do not waste more than 10 seconds in trying to feel for a pulse.
- Call the emergency number for help and send someone to get an AED.
- If alone, call for help while you simultaneously assess for breathing and pulse.
- If unresponsive, start chest compressions and provide rescue breaths.

Steps in Cardiopulmonary Resuscitation

- Place the heel of one hand on the lower half of the sternum in the middle of the chest. The other hand should be placed on top of the first hand.
- Straighten both your arms and press straight down at a rate of 100–120/min.
- Depth—at least 5–6 cm should be attained.
- The rescuer should make sure to provide adequate recoil of the chest wall after each compression. (The chest wall should be allowed to return to its natural position).
- After 30 compressions, stop and open the airway by head tilt and chin lift maneuver as necessary.
- Provide rescue breaths. Each breath should be provided over one second while watching the chest rise simultaneously.
- Note:
  - Leaning or resting on the chest wall between the compressions does not allow adequate chest recoil and prevents the heart from refilling making the CPR less effective.
  - If a neck injury is suspected, a head-tilt/chin-lift maneuver should not be

performed. Jaw thrust should be done instead.
- For the Jaw-thrust maneuver-the angles of the lower jaw should be grasped on either side and the lower jaw has to be moved forward.
- If the lips are closed, the rescuer can use his/her thumb to open the mouth.

Two Rescuer Basic Life Support for Adults

The second rescuer prepares the AED for use. While the first rescuer begins the chest compressions and counts the compressions out loud, the second rescuer applies the AED pads. The second rescuer also opens the person's airway and gives the rescue breaths.

The two rescuers can switch roles after every five cycles of compressions and two breaths. One cycle consists of 30 chest compressions and two breaths. The roles of the rescuers should be switched quickly such that the interruptions in the chest compressions are minimized. The rescuers can switch positions while the AED analyzes the heart rhythm. If a shock is indicated, minimize the interruptions; resume CPR as soon as possible.

Adult Mouth-to-Mask Ventilation

Pocket masks, if available should be used to provide rescue breaths to the victim. The mask should be sealed against the victim's face by placing four fingers of one hand across the top of the mask and the thumb of the other hand along the bottom edge of the mask in order to form a proper seal. The fingers of the bottom hand should be used to open the airway by the head-tilt/chin-lift maneuver. This allows the rescuer who is by the side of the victim to hold the mask and provide the rescue breath, especially in cases where there is a single rescuer.

If two rescuers are available, the second one is usually positioned at the victim's head while the first one provides chest compressions. The second rescuer holds the bag and mask with one hand using the "C" technique. The thumb and index finger are placed in the shape of the alphabet "C" to form a seal between the mask and the face, while the other three fingers open the airway by lifting the person's lower jaw. The second rescuer gives two breaths over one second each.

Criteria for High-quality CPR

- Chest compressions should be started within 10 seconds.
- Push hard and push fast.
- Complete recoil of the chest should be allowed between compressions.
- The interruptions in between should be minimized to <10 seconds.
- Ensure adequate chest rise while rescue breaths are delivered.
- Avoid over ventilating.
- Assessment for shockable rhythm should be done as soon as the AED is available because in witnessed arrests it is more likely a shockable rhythm.

Opening the Airway

The two methods for opening the airway include:
1. Head tilt-chin lift
2. Jaw thrust

If a head or neck injury is suspected, the jaw-thrust maneuver is done to reduce neck or spine movement.
- *Head tilt-chin lift:*
  - One hand is placed on the victim's forehead and the head is pushed back while the fingers of the other hand are placed on the bony part of the lower jaw near the chin.

- The lower jaw is lifted to bring the chin forward.
- *Jaw-Thrust maneuver:*
  - The hands are placed on either side of the victim's head and the fingers under the angles of the jaw. The lower jaw is displaced forward.
  - If the lips are closed, the thumbs can be used to push the lower lips.

Pocket Masks (Fig. 5)

Pocket masks usually have a one-way valve that diverts the exhaled air, blood, or bodily fluids away from the rescuer. The valve allows the rescuer's breath to the victim's mouth and nose and diverts the victim's exhaled air away from the rescuer. Some of them have an additional port that allows the administration of supplementary oxygen. They differ in size for adults, children, and infants.

The rescuer should position himself at the side of the victim. This position allows both chest compressions and rescue breaths to be given by a single rescuer without repositioning each time.

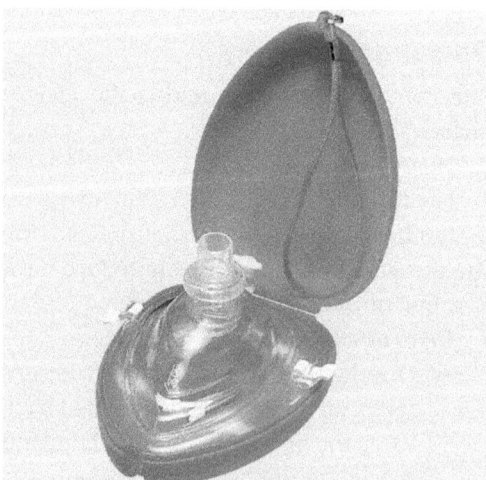

Fig. 5: Pocket masks.

Note:
- The oxygen concentration of exhaled air is about 17% oxygen.
- Each breath should be delivered over a second and visible chest rise should be confirmed.
- Chest compressions should be resumed within 10 seconds.

Bag and Mask Device

The device consists of a self-inflating bag attached to a face mask and may be used with or without an oxygen supply. It is used to provide positive pressure ventilation to the victim who is not breathing or not breathing normally. If there is no oxygen supply, the device provides 21% oxygen from room air. All BLS providers should be able to use a bag-mask device. During CPR, 2 rescuers are recommended to deliver effective ventilation, wherein one rescuer opens the airway, while the other squeezes the bag.

ADVANCED CARDIOVASCULAR LIFE SUPPORT

The BLS skills include performing effective chest compressions, use of bag and mask for ventilation, and use of an AED, and are usually provided by the emergency response team; however, health care workers and physicians require providing more advanced assessment and management **(Flowchart 2)**.

Primary Assessment

The primary assessment of the unconscious patient is done after the BLS while in conscious patients the primary assessment is done right away.

The primary assessment is done under the following heads:
- A—airway
- B—breathing
- C—circulation

- D—disability
- E—exposure

Airway

The assessment of airway and appropriate actions is summarized in **Table 1**.

Breathing

The assessment of breathing and appropriate actions is summarized in **Table 2**.

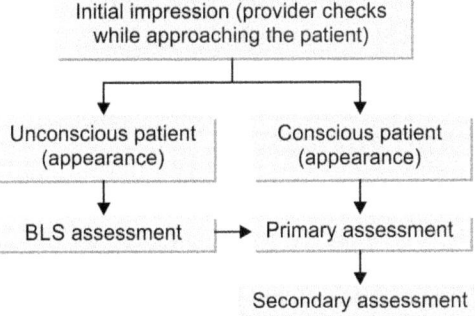

Flowchart 2: Systematic approach by the ACLS provider.

(ACLS: advanced cardiovascular life support)

Circulation

The assessment of circulation and appropriate actions is summarized in **Table 3**.

TABLE 2: Breathing.

Assessment	Actions to be taken
• Is the ventilation and oxygenation being provided adequately? • Is the oxyhemoglobin saturation and quantitative capnography being monitored continuously?	• Oxygen supplementation is to be provided as required to maintain a saturation of 94% or greater • For patients with cardiac arrest—100% oxygen is to be administered • Excessive ventilation is to be avoided • Adequacy of oxygenation and ventilation should be monitored using quantitative capnography and pulse oximetry

TABLE 1: Airway.

Assessment	Actions to be taken
• If airway is patent? • Is there an indication for an advanced airway to be placed? • Is the advanced airway placed properly? • Is the advanced airway securely placed and position reconfirmed?	• Airway patency to be maintained in unconscious by head tilt, chin lift, and nasopharyngeal or oropharyngeal airway placement • More advanced airways to be used if required • Confirm proper placement • Secure the advanced airway • Proper placement and position are to be monitored continuously by waveform capnography

TABLE 3: Circulation.

Assessment	Actions to be taken
• Assess the adequacy of chest compressions • Assess the cardiac rhythm • Is there a requirement of defibrillation or cardioversion? • IV/IO access has been established and secured? • Is ROSC present? • Is there a need to administer medication for maintenance of pulse and blood pressure?	• CPR quality can be monitored by intra-arterial pressure and end-tidal CO_2 monitoring • Provide defibrillation/cardioversion as necessary • Obtain IV/IO access • Intravenous fluids are to be administered if needed • Drugs required for maintaining the rhythm and blood pressure to be administered as needed • Glucose and temperature to be monitored

(CPR: cardiopulmonary resuscitation; IO: intraosseous; IV: intravenous; ROSC: return of spontaneous circulation)

Disability

- Check for neurologic function.
- Check for pupillary response, level of consciousness, and responsiveness.
- Alert, voice, pain, and unresponsive (AVPU).

Exposure

All clothing is removed and looked for obvious injuries, burns, bleeding, or any other signs of trauma.

Secondary Assessment

This involves a focused history and searching for the cause of cardiac arrest. A focused history is recommended by the AHA using the pneumonic SAMPLE.
- S: Signs and symptoms
- A: Allergies
- M: Medications (including last dose taken)
- P: Past medical history
- L: Last meal consumed
- E: Events

The most common causes of cardiac arrest should be kept in mind while managing cardiac arrest **(Table 4)**.

When patient shows ROSC, postcardiac arrest care should be initiated.

The cardiac arrest algorithm consists of two limbs—one is the management of a shockable rhythm while the other is regarding the nonshockable rhythm which includes asystole and pulseless electrical activity (PEA) **(Flowchart 3)**.

Following 2 minutes of uninterrupted CPR, a rhythm check which should not exceed 10 seconds should be done.
- In case of no electrical activity, epinephrine bolus is given and chest compressions should be resumed.
- If electrical activity is present, then the pulse should be palpated.
- If no pulse is palpable or even if there is a doubt regarding the pulse palpability, then without exceeding an interruption of 10 seconds the chest compressions should be resumed.

DEFIBRILLATION: PRINCIPLE AND PURPOSE

They are of two varieties: (1) monophasic and (2) biphasic.

While using a monophasic defibrillator—a single shock of 360 J is administered. The same shock dose is used for subsequent shocks.

Biphasic defibrillators use a variety of waveforms. The manufacturer's recommended shock dose should be used in such cases (120–200 J).

Defibrillation does not restart the heart; it stuns the heart and briefly terminates all the electrical activity, including ventricular fibrillation (VF) and pulseless ventricular tachycardia (pVT). If the myocardial tissue is still viable, then the normal pacemaker tissue of the heart resumes its normal electrical activity that ultimately results in a perfusing rhythm (ROSC). Following a successful defibrillation, the spontaneous cardiac rhythm achieved is too slow to provide adequate perfusion or create a palpable pulse. Therefore, CPR should be resumed for a few minutes until adequate

TABLE 4: Common causes of cardiac arrest.

H's	T's
Hypovolemia	Tension pneumothorax
Hypoxia	Tamponade
Hydrogen ions (acidosis)	Toxins
Hypo/hyperkalemia	Thrombosis (pulmonary)
Hypothermia	Thrombosis (coronary)

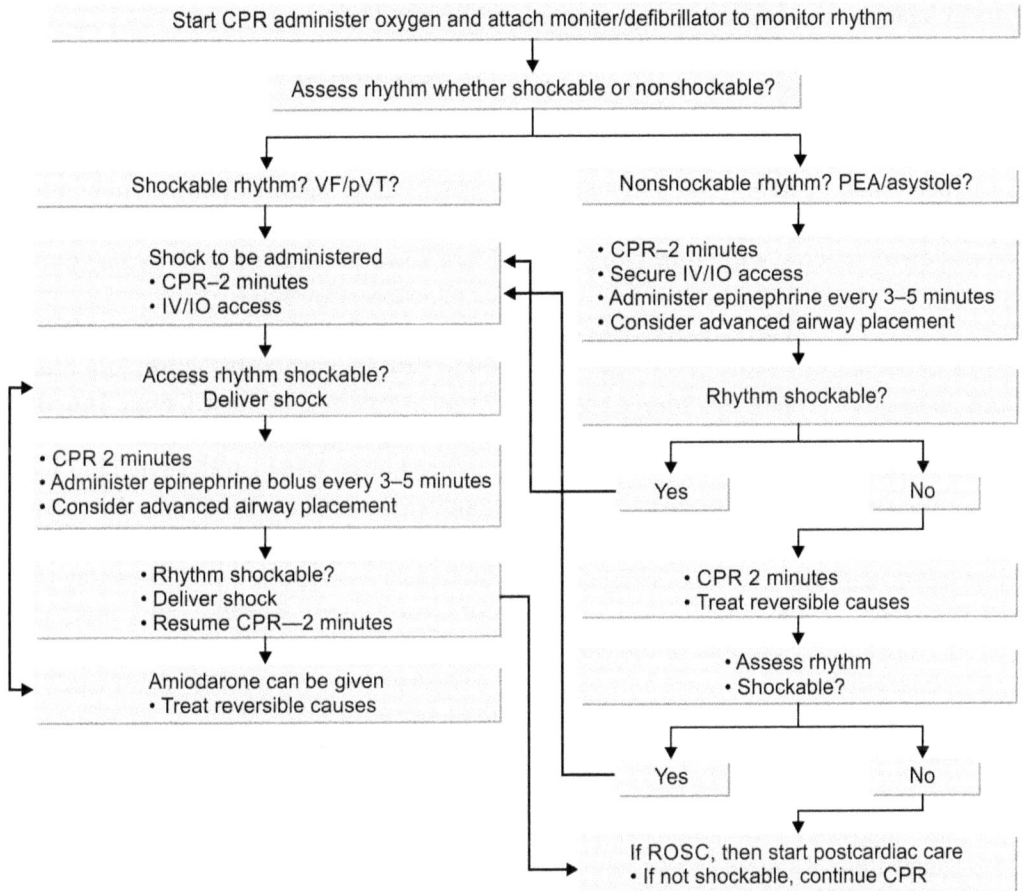

Flowchart 3: Cardiac arrest algorithm.

(CPR: cardiopulmonary resuscitation; IO: intraosseous; IV: intravenous; ROSC: return of spontaneous circulation; VF: ventricular fibrillation; pVT: pulseless ventricular tachycardia)

heart function resumes. This explains why it is imperative to resume effective chest compressions immediately after a shock.

The interval from shock to defibrillation is one of the most important determinants of survival; following a cardiac arrest, the earlier the defibrillation occurs, the higher the survival rate is. For every minute that passes between collapse and defibrillation, the chance of survival declines by 7–10% per minute if no CPR is provided. When bystander provides CPR, decline is more gradual with an average of 3–4% per minute.

To ensure safety during defibrillation, prior to providing the shock, the provider should always announce the shock warning in a very loud and firm voice. The provider also should make sure there is no one in contact with the patient, the stretcher, or other equipment. Also, oxygen should not be flowing across the patient's chest. Cardiopulmonary resuscitation should be immediately resumed after providing the shock and rhythm or a pulse check should not be performed at this point unless the patient shows signs of life or advanced monitoring indicates ROSC.

ANTIARRHYTHMICS AGENTS

Though many antiarrhythmic drugs such as amiodarone, lignocaine, and magnesium have been used during CPR, research has revealed that amiodarone is the first-line antiarrhythmic agent given in cardiac arrest. It has been demonstrated that amiodarone improves the rate of ROSC and hospital admission in adults with refractory VF/pulseless VT.

Amiodarone

Dose: 300 mg IV/IO bolus, additional 150 mg IV/IO once may be administered.

It is a class III antiarrhythmic agent, with electrophysiological characteristics of other classes as well. It blocks sodium channels (class I effect) and also exerts a noncompetitive antisympathetic action (class II effect). It also prolongs the action potential of the cardiac muscle (class III effect).

Lidocaine

Dose: 1–1.5 mg/kg IV/IO first dose, followed by 0.5–0.75 mg/kg at 5–10 minutes intervals, up to a maximum of 3 mg/kg.

It suppresses the automaticity of the conduction tissue of the heart by increasing the electrical stimulation threshold of the ventricular myocardium. Lidocaine also blocks the permeability to sodium ions which results in blockade of conduction and decreased depolarization.

Magnesium Sulfate

Dose: 1–2 g IV/IO diluted in 10 mL normal saline or 5% dextrose, given as a bolus over 5–20 minutes.

Drug of choice for Torsades de Pointes, it is a sodium/potassium pump agonist.

It has various electrophysiological effects such as suppression of atrial L and T type calcium channels and ventricular after depolarization.

Epinephrine in Cardiac Arrest

Dose: 1 mg IV/IO (can be repeated every 3–5 minutes) 2–2.5 mg diluted in 5–10 mL normal saline, can be administered directly into the endotracheal tube (ET). Endotracheal route however results in variable and unpredictable blood levels.

Epinephrine stimulates adrenergic receptors, causes vasoconstriction, increases blood pressure and heart rate, and thus improves perfusion pressure to the brain and heart. Though large studies have not been conducted to evaluate the improval of survival rate following epinephrine administration, studies have supported positive short-term outcomes such as ROSC and increased hospital admissions.

Every dose of epinephrine should be followed by at least 20 mL of normal saline flush and elevation of the extremity above the heart level for at least 10–20 seconds.

POSTCARDIAC ARREST CARE (FIG. 6)

A systematic postcardiac arrest care after ROSC has been shown to improve the likelihood of survival of the patient with a consequent good-quality life. Research has proven that the greatest number of deaths occur within the first 24 hours after resuscitation from the arrest. Thus, postarrest care has a significant potential to reduce the morbidity mortality caused by the multi-organ dysfunction and brain injury that occurs as a result of hemodynamic instability. Postcardiac arrest care emphasizes on management and optimization of cardiopulmonary function and perfusion of vital organs after ROSC.

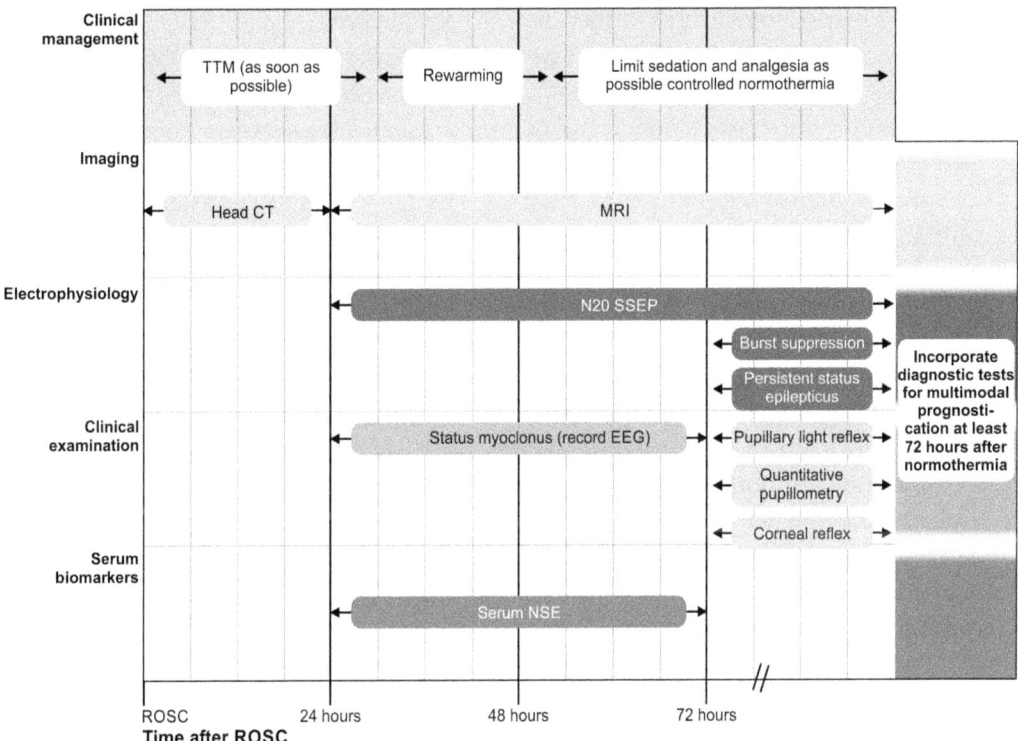

Fig. 6: Postcardiac arrest care.
(CT: computed tomography; EEG: electroencephalography; ROSC: return of spontaneous circulation)

In order to ensure a good postcardiac arrest recovery, health care providers should ensure the following:
- Adequate airway and breathing support immediately after ROSC.
- Head end elevation in order to reduce the incidence of cerebral edema, aspiration, and ventilator-associated pneumonia.
- Optimization of patient's hemodynamic and ventilation status: Proper placement and position of the advanced airway device should be monitored by waveform capnography, while oxygenation can be monitored by pulse oximetry. 100% oxygen is usually provided during initial resuscitation, however, it can be later titrated in order to achieve an arterial oxygen saturation of 94–99%. Hyperventilation decreases cardiac output by virtue of increased intrathoracic pressure and decreased preload and thus should be avoided. The low arterial CO_2 associated with hyperventilation decreases cerebral blood flow and thus a $PaCO_2$ of 40–45 mm Hg should be targeted.
- Targeted temperature management: This is usually done to protect brain and other organs, in patients who remain comatose after ROSC following a cardiac arrest. A constant target temperature between 32 and 36°C should be maintained for a period of at least 24 hours. A combination of rapid infusion of ice-cold, isotonic, nonglucose-containing fluid (30 mL/kg), endovascular catheters, surface

cooling devices, or surface interventions are common, safe, and effective methods.

Targeted temperature management (TTM) is the only intervention known to improve neurologic outcomes after cardiac arrest. Optimal duration of TTM is at least 24 hours.

ST-elevation myocardial infarction (STEMI) should be treated aggressively with interventions like coronary reperfusion by PCI if detected after ROSC. Both in and out-of-hospital medical personnel should obtain a 12-lead ECG and identify the patients with STEMI or high suspicion of acute myocardial infarction (AMI).

- Neurologic care and prognostication: The 2020 AHA guidelines recommend a multimodal approach for *neuroprognostication* in adult patients after cardiac arrest.

The prognostication of neurological outcomes should be done after 72 hours of return of spontaneous circulation in those who did not receive targeted temperature monitoring (TTM) and after 72 hours of TTM in those who received it.

Relevant differences between pediatric and adult cardiopulmonary resuscitation are given in **Table 5**.

SPECIAL SITUATIONS
Cardiopulmonary Resuscitation in Pregnancy (Table 8)

Cardiac arrest in pregnancy is rare (1:30,000).

The most common causes include:
- Bleeding
- Eclampsia
- Amniotic fluid embolism
- Drug toxicities
- Anaphylaxis
- Peripartum cardiomyopathy.

Several modifications are implemented during the cardiopulmonary resuscitation of a pregnant individual.
- Wedge is placed to give left lateral tilt.
- Hands are placed higher on the sternum for chest compressions.
- Intubation is preferred early.
- The preparation for perimortem cesarean section should be initiated and performed within 4 minutes of arrest. It is beneficial for both the baby (helps save the baby) and mother (relieves aortocaval compression).

Complications of Cardiopulmonary Resuscitation
- Chest compressions can result in fracture of the ribs and sternum.
- Artificial respiration provided using bag and mask ventilation can cause gastric insufflation, which may lead to vomiting, aspiration, and airway compromise.

Drugs in Cardiopulmonary Resuscitation
Fluid Administration

Fluid administration should be titrated along with vasoactive agents in order to optimize heart rate, blood pressure, cardiac output, and systemic perfusion with a goal to maintain a mean arterial pressure of at least 65 mm Hg. In cases of hypovolemia, normal saline or ringer lactate is used to restore the volume status and D_5 is avoided.

Epinephrine
Indications:
- *Cardiac arrest:* VF, pulseless VT, asystole, PEA.

TABLE 5: Some relevant differences between adult and pediatric CPR.

Component	Adults and adolescents	Children (age 1 year to puberty)	Infants (age <1 year and excluding newborn)
Scene safety	Make sure the environment is safe for rescuers and victims		
Recognition of cardiac arrest	• Check responsive/unresponsive • Breathing or apnea • Pulse—palpable/unpalpable		
Activation of emergency response system	• If alone—leave victim and activate emergency response team • Else, send the other person to activate response team and start CPR immediately	• Witnessed collapse—same steps as adults • Unwitnessed collapse • Give 2 minutes of CPR • Leave the victim to activate emergency response system, return and restart CPR	
Compression—ventilation ratio (without advanced airway)	One or two rescuers (30:2)	One rescuer (30:2) Two or more rescuers (15:2)	
Compression ventilation ratio (with advanced airway)	• Continuous chest compressions at 100–120/min • One breath to be given every 6 seconds		
Compression rate	100–120/min		
Compression depth	At least 2 inches (5 cm)	At least one-third of AP diameter of chest, about 2 inches (5 cm)	At least one-third of AP diameter, 1½ inches (4 cm)
Hand placement	Two hands on the lower half of the sternum	Two or one hand on lower half of the sternum	• *Single rescuer:* Two fingers in the center of the chest, just below the nipple line • *Two rescuers:* Two thumb—encircling the chest, just below the nipple line
Chest recoil	Full recoil of the chest to be allowed after each compression		
Minimizing interruptions	Interruptions should be limited to less than 10 seconds		

- *Symptomatic bradycardia:* It can be considered as an alternate to dopamine infusion.
- *Severe hypotension:* It can be used when pacing and atropine fail, when hypotension accompanies bradycardia, or with phosphodiesterase inhibitor.
- Anaphylaxis, severe allergic reactions.

Dose:
- 1 mg (10 mL of 1:10,000 dilution) was administered every 3–5 minutes, followed by 20 mL saline flush and limb elevation for 10-20 seconds after administration.
- Higher dose—up to 0.2 mg/kg is used in special conditions like β-blocker or calcium channel blocker overdose.

- Continuous infusion: 0.1–0.5 μg/kg/min, titrated to response.
- Endotracheal route: 2–2.5 mg diluted in 10 mL saline.
- Profound bradycardia or hypotension: 2–10 μg/min infusion titrated to response.

Antiarrhythmics agents used include:
- *Amiodarone:* Ventricular fibrillation or pulseless VT unresponsive to shock.
  Dose: 300 mg IV/IO push for the first dose, and if VF and pulseless VT persists, then a second dose of 150 mg IV or IO can be administered 3–5 minutes after the first dose.
- *Lignocaine:* Alternative antiarrhythmic with no proven efficacy in cardiac arrest, however, it is used when amiodarone is not available.
  Dose: 1–1.5 mg/kg IV or IO and repeated every 5–10 minutes up to a maximum dose of 3 mg/kg (endotracheal administration—2–4 mg/kg).
- *Magnesium sulfate:* To prevent or terminate torsades de pointes in patients who have a prolonged QT interval.
  Dose: 1–2 g IV or IO diluted in normal saline or D5 over 5–20 minutes.

To treat pulseless VT, immediate high energy shock is preferred, while magnesium is used as an adjunctive to prevent recurrent or persistent VT associated with torsades de pointes.

Other drugs used in ACLS and in postcardiac arrest cases:
- *Adenosine:* First drug for most forms of narrow complex supraventricular tachycardia (SVT).
  Dose: 6 mg rapid IV bolus followed by 20 mL of saline flush and extremity elevation if given via cannula in limb. Second dose of 12 mg can be given in 1–2 minutes. To be given under proper monitoring with full facility for resuscitation made available.
- *Atropine sulfate:* First drug for symptomatic bradycardia and also used in organophosphate poisoning.
  Dose: 0.5 mg IV every 3–5 minutes upto a maximum of 0.04 mg/kg (total 3 mg). In organophosphate poisoning, larger doses may be required.
- *Dopamine:* (IV infusion) second line drug for symptomatic bradycardia, after atropine. Also administered in hypotension with signs and symptoms of shock (SBP ≤70–100 mm Hg)
  Dose: 2–20 μg/kg/min infusion titrated to response.
  Hypovolemia should be corrected with IV fluids before dopamine is started.

Cardiopulmonary Resuscitation in COVID-19 Pandemic

Certain recommendations have been made by the AHA in order to balance the immediate needs of the patient without compromising their own safety. Health care workers are at highest risk for contracting this disease which is further compounded by the worldwide shortage of personal protective equipment (PPE). Basic life support and ACLS involve many aerosol-generating procedures including chest compressions, intubation, positive pressure ventilation, suctioning, etc. The aerosols generated can remain suspended and be inhaled by those nearby, which is of particular importance because resuscitation usually involves efforts of multiple healthcare workers (HCWs) who work in close proximity. The recommendations made by AHA are with regard to three main specific steps:

1. *Reduction of exposure of the HCW:*
   i. Don PPE before entering the room/scene.
   ii. Limit the number of personnel in the area.
   iii. The COVID-19 status should be communicated to any new providers to minimize errors.
   iv. Mechanical compression devices should be considered if available, and if the individual meets the height and weight criteria of the device.
2. *Prioritization of ventilation and oxygenation strategies that carry a lower risk of aerosolization:*
   i. High-efficiency particulate absorbing filter (HEPA) filter should be used for all ventilation if available.
   ii. Intubation with a cuffed tube should be done early and put on a mechanical ventilator.
   iii. The first attempt to intubate should be the best attempt with all conditions made favorable.
   iv. Chest compressions to be paused while intubating.
   v. Video laryngoscope should be used when available.
   vi. Prior to intubation, a bag and mask device with a tight seal and HEPA filter may be used. (T-piece in neonates)
   vii. Supraglottic airway device may be considered if intubation is delayed.
   viii. Circuit disconnections should be reduced to minimum.
   ix. Passive oxygenation using a non-rebreathing mask may be considered for adults, for a short duration as an alternative to bag and mask devices.
3. *Considering the appropriateness of the resuscitation:*
   i. The goals of care for the patient should be addressed.
   ii. Policies that guide the determination should be adopted while taking into account the risk factors for survival.

In case of arrest in an intubated patient:
- Patient should be left on mechanical ventilator with a HEPA filter and closed-circuit should be maintained.
- Ventilator to be adjusted to allow asynchronous ventilation.
- FiO_2 should be increased to 1.0.
- Tidal volume of 4–6 mL/kg targeted.
- Trigger to be turned "off" to prevent auto trigger from chest compressions.
- Respiratory rate to be adjusted to 10 bpm for adults and 30 bpm for neonates.
- An algorithmic approach to a patient with cardiac arrest in prone position is shown in **Flowchart 4**.

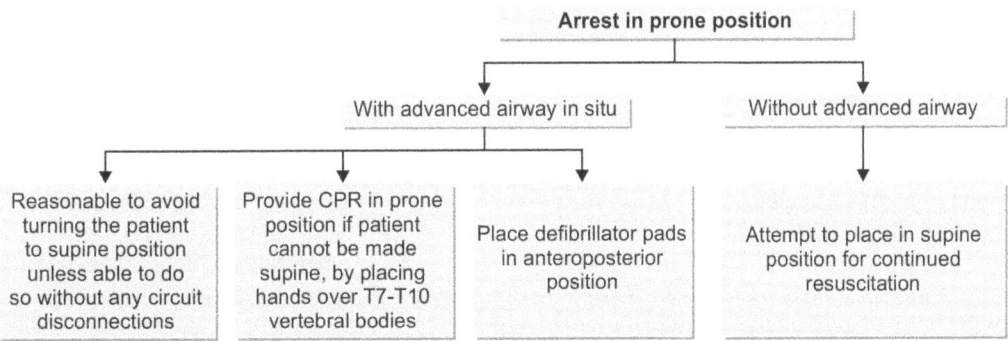

Flowchart 4: Arrest of patient in prone position.

THE 2020 UPDATE

Adult Resuscitation (Figs. 7 and 8; and Tables 6 to 8)

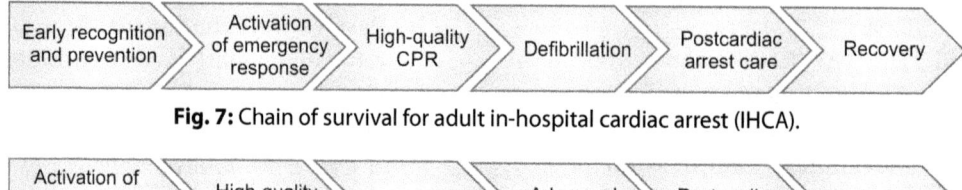

Fig. 7: Chain of survival for adult in-hospital cardiac arrest (IHCA).

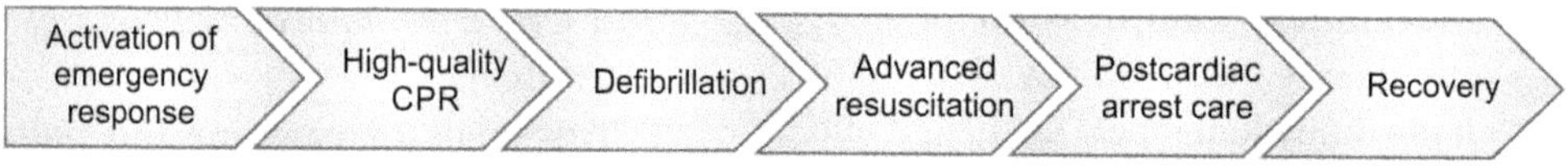

Fig. 8: Chain of survival for adult out-of-hospital cardiac arrest (OHCA).

TABLE 6: Early initiation of CPR by lay rescuers.

Older version (2010)	Update (2020)	Evidence
• Previously, it was recommended that a lay rescuer should not check for pulse and should assume an arrest if the person collapses or is unresponsive, while health care providers should not spend more than 10 seconds palpating pulse • Chest compressions to be started if no definite pulse felt	Lay persons should initiate chest compressions for any presumed cardiac arrest, as the risk of harm to the patient is low	The risk of harm to any individual receiving chest compressions even if not in cardiac arrest is low, when compared to those where lay rescues found it difficult to determine the pulse leading to a delay in initiating CPR

Early administration of epinephrine

Unchanged/reaffirmed	Unchanged/reaffirmed	Update (2020)
Nonshockable rhythm—administer epinephrine as soon as possible	Shockable rhythm—epinephrine can be administered after a failure of initial defibrillation attempts	• For nonshockable rhythms—an association was found between the early administration of epinephrine and ROSC, though improved survival rate is not confirmed • For shockable rhythms—CPR and defibrillation attempts are to be made earlier and epinephrine administered following failed attempts of CPR and defibrillation

Real-time audio-visual feedback

Unchanged/reaffirmed (2020)		Evidence
Audio-visual feedback devices may be used during CPR to optimize the resuscitation		RCT done had reported a 25% increase in survival rates of IHCA with devices providing feedback on quality of chest compressions

(CPR: cardiopulmonary resuscitation; IHCA: in-hospital cardiac arrest; RCT: randomized controlled trial; ROSC: return of spontaneous circulation)

Chapter 77: Cardiopulmonary Resuscitation

TABLE 7: Physiological monitoring of CPR.

Older version (2015)	Update (2020)	Evidence
It was not recommended but was considered reasonable to use physiologic parameters such as quantitative waveform capnography, arterial relaxation diastolic pressure, arterial pressure monitoring, and central venous oxygen saturation as a guide when feasible to monitor and guide on CPR quality, vasopressor therapy, and ROSC	It is considered reasonable to use parameters like invasive blood pressure monitoring or end-tidal carbon dioxide when feasible in order to monitor and optimize the quality of CPR	The usage of these monitoring strategies is supported by data which shows a higher possibility of ROSC when an $EtCO_2$ of at least 10 or ideally 20 mm Hg or greater was targeted. Ideal targets have not been identified yet

Double sequential defibrillation—not supported

New (2020)	Evidence
There is no recommendation on the usefulness of double sequential defibrillation for refractory VF/VT	Based on the evidence by current studies and case reports, the benefit of DSD or DCD is not known

IV access preferred over IO

Older version (2010)	New (2020)/update (2020)	Evidence
CPR providers may consider establishing an IO access if IV access is not readily available	• *New:* Providers may first attempt to establish IO access for drug administration in arrest situations • *Update:* IO access may be considered if there is no success in establishing the IV access	Administration of drugs via the intravenous route was associated with better outcomes. Thus, intravenous access is preferred, while intraosseous may be considered if IV access could not be secured

(CPR: cardiopulmonary resuscitation; DSD: dual sequential defibrillation; DCD: donor after cardiac death; VF: ventricular fibrillation; VT: ventricular tachycardia; ROSC: return of spontaneous circulation)

TABLE 8: Cardiac arrest in pregnancy.

New (2020)	Reasons
• Prioritization of oxygenation and airway management is recommended during resuscitation of a pregnant individual, because this group is more prone to hypoxia • Fetal monitoring is not recommended during resuscitation of the pregnant individual as it may interfere with the process • Targeted temperature management is recommended, in those who are comatose in the postarrest recovery phase. • Fetal monitoring is recommended during targeted temperature management of the mother due to potential complications like bradycardia	• Airway, ventilation and oxygenation are important in pregnancy because of multiple risk factors that can cause hypoxia which include an increased metabolism, decreased FRC and the potential risk of fetal brain damage during the event • Evaluating the fetal heart during maternal CPR may cause distraction from the actual process

Pediatric Resuscitation (Tables 9 to 11)

Chain of Survival for Pediatric In-Hospital Cardiac Arrest

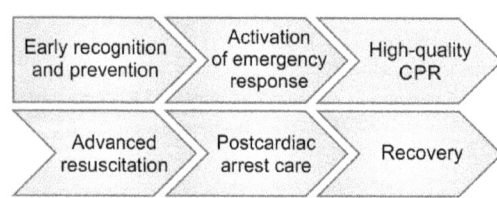

Chain of Survival for Pediatric Out-of-Hospital Cardiac Arrest

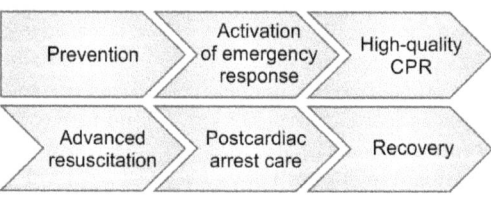

TABLE 9: Changes in assisted ventilation rate—rescue breathing.

Older (2010)	Update (2020)	Evidence
Palpable pulse 60/min or greater with inadequate breathing—rescue breaths at 12–20/min	Palpable pulse 60/min or greater with inadequate breathing—rescue breaths at 20–30/min	
Changes to assisted ventilation rate during CPR with advanced airway		
One breath every 10 seconds, i.e., 10/min	One breath every 2–3 seconds, i.e., 20–30/min	Higher ventilation rates have been found to be associated with higher rates of ROSC and survival
Cuffed ETT's		
Both cuffed and uncuffed tubes were accepted; however in certain conditions a cuffed tube may be preferred with proper precautions	The cuffed tube is recommended over the uncuffed tube, with proper consideration to size, position and cuff pressures	Studies support the safety associated with cuffed tubes and a decreased need to reintubate
Cricoid pressure during intubation		
Routine application for the prevention of aspiration during endotracheal intubation in children was supported by insufficient evidence	Cricoid pressure is not recommended as a routine practice.	Cricoid pressure decreases the rate of intubation success and also does not reduce the risk of aspiration
Early administration of epinephrine		
Epinephrine could be administered in pediatric cardiac arrest (no specific recommendation on time)	Epinephrine preferably to be administered early, within 5 minutes of starting chest compressions	Children who were administered epinephrine early (within 5 minutes), were more likely to survive to discharge than those who were administered later. For every minute delay, a significant decrease in ROSC, survival at 24 hours, survival to discharge and survival with favorable neurological outcomes was found

Contd...

Contd...

Invasive blood pressure monitoring to assess CPR quality

Older (2015)	Update (2020)	Evidence
For those who have an invasive monitoring line in situ, it is preferable to use blood pressure as a guide to CPR quality	For those who have an invasive monitoring line in situ, it is preferable to use the diastolic blood pressure to assess quality of CPR	Higher rates of survival with favorable neurological outcomes were found when diastolic pressure was at least 25 mm Hg in infants and 30 mm Hg in children during CPR

Detecting and treating seizures after ROSC

• EEG (electroencephalography) should be done for the diagnosis of seizures • EEG monitoring should be done frequently or continuously in comatose after ROSC • Anticonvulsant medications used in status epilepticus may be considered in case of seizures after ROSC	• When available, continuous EEG monitoring is recommended in postcardiac arrest with persistent encephalopathy • Clinical seizures postcardiac arrest should be treated • Nonconvulsive status postarrest may be treated with expert consultation	• Nonconvulsive epileptic activity cannot be detected without EEG monitoring, thus recommended to be done continuously in all post arrest with persistent encephalopathy • Both clinical and nonconvulsive status epilepticus are associated with poor outcomes, thus it may be beneficial to administer treatment of status epilepticus in both cases

Evaluation and support for cardiac arrest survivors

Update (2020)	Evidence
• Pediatric cardiac arrest survivors should be evaluated for rehabilitation services • Pediatric cardiac arrest survivors can be referred for ongoing neurologic evaluation for at least a year after the arrest	Recovery from cardiac arrest continues long after the initial hospitalization. Survivors require support for months to years after their arrest. Supporting these patients is important for the best possible long-term outcomes

Septic shock—fluid boluses

Older (2015)	Updated (2020)
Initial administration of bolus of 20 mL/kg was considered reasonable in conditions such as severe sepsis, severe malaria, and dengue	In septic shock a total fluid bolus of 10–20 mL/kg may be administered in aliquots, with frequent assessment

(ROSC: return of spontaneous circulation)

Prior guidelines had no recommendations regarding the choice of vasopressor or use of corticosteroids in septic shock, but later studies have proved that epinephrine is superior to dopamine as the initial vasoactive medication and that norepinephrine may also be used. Also benefit was found by corticosteroid administration in some pediatric cases with refractory septic shock.

TABLE 10: Septic shock—choice of vasopressor.

Update (2020)	Evidence
In infants and children with fluid refractory septic shock, either epinephrine or norepinephrine infusion could be used as the initial vasoactive medication	In infants and children with fluid refractory septic shock, dopamine may be considered if epinephrine and norepinephrine are not available
Septic shock—corticosteroid medication	
Stress dose of corticosteroid may be considered in infants and pediatric age group in septic shock unresponsive to fluid bolus and requiring vasoactive support	In those administered high fluid volumes rapidly, there was an increased morbidity observed secondary to fluid overload and may require mechanical ventilation. Thus it was recommended to administer fluid in aliquots with frequent assessments

TABLE 11: Hemorrhagic shock.

Update (2020)	Evidence
In infants and children with hemorrhagic shock following trauma, blood products should be preferably administered instead of crystalloids when available for resuscitation	Prior versions did not differentiate hemorrhagic shock from other hypovolemic shocks. Data supports a balance resuscitation using packed red blood cells, fresh frozen plasma and platelets

NEONATAL LIFE SUPPORT

Key Points

- Most newborns do not require cord clamping or resuscitation attempts immediately. These can be evaluated during skin contact with their mothers.
- Skin to skin contact helps to promote bonding with mother, breast feeding, and normothermia. It is also to emphasize the importance of preventing hypothermia in neonatal resuscitation.
- Ventilation is of priority (in comparison to chest compression) in newborns.
- Heart rate is the single most important indicator of effective resuscitations in this age group.
- Pulse oximetry may be used as a guide during resuscitation.
- Endotracheal suctioning in all newborn infants born with meconium stained amniotic fluid should not be a routine practice. Suctioning is recommended only when there is airway obstruction during positive pressure ventilation.
- Chest compressions are started only if heart rate does not rise in response to adequate ventilation measures (which includes endotracheal intubation).
- Heart rate response to resuscitation should be monitored using electrocardiography (ECG).
- Vascular access—umbilical vein preferred > intravenous access > intraosseous access (may be considered when IV not feasible).
- Epinephrine may be administered if there is poor response to chest compressions.
- If the infant shows no response to epinephrine and has a history or examination finding suggestive of blood loss—volume expansion should be considered.
- Despite all these resuscitative efforts, if there is no heart rate response in 20 minutes, discuss redirection of care with team and family.

Recommendations for Some Special Conditions (Flowcharts 5 and 6)

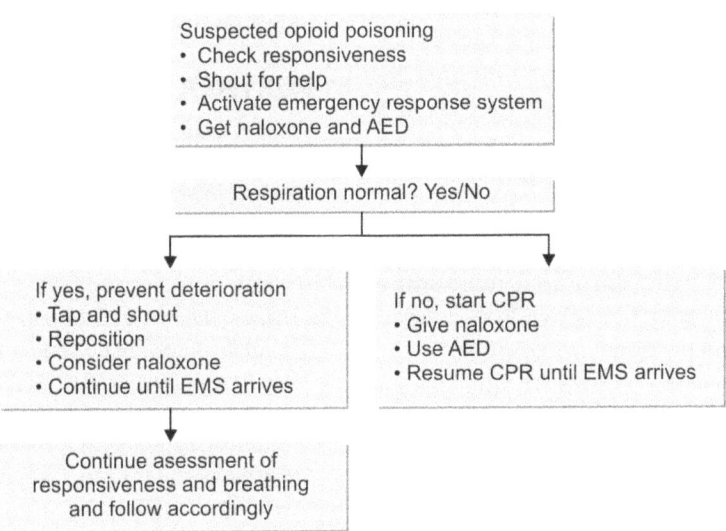

Flowchart 5: Opioid overdose: Lay responders algorithm.

(AED: automated external defibrillators; CPR: cardiopulmonary resuscitation; EMS: emergency medical services)

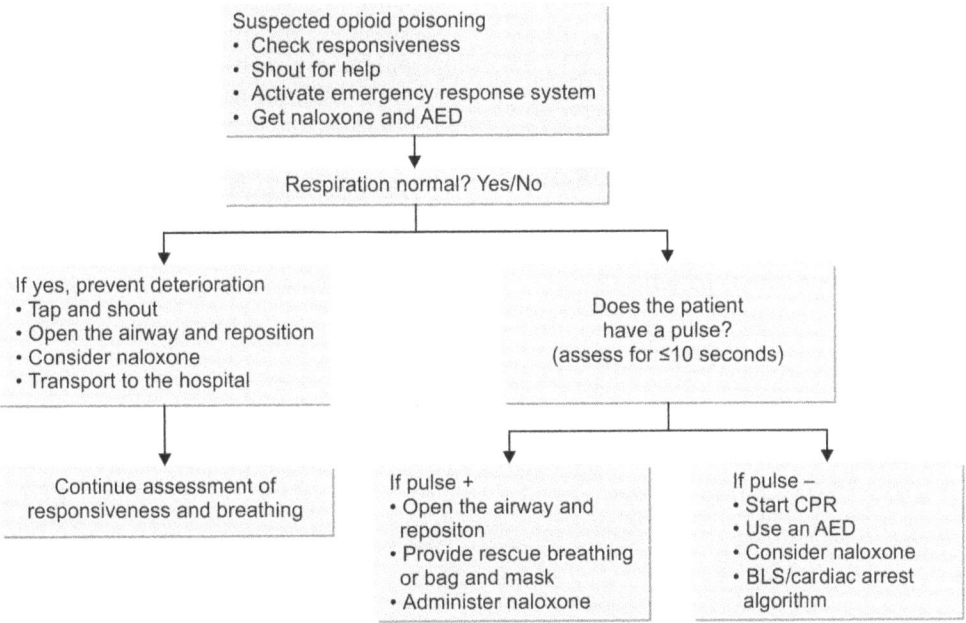

Flowchart 6: Opioid overdose—emergency healthcare providers.

(AED: automated external defibrillators; BLS: basic life support)

MYOCARDITIS

Recommendations

- In children with acute myocarditis who demonstrate arrhythmias, heart block, ST—segment changes, and/or low cardiac output—transfer to ICU, and monitoring is recommended because they have a high risk of cardiac arrest.
- In children with myocarditis or cardiomyopathy and refractory low cardiac output state—use of mechanical circulatory support or extra corporeal membrane oxygenation may help provide end organ support and prevent cardiac arrest.
- In children with myocarditis—due to high challenges to successful resuscitation, early initiation of extracorporeal CPR may be beneficial once cardiac arrest occurs.

Previous PALS guidelines did not contain specific recommendations for myocarditis in children. These recommendations are based on the 2018 AHA scientific statement on CPR in infants and children with cardiac disease.

Note:
Other new additions:
Guidelines regarding the management of conditions such as:

- *Single ventricle:* Recommendations for the treatment of preoperative and postoperative stage I palliation (Norwood/Blalock-Tausig shunt) patients
- *Single ventricle:* Recommendations for the treatment of preoperative and postoperative stage II palliation (bidirectional Glenn/hemi-Fontan) and Stage III (Fontan) palliation patients.

FURTHER READING

1. American Heart Association. American Heart Association Guidelines for CPR and ECC. (2020). [online] Available from: https://cpr.heart.org/en/resuscitation-science/cpr-and-ecc-guidelines. [Last accessed April, 2022].
2. Aziz K, Lee HC, Escobedo MB, Hoover AV, Kamath-Rayne BD, Kapadia VS, et al. Part 5: Neonatal Resuscitation: 2020 American Heart Association Guidelines for Cardiopulmonary Resuscitation and Emergency Cardiovascular Care. Circulation. 2020;142 (16 Suppl 2): S524-50.
3. Jeejeebhoy FM, Zelop CM, Lipman S, Carvalho B, Joglar J, Mhyre JM, et al. Cardiac arrest in pregnancy: a Scientific Statement From the American Heart Association. Circulation. 2015;132(18):1747-73.
4. Lurie KG, Nemergut EC, Yannopoulos D, Sweeney M. The physiology of cardiopulmonary resuscitation. Anesth Analg. 2016;122(3):767-83.
5. Merchant RM, Topjian AA, Panchal AR, Cheng A, Aziz K, Berg KM, et al. Part 1: Executive Summary: 2020 American Heart Association Guidelines for Cardiopulmonary Resuscitation and Emergency Cardiovascular Care. Circulation. 2020; 142(16_suppl_2):S337-57.

SECTION 6

Miscellaneous

- **Commonly Used Instruments in Chronic Pain**
  Samridhi Nanda
- **Physics in Anesthesia**
  T Nageswara Rao
- **Electrocardiogram and X-ray**
  Ridhima Bhatia, Puneet Khanna
- **Point-of-care Ultrasonography for the Postgraduates**
  Praveen Talawar, Vadhan Prasanna S, Sangadala Priyanka

CHAPTER 78
Commonly Used Instruments in Chronic Pain

Samridhi Nanda

INTRODUCTION

Chronic pain management is not a recent specialty. But the proportion to which it has reached now has been a very gradual process. In these past 30 years or so, the specialty has had numerous developments to get to what it has bloomed into. The incorporation of instrumental guidance has made the branch more targeted and precise. Fluoroscopes and ultrasounds have made it easy to identify and localize the structures of interest, improving the overall performance and thus results. Many advanced machines like radiofrequency generators have improved the duration of the effects even through the percutaneous approach. This chapter discusses the most used instruments in chronic pain.

NEEDLES AND CATHETERS

The entire interventional practice calls for the use of needles and catheters. From dry needling to percutaneous radiofrequency ablation (RFA), needles are the starting point of the interventions. Some commonly used needles and catheters in chronic pain management are mentioned in **Table 1**.

TABLE 1: Needles and catheters in chronic pain management.

Types	Sizes	Advantages	Uses
Spinal needle (Fig. 1)	22 G 8 cm 20 G 15 cm Chiba needle	• Commonly available • Long and sturdy • The extra length helps negotiate into deeper tissues	• All neuraxial interventions • Celiac plexus block, disk procedures, superior hypogastric plexus block, etc.
Tuohy needles (Fig. 2)	18 G	Thick and bent tip causes less design trauma to the nerve roots and other tissues	• Caudal epidural, epidural adhesiolysis, paravertebral • Block and paravertebral catheterization
Coudé tip needles (Fig. 3)	13 G, 14 G, 16 G, 18 G, 20 G, 21 G, 22 G	Coudé means elbow. These tips are even lesser traumatic due to their elbow like bend	Caudal block, caudal epidural adhesiolysis
Radiofrequency needles (Figs. 4 and 5)	16 G, 18 G, 20 G, 21 G, 22 G (straight tip/curved tip)	These needles have an insulated hub with open tip ends. The active tip length may range from 5 mm, 10 mm, 15 mm, and 20 mm. The lesion size is directly proportional to the thickness of the needles and the length of the active tip	Gasserian ganglion RFA, medial branch RFA, ganglion impar radiofrequency, etc.
Racz needles and catheters (Figs. 6A and B)	Needles—14 G, 15 G 16 G, 18 G Catheters	These rigid stainless steel, radiopaque catheters offer a sturdy, flexible-tip option for epidural neurolysis	Caudal, transforaminal, and cervical epidural adhesiolysis/neurolysis

Section 6: Miscellaneous

Fig. 1: 22 G spinal needle.

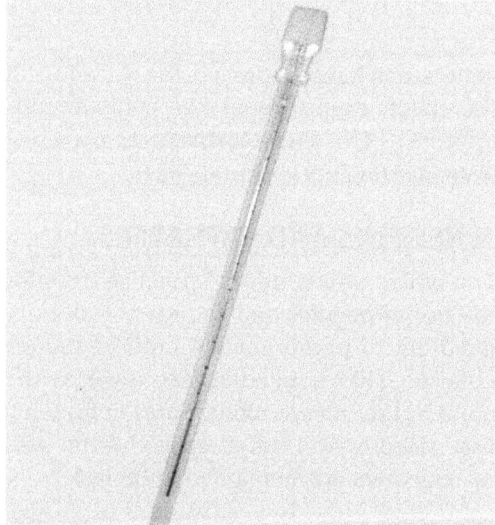

Fig. 2: 20 G 15 cm long Chiba needle.

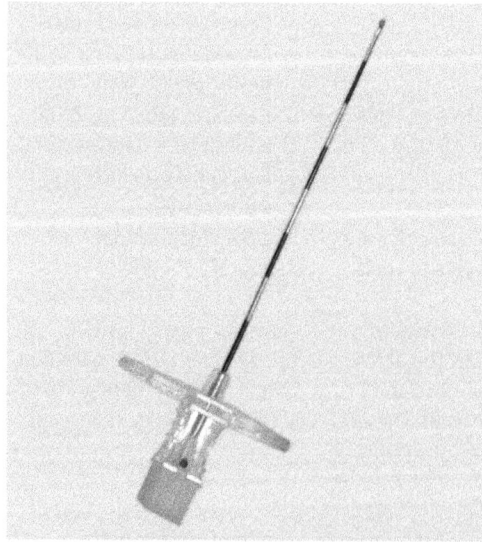

Fig. 3: 18 G Tuohy needle.

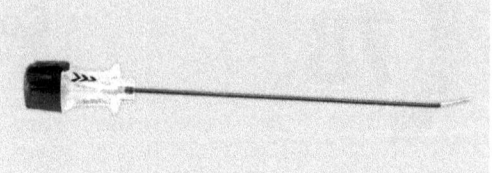

Fig. 4: 22 G and 20 G curved tip radiofrequency cannula with 10 mm active tip.

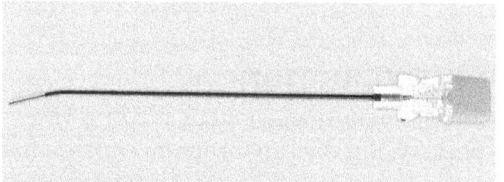

Fig. 5: Radiofrequency cannula—straight and curved tips.

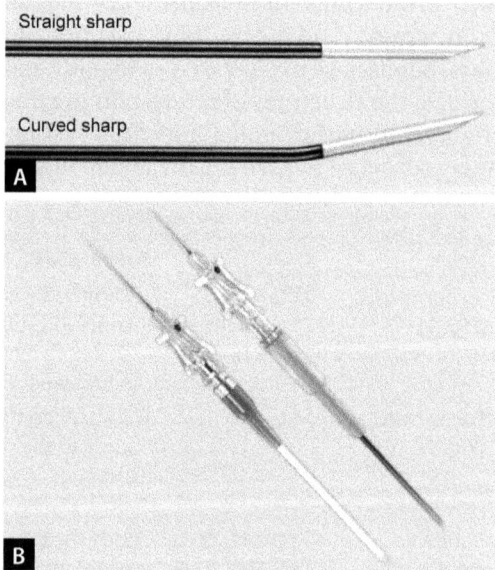

Figs. 6A and B: Radiofrequency electrode.

IMAGING TECHNIQUES IN CHRONIC PAIN

Radiography

The discovery of X-rays and their use for medical imaging led to major advances in medical practice. X-ray machines, fluoroscopes, computed tomography, and all use ionizing radiations for giving high-quality images.

Definition

Radiography is a technique of visualization of the mineralized body structures on a monitor through the use of ionizing radiation. Fluoroscopy is an imaging technique that creates images in real-time and makes the visualization of the movement of the contrast agent possible.

Principle

On passing an X-ray beam through the body, it gets absorbed in part and the rest gets scattered by the internal structures. The pattern gets transmitted to a monitor. Fluoroscopy allows real-time monitoring of the movement of the dye through the tissues.

Parts of a C-Arm

There are four main parts of a C-arm: (1) X-ray generator/X-ray tube; (2) image intensifier; (3) workstation unit; and (4) charged coupled device camera. **Figure 7** depicts the complete assembly of a C-arm.

1. *X-ray generator/X-ray tube:* It is the part that generates the ionizing radiation. It is placed at one end of the C-arm. The operation is controlled by the workstation unit.
2. *Imaging system/image intensifier tube:* It is a vacuum tube device for converting

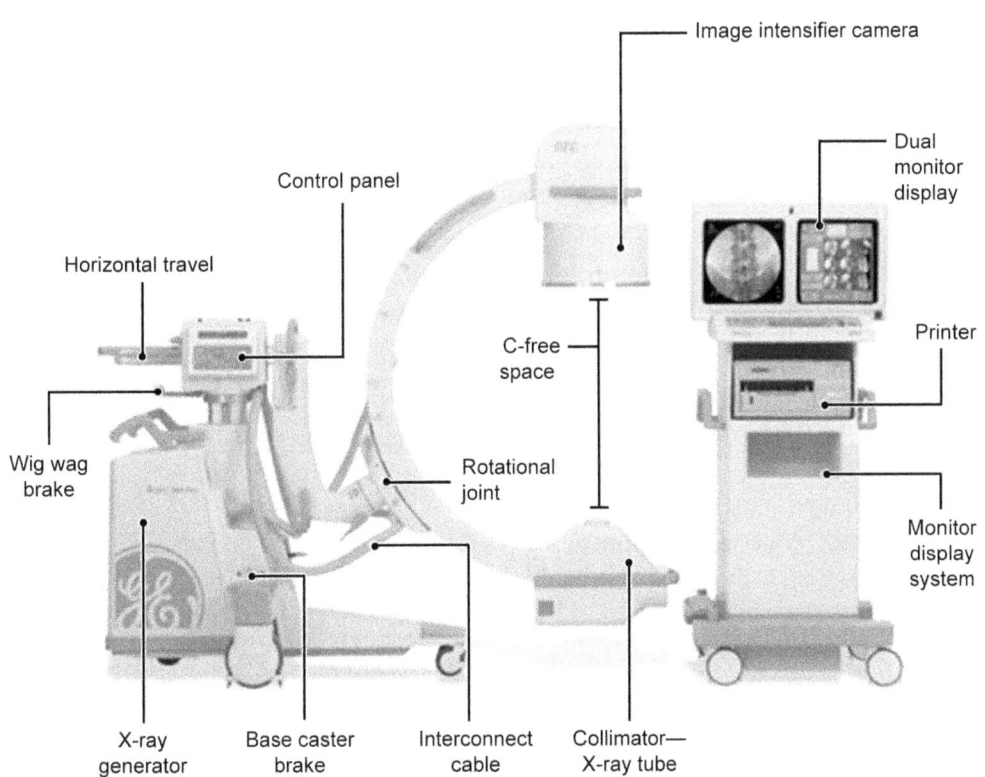

Fig. 7: Modern day image intensifier.

low-intensity ionizing radiation into visible images. The X-ray photons, after passing through the patient, are incident on the photocathode of the input screen of the image intensifier. Some photons get absorbed here, emitting photoelectrons. An electric field applied between the photocathode and the anode causes electrons to accelerate to the anode. The electrons bombard the output phosphor, producing light photons in high numbers. These eventually get caught by imaging devices (screenshot).
3. *Workstation unit:* This is the *control center* of the C-Arm. This bears controls, handles, switches and cable support systems, and a brake pedal.
4. *Charged-coupled device camera:* The camera converts a visual input into an image or video. They are quite like digital cameras.

Ergonomics

Practicing good ergonomics is an essential part of the interventional practice. This goes a long way in preventing long-term musculoskeletal disorders in operators. Chief recommendations are as follows:
- The operator should improve overall core body strength to combat long hours of axial loading.
- Assuming good posture—upright posture, not slouching forwards or bending sideways.
- Monitor straight ahead, 15° lower than the eye level. The physician's forearm, needle, and line of vision to the monitor should be in one of the same plane.
- Appropriate radiation protective garments—lead apron, lead gloves, and lead glasses should be worn and their usage should be limited to just the operating room.
- For more support, lumbar/abdominal support belts may be used. For longer procedures, intermittently, a 6-inch footrest can be employed.

Uses

Almost all chronic pain procedures can be done under fluoroscopic guidance. But with the ever-increasing use of ultrasound in chronic pain, most procedures are done under ultrasound guidance. The advantages are obvious—real-time imaging with no radiation exposure. However, fluoro guidance together with ultrasound-guided localization offers advantages of both—minimizing radiation and observing dye spread but increases the cost for the patient.

Ultrasound

Over years, ultrasound imaging has emerged as a handy modality to localize the structures of interest. In some blocks, it is considered to be superior to fluoro for guidance. However, it has its own shortcomings. The quality of the image is dependent upon the overall fat and connective tissue. Excess fat or air bubbles obscure the visibility of the targeted structures. Thus, as much as we would like to eliminate the radiation exposure completely with the use of ultrasound, fluoro is here to stay. The description of this modality is beyond the scope of the chapter.

RADIOFREQUENCY GENERATOR

Definition

A radiofrequency generator is an instrument for delivering high-frequency waves for targeted thermal damage of the neural tissue to modulate neurotransmission of pain signals.

Introduction

Radiofrequency (RF) has been in use for almost a century. It began its use in the early

19th century. For almost three decades its use was limited only to Gasserian ganglion radioablation. Later, the use expanded to percutaneous cordotomy, medial branch RFA, dorsal root ganglion RFA, and lesions of the communicating ramus and sympathetic chain. More recently, as late as 1996, RF of the nucleus of the disk was described.

The basic premise of its usage was supposed to be thermocoagulation. This concept remained unchallenged till very recently. There appeared a gap in the true understanding—one because the effect of pain relief extended way beyond the duration of sensory loss; second, the effect of 40° and 67° lesioning appeared similar and third, on creating a lesion between the peripheral nerve and DRG, that is distal to the pathology, lesioning was successful. So, with this background, pulsed radiofrequency was born.

Parts of a Radiofrequency Generator

A radiofrequency lesion generator system should have the following parts:
- Continuous impedance measurement—this enables the measurement of continuity of the electrical circuit. A break in the circuit would lead to high impedance. The acceptable impedances may vary between different tissues, they are:
  - Extradural tissues—300-600 ohms
  - Cordotomies—1,000 ohms
  - Disk lesions—up to 200 ohms
- Nerve stimulator—this helps to localize the electrodeposition at the desired site. Sensory stimulation is carried out at 50 Hz, while motor at 2 Hz
- Voltage, current, wattage monitor during interim lesioning
- Temperature monitor
- Pulsed current delivery mode.

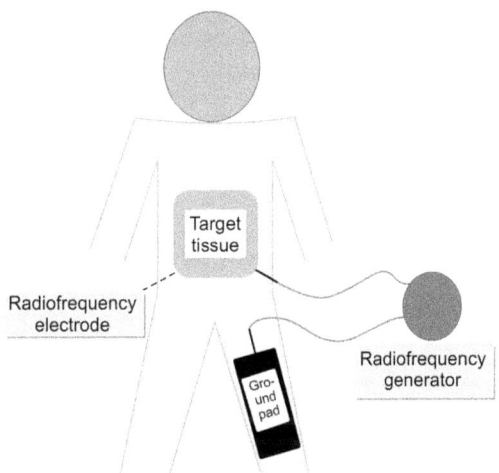

Fig. 8: A schematic diagram showing the application of the radiofrequency circuit.

Circuit

The circuit is formed by the body tissue, electrode, radiofrequency generator system, and grounding pad. A schematic diagram of the circuit formed by the radiofrequency system in the target tissue has been shown in the given figure **(Fig. 8)**.

Physiological Effects

Continuous Radiofrequency

The continuous radiofrequency produces its effects through thermocoagulation or heat lesioning. The size of the lesion depends on the temperature of the tip of the electrode.

Pulsed Radiofrequency

The pulsed radiofrequency produces both thermal and nonthermal effects in the tissues. Some destructive effects because of temperature have been described. But its most important effects are largely nonthermal. The nonthermal effects range from affecting the conductance of the various ion channels (sodium, potassium, calcium) to the death of the cell.

TABLE 2: Uses of the radiofrequency generator.

S. no.	Clinical conditions	Targeted structures
1.	Trigeminal neuralgia	Gasserian ganglion
2.	Cluster headache	Sphenopalatine ganglion
3.	Cervical brachialgia	Cervical dorsal root ganglion (of the specific cervical level)
4.	Cervical facetogenic pain/cervicogenic headache	Medial branch RF (of the specific level)
5.	Thoracic facetal pain	Thoracic medial branch RF (of the specific level)
6.	Lumbar facetal pain	Lumbar medial branch RF (of the desired level)
7.	Lumbar radicular pain	Lumbar DRG RF (of the desired level)
8.	Discogenic pain	Pulsed RF of the nucleus
9.	Intractable sacropelvic region pain/CRPS	Pulsed RF of the sympathetic chain
10.	Visceral pain (chronic pancreatitis/pancreatic cancer/liver cancer/postabdominal surgery pain	RF of the splanchnic nerves
11.	Intractable sacroiliac joint dysfunction	Cooled RF
12.	Knee osteoarthritic	Genicular nerve RF/cooled RF

(CRPS: complex regional pain syndrome; RF: radiofrequency)

Cooled Radiofrequency

The problem with the use of continuous radiofrequency is that of charring of the nearby tissues. The charred tissue acts as an insulator for further heat lesioning. Higher electrode temperature leads to more charring, thereby, limiting the lesion. This limitation led to the development of cooled RF probes that employ the use of water circulation around the tip to keep the temperature rise in check. This, in turn, causes a larger lesion size than conventional RF. A separate machine is used for this purpose.

Uses

There are various potential uses of the radiofrequency generator. Conditions in which the RFAs are commonly done are mentioned in **Table 2**.

For successful chronic pain blocks, one needs a variety of instruments. In this chapter, we stick to the most used instruments in chronic pain. It is imperative that we have a sound understanding of the different instruments and modalities used for smooth interventions. Newer and better modifications keep adding every day, however, the knowledge of these basic instruments can lead us to understand the more advanced instruments.

FURTHER READING

1. Barendse GA, van Den Berg SG, Kessels AH, Weber WE, van Kleef M. Randomized controlled trial of percutaneous intradiscal radiofrequency thermocoagulation for chronic discogenic back pain: lack of effect from a 90-second 70 C lesion. Spine (Phila Pa 1976). 2001;26(3):287-92.
2. Bellini M, Barbieri M. Cooled radiofrequency system relieves chronic knee osteoarthritis pain: the first case-series. Anaesthesiol Intensive Ther. 2015;47(1):30-3.

3. Benjamin JL, Meisinger QC. Ergonomics in the development and prevention of musculoskeletal injury in interventional radiologists. Tech Vasc Interv Radiol. 2018; 21(1):16-20.
4. Bushberg JT, Seibert JA, Jr EML, Boone JM. The Essential Physics of Medical Imaging, 3rd edition. United States: Lippincott Williams & Wilkins; 2011.
5. Erdine S, Yucel A, Cimen A, Aydin S, Sav A, Bilir A. Effects of pulsed versus conventional radiofrequency current on rabbit dorsal root ganglion morphology. Eur J. 2005;9(3):251-6.
6. Heggie JCP, Lidell NA, Maher KP. Applied Imaging Technology, 4th edition. Melbourne: St Vincent's Hospital; 2001.
7. Racz® Catheter Products. (2021). Epimed Catheters. [online] Available from: https://online.pubhtml5.com/rgkv/absw/#p=2. [Last accessed April, 2022].
8. Radiopaedia. Image intensifier. Radiology Reference Article (Murphy A, Jones J.) Radiopaedia.org. [online]. Available from: https://radiopaedia.org/articles/image-intensifier. [Last Accessed April, 2022].
9. Slappendel R, Crul BJP, Braak GJJ, Geurts JWM, Booij LHDJ, Voerman VF, et al. The efficacy of radiofrequency lesioning of the cervical spinal dorsal root ganglion in a double blinded randomized study: no difference between 40 degrees C and 67 degrees C treatments. Pain. 1997;73(2):159-63.
10. Teixeira A, Grandinson M, Sluijter ME. Pulsed radiofrequency for radicular pain due to a herniated intervertebral disc—an initial report. Pain Pract. 2005;5(2):111-5.
11. van Kleef M, Spaans F, Dingemans W, Barendse GAM, Floor E, Sluijter ME. Effects and side effects of a percutaneous thermal lesion of the dorsal root ganglion in patients with cervical pain syndrome. Pain. 1993; 52(1):49-53.
12. Weaver JC. Electroporation: a general phenomenon for manipulating cells and tissues. J Cell Biochem. 1993;51(4):426-35.

Physics in Anesthesia

T Nageswara Rao

INTRODUCTION

Understanding of physics and its clinical application allows the anesthetist to give safe anesthesia. Here in this chapter, we cover basic physics applicable to practical anesthesia only.

PRESSURE

Pressure is the force applied or distributed over a surface and is expressed as force per unit area. *Force* is that which changes or tends to change the state of rest or motion of an object. Force is measured in newtons (N).

$$N = kg \times m/s^2$$

Pressure $(P) = \frac{F}{a}$, where f = force and a = area.

Units

Pascal (SI unit), mm Hg, cmH$_2$O, psi, bar, and Torr.

Clinical Application

Pressures in anesthesia cylinders and pipelines.

FLOW

Flow is the quantity, either gas or liquid passing a cross-sectional area per unit of time.

$$F = Q/t$$

where "Q" is the quantity and "t" is the time. This flow can be laminar or turbulent.

Laminar Flow

The gas passes through a smooth tube without eddies, where central flow is high. This is directly proportional to pressure.

Clinical Application

Low flow rates in breathing systems, airways, and circulation.

Hegan–Poiseuilles Law

The velocity of the steady flow of a fluid through a narrow tube (as a blood vessel or a catheter) varies directly as the pressure and the fourth power of the radius of the tube and inversely as the length of the tube and the coefficient of viscosity. This is seen in laminar flow.

Clinical Application

Endotracheal tube (ETT), tracheostomy tube, IV catheter.

- Q Flow rate
- P Pressure
- r Radius
- η Fluid viscosity
- l Length of tubing

$$Q = \frac{\pi P r^4}{8 \eta l}$$

Turbulent Flow

In this type of flow, fluid swirls in eddies with high resistance. Here the flow is directly proportional to the square root of the pressure.

The factors that determine turbulent flow can be combined to form an equation that calculates the Reynolds number. If it is <2,000 laminar flow, 2,000–4,000 transitional flow and >4,000 turbulent flow.

Clinical Application

Sudden rise inflow through a tube, like at the origin of orifice or acute bends.

Grahams Law

Flow rate is directly proportional to the square root of the pressure gradient on either side of the tube and inversely proportional to the square root of the density of the fluid. The diffusion of a gas is inversely proportional to the square root of its molecular weight.

Viscosity

- Viscosity is a property of the fluid (blood) which reduces the flow.
- Low temperatures with smoking and elderly age increase viscosity.

Bernoulli's Principle

A gas flowing through a tube encounters a constriction, the pressure drops, and the velocity increases. This explains the Venturi effect.

Venturi Principle

Increase in the speed of a fluid/gas results in decrease in internal pressure, when passed through a cone-shaped or hourglass tube.

Clinical Application

Air entrainment devices, Venturi masks, Pethik's test.

Entrainment ratio = Entrainment flow/Driving flow

Coandă Effect

It is the tendency of the fluid jet to attach to a nearby surface. It is also called *wall attachment*. It remains attached even when the surface curves away from the initial jet direction. When a narrow tube is attached to a wide bore Y-connector, the flow unevenly divides between the two outlets and attaches to one side only.

Clinical Application

- There is an unequal gas flow to the alveoli where a slight narrowing of the bronchiole before it divides, and a mucus plug at the branching of the tracheobronchial tree, leading to unequal distribution of gases.
- Switching flow ventilator valve.

Fick Principle

Fick's law states that the rate of diffusion of a substance across a unit area (such as a surface or membrane) is proportional to the concentration gradient.

GAS LAWS

Gas laws tell how they react under altered pressure and temperature.

Standard Temperature and Pressure

Conditions, where the temperature is 273.15 K (0°C) and the atmospheric pressure is 101.3 kPa (760 mm Hg).

Avogadro's Law

Equal volumes of gases at the same temperature and pressure contain the same number of molecules.

Number of molecules = Number of moles × Avogadro's number

- *The mole:* One mole is defined as 12 g of carbon (C-12) containing 6.022×10^{23} atoms.
- *The molar mass:* The molar mass of a substance is the mass of 6.022×10^{23} particles of

the substance and is measured in grams per mole (g·mol^{-1}).

Mass of a substance = molar mass × number of moles

For example, 32 g of O_2 occupies 22.4 L at standard temperature and pressure (STP).

- *Partial pressure of a gas in solution:* Partial pressure of gas in a gas mixture that is in equilibrium with the solution.

Dalton's Law

The partial pressure of a gas in a gas mixture is the pressure that this gas would exert if it occupied the total volume of the mixture in the absence of the other components. Dalton's law for a gas, the total pressure is simply all the partial pressures added together.

$$P_T = P_1 + P_2 + P_3$$

General Gas Law or Universal Gas Law

$$PV = RT$$

(where P = pressure, V = volume, T = Temperature and R is constant)

Boyle's Law (The First Ideal Gas Law)

The volume of a gas is inversely proportional to its pressure (at a fixed temperature).

$$P \propto 1/V$$

At constant temperature, $P_1V_1 = P_2V_2$.

Clinical Application

Gas in a cylinder, work of breathing, diving.

Charle's Law (The Second Ideal Gas Law)

At a given pressure the temperature is directly proportional to the volume of a gas.

$$V \propto T$$

$V_1/V_2 = T_1/T_2$ at constant pressure.

Clinical Application

Bourdon thermometer, exacerbation of the bends (expansion of the small bubbles of nitrogen post diving)

The Pressure Law (Gay-Lussac's Law; the Third Ideal Gas Law)

The pressure of a gas is directly proportional to its temperature (within a fixed volume).

$$P \propto T$$

Clinical Application

Filling ratios (the degree to which a cylinder should be filled is partly dependent on the pressure law. The filling ratios for gas cylinders must take into account the rise in pressure in a cylinder associated with a rise in temperature. If the pressure reaches a critical level the cylinder will rupture at its weakest point and explode. For this reason, cylinders should be filled at the ambient temperature at which they are going to be stored and used. Scuba diving tanks are often filled in a water bath set to the temperature appropriate to the location of the dive.

Combined Gas Law

The gas laws (Boyle's law, Charles's law, and the pressure law) may be combined into one equation called the combined gas law. A condition for the combined gas equation is that the amount of gas must remain constant. The combined gas law simply states that the product of pressure and volume is proportional to the absolute temperature:

$$P.V \propto T$$
$$P_1.V_1/T_1 = P_2.V_2/T_2$$

Henry's Law

Concentration of gas dissolved in a liquid is proportional to its partial pressure.

$$C_x = K P_x$$

(where C is concentration and P is partial pressure).

According to this law, the partial pressure of the anesthetic agent in the blood is proportional to the partial pressure of the volatile in the alveoli. Therefore, if the inspired concentration of the volatile agents in the gas mixture is increased, then the concentration in the blood will also increase.

QUESTION

Q. 1. What is microshock and macroshock? Method to prevention.

FURTHER READING

1. Dorsch JA, Dorsch SE. Understanding Anaesthesia Equipment, 2012.

80. Electrocardiogram and X-ray

Ridhima Bhatia, Puneet Khanna

ELECTROCARDIOGRAM

- *12 lead electrocardiogram (ECG):*
  - 6 limb leads (lead I, II, and III, aVR, aVF, aVL)
  - I, II, and III—bipolar leads
  - aVR, aVF, aVL—unipolar leads
  - 6 chest leads (V1, V2, V3, V4, V5, and V6)—unipolar leads
- *Electrocardiogram paper:*
  - Runs at a standard rate of 25 mm/sec
  - 1 small square = 0.04 second
  - 1 large square = 5 small squares = 0.2 seconds
  - 5 large squares/second or 300/min
  - Vertical axis represents voltage, 1 small square = 0.1 mV
- *Normal ECG description:* Rate, rhythm, axis, components of ECG, and conclusion
- *Rate calculation:*
  - Regular rhythm—1,500/number of small squares between one R-R interval or 300/number of large squares between one R-R interval.
  - Irregular rhythm—the number of R-R intervals in 3 seconds (15 large squares) multiplied by 20.
- *Axis:*
  - Normal = –30 to +90
  - Left axis deviation = –30 to –90
  - Right axis deviation = +90 to +150
- Components of ECG **(Fig. 1 and Table 1)**.

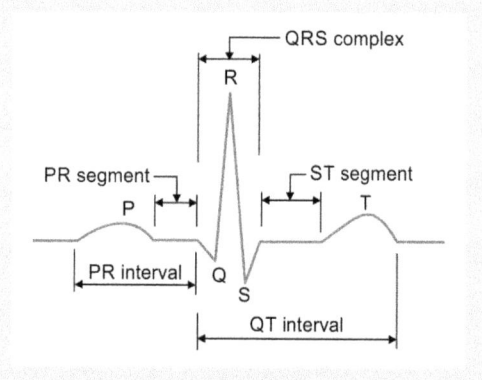

Fig. 1: Components of electrocardiogram (ECG).

Normal Electrocardiogram (Fig. 2)

- Sinus rhythm, rate 75/min
- Normal axis
- Normal PR interval, 0.12 second
- Normal QRS complex duration, 0.12 second
- Normal ST segment and T wave.

Rhythm Abnormalities

Sinus Bradycardia (Fig. 3)

- Sinus rhythm, rate 42/min
- Normal axis and normal components
- *Definition:* Rate <50/min or <60/min associated with symptoms
- *Causes:*
  - Physiological: Sleep, athlete, starvation
  - Pathological:
    - Raised intracranial pressure (ICP), hypothyroidism

TABLE 1: Components and duration of ECG.

Component		Duration
P wave	Represents depolarization through atrial myocardium	0.12 second
PR interval	• Beginning of P wave to beginning of QRS complex • Time is taken by the electrical impulse to travel from SA node to AV node	0.12–0.2 seconds/ 3–5 small squares
QRS complex	Represents ventricular depolarization	0.08–0.12 seconds/3 small squares
T wave	Ventricular repolarization	0.12–0.16 seconds
QT interval	Beginning of QRS complex to end of T wave	0.2–0.4 seconds
ST segment	Plateau phase of ventricular action potential	0.08–0.12 seconds

(SA: sinoatrial; AV: atrioventricular)

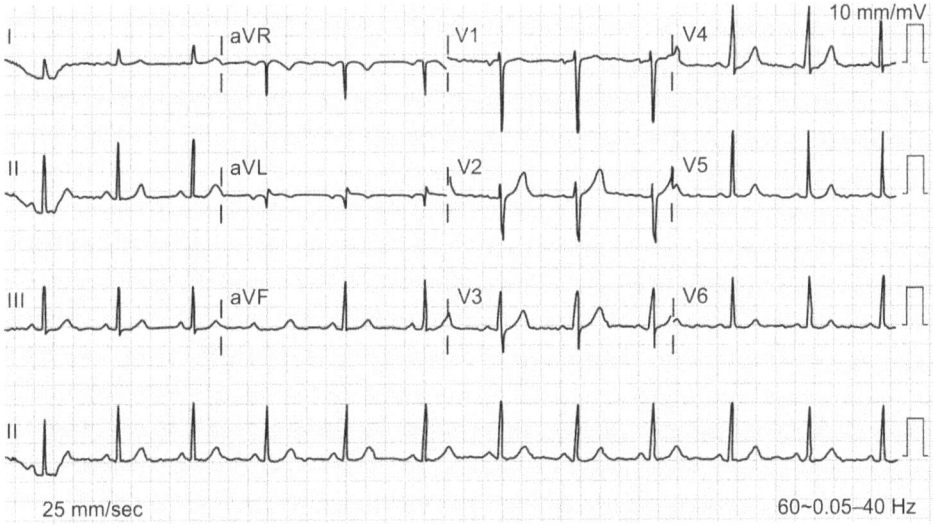

Fig. 2: Normal electrocardiogram (ECG).

- Obstructive jaundice [the action of bile salts on sinoatrial (SA) node]
- Glaucoma
- Vasovagal syncope
- Drugs—β-blockers, calcium channel blockers, digitalis
- *Treatment:* Advanced Cardiovascular Life Support (ACLS) bradyarrhythmia algorithm
  - Drugs:
    - Injection of atropine—1 mg repeated every 3–5 minutes up to 3 mg
    - Injection of dopamine—5–20 µg/kg/min
    - Injection of epinephrine—2–10 µg/min
  - Transcutaneous pacing
  - Transvenous pacing.

Sinus Tachycardia (Fig. 4)

- Sinus rhythm, rate 150/min
- Normal axis and normal components
- *Definition:* Rate more than 100/min

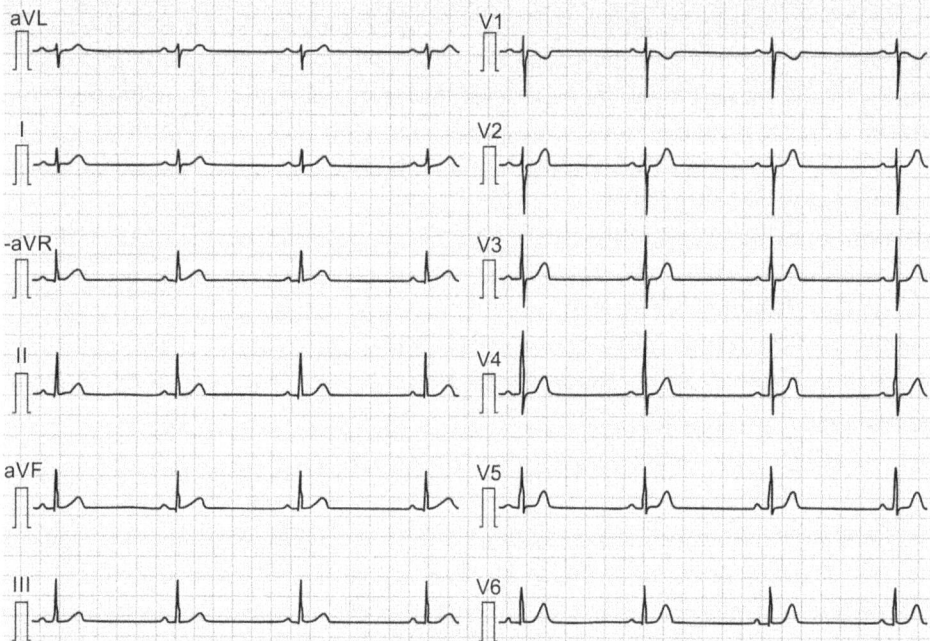

Fig. 3: Sinus bradycardia.

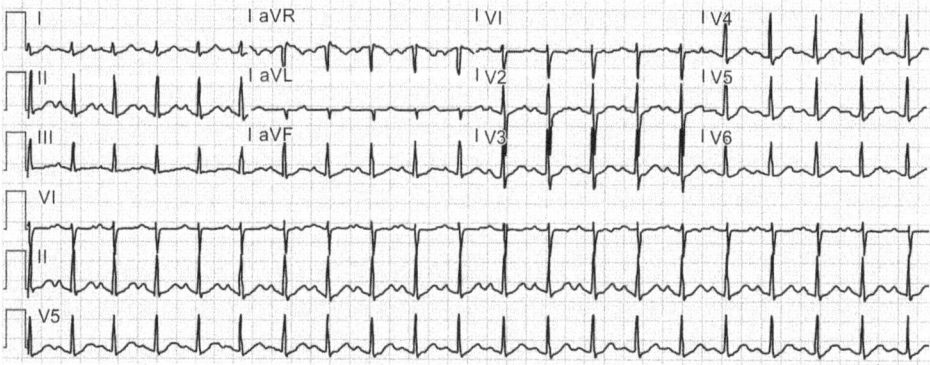

Fig. 4: Sinus tachycardia.

- *Causes:*
    - Physiological: Exercise, pregnancy, and high altitude
    - Pathological:
        - Hypermetabolic states such as thyrotoxicosis, and fever
        - Pain
        - Anxiety
        - Excessive caffeine intake
        - Hemorrhage
        - Drugs such as atropine and adrenaline
- *Treatment:* Symptomatic treatment
    - Analgesic
    - Antianxiety
    - Fluid challenge
    - Drugs–β-blocker

Conduction Abnormalities

Interference with the conduction process causes the results in the phenomenon known as "heart block".

First Degree Heart Block

- *Diagnosis*:
  - One P wave per QRS complex (regular rhythm)
  - Prolonged PR interval >0.2 seconds **(Fig. 5)**.
- *Causes*:
  - Idiopathic
  - Coronary artery disease
  - Acute rheumatic disease
  - Digoxin toxicity
  - Electrolyte disturbances
- *Treatment*:
  - No specific action is needed.

Second Degree Heart Block (Fig. 6)

- *Mobitz type I (Wenckebach phenomenon)*
  - Gradual increase in PR interval followed by failure of conduction of atrial beat.
  - Usually benign
  - Treatment not needed
- *Mobitz type II*
  - Constant PR interval
  - Intermittent block in the conduction of the P wave to the ventricles
- *Causes*:
  - Coronary artery disease
  - Acute rheumatic disease
  - Digoxin toxicity
- *Treatment*:
  - 3:1 or 4:1 block may need temporary or permanent pacing.

Third Degree Heart Block/Complete Heart Block (Fig. 7)

- *Diagnosis*
  - Normal atrial contraction but not conducted to the ventricles.
  - Ventricles excited by slow "escape mechanism".
  - Complete interruption of AV conduction—AV disassociation.
  - No relation between P waves and QRS complexes.
- *Causes*:
  - Acute myocardial infarction.
  - Fibrosis around the bundle of His.
- *Treatment*:
  - Pacemaker insertion.

Right Bundle Branch Block (Fig. 8)

- *Diagnosis*:
  - Right axis deviation
  - QRS duration >0.12 seconds
  - RSR' pattern in V1-3 ("M-shaped" QRS complex)
  - Wide, slurred S wave in lateral leads (I, aVL, V5-6)
  - RSR' pattern with normal QRS width; incomplete right bundle branch block (RBBB)

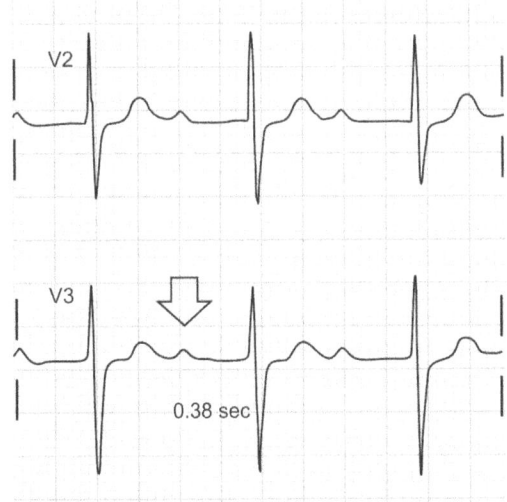

Fig. 5: First degree heart block.

Second degree AV block (Mobitz I or Wenckebach)

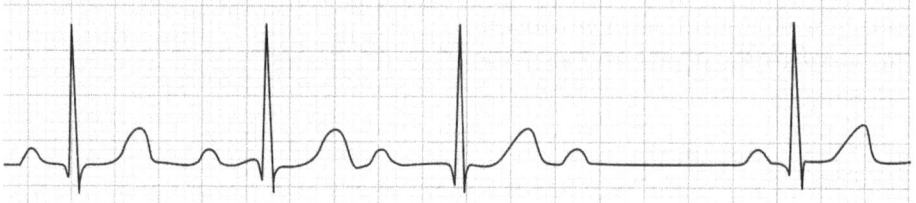

Second degree AV block (Mobitz II)

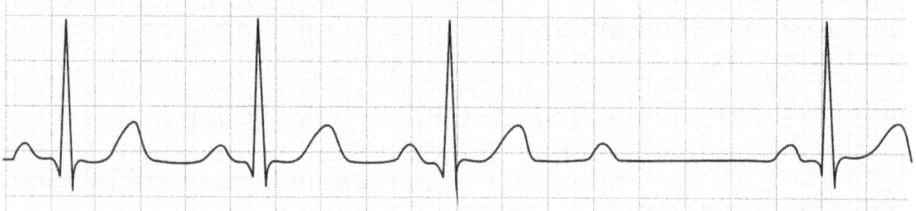

Second degree AV block (2:1 block)

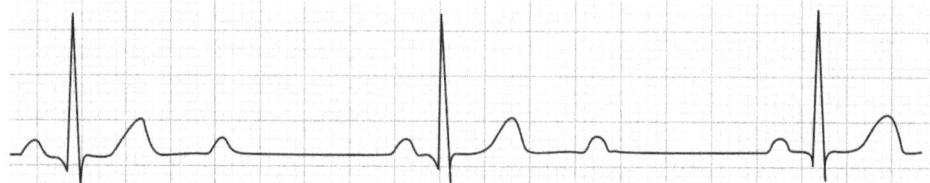

Fig. 6: Second degree heart block.

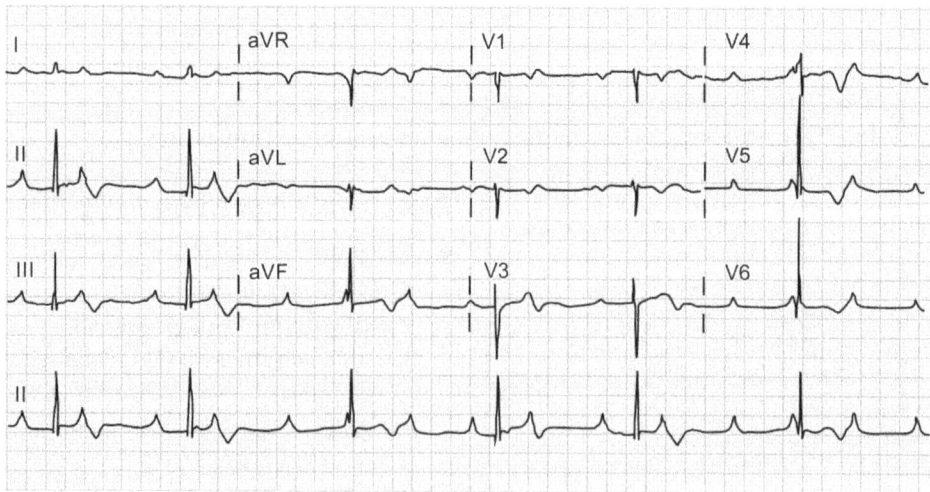

Fig. 7: Third degree heart block/complete heart block.

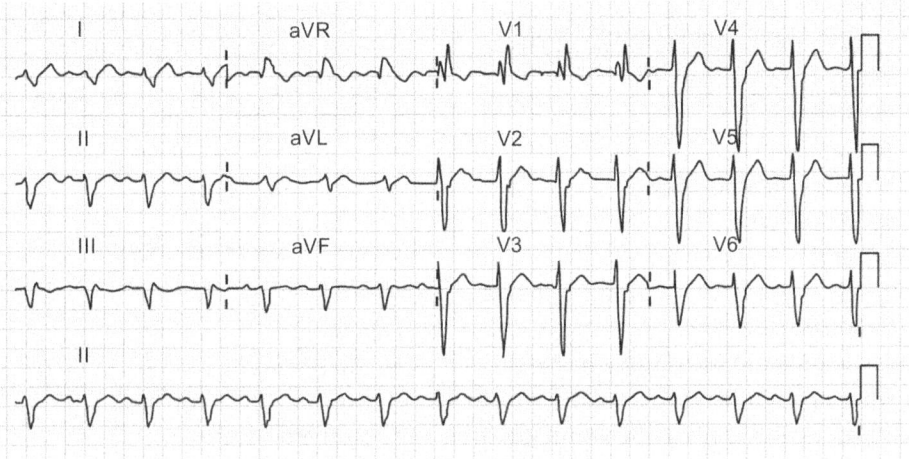

Fig. 8: Right bundle branch block.

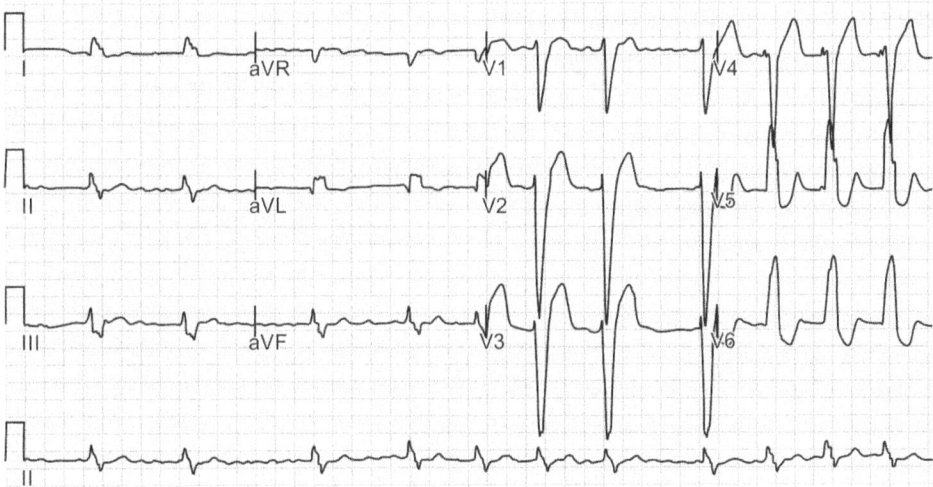

Fig. 9: Left bundle branch block.

- *Causes:*
  - Normal individuals
  - Right ventricular hypertrophy
  - Pulmonary embolus
  - Ischemic heart disease
  - Rheumatic heart disease
  - Congenital heart disease (e.g., atrial septal defect)
- *Treatment:*
  - No specific action needed.

Left Bundle Branch Block (Fig. 9)

- *Diagnosis:*
  - Left axis deviation.
  - QRS duration >0.12 seconds.
  - Dominant S wave in V1 (W pattern).
  - Broad monophasic R wave, M pattern in V6.
  - Sometimes inverted T waves lead I aVL, V5, V6.

- Causes:
  - Interior myocardial infarction (MI)
  - Dilated cardiomyopathy
  - Hypertension
  - Aortic stenosis
  - Ischemic heart disease
  - Hyperkalemia
- Treatment:
  - If the patient is asymptomatic, no action is needed.
  - If the patient has recently had severe chest pain, the left bundle branch block (LBBB) may indicate an acute MI, and thrombolysis should be considered.

Abnormal Supraventricular Rhythms

Premature Atrial Contraction (Fig. 10)

- Diagnosis:
  - Abnormal or absent P wave
  - Early QRS complex
  - Normal QRS complex and T wave
  - Next P wave is reset
- Causes:
  - Coronary artery disease
  - Hypertrophic cardiomyopathy
  - Left-ventricular hypertrophy
- Treatment:
  - Asymptomatic—no treatment
  - Symptomatic—β-blockers or anti-arrhythmic drugs.

Paroxysmal Supraventricular Tachycardia (Fig. 11)

- Diagnosis:
  - No P waves
  - Narrow QRS
  - Sudden onset
  - Stops abruptly
  - Rate >200/min
- Causes:
  - Idiopathic
  - Thyrotoxicosis
  - Excessive caffeine intake
  - Drugs—adrenaline, amphetamines
  - Sepsis
- Treatment:
  - Usually benign
  - Persistent may lead to heart failure
  - Beta-blockers or antiarrhythmic drugs
  - Vagal maneuvers.

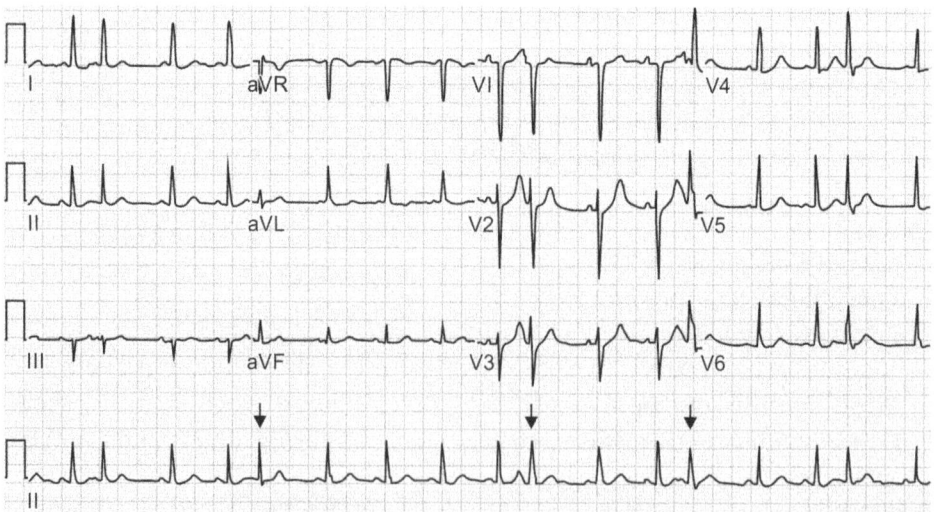

Fig. 10: Premature atrial contraction.

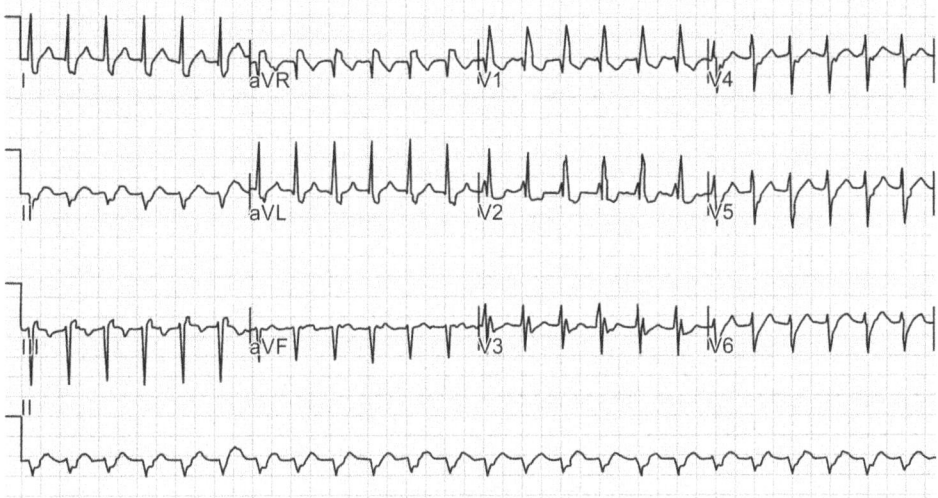

Fig. 11: Paroxysmal supraventricular tachycardia (PSVT).

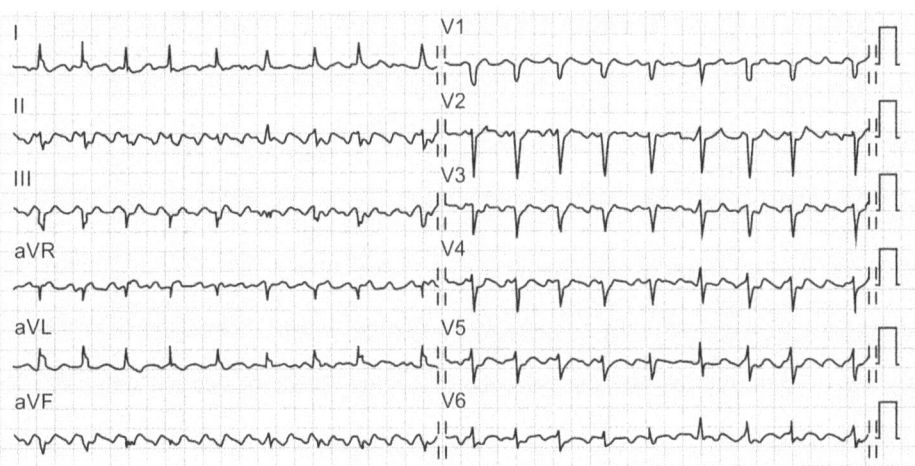

Fig. 12: Atrial flutter.

Atrial Flutter (Fig. 12)

- Diagnosis:
    - Atrial rate/P wave >250/min
    - Narrow QRS complex
    - Saw tooth pattern
    - It may be associated with 2:1, 3:1, or 4:1 block increased by vagal maneuver
- Treatment:
    - Asymptomatic—no treatment
    - Symptomatic—cardioversion may be needed.

Atrial Fibrillation (Fig. 13)

- Diagnosis:
    - Irregular rhythm
    - No P waves
    - Narrow QRS complex
    - Rate >300/min
- Causes:
    - Hypertension
    - Valvular heart disease (especially mitral stenosis/regurgitation)
    - Acute infections

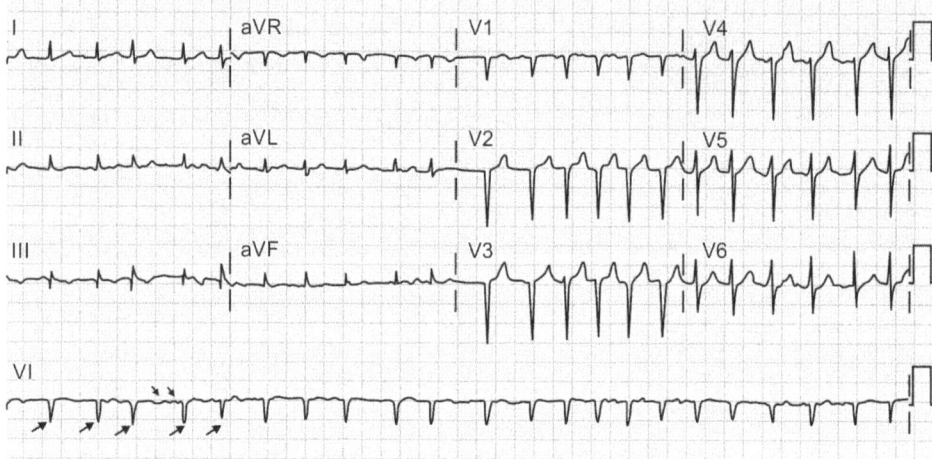

Fig. 13: Atrial fibrillation.

- Electrolyte disturbance (hypokalemia, hypomagnesemia)
- Thyrotoxicosis
- Drugs (e.g., sympathomimetics)
- Alcohol
- Pulmonary embolus
- Pericardial disease
- *Treatment:*
  - Stable patient—medical management
  - Hemodynamically unstable patient—urgent synchronized direct current (DC) cardioversion (200 J).

Ventricular Rhythms

Characteristics

- Wide QRS complex
- Abnormal axis
- Abnormal T waves.

Ventricular Ectopic (Fig. 14)

- *Diagnosis:*
  - Early and wide QRS complex
  - No P wave
  - Abnormally shaped QRS complex and T wave
  - Next P wave is on time
- Usually benign and do not need treatment.

Ventricular Tachycardia

Rhythm faster than 100/min with pacemaker distal to bundle of His.

- *Diagnosis:*
  - No P waves
  - Rate >160/min
  - Broad QRS complex with abnormal shape
  - No identifiable T waves
- *Types:*
  - *Monomorphic ventricular tachycardia (VT):* A single focus gives rise to ventricular activation; hence, morphology remains the same **(Fig. 15)**.
  - *Polymorphic VT:* Multiple focuses give rise to ventricular activation, resulting in different ECG patterns **(Fig. 16)**.
  - *Torsade-de-pointes (TdP):* A polymorphic VT associated with the long QT syndromes.
- *Causes:*
  - Ischemic heart disease
  - Cardiomyopathy
  - Polymorphic VT and TdP can be drug-induced or due to hypokalemia

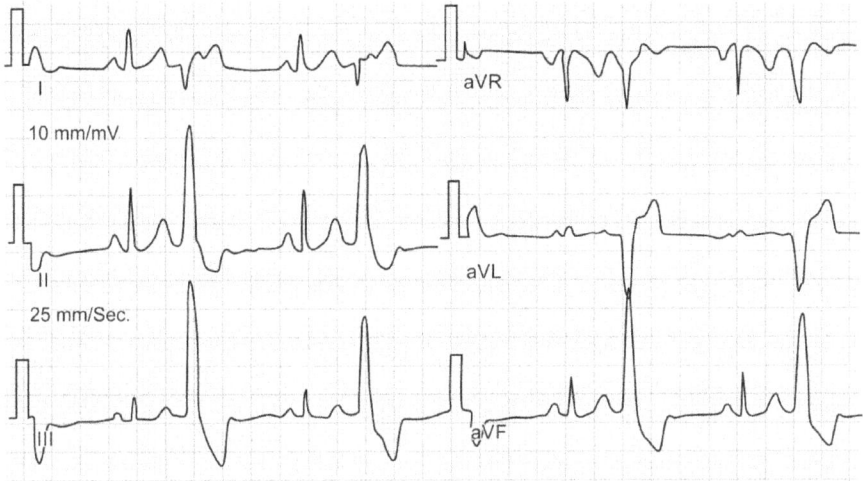

Fig. 14: Ventricular ectopic.

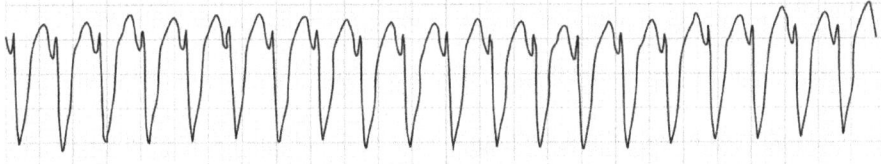

Fig. 15: Monomorphic ventricular tachycardia (VT).

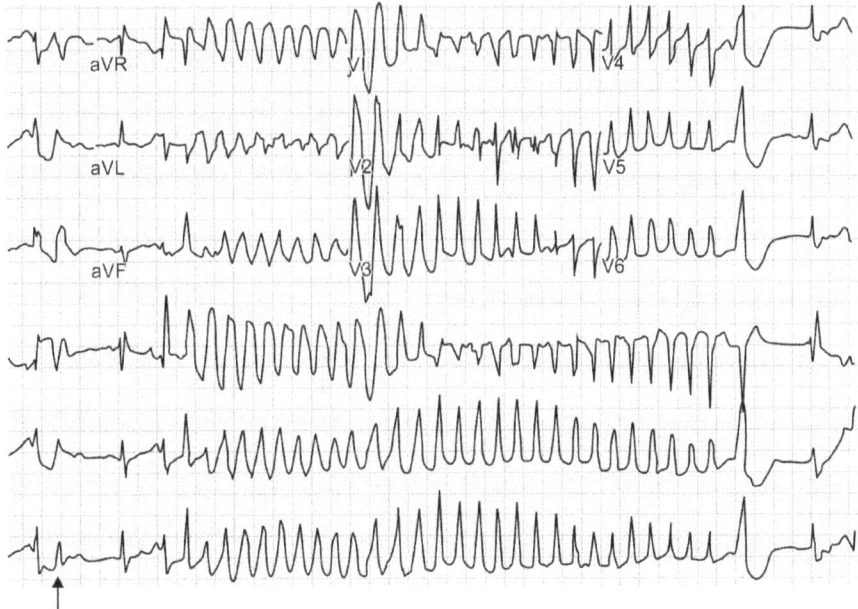

Fig. 16: Polymorphic VT.

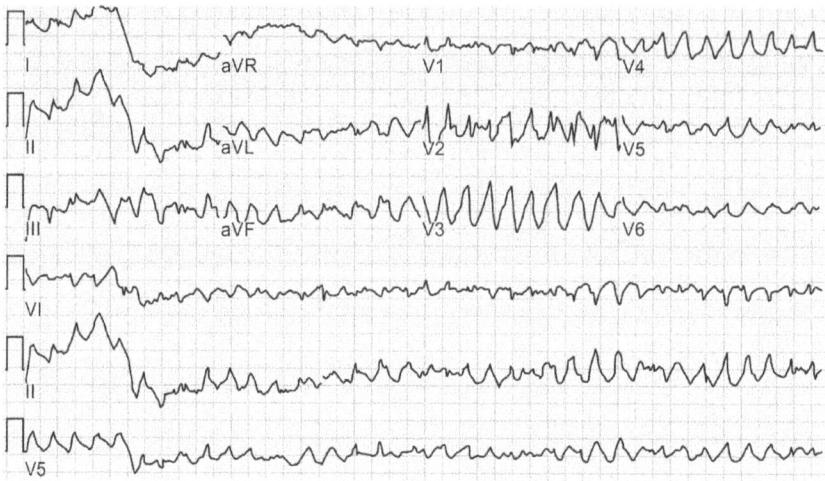

Fig. 17: Ventricular fibrillation.

- *Treatment:*
  - VT with a pulse—drugs:
    - Adenosine for monomorphic VT only
    - Antiarrhythmic drugs (amiodarone, procainamide, sotalol)
    - *Cardioversion*—100 J for unstable monomorphic VT
  - Unstable polymorphic VT to be treated as ventricular fibrillation (VF)
  - Pulseless VT—follow ACLS cardiac arrest algorithm.

Ventricular Fibrillation (Fig. 17)

- *Diagnosis:*
  - Individual ventricular muscle contracts independently resulting in disorganized ECG
  - Unconscious patient
- *Treatment:*
  - ACLS cardiac arrest algorithm.

CHEST X-RAY

Basic Interpretation and Technical Quality of the Chest X-ray

- *Label:* To confirm the name of the patient.
- *Projection:* It is defined by the direction of the X-ray beam in relation to the patient.
  - Mostly posteroanterior (PA) views (X-ray from behind and film in the front), usually not marked
  - Intensive care unit (ICU) and emergency X-rays are mostly anteroposterior (AP) view, mostly marked
  - AP view: Mediastinum appears large—difficult to comment on cardiomegaly.
- *Orientation:* Check the left/right marking. Do not miss *dextrocardia* or *situs inversus*.
- *Rotation*: In the unrotated film, the sternal end (medial ends of clavicle) are equidistant from the spinous process.
- *Exposure/penetration:* In PA view, spinous process of the first four thoracic vertebrae should be visible.
  - Overexposed film—blacker lung fields, increased chance of missing pneumothorax
  - Underexposed film—whiter lung fields.
- *Timing:* Mostly end-inspiratory films. Able to see six anterior or ten posterior ribs.

Scanning the Posteroanterior Film

- Be systematic, so that no anatomical structure is missed
- From center to periphery—mediastinum, lung fields, bones, and soft tissues, abdominal shadows, and foreign bodies.

Mediastinum

- Check size, shape, and position.
- Check if the trachea is central or not.
- *Boundaries:*
  - Right—brachiocephalic vessels, ascending aorta, superior vena cava, and right atrium
  - Left—left brachiocephalic vessel, aortic arch, pulmonary trunk, left atrial appendage, and left ventricle
- Calculate the cardiothoracic ratio. Normally <0.5.

Lung Fields

- There should be equal radiolucency.
- Costophrenic and cardiophrenic angles should be clear.
- Three parts:
  1. *Upper*—from the anterior end of the second rib
  2. *Middle*—2nd to 4th rib
  3. *Lower*—below anterior end of the fourth rib.

Pulmonary Vasculature

- Left hilum (pulmonary artery) is higher than the right
- Both hila should be concave in shape and look similar to each other
- Vessel size is more in lower areas. A reversal occurs in congestive cardiac failure.

Diaphragm

- Right higher (2.5 cm) than the left
- Smooth, curving upwards.

Bone and Soft Tissue

- Look at the ribs, scapulae, and vertebrae
- Look for the fractures
- Look for mass, calcification, subcutaneous emphysema.

Abdominal Shadows

- Look for bowel gas, free air, etc.

Foreign Bodies

- Endotracheal tube—should be above the carina
- Nasogastric tube—below the diaphragm
- Tracheostomy tube
- Central venous catheters (CVC) tip
- Intercostal drain—all eyes should be inside the chest
- Pacemaker
- Other.

Common X-ray

Pneumothorax (Fig. 18)

- The black lung
- Disappearance of vascular shadow
- See upper lobe where air will accumulate first
- Mediastinal shift suggests the development of tension pneumothorax

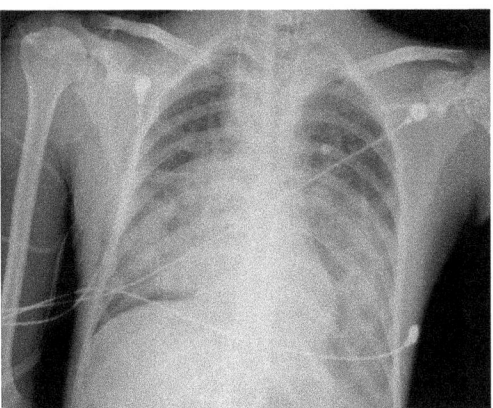

Fig. 18: X-ray of pneumothorax.

- In the expiratory film—lung becomes smaller, pneumothorax is better appreciated.

Questions:
- Causes of pneumothorax:
  - Spontaneous
  - Iatrogenic—CVC insertions, pleural tap, etc.
- Treatment—ICD (to be read in detail)
- Tension pneumothorax and management.

Emphysema/Chronic Obstructive Pulmonary Disease (Fig. 19)

- Check penetration of the film
- Both lungs appear blacker and larger in volume
- Flattened hemidiaphragm (more reliable sign)
- More than seven anterior ribs are visible
- More than 10 posterior ribs are visible
- Tubular heart (in right ventricular hypertrophy)
- Bilaterally reduced lung marking.

Questions:
- Pathophysiology of COPD, emphysema, and asthma
- Preoperative evaluation
- Bedside pulmonary function tests (PFT)
- Optimization of the patient
- Intraoperative and postoperative management.

Collapse

- Important cause of white lung on X-ray.
- Right-sided collapse—right lung smaller than the left.
- Left-sided collapse—distorted position of right diaphragm compared to left.
- Heart shadow or mediastinal shift to the side of collapse.
- Tracheal shift towards the side of collapse **(Fig. 20)**.

Questions:
- Causes of lobar collapse—luminal mass (neoplasm, mucous plug), inflammation [tuberculosis (TB), sarcoidosis], external compression (lymph node, aneurysm)
- Causes of postoperative lobar collapse
- Postoperative pulmonary complication
- Measure to prevent postoperative pulmonary complication.

Consolidation

- Alveolar spaces are filled with fluid—making them appear white whereas airways retain air and look black.

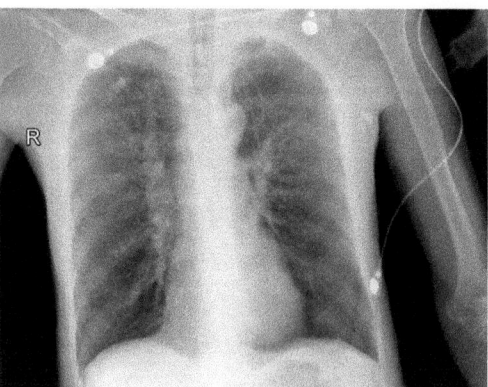

Fig. 19: X-ray of emphysema/chronic obstructive pulmonary disease (COPD).

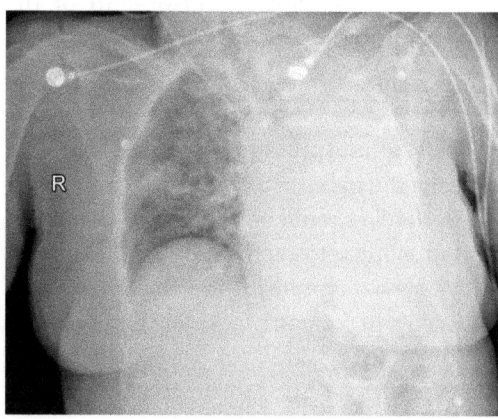

Fig. 20: X-ray of collapse.

- Appears as black small airways against white background known as an *air bronchogram*
- The better demarcated lower border
- History symptom of fever.

Questions

- Causes of consolidation
- Management of consolidation.

Bronchiectasis

- Ring shadows up to 1 cm in diameter
- Can be single or in groups, giving rise to a *honeycomb appearance*
- Tubular shadows—solid thick white shadows.

Questions

- Causes and clinical features of bronchiectasis
- Preoperative optimization
- Role of physiotherapy
- Intraoperative and postoperative management.

Pleural Effusion

- Whiteness at the base of the lung
- Absent air bronchogram
- Concave upper border.

Questions

- Causes of pleural effusion
- Management
- Intercostal drainage (ICD).

Congenital Diaphragmatic Hernia

- X-ray of a child with bowel loops in the hemithorax
- Viva follows on congenital diaphragmatic hernia (CDH).

Mitral Stenosis

- Straightened left heart border
- Enlarged pulmonary conus
- Elevation of left main bronchus—*antler sign* or *mustache sign*
- Double atrial shadow
- Kerley B lines.

FURTHER READING

1. American Heart Association. (2020). Algorithms. [online] Available from: https://cpr.heart.org/en/resuscitation-science/cpr-and-ecc-guidelines/algorithms [Last accessed May, 2022].
2. Gropper M, Eriksson L, Fleisher L, Wiener-Kronish J, Cohen N, Leslie K. Miller Anesthesia, 9th edition. Amsterdam: Elsevier; 2019.
3. Hampton JR. ECG Made Easy, 8th edition. London: Churchill Livingstone; 2013.

Point-of-care Ultrasonography for the Postgraduates

Praveen Talawar, Vadhan Prasanna S, Sangadala Priyanka

INTRODUCTION

The point-of-care ultrasonography (POCUS) is emerging as a bedside tool revolutionizing the diagnosis and patient outcomes. It is useful in bedside assessment of life-threatening conditions and drastically changing the outcomes. Day by day POCUS is substituting and finding as an extension to physical examination.

The currently available ultrasound (US) equipment are very much portable, offers excellent imaging, simple to use, and is preloaded with various clinical settings. The sound waves (>20 kHz) emanated from a transducer, passing through different densities of tissues, and are reflected back to produce an image. The concepts of ultrasound physics such as reflection, refraction, scattering, and attenuation hold a fundamental role in the interpretation of an image. The artifacts produced due to these physics concepts too play an important role in POCUS imaging and interpretation.

The selection of a proper transducer for a particular examination is important, to ensure optimal axial and lateral resolution. The high-frequency linear transducers are ideal for superficial structures such as pleura and airway due to their limited depth of imaging (good resolution and lesser penetration). The curvilinear transducers provide images of deeper structures and are best for imaging intraperitoneal and retroperitoneal organs. A low-frequency phased array transducer with a small footprint is used to image intrathoracic structures such as the heart and large vessels.

AIRWAY IN POINT-OF-CARE ULTRASONOGRAPHY

Airway management is important for Anesthesiologist.

A detailed understanding of airway anatomy is essential. The airway can be divided into the upper airway (nasal cavity, oral cavity, pharynx, and larynx) and the lower airway, which includes the tracheobronchial tree **(Fig. 1)**.

Point-of-care ultrasound was once been a tool for radiologists alone and now seeping its roots into emergency medicine and anesthesiology and many subspecialties. Among many uses of POCUS, airway ultrasound has recently gained importance.

Indications

- To predict difficult airway
- To confirm endotracheal, endobronchial, or esophageal intubation
- To confirm orogastric or nasogastric tube position

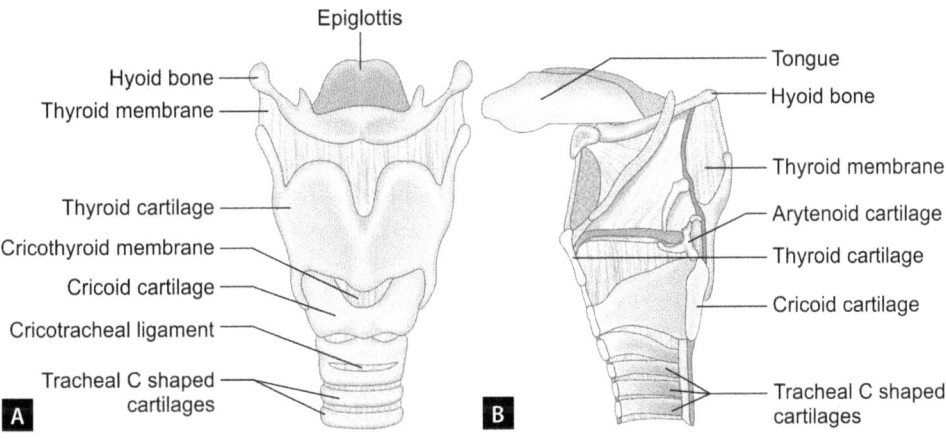

Figs. 1A and B: Airway anatomy—(A) Anterior view of the larynx; (B) Lateral view of the larynx.

- Ultrasound-guided nerve blocks of the airways for awake intubation
- Prediction of tube size in pediatric age groups
- During emergency airway protection-front of neck access.

Ultrasound Examination of the Airway Structures

The stepwise airway examination by ultrasound is explained here, the patient is placed in supine with a sniffing position, and a pillow needs to be kept below the occiput to achieve a maximum extension of the head. The assessment begins from the floor of mouth (oropharynx), then moved to supraglottic, glottic, and subglottic regions. First assessment of structures of the oropharynx is done by the curvilinear probe, followed by the airway structures in the neck by linear probe.

For the examination of the floor of mouth, the patient is asked to close the mouth; the tongue is kept in a relaxed condition. The probe is placed below the chin in the median sagittal plane (midline longitudinal and transverse views). The *tongue* is seen deep in muscles of the floor of the mouth (extrinsic muscles), with its dorsal surface as hyperechoic appearance due to air mucosal interface, the entire tongue (striated pattern) outline is noted, and the tongue thickness is noted as maximum vertical dimension from tongue surface to the submental skin. The *hyoid bone* is seen as a narrow hyperechoic curved structure with an acoustic shadow in the sagittal view, while as an inverted U-shaped hyperechoic structure on the transverse view. The probe is moved down to visualize supraglottic and glottic structures, the *epiglottis* (examined in both parasagittal and transverse view) is viewed through the *thyrohyoid membrane*, it is noticeable as hypoechoic curvilinear structure, its anterior border **(Fig. 1)** is demarcated by the hyperechoic pre-epiglottic space (PES) and its posterior border looks bright due to air-mucosal interface. The *vocal cords* are visualized through thyroid cartilage, they look like an inverted V appearance, and they are appreciated best by asking the patient to phonate.

For the examination of the cricoid cartilage, cricothyroid membrane, and tracheal rings, the scanning is started with a linear probe held transversely just cranial of the sternal notch; the *tracheal rings* are seen as an air-filled, hypoechoic dark ring-like structure marked in orange color, and the air mucosal interface is seen as hyperechoic lining just inside the tracheal lumen, the probe is moved cranially, series of such tracheal rings can be seen. As the probe is moved cranially one can see, the *thyroid gland* with both lobes on either side of trachea with isthmus in front, identification of thyroid is important during percutaneous tracheostomy to avoid its injury. The *cricoid cartilage* is seen as a horseshoe-shaped slightly larger hypoechoic ring-like structure, *cricothyroid membrane* is seen just cranial to cricoid cartilage as a sharp white line with parallel lines beneath (reverberation artifact), as the probe is moved cranially the *thyroid cartilage* is seen as upside-down V-shaped hypoechoic structure. Muscle of the vocal cords can be seen at this stage; they can be well appreciated if the patient is conscious and asked to make sounds. The probe can also be shifted slightly left, one can see the *esophagus* as a muscular structure, just lateral to the trachea and which becomes prominent if the subject makes swallowing movements **(Fig. 2)**.

The airway is again examined in the longitudinal axis in midline, beginning from sternal notch and probe is moved cranially, *tracheal rings* are seen as a *string of black pearls* with the air mucosal interface as hyperechoic line below. The cricoid cartilage and thyroid cartilages are seen as larger black pearls with cricothyroid membrane in between. A small cannula can be made to roll below the probe to mark the cricothyroid membrane if the need arises for emergency airway access **(Figs. 3A and B)**.

Difficult Airway Prediction

There are many ultrasound predictors of difficult airways were examined, like an assessment of the tongue, oral cavity, and assessment of soft tissue thickness in the neck. The most commonly used predictors that were found to correlate with difficult airway were; "thickness of anterior neck soft tissue

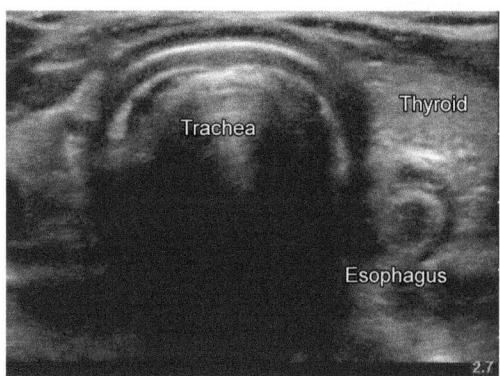

Fig. 2: Transverse view of upper airway.

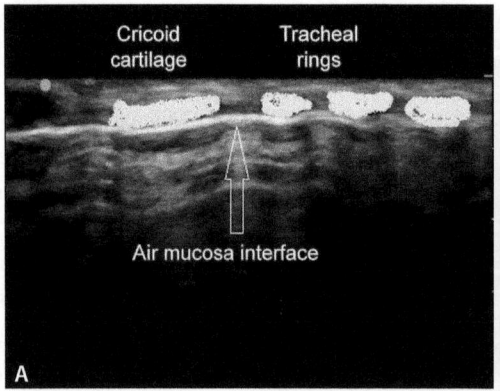

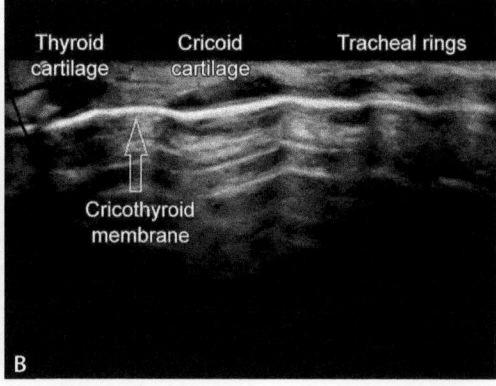

Figs. 3A and B: Sagittal view of the upper airway.

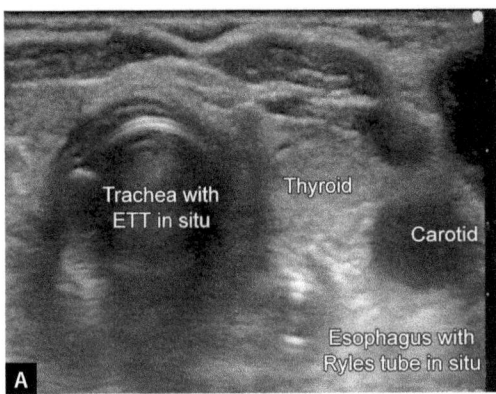 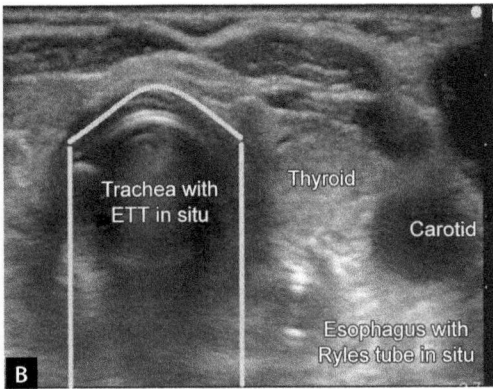

Figs. 4A and B: Endotracheal tube confirmation by ultrasonography image.

at the vocal cords", "skin to epiglottis" and "anterior neck soft tissue at the hyoid bone", HMD (hyomental distance), and hyomental distance ratio (HMDR).

Confirmation of Endotracheal/ Endobronchial/Esophageal Tube Position

Though capnography is considered as the gold standard for tube confirmation, with the help of ultrasonography (USG), one can confirm endotracheal, endobronchial, or esophageal intubation. Ultrasonography also has increased sensitivity and specificity for tube confirmation. The linear probe is placed transversely over the sternal notch; the endotracheal intubation is seen as a reverberation artifact inside the trachea, or "single comet tail" or "bullet" appearance of trachea **(Figs. 4A and B)**. Ultrasonography has more sensitivity and specificity than chest auscultation for bilateral air entry. Bilateral air entry is confirmed by bilateral pleural sliding by using USG. The endobronchial intubation is inferred from te bullet sign along with lung sliding sign on one side of the chest. The esophageal intubation is seen as a "double tract sign" as the tube is placed inside the collapsed esophagus **(Fig. 5)**.

In esophageal intubation double tract sign will be visualized.

Emergency Airway Access

During an emergency when the condition arises where one cannot ventilate and cannot intubate, and need to go for invasive methods of airway protection with cricothyroidotomy or emergency tracheostomy arises, ultrasonography helps in visualization of cricothyroid membrane and identification of tracheal rings or cartilages **(Figs. 6A and B)**.

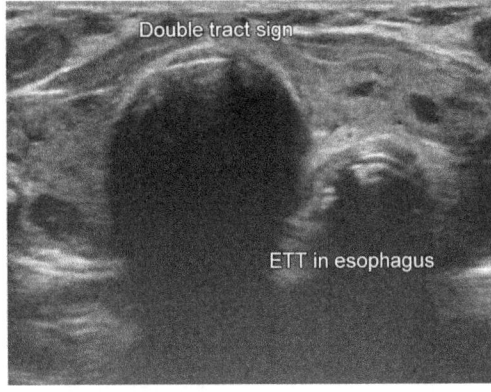

Fig. 5: Double tract sign being visualized in esophageal intubation.

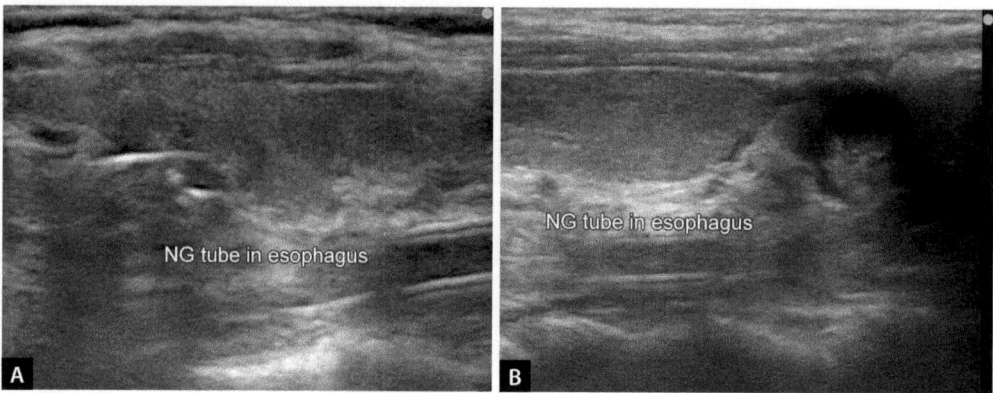

Figs. 6A and B: Position of NG tube in the esophagus. Long-axis USG images of the esophagus during nasogastric placement in the parasagittal plane in the anterior neck—(A) Insertion of a nasogastric feeding tube to the esophagus; (B) Passing of the tube through the esophagus.
(NG: nasogastric tube; USG: ultrasonography)

Confirming Nasogastric or Orogastric Tube Position

Figures 6A and B depicting insertion and passing of nasogastric tube through esophagus.

■ LUNG ULTRASOUND

The knowledge of lung ultrasound (LUS) is important for pain physicians and regional anesthesiologists. Various chronic pain and regional anesthesia procedures close to lung; [thoracic paravertebral blocks, erector spinae plane (ESP), thoracic facet injections, brachial plexus blocks, etc.] can produce respiratory insufficiency due to a pneumothorax (pleural puncture), hemothorax (puncturing any major vessels), hemidiaphragmatic palsy (phrenic nerve palsy by brachial plexus blocks above the clavicle), etc. The knowledge of normal healthy and diseased lung sonoanatomy helps in arriving early diagnosis of any complications and differentiating complications from any undiagnosed pre-existing respiratory insufficiency due to any causes.

Traditionally air is considered an enemy of ultrasound, as it does not permit sound waves to pass, and produces artifacts, interpretations of various artifacts can be used as a tool for diagnosis. The "point of care" LUS, can be used as a bedside investigation for early diagnosis and intervention with better accuracy in both sensitivity and specificity over traditional physical examination and imaging modalities. Repeated imaging can be done and used for prognosis as there is no risk of radiation exposure. Lung ultrasound is superior to auscultation and X-ray. Lung ultrasound helps in bedside diagnosis of life-threatening conditions such as pneumothorax and pleural effusion.

■ NORMAL LUNG

Identification of normal lung is a must to diagnose the lung pathologies. One must know the normal lung findings in the USG to rule out pathologies. Normal lung findings in USG shows bat sign, A lines **(Figs. 7A and B)**, seashore sign in M mode, ≤2 B lines in one segment **(Fig. 8)**.

■ PNEUMOTHORAX

In pneumothorax pleural sliding will be absent, no B lines, presence of lung point,

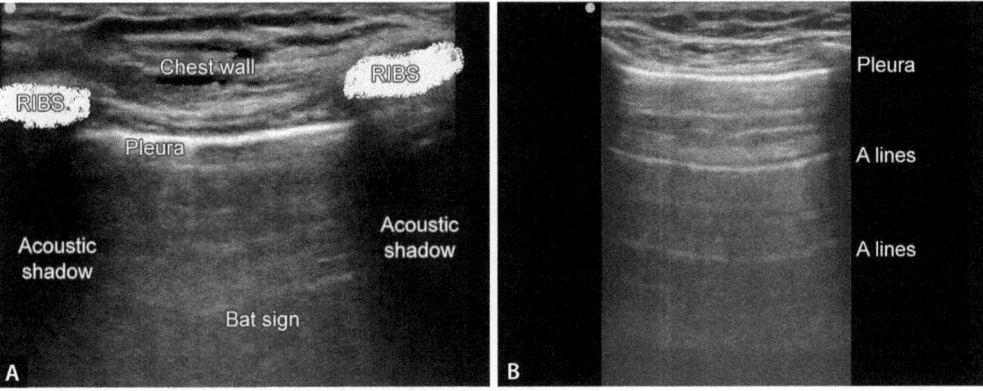

Figs. 7A and B: Hyperechoic pleural line, below pleural line shows A lines which are parallel to pleural line and perpendicular to the probe. A-lines are the reverberation artifacts.

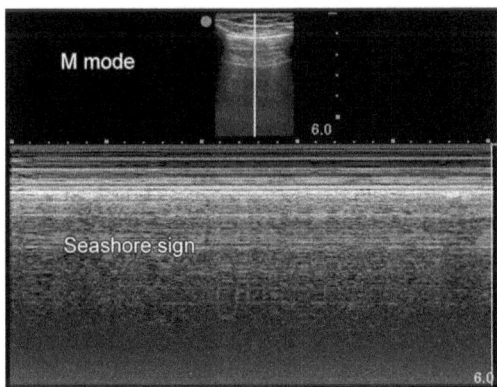

Fig. 8: Seashore sign in M mode—is a normal lung finding.

and absence of lung pulse. Visualizing lung sliding or even single B line rules out pneumothorax. Lung point is the point where two pleural lines detach from each other. Cardiac pulsations will be transmitted to lung if the pleural lines are still together; this is visualized in the M mode and is called *lung pulse* **(Figs. 9A and B)**. As B line arises from visceral pleura even the presence of a single B line rules out pneumothorax **(Flowchart 1)**.

PNEUMONIA

Consolidation is nothing but pneumonia. Pneumonia can be diagnosed by many signs depending upon the extension of the lung involvement. In translobar consolidation there will be hepatization of lung **(Fig. 10)**.

In nontranslobar pneumonia there will be a shred sign **(Fig. 11)**.

Dynamic air bronchogram is seen in pneumonia **(Fig. 12)**.

Static air bronchogram is seen in atelectasis.

In pulmonary edema >2 B lines in multiple lung fields is seen.

FOCUSED CARDIAC ULTRASOUND

Focused assessed transthoracic echocardiography (FATE) has been in practice for >25 years in critical care. Cardiac bedside ultrasonography has mainly helped in early recognition, timely management, and perioperative outcomes. Though FOCUS is not accurate and confirmatory, but it guides for further investigations to confirm the diagnosis. Focused cardiac ultrasound has helped in the timely diagnosis of aortic stenosis (AS) in old age hip fracture patients.

Focused Cardiac Ultrasound Views

Cardiac assessment is done with fundamental FOCUS views such as:

Section 6: Miscellaneous

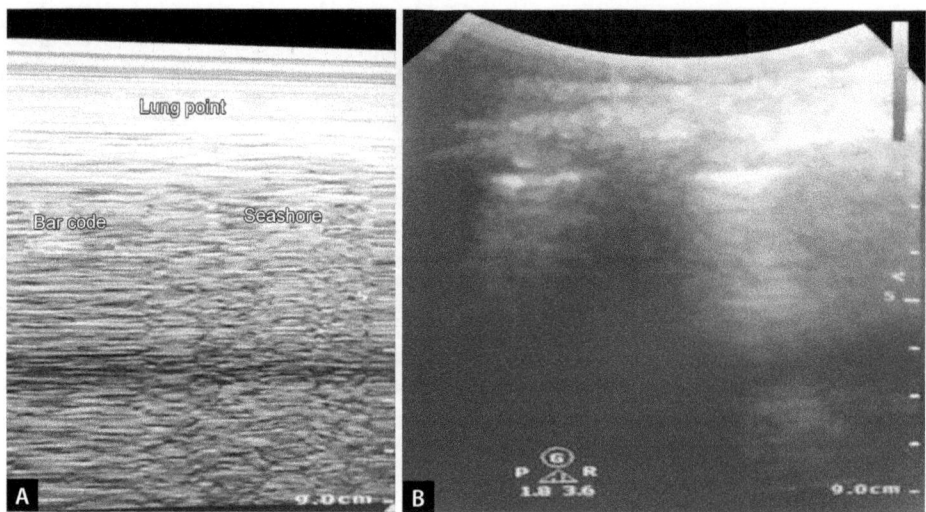

Figs. 9A and B: Bar code sign is seen in M mode of pneumothorax.

Flowchart 1: Pneumothorax identification.

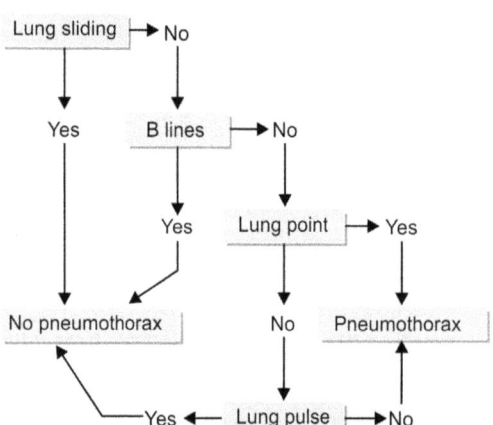

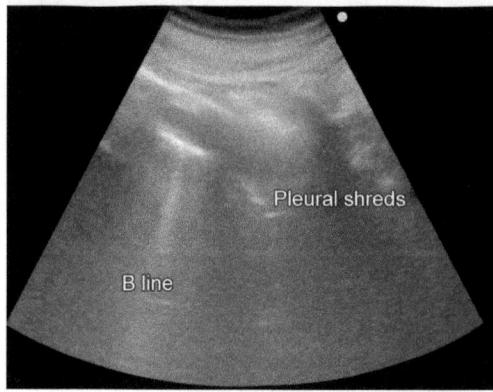

Fig. 11: Shred sign.

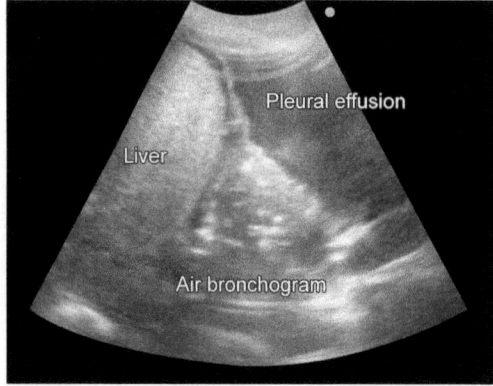

Fig. 10: Hepatization of lung.

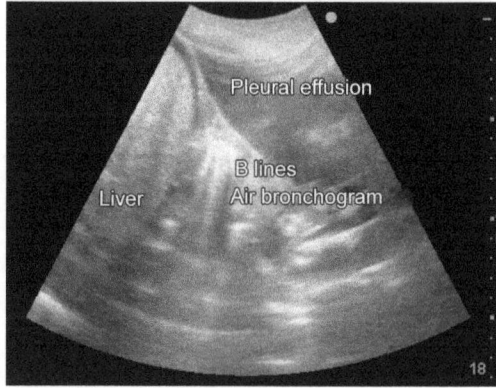

Fig. 12: Air bronchograms.

- Apical four-chamber view and five-chamber view **(Figs. 13 and 14)**
- Parasternal long axis view **(Fig. 15)**
- Parasternal short-axis view **(Fig. 16 and 17)**
- Subcostal four-chamber view **(Fig. 18)**
- Subcostal inferior vena cava view **(Figs. 19 A and B)**
- Sub costal inferior vena cava view—distended **(Fig. 20)**
- Transhepatic inferior vena cava view **(Fig. 21)**.

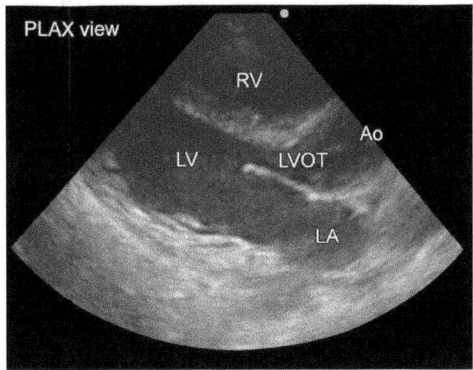

Fig. 15: Parasternal long axis (PLAX) view.
(Ao: Aorta; LA: left atrium; LV: left ventricle; LVOT: left ventricle outflow tract; RV: right ventricle)

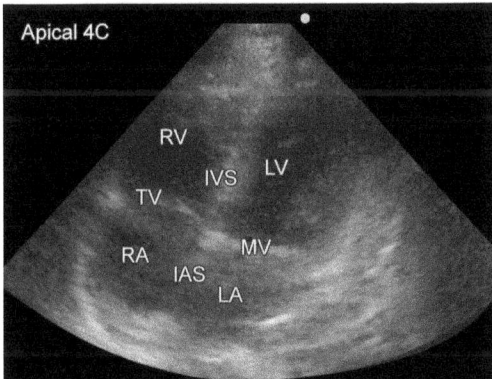

Fig. 13: Apical four-chamber view.
(IAS: interatrial septum; IVS: inter ventricular septum; LA: left atrium; LV: left ventricle; RA: right atrium; RV: right ventricle)

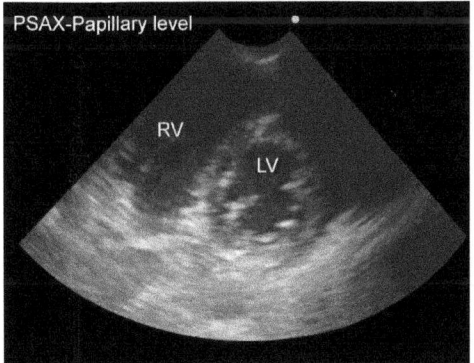

Fig. 16: Parasternal short-axis (PSAX) view—papillary level.
(LV: left ventricle; RV: right ventricle)

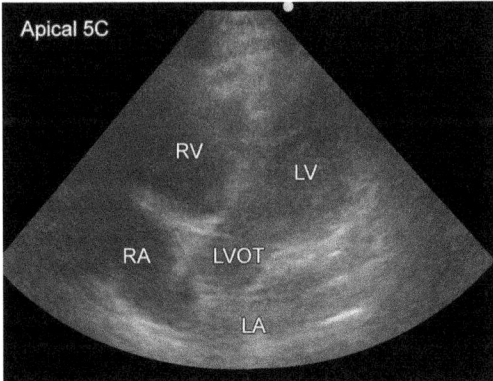

Fig. 14: Apical five-chamber view.
(LA: left atrium; LV: left ventricle; LVOT: left ventricle outflow tract; RA: right atrium; RV: right ventricle)

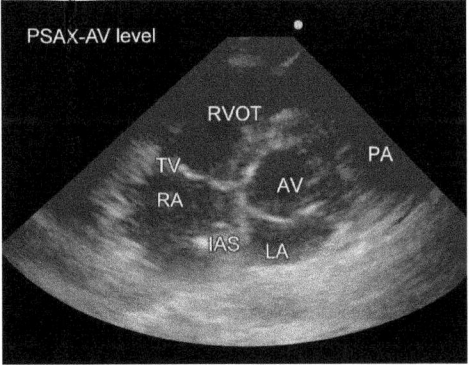

Fig. 17: Parasternal short-axis (PSAX) view—aortic valve level. (AV: aortic valve; IAS: interatrial septum; LA: left atrium; PA: pulmonary artery; RA: right atrium; RVOT: right ventricle outflow tract; TV: tricuspid valve)

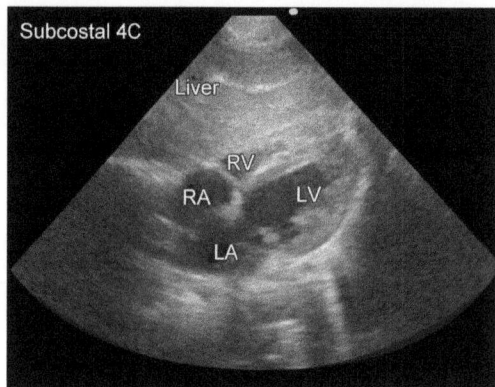

Fig. 18: Subcostal four-chamber view.
(LA: left atrium; LV: left ventricle; RA: right atrium; RV: right ventricle)

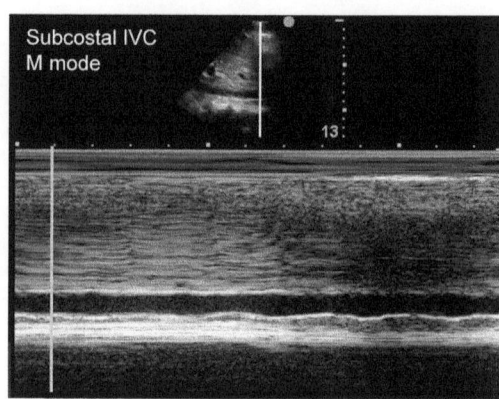

Fig. 20: Subcostal inferior vena cava view—distended.

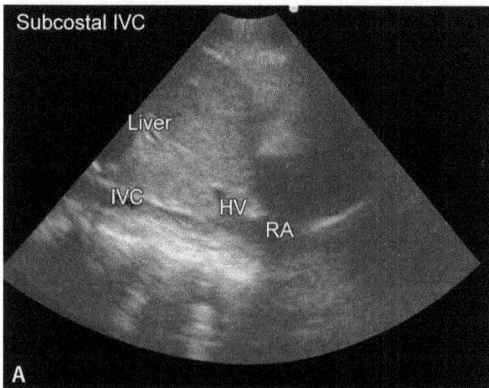

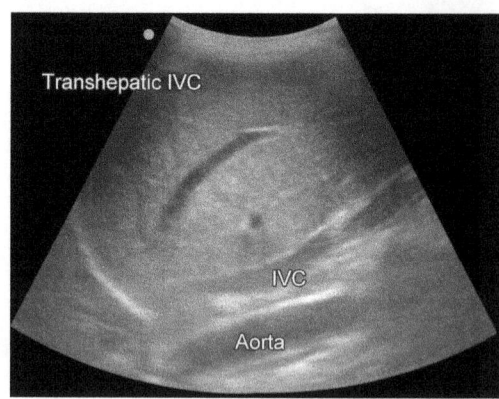

Fig. 21: Transhepatic inferior vena cava view.

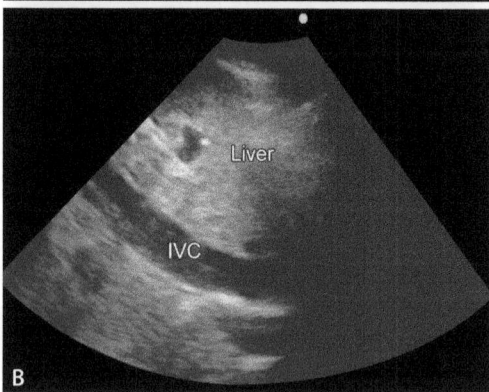

Figs. 19A and B: Subcostal inferior vena cava view. (HV: hepatic vein; IVC: inferior vena cava; RA: right atrium)

GASTRIC POINT-OF-CARE ULTRASONOGRAPHY (FIG. 22)

The use of gastric ultrasound by an anesthetist or pain physician is mainly for confirmation of nil per oral (NPO) status by visualizing or measuring gastric contents before anesthesia or any interventional pain procedure requiring sedation. By using USG and confirming NPO status we can prevent aspiration risk. Empty stomach or full stomach these two conditions have different anesthetic management and outcomes. In some conditions, even on

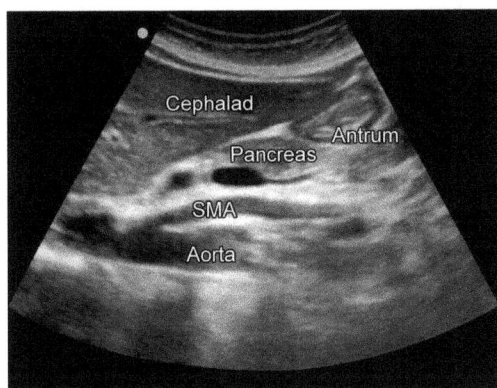

Fig. 22: Gastric POCUS.
(POCUS: point of care ultrasonography; SMA: superior mesenteric artery)

TABLE 1: Supine and/or RLD position, gastric USG is defined in a three-point grading system.

Grade	Clear fluid in supine position	Clear fluid in RLD	Implied
0	Absent	Absent	Empty stomach
1	Absent	Present	Baseline secretions
2	Present	Present	Full stomach

(RLD: right lateral decubitus; USG: ultrasonography)

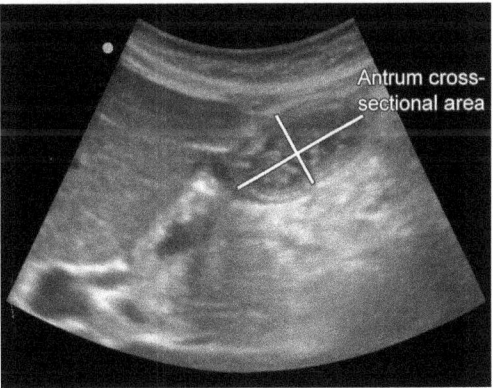

Fig. 23: Antrum cross-sectional area (CSA).

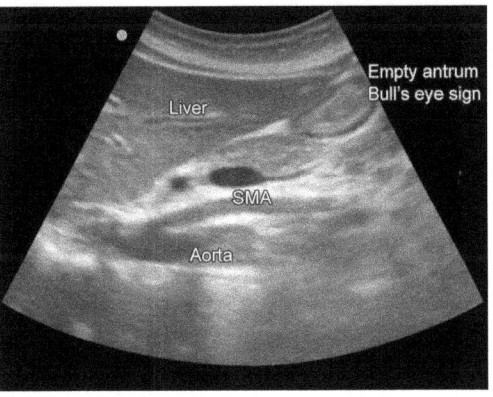

Fig. 24: Empty stomach.

fasting as per required time, there will not be an empty stomach due to delayed gastric emptying called *gastroparesis* which will be seen in diabetics, advanced liver or renal dysfunction, and neuromuscular disorders. Usually pregnant, morbidly, obese, ascites patients, abdominal tumor patients, and pediatrics are considered as a full stomach.

Gastric antrum can be visualized both in the supine position or right lateral decubitus (RLD) or semirecumbent position with 45° head elevation. As antrum size gets affected by the patient's position, it is always better to measure antrum size and contents in the RLD position. Results of gastric USG can be either empty or full stomach **(Figs. 23 and 24)**.

An empty stomach is no contents or with baseline secretions of ≤1.5 mL/kg of hypoechoic fluid.

A full stomach is also called *not empty stomach* with a volume > 1.5 mL/kg, this can be either solid particulate matter (mixed echogenicity), thick secretions (hyperechoic), or excess baseline secretions **(Figs. 25 and 26)**.

In supine and/or RLD position, gastric USG is defined in a three-point grading system **(Table 1)**.

Grade 0 and grade 1 is seen in the fasting state.

After many studies, the gastric volume measuring formula has been designed as:

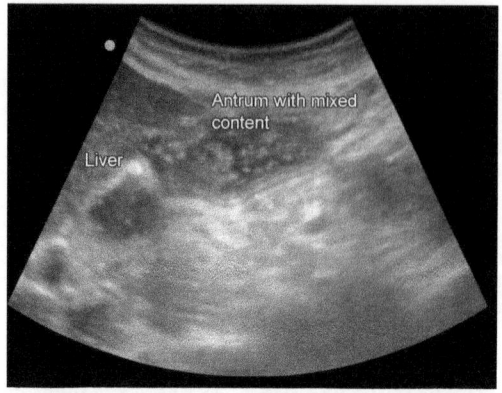

Fig. 25: Antrum with food and starry night appearance.

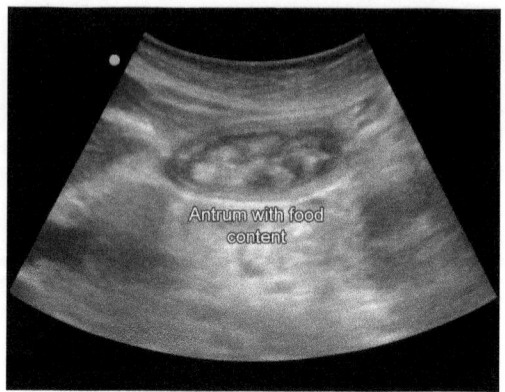

Fig. 26: Antrum with food.

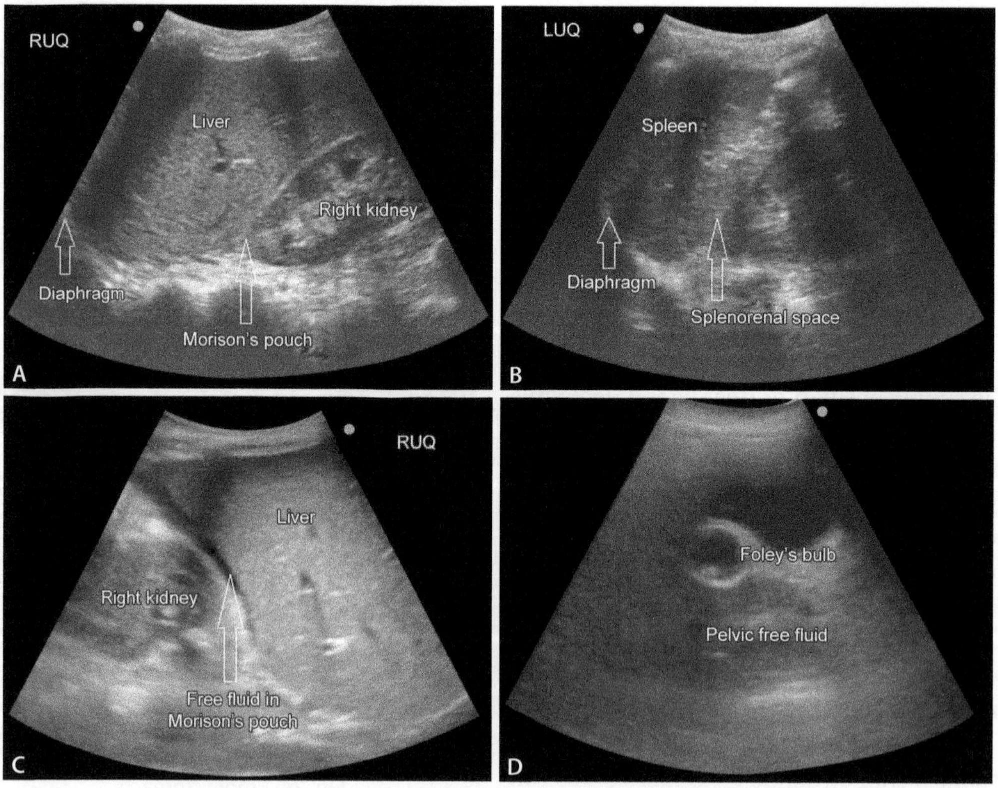

Figs. 27A to D: Focused assessment with sonography in trauma (FAST).

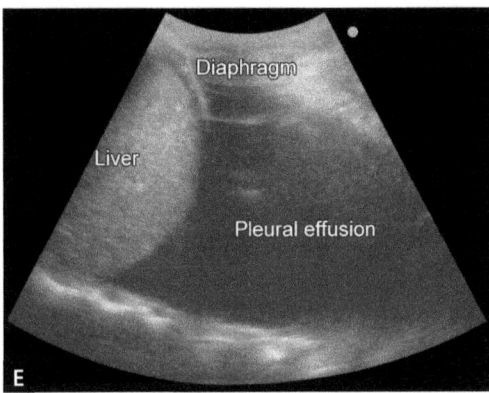

Fig. 27E: Focused assessment with sonography in trauma (FAST): Pleural effusion.

Gastric volume (mL) = 27.0 + 14.6 × cross-sectional area (CSA) − 1.28 × age

Cross-sectional area of gastric antrum at the level of the aorta only in RLD position.

FOCUSED ASSESSMENT WITH SONOGRAPHY IN TRAUMA

Focused assessment with sonography in trauma (FAST) examination is indicated in blunt or penetrating abdominal or chest trauma. In chronic pain procedures such as celiac plexus block and patients on peritoneal dialysis **(Figs. 27A to E)**.

Four views in FAST are as follows:
1. *Sub costal view:* Pericardium, heart chambers visualized.
2. *Right upper quadrant:* Morrison's pouch (hepatorenal recess), liver tip (right paracolic gutter), lower right thorax.
3. *Left upper quadrant:* Subphrenic space, splenorenal recess, spleen tip (left paracolic gutter), lower left thorax.
4. *Pelvis:* Rectovesical pouch (male), rectouterine pouch or pouch of Douglas.

Extended Focused Assessment with Sonography in Trauma

It includes a focused assessment with sonography in trauma plus examination of anterior and lateral pleural spaces to rule out hemothorax, pneumothorax or pleural effusion.

Positive Focused Assessment with Sonography in Trauma

It includes 300–500 mL of free fluid in the concerned space.
- *False positive of FAST:* Seen in apical fat pad.
- *False negative of FAST:* Small fluid collections.

FURTHER READING

1. Khanna P. Ultrasound in Critical Care, 1st edition. 2019.

Index

Page numbers followed by *b* refer to box, *f* refer to figure, *fc* refer to flowchart, and *t* refer to table.

A

Abdominal compartment syndrome 469
Absorption 50, 441
Acarbose 104
Acceleromyography 251, 257, 257*f*
Accidental intra-arterial injection 29
Acetate 456
Acetazolamide 108
Acetoacetate 276
Acetohexamide 104, 105
Acetylcholine 55, 61
Acid-base
    disorder 266, 267*t*, 268*t*, 277
    evaluation 267*fc*
    parameters 266*t*
    status 266, 270*t*
Acidemia 266
Acidic solution 75
Acidosis 75
    acute 139
    hyperchloremic metabolic 148
Acrivastine 100, 112
Actinomycin 128
Activated clotting time 116, 121
Activated partial thromboplastin time 414
Acute coronary syndrome 450
    types of 469
Acute lung injury, transfusion-related 445
Acute respiratory distress syndrome 272, 428, 437, 455
Additional venous infusion lumen 188
Adductor pollicis 253
Adenosine 492
    diphosphate 123
    monophosphate 14, 110
    side effects of 93
    triphosphate 110
    uses of 93
Adjustable pressure limiting 318-320, 332, 409

Adrenaline 75, 77, 78, 415
Advanced cardiovascular life support 484, 485, 485*fc*, 515
Advanced life support 479-481
Agranulocytosis 101, 113
Air
    bronchogram 527, 534*f*
    embolism 445, 451
    valve 434
Airtraq 358, 358*f*
Airway 335, 337, 377, 409, 484, 485, 528
    anatomy 529*f*
    assessment of 485
    classification of 337
    exchange catheter 416
    obstruction 340
    opening 483
    prediction 530
    pressure, high 426
    protection, long-term 413
    resistance 8, 281
    structures 529
    surgeries 437
    trolley, difficult 380, 380*f*, 383*f*
    uses of 337
Aladin and Aladin2 cassette vaporizers 313
Aladin cassette, advantages of 315
Albumin 151, 277, 278
    states, low 278
Alcohol 81, 84, 269, 408
    dehydrogenase dehydration 101, 113
Aldosterone blockers 107
Aldosteronism, primary 84
Alfentanil 19, 401
    ampoule 23*f*
    pharmacokinetics 19*t*
Alkalemia 266
Alkali absorbents
    free 332
    high 331
    low 331

Alkalosis 107
Alkyl chain 47
Alkylating agents 126, 127
Allen test, modified 168
Allergic reactions 103
Allergy 486
Alogliptin 104
Alpha-angle 230, 243
Alpha-blockers 80, 80*t*
    adverse effects of 79
    contraindications of 80
    use of 79
Alpha-glucosidase inhibitors 104, 105
Alpha-receptor blockers 79
Alteplase 122
Aluminum
    foil 86
    hydroxide 111
Alveolar ventilation 7
Alveolar-arterial gradient 271
Alzheimer's disease 62
Ambient atmospheric pressure 239
Ambu aScope 360*f*
American College of Cardiology 85
American Heart Association 85
American Society of Anesthesiologists 228, 377
Amides 51
Amiodarone 92, 488, 492
Amlodipine 94, 96
Amnesia 36
    anterograde 31
Amniotic fluid embolism 490
Ample novel technologies 198
Analgesia 400, 402
    dose of 396
    intraoperative 396
    postoperative 62, 394
Analgesic 516
    concentrations, minimum effective 396
    doses 401
Anaphylactoid reaction 29, 118, 152
Anaphylaxis 76, 490, 491

Index

Anesthesia 248, 249, 291, 328, 443, 510
  epidural 392
  equipment, decontamination of 409t
  general 224
  induction of 28, 34, 36, 39, 250
  instruments 287
  intravenous induction of 38
  machine 295, 301
  maintenance of 36, 39, 250
  monitoring 161
  reversal of 250
  total intravenous 43
  ventilator 409
  workstation 295
Anesthetic agents, system wise effects of 8t
Anesthetic concentration 4
Anesthetic conserving device 11
Anesthetic face mask 335, 335b
  parts of 335f
Anesthetic gas
  delivery of 342
  production of 291
Anesthetic machine 303, 304
Aneurysms, abdominothoracic 281
Angina, unstable 117, 281
Angioplasty 117
Angiotensin-converting enzymes 84
  inhibitor 72, 84, 85
Angiotensin-receptor blocker 84, 85
Anion gap 269, 276
Anistreplase 122
Antacids 110, 111
Antagonist 97, 119
Antianxiety 516
Antiarrhythmic agents 488, 492
Antiarrhythmic drugs 90-92, 520, 524
  mechanism of action of 91
  prophylactic use of 92
  therapy, goals of 90
Antibiotics 126, 270
  cytotoxic 126, 127, 129
Anticholinergic 65t
  drugs 64-67
    effects of 65t
    uses of 68
  medications 64, 66
  syndrome 67
Anticholinesterase 60, 61
  agents 66t
  drugs 60
  pharmacological properties of 62t
Anticoagulants 115

Anticonvulsants 155
  drugs 156t
Antidepressants 84
Antidiuretic hormone 17, 135, 150, 437
Antidote 122
Antiepileptic drugs 160
  classification of 155
Antihypertensive drugs 76, 84, 84t
Antimetabolites 126, 127, 129
Antimuscarinic agents, classification of 64fc
Antineutrophil cytoplasmic antibodies 433
Antiphospholipid antibody syndrome 432
Antiplatelet agents, types of 122
Antiplatelet drugs 122, 123fc, 123t
Antireflux valves 403
Antiseptic 405
Anti-spill mechanism 305
Antistatic agent, use of 303
Antler sign 527
Anxiety 81
Anxiolysis 45
Aorta 206, 535
  descending 208
Aortic coarctation 84
Aortic regurgitation 172
Aortic stenosis 171, 520, 533
Aortic valve 206, 207f, 447
  closure 170f
  level 535f
Apixaban 119, 120
Aquaporins 107
Argatroban 118, 120
Arndt bronchial blocker 375, 376f
Arndt endobronchial blocker 375
Aromatic ring 47
Arrhythmia 67, 90, 91, 187, 195, 237, 451, 500
  causes of 90
  supraventricular 81
  types of 90
Arrhythmogenicity 82
Arterial blood
  gas 266, 267
  pressure 163
    components of 163
    pressure monitoring 163
    system, components of 163
Arterial cannulation
  contraindications of 167
  indications of 167
Arterial catheter kit 163
Arterial concentration 201

Arterial oxygen saturation 227
Arterial oxygenation
  monitoring 229
Arterial pressure 165
  monitoring system 165f, 171
  waveform 164, 166f
    abnormal 171t
    distal pulse wave amplification of 171f
    normal 169, 170f
Arterial spasm 174
Arterial thrombosis 29, 174
Arterial waveform
  advantages of 204
  analysis 201, 202f
  progression of 166f
Arteries, peripheral 164, 203
Artificial manual breathing unit 325
Asepsis 405
Aspiration 327, 438
  foreign body 337
Aspirin 71, 73, 110, 122
Assisted mechanical ventilation 475
Asthma 243f
  acute severe 417
Atenolol 83
Atherosclerosis 432
Atmospheric pressure 309
Atraumatic needle 391f
Atrial fibrillation 121, 186, 521, 522f
Atrial flutter 521, 521f
Atrioventricular node 90
Atrioventricular pump-less assist device 452
Atrioventricular valves 447
Atropine 66, 67
  sulfate 492
Auscultatory method 374
Autoclave, monitoring of 406
Automated cardiopulmonary resuscitation machine 448, 449
Automated chest compressor machine 447
Automated external defibrillator 465, 466, 466f, 480, 482, 499
Auto-positive end-expiratory pressure, measurement of 475
Autopulse 448, 448f
Auxiliary oxygen cylinder 305
Avogadro's hypothesis 308
Avogadro's law 511
Axillary artery 168
  cannulation complications 174

Index

Axis 514
Ayre's T-piece 322
   modification of 316
Azelastine 99, 100, 112

B

Back pressure, effects of 311*t*
Bactericide 405
Bacteriostat 405
Bag inlet valve 325, 326
Bag refill valve 424
Bag-mask ventilation 326*f*, 379
Bag-valve mask ventilation
   complications of 327
   typical 426*f*
Bains circuit
   advantages of 321
   disadvantages of 321
Balanced salt solutions 150
Balloon
   inflation lumen 188
   mechanical properties of 475
Bar code sign 534*f*
Barbiturates 25, 27, 29, 31, 155
   adverse effects of 28
   classification of 25*t*
   drugs 25*t*
   properties of 38
Barbituric acid 25*t*
Bardex airway 340
Bare chest 466
Barotrauma 327, 426, 438
Basal nutritional requirements 131*t*
Basic anesthesia machine, pressure systems of 296
Basic life support 479, 480, 482, 482*fc*, 483, 499
Basilar artery 212
Baska mask 351, 351*f*
Basophilic granules 98
Beer and Lambert law 214, 239
Behcet's disease 433
Bell's needle 392
Belmont rapid infuser 445
Bends, exacerbation of 512
Benzene ring 31
Benzocaine 51
Benzodiazepines 27, 30, 31, 34, 36-38, 155
   effects of 32
   intravenous 30
   metabolism of 33
Berman's intubating airway 339
Bernoulli's principle 511
Beta-adrenergic antagonist 92

Beta-angle 230, 243
Beta-blockers 51, 81, 83*t*, 515, 516, 520
   adverse effects of 82
   clinical uses of 81
   toxicity 83
      clinical manifestations of 82
Beta-carboline esters 32
Beta-hydroxylase 145
Beta-lactam antibiotics, use of 273
Beta-receptor blockers 79, 81
Bicarbonate 456
Bier's needle 391
Biguanides 104, 105
Bilevel positive airway pressure 428
Bimetallic strip dial thermometer 262
Binasal airway 340
Binuria 433
Biological response modifiers 127
Biotransformation 51
Bisoprolol 83
Bispectral index 222
   monitoring 222
   values 223
Bisphosphonates 142
Bivalirudin 118
Bizzarri-Giuffrida blade 355
Bladder 75, 453
   dysfunction 470
Blades, types of 355
Bleeding
   abnormal 73
   active internal 124
   diathesis 175
Bleomycin 127, 128
Blind technique 374
Blood 4
   brain barrier 80
   vessel 115
Blood flow 75, 457
   coronary 87
   rate 458*f*
Blood gas 267
   analysis 232
   anomalies 232*t*
Blood pressure 74, 81, 124, 203
   cuff 409
   diastolic 74, 188
   noninvasive 164, 259
   systolic 39, 74, 165, 169
Body habitus 471
Body mass index 130, 130*t*, 379
Body temperature 328
Body water
   effect 458
   total 147

Boiling point 307
   low 313
Bone 525
Botulism 417
Bourdon thermometer 512
Bourdon's pressure gauge 297, 298*f*
Boyle's bottle 311
Boyle's law 299, 512
Boyle's machine 295
Brachial arteries 168
Brachial plexus 51, 53
Brachiocephalic vein 179
Brachiocephalic vessels 525
Bradyarrhythmia 515
Bradycardia 68, 101, 145
   profound 492
   symptomatic 491
   treatment of 68
Brain 7
   damage, permanent 447
   edema 457
   injury, traumatic 413
   natriuretic peptide 107
Brainstem auditory evoked potential 218, 221
Breathing 484, 485*t*
   assessment of 485
   circuit 316
   rescue 496*t*
   system 306, 316, 330, 409
   tubes 317
   work of 475
Bromochlorodifluoroethylene 333
Bronchial blocker 374, 375
   advantages of 375
   disadvantages of 375
   wire-guided 375
Bronchial disruption, major 371
Bronchiectasis 527
Bronchocath 373
Bronchoconstriction 63
Bronchodilator 76
Bronchorrhea 68
Bronchospasm 68, 243*f*
Brook's airway 338
Buccal cavity stabilizer 349
Bulk flow ventilation 436, 437
Bullard optical laryngoscope 356, 356*f*
Bumetanide 108
Buprenorphine 21
Burst suppression ratio 223
Busulfan 128
Butorphanol 401

C

Calcitonin 139, 142
Calcium 94, 131, 139
   carbonate 111
   regulation of 140*fc*
Calcium channel blockers 94, 95, 95*t*, 96, 97*t*, 455, 515
   classification of 94
   pharmacokinetics of 95*t*
Camera technology 360
Cancer pain 43
Cannulation, timing of 176
Capillary leak syndrome 451
Capnogram, normal 243*f*
Capnograph 239, 240*f*
Capnometer 239
Carbamates 60
Carbamazepine 156, 455
Carboetomidate 41
Carbohydrates 132
Carbon dioxide 34, 209, 232, 239, 276, 316, 331, 368, 386
   absorbent 306
   arterial partial pressure of 227, 232
   cutaneous 227
   partial pressure of 227, 231, 232, 242
   supercritical 227
   transcutaneous partial pressure of 227
Carbon monoxide 333
   toxicity 417
Carbonic anhydrase inhibitors 106, 107
Cardiac arrest 76, 243*f*, 274, 487*fc*, 488, 490
   causes of 486*t*
   immediate recognition of 481
   in-hospital 479, 482, 494
   out-of-hospital 479, 494*f*
   survival for
      adult in-hospital 494*f*
      pediatric in-hospital 496
      pediatric out-of-hospital 496
Cardiac cycle 206
Cardiac failure, chronic congestive 81
Cardiac function 185
Cardiac index 202
Cardiac monitoring 175
Cardiac output 7, 74, 172, 199
   measurement 196
   monitoring 198, 443
      perioperative 198

Cardiac tamponade 172, 195
Cardinal cardiovascular parameter 163
Cardiomyopathy 522
   chronic 450
   dilated 520
   hypertrophic 172
      obstructive 81
   severe 198
Cardiopulmonary bypass 116, 165
Cardiopulmonary resuscitation 447, 479, 482, 485, 487, 490, 491*t*, 492, 494, 495, 499
   complications of 490
   early initiation of 494*t*
   physiological monitoring of 495*t*
Cardiotoxicity 127
   late-onset 127
Cardiovascular system 34, 39, 41, 43, 45, 65, 72, 81, 85, 112
Cardiovascular toxicity 126
Cardioversion 465, 522, 524
   contraindications of 465
   indications of 465
Carina 371
Carlen's tubes 372, 373
C-arm, parts of 505
Carotid artery 178
   internal 212
Carotid siphon 212
Carvedilol 83
Catecholamines 74, 77
   adrenoreceptor sensitivity of 75
Catechol-O-methyl transferase 77, 78
Catheter 175, 393, 439*f*, 440, 503
   design 187
   insertion of 472
   intravenous 397
   length 189*t*
   malposition of 438
   sheath 197
   temporary 176
   types of 176*t*
Celecoxib 71
Cell cycle 125*f*
Central anticholinergic syndrome 62
Central cannula, peripherally inserted 183
Central catheter, peripherally inserted 132
Central nervous system 4, 12, 27, 39, 42, 44, 60, 64, 65, 71, 72, 82, 92, 101, 112, 271, 272
   toxicity 128
Central neuraxial catheters 397

Central venous
   carbon dioxide, partial pressure of 227
   catheter 132-134, 397, 525
      kit 177
   oxygen, partial pressure of 227
Central venous cannulation 181, 184*f*
   equipment of 177
   monitoring technique
      contraindications of 176*t*
      indications of 176, 176*b*
   technique 175
Central venous pressure 75, 175, 185, 187, 195
   components of 185*t*
   measurement of 184, 185*f*
   monitoring 175, 184
   waveform 192*f*
      abnormal 186, 186*t*
      normal 184
Cerebral artery
   anterior 212
   posterior 212
Cerebral blood flow 32, 217, 217*f*
Cerebral edema 149
Cerebral function, continuous noninvasive indicator of 216
Cerebral hypoxia 451
Cerebral ischemia 217
Cerebral oximetry 214, 214*f*
Cerebral oxygenation values 215*fc*
Cerebrospinal fluid 12, 390
Cervical spine 448
   injury 179
Cetirizine 99
C-fibers 22, 50
Channeled videolaryngoscopes 358
Charged-coupled device camera 506
Charles's law 512
Chemical
   agents, types of 406, 408*t*
   disinfection 406
   indicators 406
   sterilization 406
   structure 40, 47, 48*f*
   thermometer 262
Chemoreceptor trigger zone 16, 17
Chemotherapeutic drugs
   action of 125*f*
   classification of 126*t*
Chemotherapy 125
   toxic effects of 125
Cheng needle 392

Index

Chest
  compressions 447, 481
  pain, acute 128
  X-ray 184f, 472, 524
    technical quality of 524
Chiba needle 504f
Chlorhexidine 177
Chloride 131, 278
Chlorothiazide 108
Chlorpheniramine 100, 112
  maleate 99
Chlorpropamide 104, 105
Chlorthalidone 108
Cholinergic agonist 60, 63
Cholinergic drugs 60
  classification of 61fc
Chronic obstructive pulmonary
  disease 34, 39, 167, 236,
  271, 283, 417, 428, 433,
  438, 526, 526f
Ciaglia blue rhino single dilation
  technique 416
Cimetidine 33, 100, 112
Cinnarizine 99
Circle breathing system
  advantages of 331
  disadvantages of 331
Circle system, classic 331, 332f
Circuit 507
Circulation 484, 485, 485t
Cirrhosis 108fc, 109, 117, 129, 278
Cisplatin 126, 128, 129
Citrate 456
Clemastine 99
Clonazepam 155, 159
Clonidine 402
Closed circle system 304
Clot retraction 115
C-mac videolaryngoscope 359f,
  380f
Coagulation 151
  pathway 116f
  profile 434
Coagulopathy 187, 451
Coandă effect 511
Coaxial tube system 318
Codeine 18
Cohen tip-deflecting bronchial
  blocker 376
Cole tube 369, 369f
Collapse 526
  X-ray of 526f
Collar indexing system 291
Colloid 148, 151
  characteristics of 151t
  osmotic pressure 151

Color Doppler of radial artery
  cannulation 170f
Color-coded
  cylinders 304
  pressure gauges 304
  vaporizer 305
Coma 67
Combined spinal epidural
  needle set 394f
  technique 394
Communicating artery, posterior 212
Complementary metal-oxide-
  semiconductor 359
Complete blood count 118
Completely noninvasive
  techniques 198
Complex regional pain
  syndrome 43, 508
Compound muscle action
  potential 219, 254
Compressomyography 259
Computed tomography 434, 489
Connell's airway 337, 338
Consciousness, loss of 36
Constipation 132
Continuous arteriovenous
  hemodialysis 455
Continuous cardiac output
  measurement, methods
  of 198
Continuous central venous
  saturation 227
Continuous positive airway pressure
  426, 428
Continuous renal replacement
  therapy 457, 461
Continuous thermodilution
  technique 196
Continuous venovenous
  hemodiafiltration 131, 455, 462f
  hemodialysis 455
  hemofiltration 455
Controlled analgesia pump 399f
Convection 454
  process of 456f
Copper alloy 291
Cordotomy 507
Corning needle 391
Coronary artery disease 67, 81, 517
Corrugator supercilii muscle 253
Coudé tip needle 503
COVID-19 pandemic 492
Crawley needle 392
Cricoid cartilage 530
Cricothyroid membrane 530
Cricothyroidotomy, surgical 381, 384

Critical care
  set up 396
  ultrasonography 442
Crystalloids 148
  solutions, types of 149t
Cuff
  system 364, 365f
  types of 364
Cuffed oropharyngeal airway 338
Cuffless membranous bowl 351
Curare cleft 243f
Curved tip radiofrequency
  cannula 504f
Cushing's disease 84
Cyanide
  poisoning 417
  toxicity 88
Cyanmethemoglobin 86
Cyclic adenosine monophosphate
  99, 101
Cyclic guanosine monophosphate
  86, 87, 99
Cyclizine 99
Cyclophosphamide 127-129
Cycloplegia 66
Cyclopropane 3
Cyclopropyl-methoxycarbonyl
  metomidate 42
Cylinder pressure
  gauge 296
  test machine 299f
Cylinder valve 289, 289f
Cyproheptadine 99
Cytarabine 129
Cytosine arabinoside 128

D

Dabigatran 118, 120, 122
Dalton's law 512
Dantrolene 96
Datex-ohmeda 300, 301
D-dimer assay 434
Deep brain stimulation 249f
Deep vein thrombosis 117, 432-434
  clinical manifestations of 433
  development of 432
  diagnose 433
  pathogenesis of 432
  risk factors of 432
Defibrillation 465, 486
  contraindications of 465
  energy for 466
  indications of 465
Degludec 102
Deltex monitor 208

Deoxyhemoglobin 201
Deoxyribonucleic acid 102, 125, 126
Desflurane 3, 219, 308
Desirudin 118, 121
Desloratadine 99
Detemir 102
Dexlansoprazole 113
Dexmedetomidine 38, 44, 219, 396
Dextrans 152
Dextrose 163, 460
   solutions 150
Diabetes
   insipidus, central 135
   mellitus 103*fc*, 107, 433
Diacetylmorphine 12
Dialysate flow rate 458, 460
Dialysate solution
      composition 460
Dialysis
   fluid 456
   indications of 455
   low-effifiency 461
   setup, components of 454
   slow continuous 455
Dialyzer membrane 460
Diameter index safety system 299
Diamorphine 12, 17, 22
Diaphragm 525
Diaphragmatic hernia,
      congenital 527
Diarrhea 132
Diazepam 30-33, 35, 158
Diazepine ring 31
Dibucaine number 56
Dick formula, modified 196
Diclofenac 71
Difficult airway management 377, 379*t*, 383*fc*, 384
   devices for 377
Digoxin 97
   side effects of 93
   toxicity 517
Dihydropyridines 94
Diisopropylphenol 38
Diltiazem 94-97
Dimenhydrinate 99
Diphenhydramine 99, 100, 112
Dipipanone 20
Direct arterial pressure 165*f*
Direct cellular toxicity 127
Direct rigid laryngoscope 354
Direct thrombin inhibitors 120, 121*t*
Direct vision technique 374
Direction control valve 425
Disequilibrium syndrome 462

Disinfection 405, 406
   advantages of 407*t*
   disadvantages of 407*t*
   high-level 405, 408
   low-level 405, 408
   methods of 406
   process, high-level 406
   types of 405
Disk lesions 507
Disodium editate 38
Disorientation 67
Disposable adult bispectral index sensor 222*f*
Disposable airflow sensor 209
Disseminated intravascular coagulation 117
Distal esophagus 261
Distal lumen 187
Diuretics 106
   pharmacodynamics of 108*t*
   pharmacokinetics of 108*t*
Dobutamine 78
Docetaxel 127
Domperidone 114
Donald Miller's classification 343*t*
Dopamine 78, 107, 492
   blockers 114
      pharmacokinetics of 114*t*
   injection of 515
Doppler mode 442
Doppler principles 207
Doppler-assisted techniques 169
Dorsalis pedis 168
Double burst stimulation 248
Double lumen tube 371, 372, 375, 409
Double tract sign 531*f*
Doxorubicin 127
D-phenylalanine 13
Droperidol 396, 402
Drowsiness 36
Drugs
   class of 25, 69
   concentration 396
   effects of 67*t*
   produces sedation, class of 30
Dry baralyme 333
Dry heat sterilization 406
Dual drainage system 351
Dual gastric drainage 352
Dual sequential defibrillation 495
Duct injury, risk of 179
Dura noncutting needle 391, 391*f*
Dyes 237
Dynamic lung volumes 283, 283*f*
Dynorphins 12, 13

Dyshemoglobinemia 236
Dyslipidemia 107, 432
Dysphoria 16
Dysrhythmia 438, 465

E

Easy fill system 315
Ebastine 99
Ebstein's malformation 187
Eclampsia 490
Edema, interstitial 148
Edrophonium 60, 61
Ehrenworth formula 309
Eisenkraft formula 309
Elastic Bougie aided 379
Eldor needle 391
Electrical cardiometry 206, 208*f*
Electrical nerve stimulation, patterns of 246*f*
Electrocardiogram 127, 145, 195, 204, 481, 514
   components of 514*f*
   normal 514, 515*f*
   paper 514
Electrodes 216
Electroencephalography 35, 224, 489
Electrolytes 28, 135
   disturbance 451, 517, 522
Electromyography 224, 227, 251, 254, 257*f*
Electronic control system 312
Electronic patient-controlled analgesia pumps 399*f*
Embolectomy 376
   catheter 376
Embolization 174
Emergency response system, activation of 481
Emphysema 526
   severe 175
   X-ray of 526*f*
Empty stomach 537, 537*f*
Endobronchial tube position 531
Endocrine 7
   disease 84
   system 41
Endogenous opioid
   clinical significance of 14*b*
   peptides 12
Endomorphin 14
Endorphins 12, 13
Endoscopic face mask 336, 336*f*
Endotracheal intubation 4, 354, 359, 378, 379, 413

Index

Endotracheal stylets 380
Endotracheal tube 240, 293, 352, 362, 369, 380, 488, 510, 525, 531f
   cuff 294
   insertion of 354
   placement of 346f
   position 531
End-tidal carbon dioxide 231, 264, 438
   partial pressure of 227
Enflurane 3, 312
Enkephalins 12
Enteral nutrition 130, 131, 133
   advantages of 133t
   disadvantages of 133t
Entonox 291
Entropy 224, 225
   module 226f
Enzyme, dose-dependent reversible inhibition of 41
Ephedrine 78
Epidural catheter 393, 394, 397
Epidural needles 390, 392-394
   range of 394
   types of 392, 392f
Epidural set 393f
Epidural vessels 393
Epiglottic rest 349
Epiglottis 342, 355, 529
Epilepsy syndrome 155
Epinephrine 488, 490
   injection of 515
Epirubicin 127
Epstein Macintosh Oxford 308, 310
Erector spinae plane 532
Esmolol 83
Esomeprazole 113
Esophageal balloon, inflation of 472
Esophageal catheter 472, 473
   type of 473
Esophageal Doppler technique 209f
Esophageal intubation 528, 531f
Esophageal manometry, clinical applications of 473
Esophageal monitoring, limitations of 475
Esophageal pressure 472
   manometry 472
   measurement 472
Esophageal spasm 475
Esophageal surgery 371
Esophageal tube position 531
Esophagus 530, 532f
   drainage 351
Ethacrynic acid 108

Ether 3
Ethosuximide 158
Ethylene oxide 407, 409
Ethylenediaminetetraacetic acid 38, 52
Etomidate 38, 40, 41
Euphoria 16
European Society for Clinical Nutrition and Metabolism 130, 133
Euvolemia 135
   management of 136b
Evoked potentials 219t, 220f
   interpretation of 219
   role of 219
Expiratory pressures 281
Expiratory reserve volume 280, 281, 283
Expired carbon dioxide, monitoring of 230
External jugular vein 181, 182
Extracellular fluid 147, 273
   volume 136
Extracorporeal membrane oxygenation 450, 452f
   circuit, components of 452
   contraindications to 450
   indications of 450
   techniques of 451
   use of 450, 451
   venoarterial 451
   venovenous 451
Extrathoracic airway obstruction 285
Eye 65
   injury 337
   surgery 281
Eyepiece 360

F

Face mask 335, 337t, 409
   dead space of 335
   right size of 335
   selection of 336f
   types of 336
   uses of 336
   ventilation 337t
Facial nerve 253
Fallot tetralogy 81, 187
Famotidine 100, 112
Fatty acids 132, 133
Feeding
   formulas, composition of 132
   initiation of 131
Felodipine 94
Femoral artery 168

Femoral vein 182
   anatomy of 182f
   catheterization 178
Fenoldopam 107
Fentanyl 18, 22, 401
   ampoule 23f
Fexofenadine 99
Fiberless bronchoscopes 360
Fiberoptic bronchoscope 374, 379, 415
Fiberscope 360f
Fibrin clot 115
Fibrinolytic agents 122, 123t
Fibroblast growth factor 308
Fibromyalgia 43
Fibrosis 129
Fick's equation 210
Fick's law 511
Fick's principle 511
Film, posteroanterior 525
Fink blade 355
First-generation receptor antagonists 100
Fistula, bronchopleural 281, 371
Fixed upper airway obstruction 286
Flexible endoscopy technique 374
Flexible fiberoptic bronchoscope 354, 359
Flexible intubating video endoscopes 360
Flexible tip miller blade 355
Flow adjustment valve 300
Flow control valve 300
Flow rate 317
Flowmeter-needle valves 299
Flow-volume
   curves 284f
   loop 284, 317
Fluid 148
   administration 490
   challenge 516
   hyperoncotic 151
   intravenous 147
   management 153
   overheating of 445
   removal 457
   strategies 153, 153t
Flumazenil 32, 36
Fluorouracil 126, 127, 129
Flushing system 163
Flux, negative 400
Fogarty catheter 376
Fondaparinux 120
Forced expiratory volume 281
Forced vital capacity maneuver 281, 283

Formaldehyde 408
Fosphenytoin 156
Fractional oximetry 234
Frank-Starling
    curve 198, 444
    law 474
Fresh frozen plasma 118
Fresh gas
    flow 244, 310, 318-320
    inlet 331
Functional residual capacity 7, 232, 281, 283
Furosemide 106, 108, 142

G

Gabapentin 157
Galvanic cell analyzers 228
Galvanic oxygen analyzer 388
Gamma-aminobutyric acid 4, 17, 26, 159
Ganglion blockers 65
Gangrene 29
Gas
    cylinders 409
    exchange, failure of 451
    expansion thermometers 262
    flowmeters 304f
    flows, total 424t
    laws 511
    mixture 307
    monitoring equipment 386
    partial pressure of 512
    pipeline 291
    plasma sterilization 406, 407
    pressure of 299
    specific Schrader
        connection 299
        valve 291
    sterilization 406
Gastric acid secretion, physiology of 110
Gastric emesis 68
Gastric fluid
    production 111
    volume 111
Gastric function 110
Gastric inflation 337
Gastric lumen 110f
Gastric outlet obstruction 149
Gastric point-of-care ultrasonography 536
Gastric rupture 438
Gastric volume 539
Gastrin levels, high serum 113
Gastroduodenal perforation 14

Gastroesophageal reflux disease 113
Gastrointestinal loss 270
Gastrointestinal prokinetic agent 113
Gastrointestinal system 65, 72
Gastrointestinal toxicity 129
Gastrointestinal tract 75, 117, 133, 141, 144, 146
Gastroparesis 537
Gay-Lussac's law 512
G-cells 110
Gelatins 153
Gertie Marx needle 391
Glargine 102
Glasgow Coma Scale 428
Glaucoma 62, 66, 81
Gliclazide 104
Glidescope 358
    cobalt 359
    ranger 359
    types of 359
    videolaryngoscope 358f
Glimepiride 104, 105
Glipizide 104, 105
Global end-diastolic volume 199
Glomerular filtration rate 128
Glottic opening, percentage of 379
Glucocorticoids 142
Gluconate 150
Glulisine 102
Glutaraldehyde 408
Glyburide 104, 105
Glycoprotein 123
Glycopyrrolate 66, 67
Gordon's airway 339
G-protein-coupled receptor 98
Grahams law 511
Gravity 444, 469
Greenhouse effect 11
Guanine proteins 110
Guanosine triphosphate 14
Guanylate cyclase 86
Guedel's airway 337, 338
    parts of 340f
Guillain-Barré syndrome 271, 417

H

H_1-blockers, classification of 99t
H_1-receptor antagonist 99, 101, 112
H_2-receptor antagonist
    pharmacokinetics of 100t, 112t
    side effects of 101
H_2-receptor blocker 51
Hagen-Poiseuille law 303
Halothane 3, 312
Hanger yoke assembly 296, 298

Hard palate 342
Head tilt-chin lift 483
Head trauma 271
Headache 101
    postdural puncture 391
Healthcare workers 492
    reduction of exposure of 493
Heart 7, 60
    beat, transmission of 475
    transplant recipients 67
Heart block 101, 500, 517
    complete 517, 518f
    first degree 517, 517f
Heart disease
    congenital 519
    ischemic 41, 519, 520, 522
    structural 463
    valvular 41
Heart failure 432
    congestive 107-109, 127, 455
Heart rate 8, 66, 74, 81, 203, 207
    higher 166
Heat exchanger 452
Heat moisture exchangers 328
Heated humidifiers
    advantages of 329
    disadvantages of 329
Hegan-Poiseuilles law 510
Helicobacter pylori 72
Heliox 291
Hemagglutinin-neuraminidase 132
Hematological toxicity 129
Hematoma 174
Hemodiafiltration,
    slow continuous 461
Hemodialysis 145
    intermittent 455, 457, 460, 461
    modalities 461t
    types of 455f
    prescription writing 460
    slow continuous 461
    sub-techniques of 455t
    temporary 175
Hemodynamic parameters,
    calculation of 200f
Hemofiltration 454
    process of 456f
    slow continuous 461
Hemoglobin 414
Hemolysis 445, 451
Hemorrhage 174, 451
    intra-abdominal 443
Hemothorax 178, 532
Henderson-Hasselbalch
    equation 266
Henle loop 107

Henry Edmund Gaskin 295
Henry's law 3, 512
Heparin 116, 454
    infusion 117
    reversal of 118
    unfractionated 119, 434
Hepatic dysfunction, severe 27
Hepatic enzyme inhibitors 33
Hepatic failure 82
    fulminant 129
Hepatic system 72
Hepatic toxicity 129
Hepatic transaminase levels 101
Hepatic vein 536
Hepatitis, cholestatic 129
Hepatotoxicity 129
Heroin 17
High pressure system 296
    parts of 296, 297f
High-frequency jet ventilation 436
    physiology of ventilation during 436
High-volume low-pressure cuff 364
Histamine 98
    effects of 98
    major physiologic actions of 98t
    receptor
        antagonist 98, 112
        characteristics of 99t
Hofmann elimination 58
Honeycomb appearance 527
Hormonal therapy 432
Hormone, adrenocorticotropic 17
Huber's point 393
Humidification
    anesthetic considerations of 328
    devices, types of 328
Humidity 328
Hydantoins 155
Hydralazine
    mechanism of action of 85
    side effects of 85
Hydrochloric acid 49
    secretion 110f
Hydrochlorothiazide 108
Hydrogen-potassium adenosine triphosphatase 110
Hydromorphone 401
Hydrostatic pressure 164
Hydroxocobalamin 88
Hydroxyethyl starches, preparations of 152t
Hydroxyvitamin D plasma concentrations 134
Hydroxyzine 99, 100, 112
Hyoid bone 529

Hyomental distance 379, 531
Hyperamylasemia 152
Hypercalcemia 140, 273
    causes of 140, 141t
    evaluation of 142
    management of 140, 142b
    severe 141t
    symptoms of 141t
Hypercapnic respiratory failure, acute 429
Hyperechoic pleural line 533f
Hyperhomocysteinemia 433
Hyperkalemia 56, 76, 107, 138, 461, 520
    management of 139b
    severe 457
Hyperlactatemia 77
Hyperlipidemia 40
Hypermagnesemia 144
    severe 145
Hypernatremia 135
    hypervolemic 136, 136t
    hypovolemic 136b
    management of 136, 136b
Hyperparathyroidism 84
Hyperphosphatemia 142
    causes of 143t
    management of 143, 144b
    severe 457
Hyperprolactinemia 101
Hypertension 81, 87, 432, 451, 520
    causes of 84
    intra-abdominal 469, 471
Hyperthermia
    causes of 264
    prevention of 264
Hyperthyroidism 84
Hypertonic saline 149
Hypertrophy, benign prostatic 79
Hyperuricemia 107
Hypervolemia 445
Hypnotics
    high amount of 225
    low amount of 225
Hypocalcemia 144, 269
    causes of 141t
    management of 140
    mechanism of 141t
Hypoglycemia 103
Hypokalemia 107, 138, 144
    causes of 138t
    management of 138, 139b
    mechanism of 138t
Hypomagnesemia 144, 269
    causes of 144t
    clinical manifestations of 144t

    management of 145b
    mild 145
    severe 145
Hyponatremia 107, 136, 149
    hypervolemic 137
    hypotonic 136
    hypovolemic 136
    management of 137, 138t
Hypopharynx 342
Hypophosphatemia 141, 144
    causes of 142, 143t
    management of 143t
Hypotension 76, 101, 145, 463, 492,
    intradialytic 463f
    severe 491
Hypothermia 223, 445
    causes of 263, 264t
    prevention of 263
Hypothyroidism 84
Hypoventilation 243f, 271
Hypovolemia 151, 492
Hypoxemia, arterial 417
Hypoxemic respiratory failure, acute 429
Hypoxia 106, 417
    causes of 417
    coronary 451
    diffusion 7
Hypoxic mixture 301
    delivery of 301, 302
Hypoxic pulmonary vasoconstriction response 8

I

Ibuprofen 71
Idarucizumab 122
Ideal body weight, calculation of 131b
Ifosfamide 128
I-gel 349f
    O2 350f
Image intensifier tube 505
Iminostilbenes 160
Immobilization, prolonged 432
Immunoglobulin E 98
Implantable cardioverter defibrillator 466, 467f
Indapamide 108
Indirect noninvasive blood pressure 165f
Indomethacin 71
Indwelling arterial cannula 200
Infection 174
Inflammatory bowel disease 433

Infrared analysis
  advantages of 387
  disadvantages of 387
Infrared spectrography 239
Infrared tympanic membrane
    thermometers 263
Infundibular spasm 187
Infusion pump 396, 444
Inhalational agents
  alveolar concentration of 7
  mechanism of action of 4
  pharmacodynamics of 7
  pharmacokinetics of 4
Inhalational anesthetics,
    pharmacokinetics of 6f
Inspiratory capacity 281, 283
Inspiratory reserve volume 280, 283
Inspired carbon dioxide,
    monitoring of 230
Inspired oxygen
  concentration, monitoring
    of 228
  fraction of 331
Insulin 102
  deficiency 139
  lispro 102
  preparations 102, 104, 104t
  regular 102
  resistance 103
Intensive care unit 3, 130, 234, 443,
    454, 481, 524
Interatrial septum 535
Intercostal drain 525, 527
Interlock system 305, 311
Intermediate pressure system 296,
    300
Intermittent positive-pressure
    ventilation 437
Intermittent renal replacement
    therapy, prolonged 455
Intermittent thermodilution
    technique 196
Internal jugular vein 179, 181, 188
  cannulation 178, 179
    anatomy of 178f
International League Against
    Epilepsy 155, 155fc
Intra-abdominal pressure 469, 470
  management of 471f
  monitoring 469
  normal 469
  technique of measuring 470f
Intra-aortic balloon pump
    placement 168
Intracranial pressure 28, 66, 107,
    514

Intraoperative floppy iris
    syndrome 80
Intrathecal midazolam 31
Intrathoracic airway obstruction 285
Intrauterine growth retardation 73
Intrinsic pathway, test of 117
Intubating laryngeal mask airway
    343, 346f
  removal of 347f
Invasive ventilation 428
Iodophores 408
Ion
  channels modulation 160
  difference, strong 275, 276
  gap, strong 276
Iron deficiency 145t
Ischemia, detection of 213
Ischemic tissues, reperfusion of 139
Isoflurane 3, 219, 312
Isoprenaline 75, 78
Isosorbide dinitrate 86, 89
Isotonic saline 142
Isradipine 94

J

Jackson Rees circuit 323
Jaundice
  cholestatic 39
  obstructive 515
Jaw pain, postoperative 337
Jaw-thrust maneuver 484
Jet ventilation 436, 438
  advantages of 437, 438t
  complications of 438
  contraindication of 437
  disadvantages of 438, 438t
  equipment used for 438
  indications for 437
  low-frequency 436
  types of 436

K

Kerley B lines 527
Ketamine 38, 42, 43, 219, 396
  doses of 43t
  uses of 43t
Ketoacidosis, diabetic 149
Ketorolac 71, 402
Key fill system 315
Kidney 7
  disease, chronic 454
  injury, acute 454
Kinemyography 258
Kirschner needle 391

L

Labetalol 83
Labor analgesia 397, 398
Lack's system 318, 318f
Lacosamide 156
Lacrimation 68
Lactate 456
Lactic acidosis 269
Lambert's law 214
Lambert-Beer law 234
Laminar flow 317, 510
Lamotrigine 156
Lansoprazole 113
Laryngeal mask airway 343, 345,
    366, 409
  blockbuster 351
  classic 344f
  insertion of 346f
  protector™ airway 351
  supreme 348
Laryngectomy tube 368, 369f
Laryngopharynx, right lateral
    view of 344f
Laryngoscope 354, 380
  blades 380, 409
  indirect 356, 359
Laryngoscopy 356, 377
  technique of 354, 356
Larynx 529f
  visualization of 354
Laser surgery, tubes for 368
Last meal consumed 486
Latex allergy 337
Leak test 334
Left atrium 535, 536
Left bundle branch block 196, 519,
    519f, 520
Left sided double lumen tube 373f
Left upper quadrant 539
Left ventricle 535, 536
  outflow tract 535
Left ventricular
  ejection time 207
  end-diastolic pressure 190, 195
Leg vein, thrombosis of 435
Lemon law 378, 378f
Lepirudin 118, 121
Leucine 12
Leuconostoc mesenteroides 152
Leukocyte dysfunction 142
Levetiracetam 157
Levocetirizine 99
Lewis triple response 98
Lidocaine 51, 92, 402, 488
Lifeflow rapid infuser 445

Light amplification 437
Light emitting diode 229, 313
Lignocaine 396, 415, 492
Limb ischemia 168
Limbic system 12, 31
Linagliptin 104
Linder nasopharyngeal airway 340
Linear array probes 442
Lipodystrophy 103
Lipoprotein, high-density 82
Liquid expansion thermometer 262
Liquid-crystal display 359
Lithium
    chloride 200
    concentration 200
    dilution technique 200
    hydroxide 332
    plasma concentration 200
Liver 7
    enzymes 129
    failure 72
    tip 539
    transplant 187
Local anesthesia systemic
    toxicity 53
Local anesthetic 47, 49, 96
    agent 51
    chemical structure of 47, 48f
    classification of 47
    contraindications of 51
    eutectic mixture of 50
    indications of 51
    mechanism of 48
    pharmacokinetics of 50
Locking device 399
Loop diuretics 107
Loratadine 99, 100, 112
Lorazepam 30-32, 34, 35
Low molecular weight heparin 119, 434, 456
Low pressure system 296, 302
    component of 302
Low serum potassium 270
Low-density lipoprotein 82
Lower limb 218
    bones, fracture of 435
Low-flow devices 418, 419
Low-volume high-pressure cuff 364
Lung
    abscess 371
    capacities 283
    cyst, unilateral 371
    diffusing capacity of 281
    disease
        interstitial 271
        obstructive 283, 284

    fields 525
    hepatization of 533, 534f
    injury, ventilator-induced 472
    isolation devices 371
    normal 532, 533f
    protective mechanical
        ventilation 430
    pulse 533
    ultrasound 532
    ventilation 371
    volume 282f
        reduction surgery 371

M

M mode 533f
MacIntosh blade 355f
Macrolide antibiotics 114
Magill's circuits 321
Magill's forceps 380
Magnesium 131, 143, 396, 402, 460
    hydroxide 111
    preparations 144
    sulfate 488, 492
Magnetic resonance imaging 289, 308, 321
Magnetic sensors 314
Magnetic stimulation 249
    advantages of 249
    disadvantages of 250
Mainstream capnograph 240
Mainstream sensors
    advantages of 386
    disadvantages of 386
Malignant transformation 129
Malleable stylet 356
Mallinckrodt laser-flex tracheal
    tubes 368, 368f
Mammalian neuromuscular
    junction 55
Manual resuscitator 325
    bag 424
    components of 325
    disadvantages of 426
    uses of 325
Manual syringe infusion 444
Manual trigger device 439f
Manual ventilators 325
Mapelson circuit, modified 318
Mapelson's B circuit 320, 320f
Mapelson's breathing circuit 318
    advantages of 320
    arrangement of 317
    components of 317
    disadvantages of 320

Mapelson's C circuit 320, 320f
Mapelson's circuit 318f
    functional analysis of 319f, 322f
Mapelson's D circuit 320f, 322f, 323
    Bains modification of 320
Mapelson's E and F system
    advantages of 323
    disadvantages of 323
Mapelson's E circuit 322, 323f
Mapelson's system 318
    advantages of 323
    disadvantages of 323
Masimo pulse oximeter 236f
Mask ventilation 377
    techniques of 337
Mass spectrography 239
Masseter spasm 57
Massive hemorrhage 371
Mast cells 98
Master and Slave mechanism 301
Maternal-child relations 398
Mathew's blade 355
Maximal inspiratory 281
Maximal sterile barriers 174
Maximal voluntary ventilation 281
Maximum expiratory flow-volume
    curve 281
McCoy laryngoscope 355
McGrath series 359
McGrath videolaryngoscope 359f
Mean arterial pressure 74, 201, 219
Mean flow velocity 212
Mechanical indicators 406
Mechanical methods 434
Mechanical pump 432
Mechanical ventilation 272
    indications for 428
    mode of 429
Mechanomyography 251, 254, 257f
Meclizine 99
Mediastinal mass reduction 371
Mediastinum 525
Medical gas 300, 328
    cylinder 289
    parts of 289
Medical vacuum 291
Medication chamber 398
Meglitinides 104, 105
Meloxicam 71
Membrane oxygenator 452
Memory, random-access 466
Meniere's disease 99
Meperidine 401
Mephentermine 78
Mepivacaine 51
Meptazinol 21

Mesenteric artery, superior 537
Metabolic acidosis 107, 232, 267, 268, 270t, 273, 274, 278
 evaluation 268fc
 severe 457
Metabolic alkalosis 232, 267, 269, 272, 275, 278
 evaluation 273
 causes of 274t
Metformin 104
Methadone 12, 19, 23f
Methemoglobinemia 88, 233
Methionine 12
Methohexital vial 26f
Methotrexate 128, 129
Methoxycarbonyl-etomidate 41
Methoxyflurane 3
Metoclopramide 114
Metoprolol 83
Microalbuminemia 433
Microcontroller unit 434
Microlaryngeal tracheal surgery tube 367, 368f
Microporous hollow-fiber membranes coated 452
 oxygenators 452
Microstream technology 387
Midazolam 30-36, 219
 intravenous 36
Middle cerebral artery 211, 212
Miglitol 104
Migraine 81
Miller blade 355, 355f
Mineralocorticoid blockade-spironolactone 139
Mineralocorticoid deficiency 139
Minerals 135
Minimally invasive cardiac output monitoring 198
Minimum alveolar concentration 4, 217, 219, 223, 307, 312
Mitomycin 128
 C 127, 128
Mitral stenosis 194, 527
Mitral valve prolapse 81
Mixed gas flow 304
Mixed venous
 carbon dioxide, partial pressure of 227
 oximetry pulmonary artery catheter 196
Mixed venous oxygen
 partial pressure of 227
 saturation 227
 tension 227
Mizolastine 99
Modern day image intensifier 505f

Moisture exchanging filters 329
Molar mass 511
Mole 511
Molecular size and weight 456t
Molecular weight 152, 459
 basis of 152
Molecules, number of 511
Monitoring system, characteristics of 165
Monoamine oxidase 18, 56, 77, 78
Monomorphic ventricular tachycardia 523f
Morphine 14, 22, 23f, 401
 ampoule 23f
 metabolism 18fc
 milligram equivalents 17t
 pharmacological effects of 16t
Morrison's pouch 539
Motion sickness, prevention of 66
Motor evoked potentials 218, 219, 219t
 limitations of 220
Motorized piston 448, 448f
Mouth-to-mask ventilation 483
Mucous membrane 75
Multidisciplinary postcardiac arrest care 481
Multimodal analgesia 402
Multiple sclerosis 271
Murphy's eye 363, 363f, 366
Muscarinic receptor 4, 64, 65
Muscle
 action potential 218
 relaxant 25, 55
 weakness 63
Mustache sign 527
Myalgias 57
Myasthenia gravis 62
Mycobacterium tuberculosis 405
Mydriasis 66
Myocardial infarction 87, 120, 198, 463, 520
 acute 490
Myocardial ischemia 194
Myocardial oxygen demand 81
Myocardial relaxation 81
Myocarditis 127, 500
 acute 450
Myocardium 465
Myoglobinuria 56
Myxedema 271

N

Nail polish 237
Nalbuphine 401
N-allyl-normorphine 23

Nalorphine 23
Naloxone 23, 24, 402
Naltrexone 24
Naproxen 71
Nasal airway 340
Nasal breathing, normal 328
Nasal cannula 418, 419, 419f
 high-frequency 426, 426f
Nasogastric feeding tube 532f
Nasogastric tube 354, 525, 532
 position 528, 532
Nasopharyngeal airway 340, 341, 341f, 341t
 types of 340t
Nasopharyngeal catheter 420, 420f
Nasopharyngeal temperature probe 261f
Nasopharynx 261
Nateglinide 104
Natriuretic peptides 109
Natural catecholamines 78
Nausea 30, 35, 36, 63
Near-infrared spectroscopy 227
Nebivolol 83
Nebulizer 330
 types of 330
 ultrasonic 330, 330f
Necrotizing tracheobronchitis 438
Needle 503
 and catheters 503t
 cricothyroidotomy 381, 384f
 electrodes 254
 gauge 390, 391f
 tip 391, 391f
 types of 392
Neonatal life support 498
Neonatal metabolic acidosis 73
Neonatal resuscitation 369
Neostigmine 60, 61, 63
Nephritis, interstitial 101, 113
Nephrotic syndrome 72, 108fc, 117, 278, 433
Nephrotoxicity 152
Neprilysin antagonists 109
Nerve
 blocks, ultrasound-guided 443
 damage 174
 injury 337
Nerve stimulation
 patterns of 245, 248f
 sites of 250, 253
Nerve stimulator 253, 253f, 255t, 507
 essential features of 245, 253
Neuraxial anesthesia 261
Neuraxial blockade 398

Neuromuscular blockade,
	reversal of 61
Neuromuscular blockers 65
Neuromuscular blocking
	agents 55, 58, 59t, 94, 246f, 249f
	drugs, effects of 225t
Neuromuscular disorders 417
Neuromuscular electrical
	stimulation 434
Neuromuscular junctions 64
Neuromuscular monitoring 250, 251
	clinical significance of 250
Neuromuscular stimulation,
	patterns of 245
Neuroprognostication 490
Neurotoxicity 11
Neutral protamine Hagedorn 102
Nicardipine 94-97
Nickel 392
Nicotinic acetylcholine receptor 55f
Nicotinic ACh receptors 55
Nicotinic receptor 4, 60, 65, 68
Nifedipine 94-97
Nightmares 30
Nimodipine 94-96
Nitrazepam 155
Nitric oxide 86
Nitrodilators 86
Nitrogen-filled vials 26
Nitroglycerin 86, 89
	compounds 86
	infusion 117
Nitrosoureas 127-129
Nitrous
	cylinder 297
	oxide 3, 219, 291, 296, 300
Nizatidine 100, 112
N-methyl-D-aspartate 17
	receptors 42
Nociceptin 12, 14
Nonanion gap metabolic
	acidosis 270
Nonbarbiturate intravenous
	anesthetic agents 38
Non-blood pressure 295
Noncalibrated techniques 201
Noncardiac surgery 215
Noncardiogenic pulmonary
	edema 128
Noncatecholamines 74
Nonchanneled videolaryngoscopes 358
Noncritical items 408
Nondepolarizing muscle 55
	relaxants 57, 57t, 58

Nondepolarizing neuromuscular
	block 248f, 251t
	agents 58
	drugs 57t
Nonelectrical methods 262
Nonglucose-containing fluid 489
Noninflatable cuff 349
Noninterchangeable screw
	thread 299
Noninvasive finger arterial pressure
	waveform analysis 202
Noninvasive ventilation 428
	modes of 428
Nonprotein calories 132
Nonrebreathing
	mask 422, 422f, 422t
	valve 325, 326, 424, 425
Nonsteroidal anti-inflammatory
	drugs 69, 72t, 110
	adverse effects of 72
	classification of 69fc
	concerns of 73
	use of 72
Noradrenaline 75, 78
Nutrition 113

O

Obstructive disease 284
Oddi spasm 16
Ohm's law 296
Oliguria 451
Omeprazole 113
Oncotic pressure 148
One-way check valve 300
Open face mask 335
Ophthalmic artery 212
Opioid 12, 219, 401
	analgesic drugs 14, 15t
	antagonists 23
	drugs 13t
	epidural 22
	mechanism of action of 14fc
	overdose 499, 499fc
	pharmacokinetics of 17t
	sparing effects 45
	withdrawal 81
Optical plethysmography 229
Optimized cardiac output 198
Oral anticoagulants 121t
Oral cavity 294
Oral contraceptive 84
	drugs 102, 103, 104t
	pills 432
Oral pyridostigmine 62
Organ dysfunction 470

Organophosphates 61, 68
Organophosphorus poisoning 63, 68
Orifice location 391
Orogastric tube 352
	position 532
Oropharyngeal airway 337, 338, 338t, 339, 340
	parts of 340
Oropharynx 359
	anterior view of 344f
Orphan receptor 12, 14
Orthophthaldehyde 408
Osmolal gap 270
Osmolality 148
Osmolarity 140, 148
Osmoles, number of 148
Osmolite 132
Osmosis 147
Osmotic diuretics 107
O-toluidine 51
Ototoxicity 107
Out-of-hospital chain 479f
	pediatric 480f
Ovassapian airway 339
Over transfusion 445
Oxazepam 33
Oxazolidinediones 155
Oxford miniature vaporizer 308
Oxford tube 367, 367f
Oximetry lumen 188
Oxiport miller blade 355
Oxycodone ampoule 23f
Oxygen
	analysis, use of 388
	analyzer 302, 388
	arterial partial pressure of 227
	concentration, low delivered 426
	consumption 130
	delivery 417
		devices 417
	enrichment device 325, 326
	face mask 420, 421f
	fail-safe system 299
	failure protection device 300, 301
	flow 421
		decrease 301
	flush 299
	high partial pressure of 236
	masks 409
	partial pressure of 88
	pressure
		fail safe system 301
		regulator 300
	ratio monitor controller 302
	ration proportioning systems 301

reservoir 327
saturation 204
  peripheral 227
supplementation 425
therapy 328
  devices 418
  goal of 418
  indications of 417
Oxygenation 342
Oxyhemoglobin 201, 229, 234

P

Paclitaxel 127
Pain
  chronic 43, 397, 443, 503, 503t, 504
  management 43
  mild-to-moderate 69
Palate surgery 367
Palsy, hemidiaphragmatic 532
P-aminobenzoic acid 51
Pancreatitis 40
  acute 101, 113
Pantoprazole 113
Pap waveform 190
Papaveretum 15
Parallel tube system 318
Paramagnetic oxygen analyzer 388
Parasternal long axis 535, 535f
Parasternal short-axis 535, 535f
Parathyroid hormone 140-142
  control of 139
Parenteral nutrition 130, 132, 133, 183
  advantages of 133t
  disadvantages of 133t
Parietal cells, stimulation of 110f
Paroxysmal nocturnal hemoglobin 433
Paroxysmal supraventricular tachycardia 520, 521f
Partial carbon dioxide rebreathing technique 209
Partial enteral nutrition 132t
Partial pressure 307
Partial rebreather mask 421, 421t
Partial thromboplastin time 121
Pascal 510
Past medical history 486
Pasteurization 406
Patent ductus arteriosus 71
Patient valve 425
Patient-controlled analgesia 396, 397, 398
  monitoring of 403, 404b

pumps 396, 397f, 398, 402b
regimens 401
side effects of 403
Patil-Syracuse airway 339
Peak expiratory flow rate 283, 284
Pediatric patients 470
Pediatric pulse oximeter probe 235f
Pediatric resuscitation 424, 496
Peel away cannula technique 183
Pelvis 539
Pencil-point needle 391, 391f
Pendelluft ventilation 436
Pentamidine 270
Pentax airway scope 358
Pentax videolaryngoscope 358f
Pentazocine 20, 401
Perampanel 159
Percutaneous tracheostomy 413, 415
  advantages of 413
  complications of 414
  contraindications for 413
  disadvantages of 413
  indications of 413
  techniques of 415
Percutaneous transluminal coronary angioplasty 121
Percutaneous transtracheal oxygenation 381
Perforated hollow viscus 443
Perfusing rhythm 486
Perfusion pressure, abdominal 469
Pericardial disease 522
Pericardial effusion 443
Pericarditis, hemorrhagic 127
Pericardium 539
Peripartum cardiomyopathy 490
Peripheral monitoring 166f
Peripheral nerve
  automated 295
  catheter 396
  stimulation
    principle of 245
    types of 249
Peripheral neuropathy, chemotherapy-induced 128
Peripheral vasculature 65
Peripheral venous
  blood gas 266
  catheter 397, 200
Peroneal nerve 253
Peroxide-based compounds 408
Personal protective equipment 482, 492
Pethidine 12, 18
Pethik's test 511

Pharmacodynamics 55, 108t
Pharmacokinetics 15, 55, 95t, 100t, 116, 119
Pharmacological agents 402, 434
Pharynx 294, 342
  posterior view of 344f
Phenacemide 155
Phencyclidine group 396
Pheniramine 99
Phenolics 408
Phenoxybenzamine 79
Phentolamine 79
Phenylalkylamine 94
Phenylephrine 75, 78
Phenylpropylamine 12
Phenytoin 92, 156, 160
Pheochromocytoma 81, 84
Phonomyography 251, 259
Phosgene 333
Phosphate 131, 460
Phosphorus 140, 141
  regulation of 140fc
Photo-acoustic spectrography 239
Physiological effects 507
Physostigmine 60
Piezoelectric absorption 388
Piezoelectric crystals 441
Piezoelectric neuromuscular monitor 251
Pilocarpine 63
Pin index safety system 289, 290, 290f, 296, 297t
Pinch-off syndrome 179
Pioglitazone 104
Pipeline connection, isolation of 291
Pipeline failure, mock drills of 292
Pipeline inlet connections 299
Pipeline pressure
  gauges 299
  surges 299
Pipeline system 291
  safety maneuvers for 292
Pipeline testing, modalities of 292t
Piston pump 293
Pitkin needle 391
Placing esophageal catheter 472
Plant alkaloids 127
Platelet 122
  function 97
  plug 115
Platinum compounds 129
Plenum 308
  vaporizers 312, 315
Plethysmography 168
Pleural effusion 443, 527, 539, 539f
  large 475

Pleurisy 128
Pneumatic compression device 434
  contraindications of 435
  parts of typical 434f
Pneumatic gas appliance 295
Pneumatic nebulizer 330, 330f
Pneumatic pump 434
Pneumatic system 301
Pneumomediastinum 438
Pneumonectomy 371
Pneumonia 272, 533
Pneumonitis
  acute interstitial 128
  hypersensitivity 128
Pneumopericardium 438
Pneumoperitoneum 438
Pneumothorax 175, 179, 281, 438, 525, 532, 534f, 539
  identification 534fc
  incidence of 179
  X-ray of 525f
Pocket masks 484, 484f
Point-of-care
  testing 227
  ultrasonography 528, 537
Polarographic oxygen analyzer 228, 388
Polio blade 355
Polycystic ovary syndrome 433
Polycythemia vera 433
Polymorphic tidal volume 523f
Polymorphic ventricular tachycardia 522
Polysulfone 335
Polyvinyl chloride 325, 362, 393, 453
Porphyria 417
Portal hypertension 81
Positive deflection 473
Positive end-expiratory pressure 176, 424-426, 470, 473
Postcardiac arrest care 488, 489f
Post-tetanic count stimulation 248
Post-tracheostomy patient, care for 416
Post-traumatic stress disorder 80
Potassium 137
  chloride 25, 139
  depletion 138
  hydroxide 331
  phosphate 143
  sparing diuretics 107, 109
  titanyl phosphate 368
Prazosin, use of 79
Pre-epiglottic space 529
Pregabalin 157
Pregnancy 432

Premature atrial contraction 520, 520f
Preprocedural assessment 414
Preprocedural optimization 414
Pressure 510
  displayed, interpretation of 473
  infusion 444
  law 512
  limiting device 326
  monitoring
    lumens 189
    system 166, 167f
  regulator 296
  relief devices 290
  relief valve 289, 302
  sensor 312
  targeted 429
  transducer 163, 165f
  waveform oscillates 167f
Prilocaine 51
Primidone 158
Prismatic slide glass 314
Prokinetics 110
Promethazine 99
Propofol 219
  infusion syndrome 40
  pharmacokinetics of 38fc
Propranolol 81, 83
ProSeal laryngeal mask airway 343, 347, 348f
Prostaglandin 70fc, 110
  synthesis of 72
Prostatic hyperplasia 67
Protamine 103, 118, 119
Protein binding 50, 160
Prothrombin complex concentrate 118
Prothrombin time 118
Proton pump inhibitors 113
  pharmacokinetics of 113t
Proximal infusion lumen 187
Proximal injectate lumen 187
Proximal tubule 107
Pseudoaneurysm 168
  formation 174
Pseudocholinesterase activity 56
Pseudomonas aeruginosa 329
Pulmonary alveolar blood flow 7
Pulmonary alveolitis 93
Pulmonary arterial wedge pressure 195, 438
Pulmonary artery 175, 191, 193, 195, 261, 535
  abnormal 192
  catheterization 175
  wedge pressure 191

Pulmonary artery catheter 187, 188f, 189f, 195
  monitoring 187, 192, 196
    complications of 196b
  position 189, 189t, 190f
  removal of 197
  use of 198
Pulmonary artery pressure 74, 172, 187, 192f, 195
  normal 189
Pulmonary capillary wedge pressure 187, 189, 192f
Pulmonary conus, enlarged 527
Pulmonary edema, severe 274
Pulmonary embolism 271, 432, 450
Pulmonary embolus 519, 522
Pulmonary endarterectomy 450
Pulmonary fibrosis 128
Pulmonary function test 280, 526
Pulmonary thromboembolism 186
Pulmonary toilet 413
Pulmonary toxicity 127
Pulmonary vascular permeability index 200
Pulmonary vasculature 525
Pulmonary vasoconstriction 266
Pulmonic stenosis 187
Pulsatility index 212
Pulsating finger artery 203
Pulse
  contour analysis 202
  Doppler probe 211
  dye densitometry 201, 201f
  pressure variation 173, 173f
  radiofrequency 507
  rate 166
  volume 234
  wave transit time 204, 204f
Pulse oximeter
  limitations of 236, 238t
  uses of 237
Pulse oximetry 229, 234, 415
  complications of 238
  physics of 234
  principle of 235f
  types of 229
Pulseless electrical activity 486
Pulseless ventricular tachycardia 486, 487
Pump 452
  failure 451
Push button 401
Pyridostigmine 60

Index

Q

Quantitative monitors, types of 254
Quantitative neuromuscular monitoring 251*t*
Quaternary ammonium 67
  alcohol 60
  compounds 408
Quincke-Babcock needle 391
Quinidine 92

R

Rabeprazole 113
Racemic epinephrine 77
Racz needles 503
Radial artery 168
  direct cannulation 170*f*
Radiation
  sterilization 407
  stimulated emission of 437
Radiofrequency 506, 508
  ablation 503
  cannula 504*f*
  circuit, application of 507*f*
  electrode 504*f*
  generator 506
    parts of 507
    uses of 508*t*
  needles 503
Radiography 504
Raman's spectrography 239
Ranitidine 100, 112
Rapid defibrillation 481
Rapid eye movement 17
Rapid fluid
  infusers, types of 445
  infusion, methods of 444
Rapid high pressure flush test 167*f*
Rapid infusion 445
  complications related to 445
  devices of 445
  of ice-cold, combination of 489
  pumps 444
  system 445
Rapid sequence intubation 56, 57
Rapid shallow breathing index 430
Rebreathing 426
Receptor antagonists, second-generation 100
Rectovesical pouch 539
Red blood cell 206, 211, 263, 458
  alignment of 207*f*
  effect 458
  packed 150
Red rubber tubes 362
Reference junction 262
Reflectance pulse oximetry 230
Reflex tachycardia 79
Refractometry 389
Regional anesthesia 40, 73, 443
Regional citrate anticoagulation 462
Remifentanil 19, 23*f*, 401
Remimazolam 32, 34
Renal artery stenosis 84
Renal blood flow 28
Renal disease 72, 84
Renal dose dopamine 77
Renal dysfunction 152
Renal failure 82, 269, 433
  chronic 108*fc*, 451
Renal parenchymal disease 84
Renal replacement therapy 454
  complications of 462
  types of 454
Renal system 72
Renal toxicity 128
Renal transplantation 433
Rendell-Baker-Soucek masks 336, 336*f*
Renin-angiotensin-aldosterone system 84, 106
  inhibitors 84
Repaglinide 104
Reservoir
  bag 331, 409, 422
  system 424
Resistive index 213
Respirable gas inlet 424
Respiratory acidosis 232, 267, 270, 274, 277
  evaluation 271*fc*
  concomitant 269
Respiratory alkalosis 232, 267, 272
  evaluation 272
  concomitant 269
Respiratory center depression drugs 417
Respiratory depression 36
Respiratory failure 142
Respiratory mechanics 475
Respiratory monitoring techniques 227, 227*f*
Respiratory rate 8, 227
Respiratory support, indications for 450
Respiratory system 34, 39, 41, 42, 44, 65
Respiratory tract 328
Restrictive lung disease 284, 285
Resuscitation 477, 493, 494
  advanced 481
  airways 337
Reteplase 122
Retigabine 159
Reynold's number 303, 317
Rhabdomyolysis 142
Rheumatic disease, acute 517
Rheumatic heart disease 519
Rheumatoid arthritis 433
  active 72
Rhodanese 86
Rhythm abnormalities 514
Ribonucleic acid 126
Right atrium 535, 536
Right bundle branch block 196, 517, 519*f*
Right lateral decubitus 537
Right upper quadrant 539
Right ventricle 195, 535, 536
Right ventricular
  hypertrophy 519
  ischemia 194
Ring-Adair-Elwin tubes 366, 367*f*
Ringer acetate 150
Ringer lactate 150
Ringer solutions 150
Rivaroxaban 119, 120
Robertshaw double-lumen tube 373
Ropivacaine 51
Rosiglitazone 104
Rotameter flow scales glows 303
Rovenstine needle 391
Rufinamide 99, 159
Runaway pumps 403
Ruptured tympanic membrane 281
Rusch tubes 368, 369*b*
Ryle's tube 293, 294

S

Safar's airway 338
Saline lock 177
Salivation 68
Sanitization 405
Sanitizer 405
Saturated vapor
  generator 313
  pressure 307, 312
Saxagliptin 104
Scavenging system function 306
Scopolamine 67
Seashore sign 533*f*
Second degree heart block 517, 518*f*
Second ideal gas law 512
Sedation 35, 66, 76
Sédillot's triangle 178
Seizures 67, 142, 217
  classification of 155*fc*

Index

Seldinger technique 175, 415
   modified 169, 183
Selectatec systems 305
Self-inflating bag 326, 424
Self-refilling bag 325, 326
Self-sealing valve 363f
Semicritical items 408
Septic shock 76, 187, 498t
Serum potassium, normal 270
Sevoflurane 3, 219, 312
Shear deformation 469
Sheridan tube 368, 369b
Shock 76, 417, 444
   cardiogenic 76
   hemorrhagic 41, 498t
   management of 444
Shred sign 534f
Shunted venous blood 190
Sidestream
   capnograph 241, 241f
   monitoring 386
Sidestream sensors
   advantages of 386
   disadvantages of 387
Signal quality index 223
Silicone 335, 363
   rubber 325, 363
Silver alloy 392
Simple airway tubes 343
Single lumen
   bronchial tubes 376
   endobronchial tubes 371
Single twitch stimulation 245
Sinoatrial node 90
Sinus
   bradycardia 514, 516f
   rhythm 465, 514, 515
   tachycardia 515, 516f
Sinusoidal blockage 129
Sitagliptin 104
Sjogren's syndrome 63
Skeletal muscle 75
Skin 65, 75
   electrodes 205
   problems 337
   rashes 30
   temperature probe 262f
Sleeve 434
Slim camera chips 357
Small-bore nipple 424
Soda lime
   components of 332
   reaction of 333
Sodium 131
   bicarbonate 111
   chloride 148

citrate 111
   loss 135
   nitrate 88
   nitroprusside 86
      metabolism 87fc
   phosphate 143
   thiosulfate 88
Soft palate 342
Soft silicone inflatable mask 342
Soft tissue 525
Somatosensory evoked potential 218, 219, 219t
   limitations of 220
Somnolence 101
Sonography, focused assessment with 538f, 539
Sore throat 370
Spectrophotometery 229
Spinal catheter insertion 392
Spinal epidural
   hematoma, risk of 73
   set 394
Spinal injuries polio 417
Spinal needle 390, 392, 503, 504f
   features of 390
   parts of 390, 390f
   range of 394
Spinal opioid analgesia 22
Spiral wound silicone-membrane oxygenator 452
Spirometry 280, 282f
Spironolactone 108
Splanchnic blood flow 8
Spontaneous breathing 318, 319f, 322f
   trial 431
Spontaneous circulation, return of 243f, 481, 485, 487, 489, 494, 495, 497
Spontaneous respiration 320, 321
Sprotte needle 391
Sprotte spinal needle 392
Standard base excess 267, 275
Standard temperature and pressure 511, 512
Standard wire gauge 390
Staphylococcus aureus 39
Starvation 269
Static lung volumes 282
Status asthmaticus 271
Steam sterilization 406
ST-elevation myocardial infarction 490
Sterile products 177
Sterilization 405, 406
   advantages of 407t

   disadvantages of 407t
   methods of 406
Sterilizers, automatic 407
Sternoclavicular joint 179
Sternocleidomastoid muscle 181
Steroids 31
Stethoscopes 409
Stewart approach 277
Stewart method 278
Stewart strong ion difference 275
Stewart-Hamilton equation 200
Stimulating electrode 254
Streptokinase 122
Stroke
   distance 208
   volume 201, 203, 206
Styrene-ethylene-butadiene-styrene 349
Subarachnoid block 394
Subclavian artery 179
   puncture 179
Subclavian pinch-off syndrome 179
Subclavian vein 179
   anatomy of 181f
Subcostal four-chamber view 535, 536f
Subcutaneous emphysema 438
Subcutaneous implantable cardioverter-defibrillator 467, 467f
Subglottic approach 438
Subglottic granulation tissue 370
Subglottic regions 529
Subglottis 365
Subphrenic space 539
Substance, mass of 512
Succinylcholine 55, 139
Succinylcholine
   block 56t
   dose of 56t
   side effects of 56
Suction apparatus 293, 293f
   internal resistance of 294
   uses of 294
Suction catheter 380
Sudden cardiac arrest 467
Sufentanil 401
Sulfonylurea oral hypoglycemic
   classification of 105t
   pharmacokinetics of 105t
Sulfonylureas 104, 105
Sulfur donors 86
Supraglottic airway device 342, 343t, 377
   classification of 342
Supraglottic approach 438

Index

Supraglottic device, second-generation 381
Supraventricular rhythms, abnormal 520
Surface electrode 254
Surgery, cardiac 117
Sympathomimetics 74, 78t
  effects of 74
  indications of 76
Syndrome of inappropriate antidiuretic hormone secretion 107, 109, 137, 137fc
Synthetic noncatecholamines 78
Systemic lupus erythematosus 433
Systemic vascular resistance 8, 41, 74, 201, 202
Systemic vasodilatation 266
Systolic pressure 188
  variation 171, 173f

T

T waves, abnormal 522
Tachycardia 29
  supraventricular 465, 492
Tamoxifen 127
Targeted temperature management 490
  monitoring 490
Taxanes 128
Taxol 126, 127
Taylor dispersion 437
Temazepam 32, 33
Temperature
  compensation methods 308, 311
  measurement of 261
  sensor 312, 314
Tetanic stimulation 246, 247f
Thermal conductivity 307, 308
Thermistor connector lumen 188
Thermistor semiconductors 263
Thermocompensation 311, 312
Thermometers, types of 262
Thermoplastic elastomer 335, 349
Thermoregulation, control of 260fc
Thermoregulatory effector responses, activation of 261f
Thiamylal 27
Thiazide 107
  diuretic 106, 108
Thiazolidinediones 104, 105
Thin siloxane layers 452
Thiobarbiturates, metabolism of 27, 27fc

Thiocyanate toxicity 88
Thiopental
  pharmacokinetics properties of 26t
  sodium vial 26f
  solution 26
Thiopentone 219
Third degree heart block 517, 518f
Third ideal gas law 512
Thoracic bioimpedance 204
  measurement 205f
Thoracic bioreactance 205
  measurement 206f
Thoracic cage facilitates 447
Thoracic duct 179
Thoracic gas volume 281
Thoracoscopic surgery, video-assisted 371
Thorpe's tubes 302
Three-point grading system 537t
Thromboangiitis obliterans 168
Thrombocytopenia 101, 113
  heparin-induced 117, 118, 118t, 121
Thromboembolic event, history of 432
Thromboembolism 451
Thrombolytic agents 122, 123t
Thromboxane synthesis 70fc
Thumper 447
Thyrohyoid membrane 529
Thyroid
  cartilage 530
  gland 530
  notch 415
  storm 81
Thyrotoxicosis 520, 522
Tiagabine 158
Tibial artery, posterior 168
Tibial nerve 253
Tidal volume 280, 282
Tissue 98
  mass 51
  necrosis 29
  solubility 7
  toxicity 363f
Tocolytics 76
Tolazamide 104, 105
Tolbutamide 104, 105
Topiramate 157
Torsade-de-pointes 522
Total lung capacity 283
Total opioid requirement 402
Toxicity 122, 124
  chronic 127
Trachea 409, 415, 418

Tracheal cannula 413
Tracheal cuff 363f
Tracheal dilation 415
Tracheal intubation 353, 379
Tracheal rings 529, 530
Tracheal stoma 415
Tracheal tube 365, 425
  channels for 358
Tracheobronchial tree 511
  anatomy of 372f
Tracheostomy
  advantages of 413
  surgical 413
  tube 413, 510, 525
Train-of-four stimulation ratio 246
Tramadol 20
Transcellular shift 138, 139
Transcranial Doppler 211, 211f, 213
Transdermal opioids 21t
Transesophageal echocardiogram 153, 195
Transesophageal echocardiography 443
Transfixation 169
Transmission pulse oximetry 229
Transnasal humidified rapid insufflation ventilatory exchange 384
Transpulmonary thermodilution technique 199, 199f, 200f
Transthoracic echocardiograms 153
Transthoracic echocardiography 443
Transtracheal approach 438
Transvenous cardiac pacing 175
Trastuzumab 126, 127
Trauma 124
  sonography in 539f
Tremors 81
Tricuspid stenosis 187
Tricuspid valve 535
Trimethoprim 139, 270
Triprolidine 99
Trophic feeding 131
Tube
  feedings 132, 133fc
  occlusion 132
  passing of 532f
  X-ray 505
Tuberculosis 526
Tubular heart 526
Tubular shadows 527
Tubulointerstitial nephritis 139
Tug tests 292
Tuohy's needle 392, 393f, 394, 503, 504f
  parts of 392

Index

Turbulent flow 317, 510
Tympanic membrane 261
   temperature probe 263f
   thermometers 263

U

U waves 138
Ulnar arteries 168
Ulnar nerve 253
Ultrafiltration, slow continuous 455, 457, 461
Ultrasonography 434, 531, 532, 537
Ultrasound 169, 384, 506, 528
   dilution technique 210, 210f
   guidance 181
   guided central venous cannulation 183
   machine 441, 442
   scanner, components of 442
   sonography 384
      role of 384
   waves, generation of 441
Uniform compression 469
Univent bronchial blocking tubes 375, 376f
Universal gas law 512
Universal precautions 405
Upper airway 530f
   lateral view of 344f
   transverse view of 530f
Upper limb 218
Upper lobectomy 371
UpsherScope 356, 357f
Urea
   clearance 457
   inbound 459
   rebound 459
   reduction rate 459
Urination 68
Urokinase 122
Uterus 75

V

Vacuum
   degree of 293
   source 293
Valproate 157
Valves 305f
   reduction 298
   types of 290
Valvular heart disease, severe 198
Vanillylmandelic acid 77

Vapor 307
   pressure 3
Vaporization, latent heat of 307
Vaporizer 304f, 307
   Dorsch's classification of 308
   functioning 311
   inside circuit 309, 310
   outside circuit 309, 310
Variceal bleed, prophylaxis for 81
Varicose vein 432
Vascular access 498
   ultrasound guidance for 443
Vascular injury 432
Vasoconstriction
   endothelial-independent 127
   severe 29
Vasoconstrictors 51
Vasodilatation 60
Vasodilators, peripheral 86
Vasopressin 107
   receptor antagonist 109
Vasospasm, detection of 212, 213t
Vasovagal syncope 515
Vaughan-Williams classification 90
Vena cava
   inferior 535, 536f
   superior 178
   transhepatic inferior 535, 536f
Veno-occlusive disease 129
Venous air embolism, risk of 175
Venous blood gas 267
Venous oxygen saturation 227
Venous stasis 432
Venous thromboembolism 121
Ventilation 7, 342
   pressure control mode of 429
   volume control mode of 429
Ventilator 428-430, 438, 439f
   dependent patients 424
   disconnection alarm 305
   graphics 428
   power outlets 299
   support 431
Ventricular fibrillation 486, 487, 495, 524, 524f
Ventricular rhythms 522
Ventricular tachycardia 495, 522
Venture mask 422, 423, 423f, 423t, 511
Venturi principle 293, 511
Venturi pump 293
Verapamil 93-95, 97
Vertebral arteries 212
Vertigo 99

Videolaryngoscopes 354, 357, 377
Vigabatrin 158, 160
Vildagliptin 104
Vincristine 128, 129
Virchow's triad 432
Viscosity 511
Visual alarms 305
Visual evoked
   potential 221
   response 218
Vitamin
   D_3 134
   K 118
      antagonists 434
Vocal cords 354, 529
Volume clamp method 203f
Volume pressure curve 232f
Volumetric capnography 241, 241f
Vomiting 35, 36, 63

W

Wagner's needle 392
Warfarin 118, 120t
Waters' airway 337, 338
Weak acids 275, 276
   total concentration of 276
Wedge pressure waveforms 192, 193
Wells scoring system 433
   criteria description of 433
Wenckebach phenomenon 517
Whitacre needle 391
Williams airway intubator 339
Wisconsin blade 355
Wolff-Parkinson-White syndrome 93
Workstation unit 505, 506
Wuscope 356, 357f

X

Xenon 11
X-ray 514
   common 525
   generator 505

Y

Y-adapter 372
Yoke block 296
Yoke plug 298

Z

Zonisamide 159

EU GSPR Authorised Reprsentative
Logos Europe, 9 rue Nicolas Poussin
1700, La Rochelle, France
Phone: +33 (0) 6 67 93 73 78
E-mail: contact@logoseurope.eu

www.ingramcontent.com/pod-product-compliance
Ingram Content Group UK Ltd.
Pitfield, Milton Keynes, MK11 3LW, UK
UKHW050455150426
5217IPUK00025B/1704